MASTERING MEDICAL CODING

Evolve Student Learning Resources for Diamond: Mastering Medical Coding, *Fourth Edition, offer the following features:*

- **Case Studies for Practice:** Practice your skills with these real-life cases, complete illustrations, procedure videos, and self-assessment questions
- **Certification Examination:** Prepare yourself for coding certification with this mock examination
- **Chapter Review Exercises:** Reinforce your skills by completing these exercises
- **Content Updates:** Easily access the latest coding information
- **ICD-9-CM Official Guidelines for Coding and Reporting:** Refer to the latest guidelines for the most accurate codes
- **Godfrey Regional Practice and Sample Forms:** Use these forms to work through the book exercises and for later practice
- **Putting It All Together:** A Day in the Life of Godfrey Regional: Complete all of these exercises to simulate an entire day at a medical practice

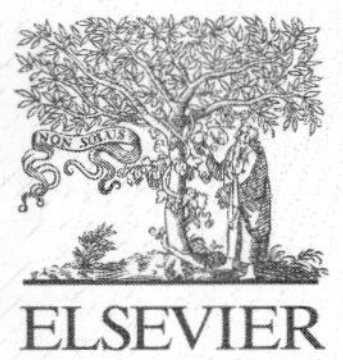

FOURTH EDITION

MASTERING MEDICAL CODING

Marsha S. Diamond, CPC, CPC-H, CCS

Instructor, Former Department Chair
Health Information Technology
Central Florida College
Orlando, Florida

Past National Advisory Board Member
American Academy of Professional Coders
Salt Lake City, Utah

Senior Consultant/Auditor
Medical Audit Resource Services, Inc.
Orlando, Florida

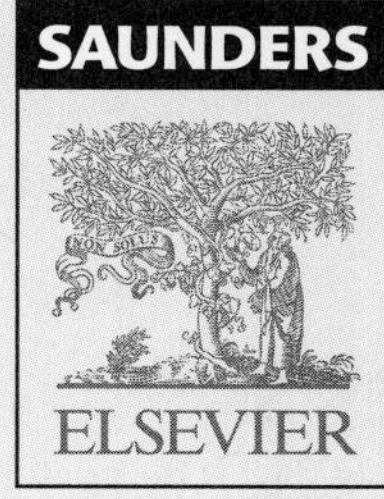

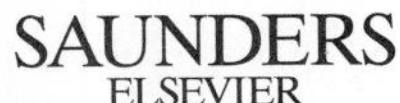

3251 Riverport Lane
Maryland Heights, Missouri 63043

MASTERING MEDICAL CODING 978-1-4160-5035-3

Notice

Knowledge and best practice in this field are constantly changing. As new research and experience broaden our knowledge, changes in practice, treatment and drug therapy may become necessary or appropriate. Readers are advised to check the most current information provided (i) on procedures featured or (ii) by the manufacturer of each product to be administered, to verify the recommended dose or formula, the method and duration of administration, and contraindications. It is the responsibility of the practitioner, relying on their own experience and knowledge of the patient, to make diagnoses, to determine dosages and the best treatment for each individual patient, and to take all appropriate safety precautions. To the fullest extent of the law, neither the Publisher nor the Author assumes any liability for any injury and/or damage to persons or property arising out of or related to any use of the material contained in this book.

Library of Congress Cataloging-in-Publication Data

Diamond, Marsha S.
Mastering medical coding / Marsha S. Diamond. — 4th ed.
p. ; cm.
Includes index.
ISBN-13: 978-1-4160-5035-3 (pbk. : alk. paper)
ISBN-10: (invalid) 1-4160-5035-X (pbk. : alk. paper)
1. Nosology—Code numbers. I. Title.
[DNLM: 1. Relative Value Scales—Problems and Exercises. 2. Forms and Records Control—methods—Problems and Exercises. 3. Insurance Claim Reporting—Problems and Exercises. 4. Insurance, Health, Reimbursement—Problems and Exercises. 5. Practice Management, Medical—Problems and Exercises. W 18.2 D537m 2010]
RB115.D535 2010
616.001′2—dc22

2009034669

Vice President and Publisher, Health Professions: Andrew M. Allen
Executive Editor: Susan Cole
Developmental Editor: Beth LoGiudice
Publishing Services Manager: Patricia Tannian
Project Manager: Carrie Stetz
Designer: Teresa McBryan
Producer: Bruce Siebert

Printed in Canada

Last digit is the print number: 9 8 7 6 5 4 3 2 1

If you want to be successful,
KNOW what you are doing,
LOVE what you are doing, and
BELIEVE in what you are doing.

WILL ROGERS

For those who love what they do, they can only hope to have the opportunity to pass the passion for their profession along to others in the field. By writing about and teaching in the field of medical coding, I have achieved that golden opportunity. My special thanks to the many students who have passed through my classroom, who have entered the coding field, and who share that same passion; they are the continuum for the coding profession.

For those outside the classroom who support my endeavors on a never-ending basis: my constant companions during my endless hours of writing, Charlotte and Cassie, and those companions in the past, Oreo and Charlie, whose wagging tails and sparkle in their eyes have held fast despite the long hours of writing and rewriting.

My grandchildren, Tavious and Jaylen, who, I hope, will one day look at their grandmother as an educator and motivator in the coding profession.

My loving daughter, Jennifer, who understands and shares the work ethic of dedication and perseverance in all her endeavors.

To Stan, who endures it all, assisting in improving the clinical accuracy of the medical information and supplying the endless amounts of paper, paper, and more paper.

And, of course, Mom and Dad, who are my lifelong inspirations of work ethic and perseverance—something I hope I successfully pass along to all who learn from me.

Development of This Edition

This book would not have been possible without the following team of educators and professionals, including practicing coders and educational consultants.

Editorial Review Board

Angie Brown, CMA, CMOM, CMC, OMA, AHI, CMIS
Department Head
Indirect Patient Care
CE Health Sciences/Nursing
Greenville Technical College
Greenville, South Carolina

Ila Callagan, CPC
Instructor—Medical Secretary Program
Northwest Technical College Bemidji
Bemidji, Minnesota

Carolyn Fuller
South Puget Sound Community College
Olympia, Washington

Ellie Halibozek, MAE
Curriculum Manager
Corinthian Colleges, Inc.
Santa Ana, California

Jessica Holtsberry
Student Services Coordinator
Ohio Institute of Health Careers
Columbus, Ohio

Marsha Holtsberry, CMA/AAMA
Medical Administrative Specialist Program Manager
Ohio Institute of Health Careers
Columbus, Ohio

Amy Kalieta, CPC
Medical Billing and Coding Specialist
Cardiology Center of North Jersey
Medical Billing and Coding Instructor
Lincoln Tech
Bergen Community College
Clifton, New Jersey

Susan Lewis, MBA
Associate Lecturer
University of Akron
Wayne College
Akron Institute
Malone College
Navarre, Ohio

Linda A. Poulos, MA, CPC, CPC-H, CCP
President
Coder Co-op
San Diego, California

Deborah Roundy, RN, RHIT, CPC, CCS-P
Coding Specialist
Spokane, Washington

Pam Ventgen, CMA, CCS-P, CPC
Professor
University of Alaska Anchorage
Anchorage, Alaska

Lori Warren, MA, RN, CPC, CCP, CLNC
Medical Department Co-Director
Medical Coding/Healthcare Reimbursement Program Director
Spencerian College
Louisville, Kentucky

Preface

Both as an experienced instructor of medical coding and billing and as a user of the medical coding texts that are available in the market, I have come to the conclusion that these texts do not help teach the student *how* to code. Although most of these texts specifically present the many idiosyncrasies of coding for specialty cases, few, if any, explain the actual process of selecting the diagnosis and the corresponding codes.

Mastering Medical Coding provides an accurate picture of the real world of medical coding by illustrating all types of medical records within a medical practice and highlighting the role of the medical coder in the entire reimbursement process. As you will learn, medical chart documentation drives the coding process. As a result, this text extensively discusses documentation and provides suggestions for enhancements to maximize coding and reimbursement. Most other texts begin by introducing diagnostic and/or procedure coding without offering an explanation of what part of the documentation can be used. *Mastering Medical Coding* provides instruction on the selection of information that is codeable from the documentation, which is perhaps the most important step in the coding process.

Mastering coding is a building-block process. It is building on the knowledge learned from previous steps. The basic rules remain the same, even in the most complex coding scenarios. Coding encompasses a multitude of rules and guidelines that are built from basic ground rules. With basic rules or building blocks, the process of coding becomes much simpler. *Mastering Medical Coding* introduces coding step by step, providing an explanation of each step of the process as well as coding examples and practice exercises along the way to make certain the student has captured each concept before proceeding to the next.

Prerequisite Instruction

To learn effectively from this text, you must have a comprehensive knowledge of medical terminology, anatomy and physiology, and disease processes. It is recommended that you complete courses in these areas before undertaking any comprehensive coding education.

Organization of This Textbook

Mastering Medical Coding provides a solid foundation in coding principles with an emphasis on teaching through actual physician documentation that prepares students to tackle any coding scenario, from routine to complex. The 24 chapters are divided into the following seven sections.

Section 1, Crucial Role of Documentation in the Coding Process, emphasizes the unique approach of *Mastering Medical Coding* by discussing the importance of the medical record and medical documentation in the coding and reimbursement process. It also reinforces the need for a solid background of medical terminology to become a successful coder by providing an overall review to evaluate the student's level of knowledge in this area.

Section 2, ICD-9-CM Diagnostic Coding, has been expanded from the previous edition to include even more coverage of ICD-9-CM coding. A full chapter on V and E codes is also included as well as a separate chapter on ICD-10-CM. Additional coding exercises and practical application exercises have been provided in this new edition of *Mastering Medical Coding.*

Section 3, CPT and HCPCS Procedural Coding, covers all aspects of procedural coding, from assigning CPT codes to using modifiers to HCPCS coding. Content is split into short, manageable chapters that can be covered quickly and can be easily reinforced. In addition to a chapter on the basic understanding of surgical coding, an additional chapter has been added to delve more deeply into the coding complexities of each anatomic system of procedural coding. Again, additional coding exercises and practical application exercises provide the student with step-by-step learning techniques.

Section 4, The Reimbursement Perspective, focuses on the guidelines and rules of different third-party carriers and promotes a thorough understanding of the effect of coding on all aspects of the reimbursement process.

Section 5, Facility Coding and Reimbursement Processes, discusses both coding and billing for hospital services, including guidelines for inpatient coding and proper APC and DRG assignment. An explanation regarding the primary differences of inpatient, outpatient, and physician coding is discussed. Thus *Mastering Medical Coding* is a truly comprehensive coding textbook.

Section 6, Monitoring, Compliance, Certification, and Career Development, reemphasizes the importance of proper medical documentation and discusses the legislation regarding fraud and abuse as well as a comprehensive monitoring process to ensure compliance.

A new chapter of the fourth edition of *Mastering Medical Coding,* "You Learned It, You Earned It: Get That Coding Job!" helps students with techniques for marketing their skills, interviewing, and networking. This chapter includes information for the student to use while completing a coding program and preparing for the world of coding.

Also in this section is a certification review that contains review materials, practice examinations, and a 50-question mock certification examination, which is a culmination of the textbook content. These questions provide valuable practice for an actual examination and will give you a chance to test your retention of the information in the book.

Distinctive Features

This book was designed to be the start of your coding education, and it has many unique features to assist you.

Learning objectives, numerous examples, chapter reviews, and coding reference tools throughout *Mastering Medical Coding* provide the necessary educational aids to fully master basic and advanced coding concepts. In addition to fully updated content, the new edition has an expanded discussion of the medical record and a simulated medical practice, Godfrey Medical Associates, which is followed throughout the book in different documentation examples. The reinforced focus truly makes it clear that documentation drives the coding process. This book contains the tools you need to develop the necessary skills to succeed in the workplace.

Key Features

Several key features have been included to assist you through your coursework:

- **Anatomy, Physiology, and Medical Terminology Review** is provided to assess student preparation for reading and comprehending medical reports that are required for coding.
- As stated in Chapter 2, the main emphasis of *Mastering Medical Coding* is on proper review of **actual physician documentation** in the medical record and on application of basic coding rules—the key steps in the coding process.
- **Godfrey Medical Associates,** a simulated medical practice used throughout the text and explained in the Introduction, reinforces the focus of the text by providing a standard list of physicians and records for explanation and understanding.
- **Explanatory illustrations** of different types of medical records and physician documentation provide visual examples and practice opportunities in every chapter.
- Each chapter contains specialized **coding reference tools,** which put together key information from the text discussion into an easy-to-use format for quick reference and everyday use.
- **Key terms, learning objectives,** and **coding reference tools** are listed at the beginning of every chapter to highlight important information to improve comprehension when reading the material.
- In-text **Stop & Practice exercises** appear in every chapter to provide immediate reinforcement of concepts and procedures just discussed in the text.
- **Chapter Review exercises** at the end of each chapter provide more reinforcement and practice for chapter concepts with several different types of questions, including sample medical charts for practical application of the skills learned.
- **Practical Application exercises** in each chapter give the student the opportunity to experience the world of real coding with exercises that are actual medical reports taken from a variety of providers and facilities. They are unedited and contain omissions, errors, and the other issues the coder will encounter in the real world of coding.
- Concepts necessary for preparing for the coding **certification examination** are included at the end of each chapter in a bulleted list.
- The **Student Study Guide** at the end of each chapter lists suggested activities for continued success while the textbook and its ancillaries are used.
- **Online activities** are provided on the companion Evolve Web site to give the student additional practice, including some representative actual operative sessions that illustrate the information found in some of the operative reports. Also included on the companion Evolve site are **Chapter Review** exercises and a mock certification examination for the student to complete in preparation for the certification exam. There is no need to purchase additional texts for certification preparation; *Mastering Medical Coding* provides all the student will need.
- To bring together all the coding concepts in simulated practice, **the companion Evolve site** contains all the documentation for a full "day in the life of Godfrey Medical Associates." By completing these activities, you will see how information flows in the medical office and how to code multiple cases for multiple physicians with a variety of responsibilities.

Extensive Supplemental Resources

Student Workbook

The Workbook for *Mastering Medical Coding* provides extra practice with medical record documentation. All the content has been fully updated to reflect the latest coding information, and the cases have been tailored to the new edition of the textbook.

The simulated medical practice, Godfrey Medical Associates, is carried through the Workbook to provide consistency with the text and offer the opportunity for fully integrated assignments.

Exercises previously contained in the supplemental text *Medical Coding Practice and Review* have now been incorporated in this text and workbook to eliminate the need for a separate text to purchase. The extensive incorporation of medical reports makes *Mastering Medical Coding* and the accompanying Workbook perhaps the most all-in-one coding text package available.

Evolve Resources

In addition the exercises previously mentioned. The companion Evolve Web site also contains important resources. The latest version of the ICD-9-CM *Official Guidelines for Coding and Reporting* is included, along with the reference documents related to Godfrey Medical Associates. These resources can be used by the student for reference while completing exercises in the text or Workbook.

A course management system is also available as an option for instructors who adopt the textbook. This Web-based platform gives instructors yet another resource to facilitate learning and to make medical coding content accessible to students. Instructors who choose this option can manage their entire course online, with online assessments, chat functionality, threaded discussions, and an online grade book.

If your instructor has chosen to use this comprehensive online resource, simply go to the Evolve home page at http://evolve.elsevier.com and enter the user name and password provided by your instructor. If your instructor has not set up a course management system, you can still access the free Evolve resources at http://evolve.elsevier.com/Diamond coding.

TEACH Instructor Resources

TEACH Lesson Plans for *Mastering Medical Coding* are based on chapter-by-chapter learning objectives in 50-minute building blocks. Instructors can customize the Lesson Plans to match their course sequence and add their own content. The Lesson Plans follow chapter content and link all resources of the educational package: PowerPoint slides, the Workbook, and class activities. Also included are Background Assessment Questions and Critical Thinking Questions to spur class discussion. Lecture Outlines present the PowerPoint slides with practical talking points and thought-provoking questions to spur classroom discussion.

In addition to the Lesson Plans and Lecture Outlines, the Instructor Resources for *Mastering Medical Coding* include a test bank, answers to the Stop and Practice, Chapter Review, and Workbook exercises for each chapter. All of the Instructor Resources can be accessed through the companion Evolve Web site.

Coding References and Sources

Although *Mastering Medical Coding* is intended to provide knowledge of concepts for hospital, outpatient, and provider practice coding, it is not intended to be the resource for third-party carriers in the assignment of codes for services. This book is intended for educational purposes only. The only code books that should be references for third-party justification are the ICD-9-CM and CPT.

Coding Updates and Changes

The coding world is constantly changing. Every attempt has been made to ensure that all references to CPT, ICD-9-CM, and DRG code assignments are current at the time of publication. Changes that occur after the printing of *Mastering Medical Coding* may affect the assignment of codes. Reference should always be made to the current coding manuals and to any available code books updated to the current year ICD-9-CM and CPT. Updates to this text will be made available to instructors through the Evolve companion site when yearly coding updates necessitate change.

Acknowledgments

Many thanks to the editorial staff at Elsevier who made the publication of this textbook possible.

To Beth LoGiudice, Developmental Editor, for her diligence in reviewing, editing, and critiquing the manuscript. Her insights into the medical coding field and her extraordinary vision for this text have been exemplary.

To Susan Cole, Executive Editor, for her foresight in the unique concept of this coding text compared with other coding textbooks and the development and design of this textbook. Many thanks for her faith and patience in supporting new ideas and new concepts and thinking outside the "norm."

Thanks also to Jill L. Brown, RN, CPC, CPC-H, MPA, for introducing me to the Elsevier editorial staff, which resulted in the publication of this textbook.

Marsha S. Diamond, CPC, CPC-H, CCS

Contents

Contents

Introduction

Welcome to the world of coding! You have chosen your career wisely. The field of medical coding has evolved over the past few decades to a profession all its own. From the 1970s and 1980s, when coding was only one small facet of the business office, to a career that demands top pay and is recognized as a distinguished profession, coders today represent the professional expertise that promotes a successful practice or facility.

The real world of coding extends beyond the idea that coders are positioned in their cramped cubicles buried in their own little world of code books and medical charts. The coder of today is the key to successful reimbursement for the practice or facility. Having worked in the medical field for well over 30 years, I have seen firsthand that the financial success of practices and facilities always comes back to coding. As a Practice Manager, Billing/Reimbursement Manager, and A/R Manager, I quickly learned that the practice's timely and accurate reimbursement revolved around CPT and ICD-9-CM coding and the accompanying documentation that supported those codes. Many a practice has come and gone despite the wonderful interpersonal skills of the staff or physicians of the practice.

As a consultant working for practices with reimbursement issues, I came to understand that if the appropriate coding processes had been followed to support the documentation, there would be no need for any assistance in securing reimbursement. And so, over time, my world eventually revolved around coding.

What Exactly Is Medical Coding?

Medical coding has been defined as the systematic classification of data and assignment of a number system to that service for identification purposes. When these numbers are assigned for diagnoses and procedures, codes are from a predefined classification system, or a grouping together of similar items. In the case of disease classification, the *International Classification of Diseases, Ninth Revision, Clinical Modification* (ICD-9-CM) is used. When procedures are coded, the *Current Procedural Terminology* (CPT) is used.

Coding serves a number of purposes, including the retrieval or reporting of information according to diagnosis and procedure. It also plays an integral role in reimbursement because it is the primary tool of communication between the provider of care and the third-party carrier (insurance).

Coding, however, involves much more than just the systematic assignment of codes. Perhaps more complex is extracting the necessary information from the documentation that is required to assign the correct codes. From the history and physical examination form to the surgical operative report, the interpretation of data for coding purposes can often be more involved than the actual code assignment process.

This text covers several types of coding. The use of these classifications is based on the location and type of service being reported, as follows:

Facility/Provider Type	Coding System(s) Used
Facility Inpatient	ICD-9-CM (Diagnosis/Procedures)
Facility Outpatient	ICD-9-CM (Diagnosis/Procedures) CPT/HCPCS (Procedures)
Physician/ Professional	ICD-9-CM (Diagnoses) CPT/HCPCS (Procedures)

The world of medical coding has become complex. From significantly different guidelines for physicians, inpatient facilities, and outpatient facilities to different coding systems for diagnostic coding and procedural coding, the coder of the twenty-first century is faced with many challenges.

In addition to yearly changes in diagnostic and procedure coding, third-party carriers continue to apply individual caveats on common guidelines that are available. Ambulatory Payment Classifications (APCs) are relatively new to the scope of coding. Next on the horizon, the coder faces the implementation of ICD-10-CM and possible ICD-10-PCS. Needless to say, the world of the coder is an environment of constant change.

As a result, the successful coder of today needs to remain flexible and informed regarding changes in the coding world. Constant updates, literature, and third-party bulletins make the coder's job a never-ending educational process. For this reason national certification organizations require coders to maintain continuing education units (CEUs) each year to make certain that the strive for excellence in coding continues long after the certification process.

The practice or facility coder has a number of responsibilities extending beyond the coding arena. As the "expert" in the practice or facility, the coder also is responsible for the education of the entire medical staff on coding issues and the success of the practice through effective coding and monitoring techniques. Although these techniques center on the coder, the office staff (clerical, clinical, and medical) must understand that the practice's success hinges on many individuals in the practice understanding the coding and reimbursement process.

With third-party carriers imposing additional guidelines in their individual contracts with physicians and facilities comes the need for an initial **clean claim,** an insurance claim that is free (clean) of errors. Although this may sound like the job of the billing department, the culmination of this clean claim process begins with the accurate and timely coding for services that you will learn about in this textbook.

Because of the large number of **dirty claims** (not clean), reimbursements are not paid promptly or services are denied. The annual cost for reprocessing claims is well into the billions of dollars. As a result, some state and federal organizations have recommended legislation that some carriers require claims be reviewed by professional certified coders only. Laws regarding this requirement have passed in a few states and remain on the agendas of several states and the federal government; hence the need for certified coders continues to grow.

What About Certification?

As with any profession, an attempt to identify individuals who have mastered the skill has been made in the field of coding, much like the CPA (certified public accountant) in the business world.

The two main organizations for nationally recognized certification are the American Academy of Professional Coders (AAPC) and the American Health Information Management Association (AHIMA).

The following are the four certification examinations available:

CPC	Certified Professional Coder
CPC-H	Certified Professional Coder/Hospital

These two certifications are granted through the AAPC. The CPC credential is intended for the professional/physician coder, whereas the CPC-H is intended for the coder who performs outpatient facility coding.

CCS	Certified Coding Specialist
CCS-P	Certified Coding Specialist/Physician

These two certifications are offered through AHIMA. The CCS-P examination, intended for physician/professional coders, is similar in intent to the CPC offered by AAPC, whereas the CCS offers testing in the mastery of inpatient hospital coding.

Statistics available from these two credentialing organizations indicate that certified coders should expect to receive a salary that is 10% to 15% higher than their noncertified peers.

Testing for all these examinations is available throughout the year at various locations in the United States and in other countries.

Additional information regarding the AAPC and AHIMA and their certification processes is available at their respective Web sites: www.aapc.com and www.ahima.org.

Roles of the Coder in the Twenty-First Century

Coders initially worked within the medical record or health information department of the facility or physician's office performing ICD-9-CM coding, CPT coding, or both. Their jobs seemed rather regimented, and they ranked among the many other staff who prepared for a rather bland, tedious job.

Many physician offices did not even employ full-time coders but instead used a billing office staff to perform both the coding and billing functions. Physicians, too, have now realized the necessity of professional coders and the benefits they add to the organization.

"Traditional" Coder

The traditional role of the coder in the medical practice, outpatient facility, or inpatient facility remains the same in title only. Although the coder continues to perform the functions of ICD-9-CM and CPT coding, the job has developed additional complexities and responsibilities.

Initially, this position assigned appropriate coding to services performed; however, as coding rules became more complex and individual carriers began to implement coding guidelines specific to individualized contracts, specific guidelines continued to increase, and the specialization of the coder in the traditional sense began to change.

With the rising prominence of managed care contracts came coding restrictions inherent in each individual third-party contract. It is now imperative that the coder be educated on the content of these third-party contracts for effective coding. Most of the answers for nonpayment or denial of claims can be found in the contract.

The traditional coder may assign codes in myriad settings. From hospital coders, who perform inpatient facility coding and statistical coding such as tumor registry, to physician coders, who perform coding in the physician practice, medical staff organization, or group practice, the traditional coder performs an array of coding functions in a number of settings. In addition to these settings, many other entities, such as insurance carriers, managed care companies, third-party administrators, and attorneys, are employing coders.

Medical Billing Specialist

Although the medical biller or business office is typically responsible for sending claims, receiving payments or denials, and working accounts receivable, the successful medical biller should be equipped with the coding knowledge to prepare clean claims and determine coding discrepancies that have created delays or denial of claims.

Most states have some legislation that requires clean claims to be paid within a specified period (sometimes 30 days). This means that when claims are submitted free of errors, the practice should expect payment within a 30- to 60-day period from the date of service. Claims that are missing codes or have incorrect or incomplete information, however, will be delayed by many weeks or months. Thus an accounts receivable that is older than 90 days is created. Statistics reflect that accounts receivable older than 90 days are collected at the rate of 50% or less.

Chart Auditing

A somewhat new field for the medical coder is the area of chart auditing. With the growing problem of fraud and abuse, many facilities need in-house chart auditing or employ an outside entity to routinely audit charts prospectively for potential fraud and abuse scenarios.

Keep in mind that fraud and abuse may happen even in the best facilities or practices. For instance, services that are billed but not performed may constitute the definition of fraud. This can happen in a practice as a result of the charge document being marked with a service or a decision made to not perform the service, perhaps because of time restraints. The oversight involves not removing that service from the billing documents, which results in fraudulent billing for services not performed. Because fraud and abuse cost billions of dollars a year, the federal government and other third-party carriers are constantly reviewing documentation for medical necessity to make certain that guidelines have been met.

Chart audits performed within the medical practice or facility can ensure that fraud and abuse do not occur, even by oversight, in the practice. Fraud and abuse resulting from oversights can be staggering.

For instance, in a practice that incorrectly bills Medicare for two urinalyses per week that are not actually performed, the fines (an average of $5000 per item) will total $10,000 per week, or $40,000 per month, culminating in an annual penalty of approximately $480,000. If a carrier conducts an audit, proof that internal auditing has been performed may eliminate the charge of abuse in that the intent to defraud cannot be proven.

Compliance

The fastest growing field for coders is probably the compliance field. This is a direct result of the continually growing investigation of fraud and abuse. This aspect of medical coding typically requires an experienced coder to be certified. The compliance officer, compliance coordinator, or coder responsible for compliance must ensure that the entity follows federal, state, and other regulatory guidelines for coding and billing. Compliance staff often formulate a written compliance program and monitor its enforcement. Chart audits at regularly scheduled intervals are a part of the responsibility of the coder in charge of compliance.

The compliance field has also opened up additional opportunities outside the traditional inpatient, outpatient, and physician arena. Many organizations such as insurance carriers have employed compliance individuals to organize and enforce compliance programs for their organizations. In addition, third-party carriers often employ these individuals for monitoring claims for payment.

Educator

The need for coding educators grows with the continuing need for qualified expert coders. Many coders who have experienced the real world of coding have chosen to use their experiences to educate the new coding student.

Conclusion

It should now be obvious that the coder holds a number of responsibilities within the practice, and each facility will expect some or all of these duties from the coder it employs. The facility coder may be responsible for tumor registry, inpatient or outpatient coding, and a number of other coding and management functions within the facility's health information department (also called *medical records*). The provider/physician coder often is responsible for coding services provided in an outpatient/inpatient setting for the providers within the group as well as for the education and training of staff on coding-related issues.

The salary that the coder should expect will obviously be determined by the extent of responsibilities and the individual's credentials and experience.

The role of the coder offers many opportunities to the coding student. Positions such as those outlined can be obtained in a number of facilities such as hospitals, physician offices, insurance carriers, consulting groups, and third-party audit organizations. The opportunities are numerous, diverse, and rewarding. The success of the practice or facility rests in large part with coders and their ability to provide accurate coding assignment and coding education within their organizations.

SECTION 1

Crucial Role of Documentation in the Coding Process

Most coding texts begin instruction with an introduction of the coding process. This text begins at the beginning—with documentation. As the student will learn, documentation drives the coding process; without proper documentation, coding cannot be successful.

It is also appropriate that this text ends with the same process that drives coding—documentation. Accurate documentation is maintained throughout the monitoring process, which ensures that documentation is complete and is in compliance with third-party requirements.

In Section 1 the student begins to learn about the important role of documentation. It begins with a review of medical terminology, focusing specifically on terms encountered on a regular basis in the coding process. Whether your school curriculum encompasses a detailed or basic medical terminology program, it is important to make certain you have the essential tools to begin your coding instruction. Chapter 2 contains an explanation of the importance of the documentation process as well as a breakdown of the many types of medical chart documentation that drive the coding process. Final discussion focuses on improvement of the documentation process through the use of effective tools and techniques.

The student will have the opportunity to review different medical chart documents and formats and to become familiar with the many types of documents that can be used in the coding and documentation process. The charts contained in this text are real; they range from the incomplete to the complete, from the difficult-to-read to the dictated, well-organized record. Such charts represent ones you will encounter, whether in the physician's or provider's office or within the hospital setting. ■

1

Anatomy, Physiology, and Medical Terminology Review

LEARNING OBJECTIVES

After completing this chapter, the student will be able to:

- Identify key words in medical documentation for coding purposes.
- Determine the appropriate system for identifying surgical procedures.
- Define key medical terms.
- Understand standard medical abbreviations used in medical documentation.

KEY TERMS

Key terms are identified within each subsection of this chapter.

Introduction

By now, your studies have probably included medical terminology and anatomy, physiology, or both. A thorough understanding of the terminology needed to interpret and code diagnoses and procedures is necessary to understand the coding process. As you will learn, documentation is the basis for the coding process. Therefore, to understand the coding process, the student must have knowledge of medical terms and be capable of applying these terms to the medical documentation that is used for coding purposes.

This text assumes that the student has already undertaken a study of medical terminology and anatomy, physiology, or both before studying medical coding. If not, it might be appropriate to spend some time studying the terms and conditions that will be needed to code for services and diagnoses.

This introductory chapter is intended only as a review of the terms needed to interpret medical documentation for the purposes of coding. It is not intended to replace the complete study of medical terms, suffixes, prefixes, abbreviations, anatomy, and physiology.

The chapter will provide (1) a basic review of each body area and organ system, (2) a key word list, and (3) a medical document representative of that body system to review knowledge of that system.

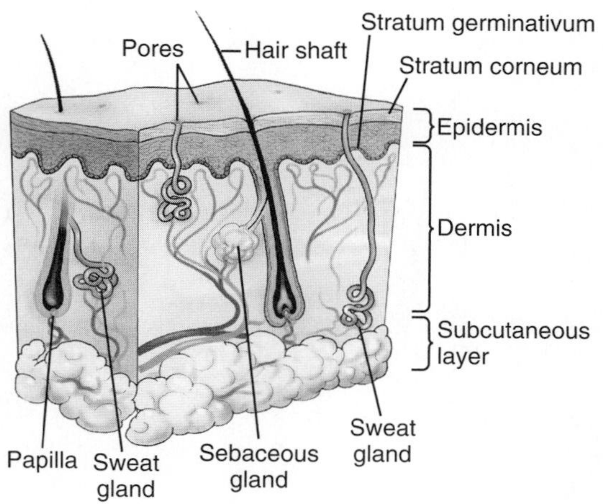

FIGURE 1-1. Diagram of the skin.

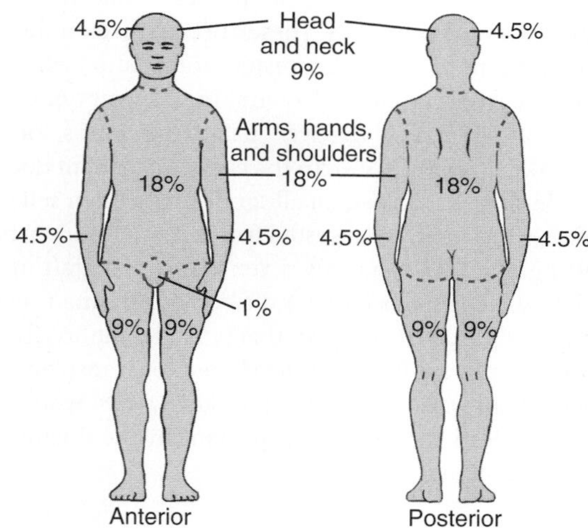

FIGURE 1-2. Rule of Nines estimating extent of burns.

Integumentary System

GENERAL OVERVIEW

The most important function of the integumentary system is to protect the body by providing an external barrier to disease. As the largest organ of the body, the skin also serves to regulate temperature and water and fluid balance in the body.

The skin accomplishes these functions with the aid of the other components of the integumentary system, the accessory structures, the hair, nails, and the sebaceous and sudoriferous glands. For purposes of procedure coding, the breast is also included in the integumentary system.

The skin is composed of two layers: the epidermis (the outer layer) and the dermis (the inner layer) (Fig. 1-1). The dermis is then attached to connective tissue known as the *subcutaneous layer.* The epidermis, although it has a limited blood supply, is constantly making new skin cells that are formed in the basal layer of the epidermis. The dermis, or underlying layer of the skin, houses the blood supply for the skin as well as lymphatics, glands, and hair follicles.

CONDITIONS OF THE SKIN

Burns

Burns are the result of injury or trauma to tissue usually caused by exposure to fire, chemicals, or electrical materials. In addition to classifying burns by depth (i.e., superficial, partial thickness, full thickness), burns are also classified by percentage of body surface area. Body surface area is classified by the Rule of Nines (Fig. 1-2), a system that roughly divides the body into 9% increments. For example, each arm is 9% and each leg is 18%.

Degrees of burns (Fig. 1-3) are classified as follows:

Superficial burn	Extent of burn only involves the epidermis (previously called *first-degree burn*)
Partial-thickness burn	Burn involves both the epidermis and/or dermis; categorized as superficial or deep (previously called *second-degree burn*)
Full-thickness burn	Involves the epidermis, dermis, and subcutaneous tissue (previously called *third-degree burn*)

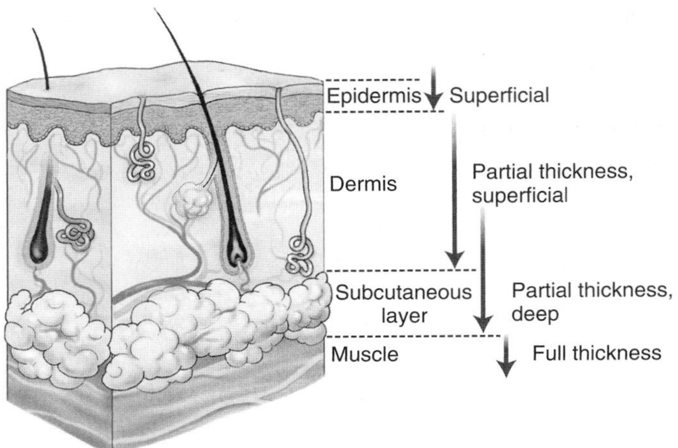

FIGURE 1-3. Depth of burns and tissue involvement.

Loss of skin from burns or other processes may necessitate the application of a skin graft. These are classified on the basis of where the skin or graft is harvested from. Auto (self) grafts are harvested from the patient's own skin. They may be categorized as split-thickness (STSG), partial-thickness, or full-thickness skin grafts (FTSG). In the event the patient does not have viable skin to transfer, an allograft (other than self) may be used, in which skin is harvested from another human being for grafting. In other instances, a xeno (foreign) graft may be utilized, in which skin is harvested f™rom nonhuman species. Often this is a porcine (pig) graft that is used temporarily until skin from the patient has been developed for transplanting.

Table 1-1 shows some of the other key words, word parts, and abbreviations that will be important in the documentation of integumentary conditions.

Lesions

Any abnormal or pathologic change in tissue is referred to as a *skin lesion.* Lesions are further classified by the nature and presentation of their appearance. Some examples are as follows:

Bulla	Vesicle, usually larger than 0.5 cm
Cyst	Lesion filled with semisolid material
Nodule	Small, solid lesion that may be elevated
Pustule	Elevated lesion that contains pus
Tumor	Larger nodule, mass, or swelling
Neoplasm	New growth
Malignant	Cancerous
Benign	Noncancerous
Carcinoma	Tumor that is carcinogenic (cancerous)
Basal cell carcinoma	Malignant tumor of the skin
Squamous cell carcinoma	Malignant tumor of the skin
Malignant melanoma	Carcinogenic lesions of epithelial tissue with tendency toward malignancy

These terms will become very important in properly assigning diagnostic codes and procedure codes for services.

TABLE 1-1 INTEGUMENTARY SYSTEM WORD LIST

Prefixes	
Allo	Other
Auto	Self
Blepharo	Eyelid
Dermo	Skin
Hidro	Sweat
Hyper	Over
Hypo	Under
Kerato	Horny, hard
Lipo	Fat
Melano	Black
Onycho	Nails
Pedis	Foot
Squamo	Scaly
Sub	Beneath, below
Tinea	Fungus
Tricho	Hair
Vasculo	Vessel
Xeno	Foreign
Terms	
Allo/graft	Harvest of skin from another human donor, usually cadaver
Auto/graft	Harvest of skin from patient's own skin
Blepharo/plasty	Surgical repair of eyelid
Cellul/itis	Inflammation of cells/tissues
Contact dermat/itis	Contact inflammation of the skin
Cyst	Nodule filled with semisolid material
Decubitus ulcer	Inflammation, sore, ulcer in skin over bony prominence
Hemat/oma	Bloody tumor, also known as *contusion*
Lip/oma	Fatty tumor
Nodule	Palpable, solid lesion
Skin tags	Small, soft, pedunculated lesions, harmless outgrowths of skin
Tinea pedia	Foot fungus
Tumor	Nodule over 2 cm, any mass or welling, including neoplasms
Xeno/graft	Graft from another species, usually pig
Abbreviations	
FTSG	Full-thickness skin graft
STSG	Split-thickness skin graft

STOP AND PRACTICE

Using your knowledge of the integumentary system, review the following operative report and answer the questions that follow.

OPERATIVE REPORT

Patient information:

Patient name:
DOB:
MR#:

Preoperative diagnosis:

Question of basal cell carcinoma of the left nare

Postoperative diagnosis:

Basal cell carcinoma of the left nare

Procedure(s) performed:

Wide excision basal cell carcinoma nare

Split thickness skin graft from neck to left nare

Anesthesia:

Assistant surgeon:

Description of procedure:

Admitted for surgery today. Because the lesion could not be closed by primary repair, advised **wide excision** and skin graft.

Patient was properly positioned and left **nare** was cleaned with Hibiclens and draped. The donor site of the left neck was also cleaned with Hibiclens and draped. The graft was first harvested from the left neck. This was a full thickness segment. Next the tumor site was marked, **infiltrated** with 2% Xylocaine, and after anesthetic proved successful, the lesion was excised adequately with margins. It was submitted for frozen section which confirmed **basal cell** carcinoma and all margins clear. The **FTSG** was then prepared and sutured into place. The patient was then taken to the Recovery Room in satisfactory condition.

Adam Westy, MD

GODFREY REGIONAL HOSPITAL
123 Main Street • Aldon, FL 77714 • (407) 555-1234

STOP AND PRACTICE—cont'd

1. Where was the skin lesion located? left nare
2. What was the final diagnosis of the skin lesion? basal cell carcinoma of left nare
3. Was the neoplasm benign or malignant? malignant
   What do "benign" and "malignant" mean? non cancerous - cancerous
4. What key words did you use to make your decision? carcinoma
5. What procedure or technique was used on the lesion for treatment?
   wide excision of basal cell carcinoma nare / STSG from neck to Lt nare
6. Define the bolded terms in the operative report.
   wide excision = whole segment
   nare = nostril / nose
   infiltrated = penetrate thru/within skin
   basal cell = skin cell
   FTSG - full thickness skin graft

Musculoskeletal System

GENERAL OVERVIEW

The musculoskeletal system is composed of bones, joints, cartilage, muscle, fascia, and tendons. Its primary component, the bones, serves as the framework of the body, protecting internal body parts. It also supports and shapes the body (Fig. 1-4).

The long bones of the body are composed of the following (Fig. 1-5):

Diaphysis	Shaft, main portion of the bone
Distal epiphysis	End farthest from the trunk
Proximal epiphysis	End closest to the trunk

When you begin reviewing medical documentation, it will become obvious how important it is to know the major bones and joints of the musculoskeletal system (Figs. 1-4 and 1-6). Take a look at the skeletal system and note the skeletal structures that have been identified.

COMMON DISORDERS OF THE MUSCULOSKELETAL SYSTEM

Fractures, or breaks, are perhaps the most common disorder of bones (Fig. 1-7). They are classified on the basis of the extent of damage, as follows:

Simple fracture	Closed with no other involvement
Closed fracture	Fracture is contained within
Open fracture	Fracture extends to the outside, through the skin
Compound fracture	Fracture extends to the outside, through the skin
Comminuted fracture	Bone is splintered or broken into pieces
Greenstick fracture	One side of bone is broken, other side is bent
Pathologic fracture	Spontaneous; usually caused by disease

The muscles contribute to appropriate posture, produce body heat, and serve as a protective covering for internal organs. The primary responsibility of muscles is movement, such as walking and talking.

To allow for this body movement, bones must have points at which they converge or articulate; these points are known as *joints* (Fig. 1-8). Synovial joints are joints that allow this movement.

The key words in Table 1-2 will prove important when you begin to review medical documentation for the components necessary for assigning appropriate diagnosis and procedure codes for the musculoskeletal system. Review them and spend additional time as necessary to master these key terms.

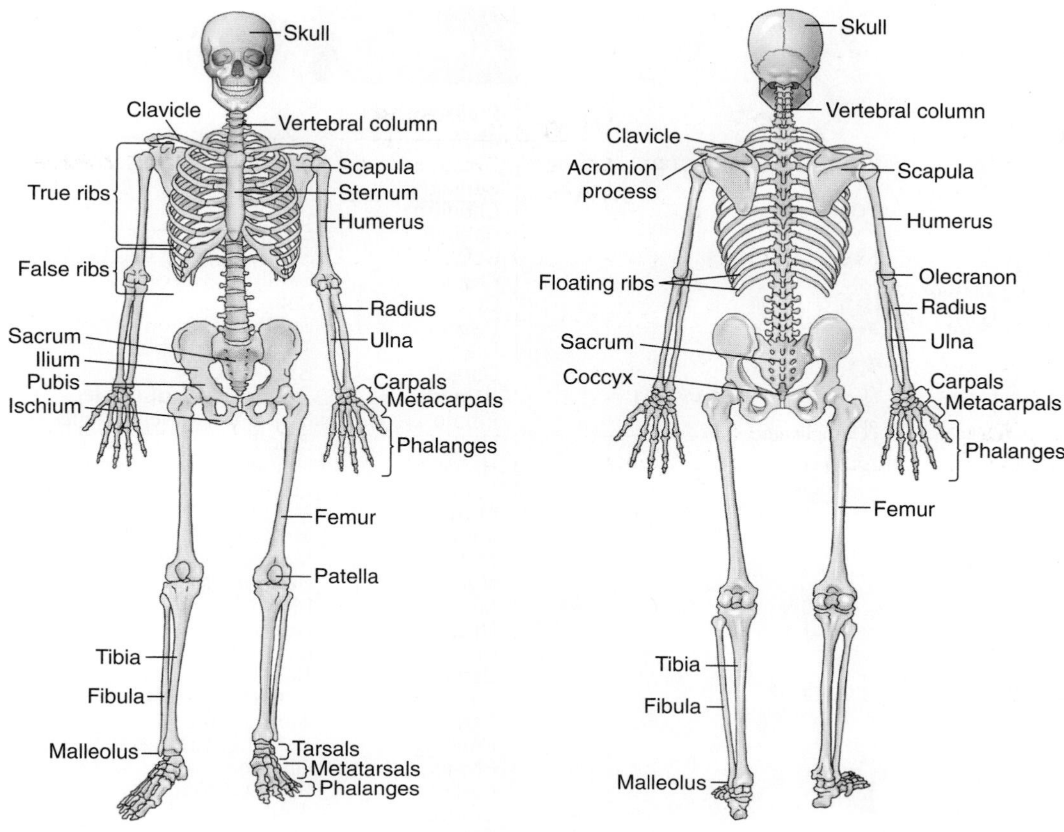

FIGURE 1-4. Axial and appendicular skeleton.

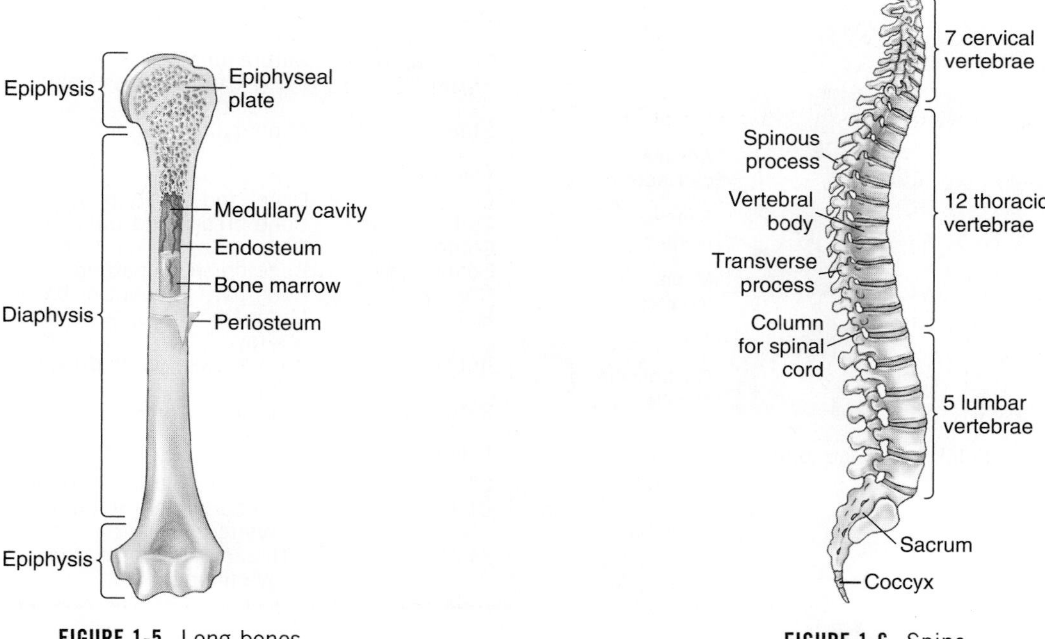

FIGURE 1-5. Long bones.

FIGURE 1-6. Spine.

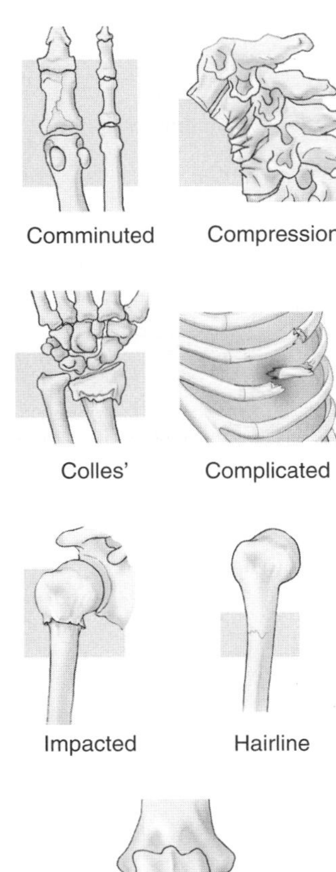

FIGURE 1-7. Fractures.

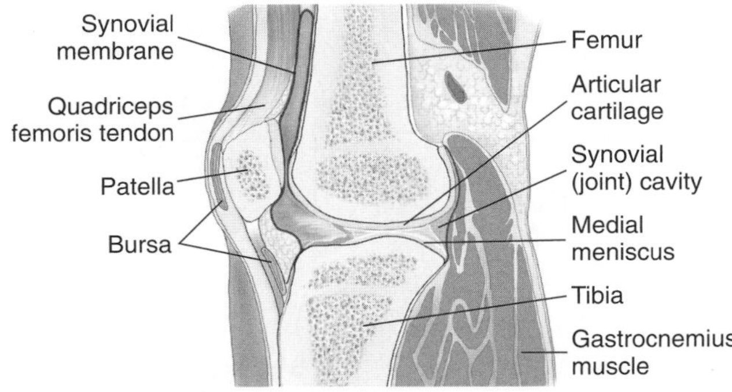

FIGURE 1-8. Knee joint.

TABLE 1-2 MUSCULOSKELETAL SYSTEM WORD LIST

Prefixes	
Arthro	Joint
Carpo	Carpal (wrist)
Cervico	Neck
Chondro	Cartilage
Condylo	Condyle
Costo	Rib
Cranio	Skull
Cyte	Cell
Desis	Surgical fixation
Dia	Through, complete
Dorso	Back of body
Femoro	Femur (long, upper leg)
Fibulo	Fibula (lower leg) (front)
Hemato	Blood
Humero	Humerus (upper arm)
Lumbo	Lower back
Maxillo	Maxilla
Metacarpo	Metacarpal (knuckles/fingers)
Metatarso	Metatarsals (knuckles/toes)
Myelo	Bone marrow
Myo	Muscle
Naso	Nose
Occipito	Occipital
Osteo	Bone
Patello	Patella (kneecap)
Peri	Surrounding
Phalango	Phalanges (fingers/toes)
Physis	Growth
Radio	Radius (wrist)
Sinuso	Sinus
Tarso	Tarsal (foot)
Tendo/tendino	Tendon
Thoracic	Thorax, chest
Tibio	Tibia (lower leg, back)
Ulno	Ulna (lower arm)
Terms	
Arthro/centesis	Surgical puncture to aspirate/joint
Arthro/desis	Surgical fixation/joint
Arthro/scopy	Scope of the joint
Distal	Most distant to point of origin (trunk)
Fibro/my/algia	Fibrous muscle pain
Myorrhaphy	Suture/muscle
Proximal	Closest proximity to point of origin (trunk)
Sten/osis	Abnormal condition, curvature
Fractures	
Colles'	Distal end of radius at the epiphysis
Complicated	Bone breaks and punctures an organ
Compression	Bone collapses on itself
Comminuted	Bone crushed/shattered
Greenstick	Bone partially bent or broken
Hairline	Minor fracture appears as a thin line on x-ray
Impacted	Bone broken, ends driven into each other
Pathologic	Fracture occurring spontaneously
Abbreviations	
C1-C7	Cervical (neck) vertebrae
L1-L5	Lumbar vertebrae (lower back vertebrae)
T1-T12	Thoracic vertebrae (thorax, middle vertebrae)

STOP AND PRACTICE

Read the following operative report and answer the questions that follow.

OPERATIVE REPORT

Patient information:

Patient name:
DOB:
MR#:

Preoperative diagnosis:

Knee Pain, possible meniscal tear

Postoperative diagnosis:

Medial Meniscal Tear, Old Bucket Tear

Procedure(s) performed:

Diagnostic Arthroscopy with Medical **Meniscectomy**

Anesthesia:

Assistant surgeon:

Description of procedure:

Examination of the knee under anesthesia revealed full range of motion with no effusion, or instability. The **arthroscope** was inserted for arthroscopic evaluation of the knee which revealed normal **ACL, PCL,** minimal synovitis and normal lateral meniscus. The **medial** compartment showed an old bucket medial meniscus tear which was resected and the remaining meniscus shaved back to a stable rim. The arthroscope was removed and the patient returned to the PACU recovery area in stable condition.

GODFREY REGIONAL HOSPITAL
123 Main Street • Aldon, FL 77714 • (407) 555-1234

STOP AND PRACTICE—cont'd

1. What technique was used to perform this procedure? Scope
2. What is the approach for this technique? arthroscope inserted for full evaluation of Knee
   What key words provided this information? arthro, meniscus, arthroscopy
3. What was determined to be the abnormality of the knee? medial meniscal tear
4. How was this resolved? medical meniscectomy
5. What medical terminology was used to describe the technique?
   arthroscope,
6. Define the bolded terms.
   arthroscope = visually examine of joint
   ACL = anterior cruchiet ligament
   PCL = posterior cruchiet ligament
   medial = middle
   meniscectomy = removal of meniscus

Respiratory System

GENERAL OVERVIEW

The organs of the respiratory system allow the transportation of oxygen into the body throughout the cells and the removal of carbon dioxide (Fig. 1-9). The breathing process (Fig. 1-10) begins with the nose; therefore the nose is included in the respiratory system.

The upper respiratory tract is composed of the nasal cavity and the pharynx, which is a passage for food and air (Fig. 1-11). There are three sections of the pharynx: nasopharynx, oropharynx, and laryngopharynx. This includes the tonsils, larynx, trachea, and epiglottis as part of the upper respiratory system.

The lower respiratory tract is composed of the bronchi and lungs. Each bronchus is divided into smaller branches, called *bronchioles,* that terminate into tiny air sacs called *alveoli.*

Of interest, there are three lobes in the right lung and only two in the left lung, the side of the chest where the heart is located. The pleura is the serous membrane that covers the walls of the thoracic cavity.

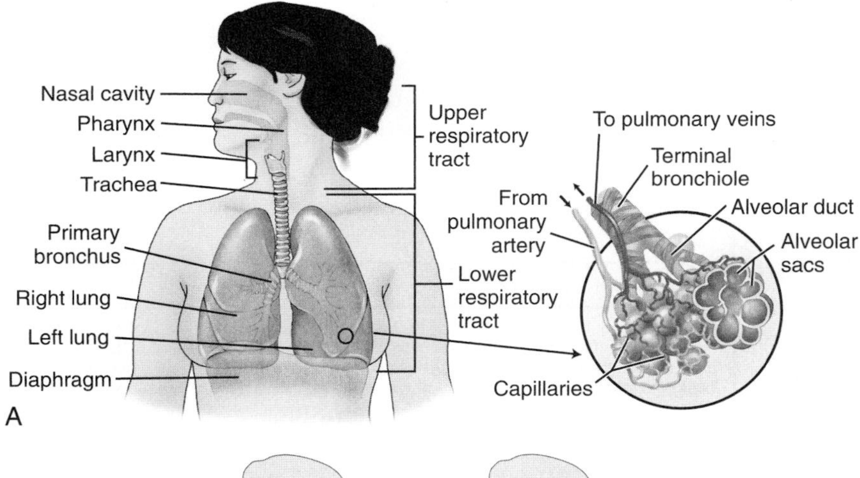

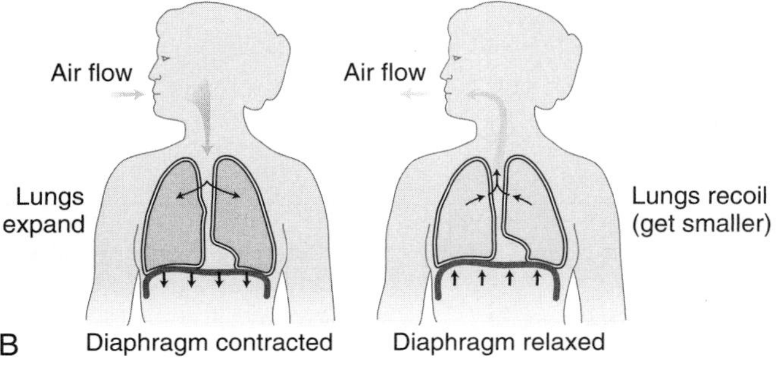

FIGURE 1-9. A, The respiratory system showing a bronchial tree *(inset).* **B,** Inspiration and expiration.

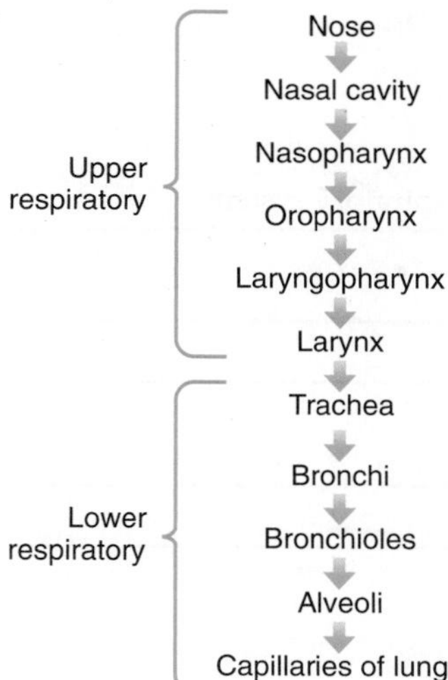

FIGURE 1-10. Schematic of the order in which air passes through the upper respiratory and into the lower respiratory system.

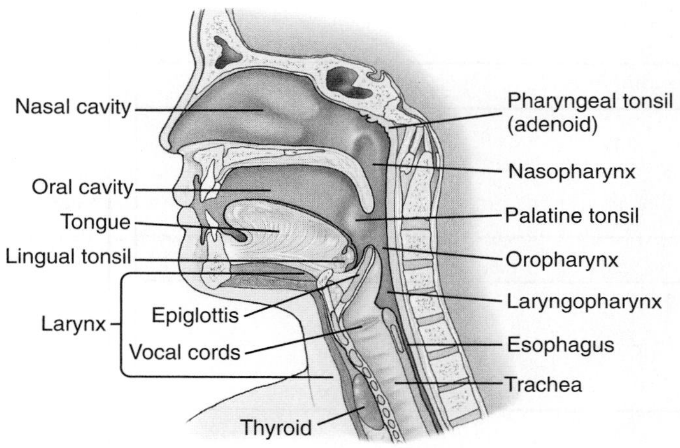

FIGURE 1-11. The upper respiratory system.

COMMON RESPIRATORY DISORDERS

Chronic Obstructive Pulmonary Disease

Chronic obstructive pulmonary disease includes respiratory disorders characterized by chronic partial obstruction of air passages and includes other major disorders such as asthma, chronic bronchitis, and emphysema.

Asthma

Asthma produces spasms in the bronchial passages known as *bronchospasms.* When bronchospasms are not controlled by treatment, the patient's condition is referred to as *status asthmaticus.*

Pleural Effusions

Any abnormal accumulation of fluid in the pleural cavity is referred to as *pleural effusion.* This increase in fluid may be caused by heart failure, ascites, hemothorax, pneumothorax, or other infectious lung diseases. It may be necessary to perform a thoracentesis, which involves the aspiration of fluid from the thorax.

Review the key words, terms, and abbreviations for the respiratory system in Table 1-3 and determine whether you are familiar with these terms.

TABLE 1-3 RESPIRATORY SYSTEM WORD LIST

Prefixes	
A	Without
Adenoido	Adenoids
Broncho	Bronchus
Costo	Rib
Dys	Difficulty
Laryngo	Larynx
Oro	Mouth
Pnea	Breathing
Pneumo	Air
Pneumo	Lung
Rrhea	Discharge
Salpingo	Tube (in this case, eustachian tube)
Spiro	Breathe
Stomato	Mouth
Thoraco	Thorax/chest
Tracheo	Trachea
Terms	
Adenoid/ectomy	Excision of adenoids
A/pnea	Without breathing/breath
COPD	Chronic obstructive pulmonary disease
Cyan/osis	Abnormal condition of blue color
Dys/pnea	Difficulty breathing
Hemo/thorax	Blood in the thorax
Hypo/xemia	Deficient/low oxygen in blood
Laryng/itis	Inflammation of larynx
Ortho/pnea	"Straight" breathing, unable to breathe unless in upright position
Rhino/plasty	Surgical repair of nose
Rhino/rrhea	Nasal discharge
Trache/ostomy	New opening into trachea
Trache/otomy	Incision into trachea
Thora/centesis	Surgical puncture to aspirate fluid from thorax (chest)
Abbreviations	
CXR	Chest x-ray
DOE	Dyspnea on exertion
LLL	Left lower lobe
LUL	Left upper lobe
PA	Posterior/anterior (back/front)
RLL	Right lower lobe
RUL	Right upper lobe
RML	Right middle lobe
SOB	Shortness of breath
URI	Upper respiratory infection

STOP AND PRACTICE

Read the following report and answer the questions that follow regarding the respiratory system.

OPERATIVE REPORT

Patient information:

Patient name:
DOB:
MR#:

Preoperative diagnosis:

Postoperative diagnosis:

Procedure(s) performed:

Bronchoscopy

Rule out recurrent bronchogenic carcinoma

Anesthesia:

Assistant surgeon:

Description of procedure:

The patient was identified and topical lidocaine was administered via nares and oropharynx. 8 mg of IV Versed was given in 1 mg titrations.

The **bronchoscope** was passed via the left nare without difficulty. The **epiglottis** folds were normal in appearance and color. The vocal cords moved easily and approximated with phonation. Bronchoscope was passed into the tracheobronchial tree. Right upper lobe, right middle lobe, right lower lobe as well as left upper and lower lobes were seen and significant mucus cleared. All appeared patent with no **endobronchial** lesions seen.

The bronchoscope was passed through the right upper lobe **transbronchially**. With fluoroscopic guidance, **biopsies** were obtained on the density in the right upper lobe.

The patient tolerated the procedure well and the patient was returned to the recovery room in satisfactory condition.

Adam Westgate MD

GODFREY REGIONAL HOSPITAL
123 Main Street • Aldon, FL 77714 • (407) 555-1234

STOP AND PRACTICE—cont'd

1. What was the approach for the procedure? Bronchoscopy (SCOPE?)
2. What is the preoperative diagnosis? R/O recurrent bronchogenic carcinoma
   What does this term mean? cancer in the bronchus
3. Were any surgical specimens obtained? mucus / biopsies on density RUL
   What terminology describes this information? biopsies
4. What approach was used for obtaining any specimens? transbronchial
5. Was bronchogenic carcinoma confirmed? no
6. Define the bolded terms.

bronchoscope = visual examine bronchus transbronchially = through bronchus
epiglottis = separates the esophagus/trachea biopsies = specimen obtained for diagnostic testing
endobronchial = within the bronchus

Cardiovascular System

GENERAL OVERVIEW

The heart and the blood vessels circulate blood throughout the body. Arteries pump blood from the heart to the body, whereas veins return blood to the heart for repumping and recirculation to the body (Fig. 1-12).

The heart is contained within a sac known as the *pericardium,* which is composed of three layers of tissue:

Endocardium	Lines the chambers of the heart
Myocardium	Muscular layer of the heart
Epicardium	Outer layer of the heart

The heart is composed of four chambers (Fig. 1-13) with an electrical conduction system that propels blood through the body (Fig. 1-14). Refer to Fig. 1-15 for a full illustration of the cardiovascular system and the cycle of blood flow.

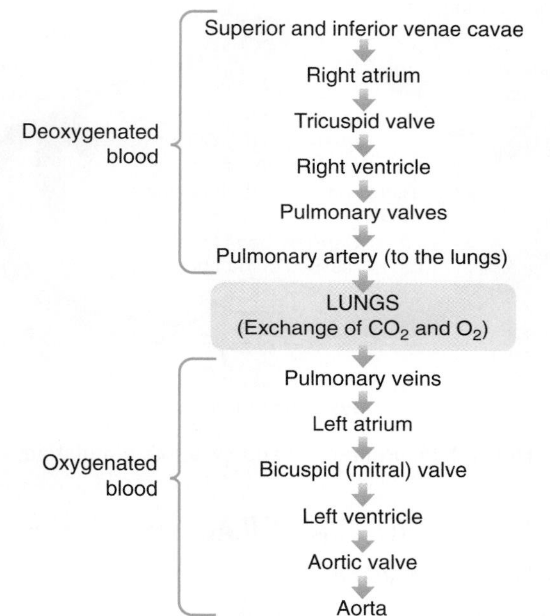

FIGURE 1-12. Oxygenated/deoxygenated status of blood.

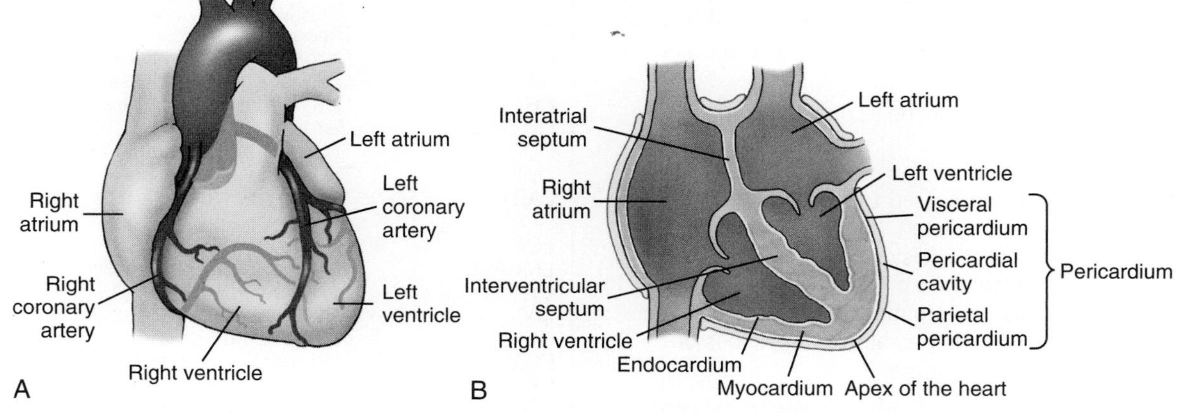

FIGURE 1-13. A, Location of the coronary arteries. **B,** Chambers of the heart.

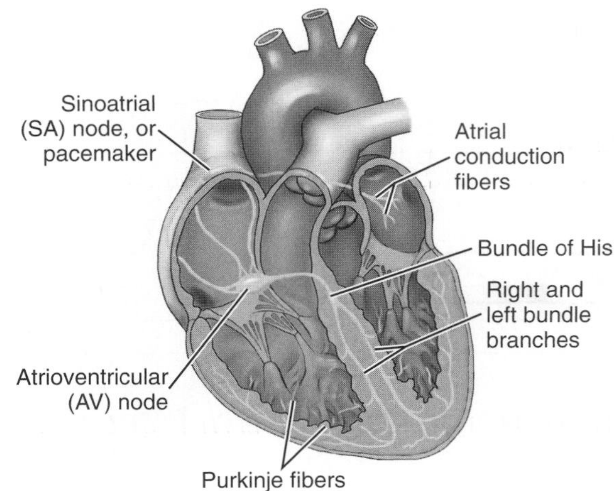

FIGURE 1-14. Electrical conduction pathways of the heart.

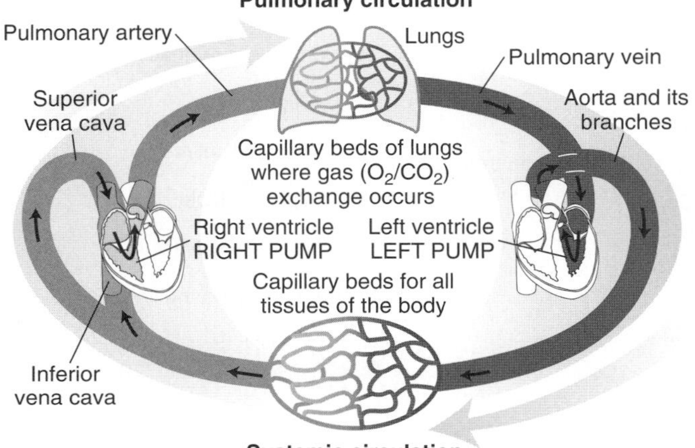

FIGURE 1-15. Pulmonary and systemic circulation.

COMMON CARDIOVASCULAR DISORDERS

Coronary Artery Disease

Any disease that results in the inability of coronary arteries to deliver sufficient blood to the heart is referred to as *coronary artery disease.* The main cause of coronary artery disease is arteriosclerosis, or hardening of the artery walls. When the plaque that causes arteriosclerosis hardens, a disorder known as *atherosclerosis* develops.

A number of procedures may be performed to treat coronary artery disease:

Angioplasty	Balloon passed to the narrowed vessel and inflated
Atherectomy	Surgical excision of the atherosclerotic plaque from the vessel wall
Coronary artery bypass graft	Surgical rerouting of blood around the occluded area(s) using venous or arterial grafts

Review the terms in Table 1-4, which relate to the cardiovascular system.

TABLE 1-4 CARDIOVASCULAR SYSTEM WORD LIST

Prefixes	
Angio	Vessel
Aorto	Aorta
Cardio	Heart
Corono	Heart
Endocardio	Endocardium
Myo	Muscle
Myocardio	Myocardium
Pericardio	Pericardium
Phlebo	Vein
Pulmono	Lung
Septo	Septum
Veno	Vein
Ventriculo	Ventricle
Terms	
Aneurysm	Dilation of an artery caused by weakness in wall
Atherectomy	Excision of plaque from coronary artery
Arrhythmia	Abnormal variation from normal heart rhythm; also known as *dysrhythmia*
Atrial fibrillation	Series of rapid and irregular heart contractions
Bradycardia	Slow heartbeat
Bundle branch block	Incomplete electrical conduction in bundle branches
CABG	Section of blood vessel from one location is grafted to reroute blood around blockage
Cardiomegaly	Enlargement of the heart
Congestive heart failure	Inability of heart muscle to pump blood efficiently
Coronary artery disease	Accumulation and hardening of plaque in coronary arteries
Diaphoresis	Profuse sweating
Hypertension	High or elevated blood pressure
Myocardial infarction	Cardiac tissue death
PTCA	Balloon inserted through a catheter to blocked vessel to push plaque against side of vessel wall and clear blockage
Sick sinus syndrome	Abnormality of sinus node
Tachycardia	Fast heartbeat
Abbreviations	
AMI	Acute myocardial infarction
ASHD	Arteriosclerotic heart disease
BBB	Bundle branch block
BP	Blood pressure
CABG	Coronary artery bypass graft
CAD	Coronary artery disease
CHF	Congestive heart failure
CV	Cardiovascular
DOE	Dyspnea on exertion
DVT	Deep vein thrombosis
LAD	Left anterior descending coronary artery
LCA	Left circumflex artery
LMCA	Left main coronary artery
LV	Left ventricle
MV	Mitral valve
NSR	Normal sinus rhythm
PICC	Peripherally inserted central catheter
PVC	Premature ventricular contraction
PTCA	Percutaneous transluminal coronary angioplasty
RCA	Right coronary artery
VAD	Ventricular assist device

STOP AND PRACTICE

Read and answer questions based on the following cardiovascular scenario.

OPERATIVE REPORT

Patient information:

Patient name:
DOB:
MR#:

Preoperative diagnosis:

Metastatic Colon Cancer

Postoperative diagnosis:

Same

Procedure(s) performed:

Placement of right internal **jugular** Port-A-Cath on right anterior chest wall

Anesthesia:

Assistant surgeon:

Description of procedure:

The patient is a pleasant 65 year old male who presented to my office with history of colon cancer undergoing chemotherapy. He has poor peripheral access and presents for the above procedure.

Patient taken to the OR and placed in supine position. After adequate IV sedation is achieved, the patient's right neck and upper chest were prepped and draped. Using 1% Lidocaine anesthetized an area over the anterior border, **sternocleidomastoid** muscle as well as the anterior chest wall. Using Seldinger technique, a guidewire was placed into the right jugular vein to the superior vena cava. Pocket was made under the right anterior chest wall so that the Infuse-A-Port would fit comfortably into the pocket. Using the dilator introducer system these were placed over the guidewire and into the internal jugular vein. Guidewire was removed and catheter itself threaded into the **superior vena cava**. Position was verified with fluoroscopy. Used the tunneling device to tunnel the catheter onto the anterior chest wall, hooking up the Infuse-A-Port and then placing in the pocket created. Pocket was closed after testing to insure working properly. Skin was closed with **subcuticular** 4-0 Monocryl. Neck incision was also closed with subcuticular 4-0 Monocryl. Benzoin and steri-strips were placed over the incision. The patient was awakened and returned to the recovery room in satisfactory condition.

GODFREY REGIONAL HOSPITAL
123 Main Street • Aldon, FL 77714 • (407) 555-1234

STOP AND PRACTICE—cont'd

1. What condition necessitated the procedure? metastatic colon CA
   Explain this condition. veins are not good for chemotherapy
2. In what type of vessel was the catheter placed? superior vena cava
3. What technique was used for placing the guide wire into the internal jugular? Seldinger technique
   Explain the technique. Guidewire was placed in (R) jugular vein into SVC
4. What other medical equipment was attached to the catheter? dialator introducer
5. What will the equipment be used for? ~~chemotherapy~~ introduce catheter
6. Define the bolded terms.

jugular - SVC | Superior Vena Cava = major artery to heart
sternoid cleidomastoid = muscle in neck | Subcuticular = skin protector / drsg

Digestive System

GENERAL OVERVIEW

The digestive system processes foods and eliminates solid wastes from the body. This process begins in the mouth, or oral cavity, and ends with the removal of wastes through the rectum and anus (Figs. 1-16 to 1-18).

The small intestine is composed of three parts:

1. Duodenum
2. Jejunum
3. Ileum

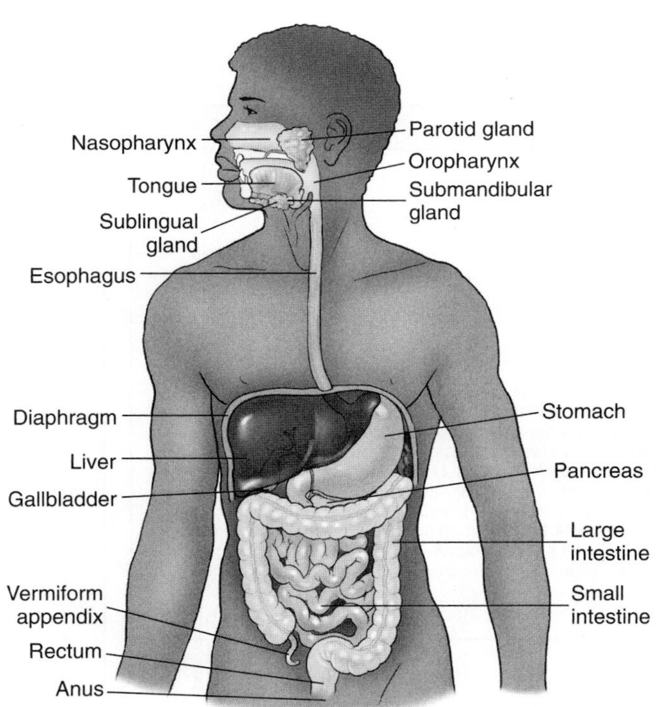

FIGURE 1-16. The gastrointestinal system.

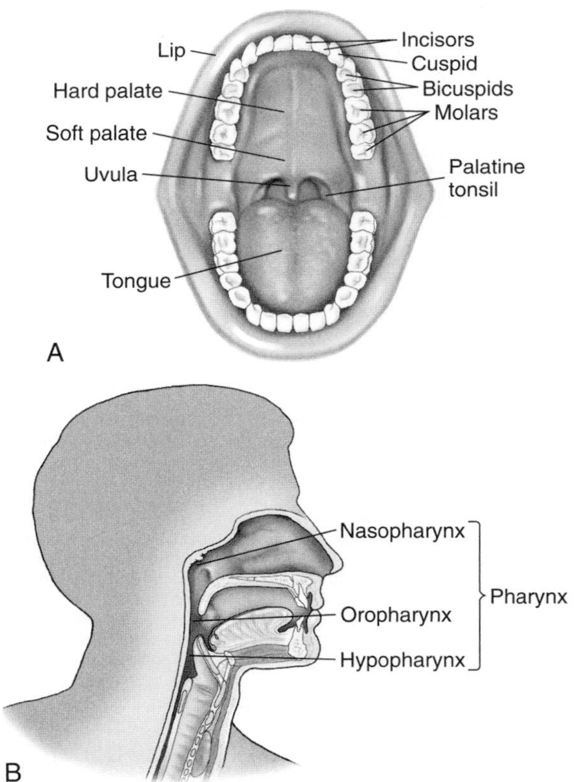

FIGURE 1-17. **A,** The oral cavity. **B,** The pharynx.

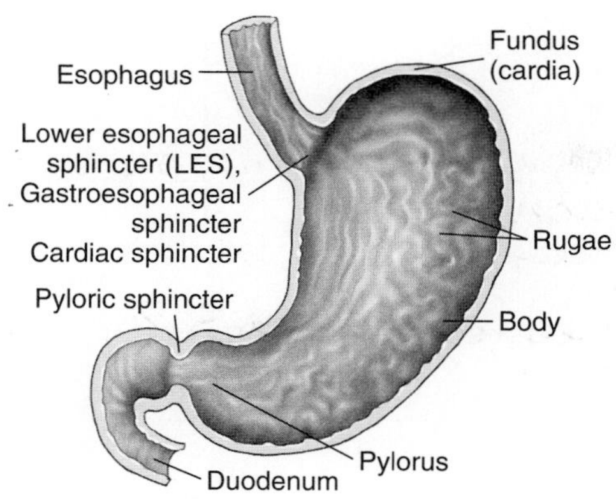

FIGURE 1-18. The stomach.

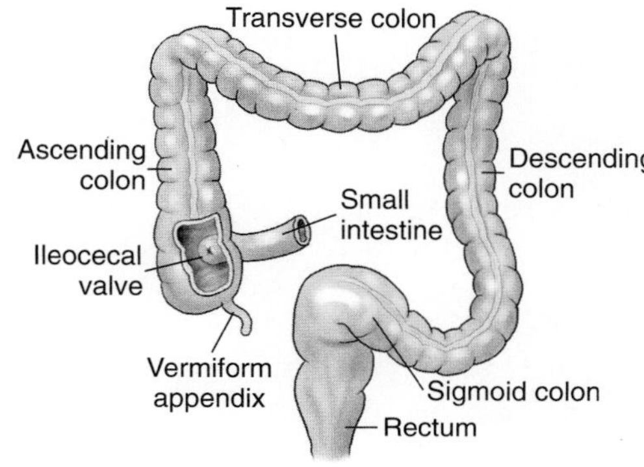

FIGURE 1-19. The large intestine (colon).

The large intestine is divided into four major regions (Fig. 1-19):

1. Cecum
2. Colon
3. Rectum
4. Anus

In addition to the primary organs of the digestive system, the accessory organs, which are outside the digestive tract, also aid in the process of digestion and absorption of nutrients for the body. These organs are the liver, pancreas, gallbladder, and appendix.

Many procedures on the digestive system are performed endoscopically, or by visual examination with an endoscope. Whereas colonoscopies are performed to visually examine the entire colon, proctosigmoidoscopies and sigmoidoscopies allow visualization of only part of the colon. Scopes may also be used to examine the esophagus (esophagoscopy), along with the stomach (gastroscopy), duodenum, and jejunum.

COMMON DIGESTIVE SYSTEM DISORDERS

Ulcer

Ulcers in the digestive tract, or peptic ulcers, usually occur as one of two types: gastric ulcers, which develop in the stomach, or duodenal ulcers, which develop in the duodenum. Colitis is an inflammation that develops in the colon and forms ulcerations within that organ.

Hernia

A protrusion of any organ, tissue, or structure is referred to as a *hernia.* Most commonly these protrusions are segments of colon through the abdominal wall. A number of hernias occur in the digestive tract:

Inguinal	Groin area
Umbilical	Umbilicus
Hiatal	Lower part of esophagus and top of stomach
Diaphragmatic	Congenital in the diaphragm

Hemorrhoids

Enlarged or varicose veins in the mucous membranes of the anus are referred to as *hemorrhoids.* Although often asymptomatic, hemorrhoids can become inflamed, prolapsed, or hemorrhagic and may need to be surgically removed or treated.

Diverticulosis

Diverticulosis is the development of small pockets, known as *diverticula,* in the lining of the large intestine. When they become inflamed, the condition is referred to as *diverticulitis.*

Refer to the illustrations in this chapter to review the structure and organs of the digestive system. Then review the word list for the digestive system in Table 1-5.

TABLE 1-5 DIGESTIVE SYSTEM WORD LIST

Prefixes	
Appendo	Appendix
Cheilo	Lips
Cholecysto	Gallbladder
Choledoco	Common bile duct
Choleo	Bile
Colo	Colon
Colono	Colon
Dys	Difficult
Entero	Small intestine
Esophago	Esophagus
Gastro	Stomach
Gingivo	Gums
Glosso	Tongue
Gluco	Sugar, sweet
Hepato	Liver
Jejuno	Jejunum
Linguo	Tongue
Lipo	Fat
Naso	Nose
Oro	Mouth
Pancreato	Pancreas
Phago	Eat or swallow
Pharyngo	Pharynx
Procto	Rectum and anus
Recto	Rectum
Sigmoido	Sigmoid colon
Stomo	Mouth
Stomato	Mouth
Terms	
Anastomosis	New connection between two structures
Appendicitis	Inflammation of the appendix
Cholecystitis	Inflammation of the gallbladder
Cholelithiasis	Formation of stones (calculi) in the gallbladder
Crohn's disease	Inflammation of the ileum; also called *regional enteritis*
Diverticulosis	Formation of pouches of diverticula in lining of colon
Diverticulitis	Inflammation caused by the formation of diverticulosis
Dyspepsia	Epigastric discomfort; also called *indigestion*
Dysphagia	Difficulty swallowing
Fistula	Abnormal channel from one organ to surface of body
Gastritis	Inflammation of the stomach
Gastric ulcer	Erosion of protective mucosal lining of stomach; also known as *peptic ulcer disease*
GERD	Return of stomach contents to the esophagus
Hematochezia	Bright-red lower gastrointestinal bleeding
Hemorrhoid	Varicose veins in the lower rectum or anus
Hepatitis	Inflammation of the liver
Hiatal hernia	Protrusion of portion of stomach through the diaphragm
Laparotomy	Incision into the abdominal wall
Melena	Black, tarry stools
Paracentesis	Surgical puncture to aspirate fluid from the abdominal cavity
Regurgitation	Return of swallowed food to mouth
Abbreviations	
BE	Barium enema
EGD	Esophagogastroduodenoscopy
GERD	Gastroesophageal reflux disease
IBD	Inflammatory bowel disease
IBS	Irritable bowel syndrome
PUD	Peptic ulcer disease

STOP AND PRACTICE

Read the medical documentation for an esophagogastroduodenoscopy and answer the following questions regarding this procedure.

OPERATIVE REPORT

Patient information:

Patient name:
DOB:
MR#:

Preoperative diagnosis:

Abdominal Pain, Epigastric

Postoperative diagnosis:

Gastritis, **Duodenitis**

Procedure(s) performed:

Esophagogastroduodenoscopy with biopsy

Anesthesia:

Assistant surgeon:

Description of procedure:

The patient was sedated with 50 mg Demerol **intravenously** plus 4 mg of Versed intravenously throughout the procedure.

The scope was inserted via the esophagus and advanced to the stomach and second portion of the duodenum.

The esophageal mucosa appear normal, with no evidence of esophageal **varices**. In the stomach, there was diffuse **erythema**, however, no ulcerations, erosions or fresh bleeding were noted. A biopsy was obtained.

Additional erythema was noted in the duodenum. An additional biopsy was obtained from the duodenum. The second portion of the duodenum appeared normal.

Rachel Perez MD

GODFREY REGIONAL HOSPITAL
123 Main Street • Aldon, FL 77714 • (407) 555-1234

STOP AND PRACTICE—cont'd

1. What conditions were found upon examination? diffuse erythema, Gastritis, Duodenitis
   Explain what these conditions are. inflammation
2. A scope was inserted and evaluation was performed on what areas? esophagus, stomach and 2nd portion of duodenum
3. How were you able to determine the extent of the procedure? the scope was advanced into duodenum
4. In addition to the visual examination, what other procedure(s) were performed? biopsies of stomach + duodeum
5. Through what orifice was the scope inserted? esophagus
6. Define the bolded terms.
   Duodenitis = inflammation of duodenum
   EGD = visual examination (via scope) of EGD
   intravenously = within vein
   varices = abn. large vein
   erythema = redness

Male and Female Genitourinary Systems

GENERAL OVERVIEW

The genitourinary system is composed of the urinary and reproductive systems. In the case of the male reproductive system, some of the urinary structures also serve reproductive functions. For purposes of review, male and female urinary and reproductive systems are reviewed here.

The urinary system filters blood to remove waste, maintains electrolyte balance, and regulates fluid balance within the body (Fig. 1-20). This is accomplished through the main structures of the urinary system: the kidneys, ureters, bladder, and urethra.

The kidneys are located outside the peritoneum, which is referred to as the *retroperitoneal area* or *cavity* (Fig. 1-21). The renal artery carries blood-contained waste products to the kidneys for processing; the waste products leave the kidneys by the renal vein. Those waste products, now in the form of urine, enter the renal pelvis, a cavity extension of the ureters, into the ureters to the urinary bladder. The urethra discharges urine from the bladder and the urinary meatus expels urine from the body.

The main function of the male reproductive system is to produce, maintain, and transport sperm (Fig. 1-22). The system also produces the hormone testosterone, which aids in the development of sperm and male sex traits.

The testes comprise the primary male reproductive organ and are located in an external sac called the *scrotum*. Under the upper surface of each testis is the epididymis, the first structure to store the sperm after its production in the testes. The sperm then enters the vas deferens, where it joins the seminal vesicles, forming the ejaculatory duct. The penis encloses the urethra, which expels both semen and urine from the body.

Kidney
Ureter
Bladder
Urethra
Female

FIGURE 1-20. Female urinary system.

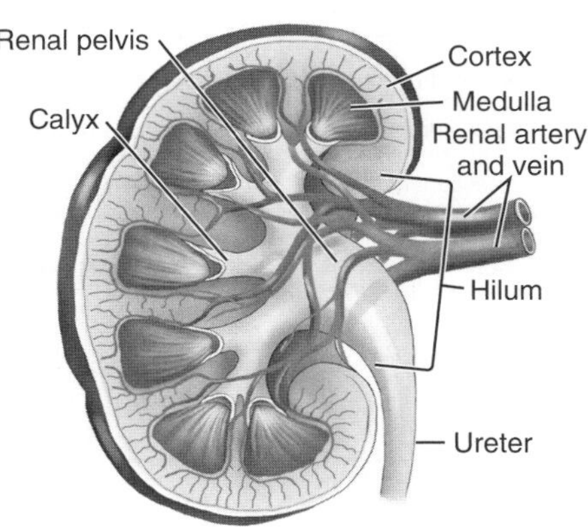

FIGURE 1-21. Cross-section of a kidney.

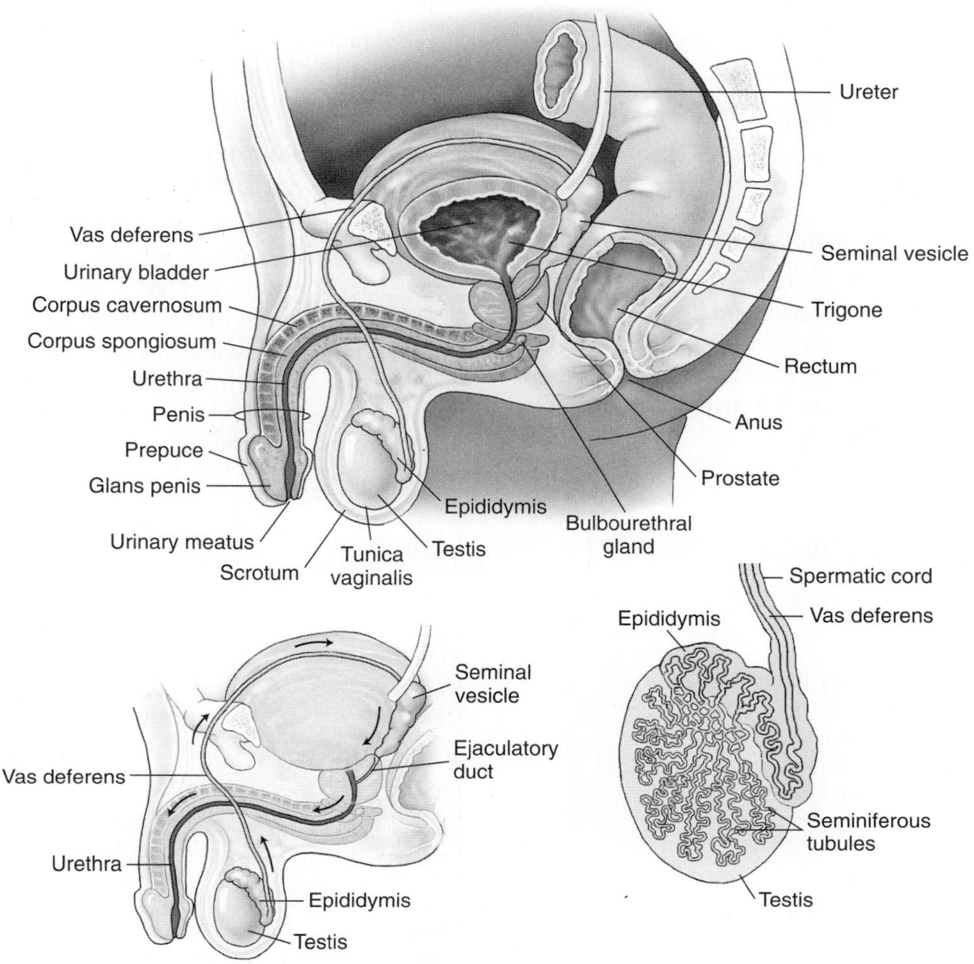

FIGURE 1-22. Male reproductive system and sperm production.

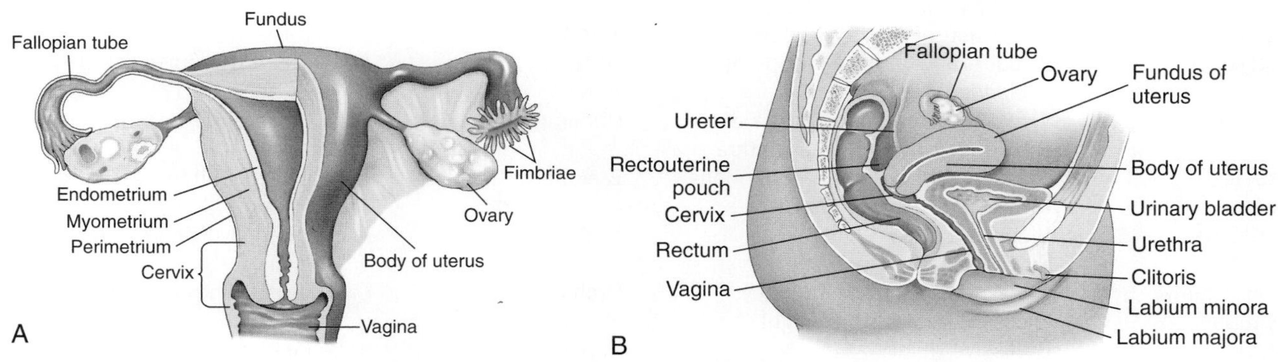

FIGURE 1-23. Female reproductive organs. **A,** Frontal view. **B,** Sagittal view.

The main organs of the female reproductive system are designed to produce ova (female reproductive cells) to transport to the site of fertilization (Fig. 1-23). The internal organs (the ovaries, fallopian tubes, vagina, and uterus) are joined by the external genitalia (the labia minor and majora, clitoris, and Bartholin glands), collectively known as the *vulva*.

The ovaries contain follicles, which contain ovum. If the egg unites with a spermatozoon, fertilization or conception will take place. The uterus stores and nourishes the embryo from the time the egg is fertilized until the fetus is expelled, or born. If fertilization has occurred outside the uterus, it is known as an *ectopic pregnancy.*

COMMON MALE AND FEMALE GENITOURINARY DISORDERS

Pyelonephritis

When a routine urinary tract infection invades the renal pelvis and kidney, it is referred to as *pyelonephritis* or *kidney infection.*

Nephrolithiasis, Cholelithiasis, and Ureterolithiasis

Stones that form in the kidney are referred to as *nephrolithiasis.* When these stones form in the ureter they are referred to as *ureterolithiasis* or *ureteral stones.* Stones may also form in the gallbladder, in which case they are referred to as *cholelithiasis.* Extracorporeal shockwave lithotripsy is often necessary to pulverize these stones.

Endometriosis

When endometrial tissue develops outside the uterus, the tissue develops into implants, or lesions, known as *endometriosis.* This condition may cause pain or infertility.

Pelvic Inflammatory Disease

General inflammation of the uterus, fallopian tubes, ovaries, or pelvic structures is referred to as *pelvic inflammatory disease.* This condition is usually caused by inflammation from bacteria, a virus, or yeast.

Review the figures in this chapter to make certain you are familiar with the various components that comprise the female, male, and urinary systems. Table 1-6 contains key terms, suffixes, prefixes, and abbreviations for the female, male, and urinary systems.

TABLE 1-6 MALE AND FEMALE URINARY SYSTEMS WORD LIST

Urinary System	
Prefixes	
Cysto	Urinary bladder
Nephro	Kidney
Oligo	Scanty
Peritoneo	Peritoneum
Pyelo	Renal pelvis
Poly	Many, excessive
Pyo	Pus
Reno	Renal
Stasis	Controlling, stabilizing
Uretero	Ureters
Urethro	Urethra
Uro	Urine, urinary system
Terms	
Cystitis	Inflammation of the urinary bladder
Cystocele	Herniation of urinary bladder
Cystoscopy	Visual examination by scope of bladder
Cystourethroscopy	Visual examination by scope of bladder by way of the urethra
Diabetes	Deficiency of antidiuretic hormone
Dysuria	Difficulty or painful urination
Hematuria	Blood in urine
Lithotripsy	Crushing of urinary stone
Nephrectomy	Excision or removal of kidney
Nocturia	Excessive urination at night
Polydipsia	Excessive thirst
Polyuria	Frequent, excessive urination
Pyelonephritis	Infection of the renal pelvis
Abbreviations	
BUN	Blood urea nitrogen
CRF	Chronic renal failure
DM	Diabetes mellitus
ESRD	End-stage renal disease
IUP	Intrauterine pregnancy
IVP	Intravenous pyelogram
KUB	Kidneys, ureters, bladder
STD	Sexually transmitted disease
UTI	Urinary tract infection
Male Genital System	
Prefixes	
Balano	Glans penis
Epididymo	Epididymis
Orchido	Testicles
Peni	Penis
Phallo	Penis
Prostato	Prostate
Testo	Testicles
Scroto	Scrotum
Vaso	Vas deferens
Terms	
BPH	Abnormal enlargement of prostate gland
Circumcision	Removal of all or part of the foreskin
Erectile dysfunction	Repeated inability to get or keep an erection
Hydrocele	Accumulation of fluid in tunica vaginalis testis
Orchiectomy	Excision or removal of one or both testes
Prostatis	Inflammation of prostate
Vasectomy	Excision or removal of vas deferens
Abbreviations	
BPH	Benign prostatic hypertrophy
DRE	Digital rectal examination
PSA	Prostate-specific antigen
TURP	Transurethral resection of the prostate

Continued

TABLE 1-6 MALE AND FEMALE URINARY SYSTEMS WORD LIST—cont'd

Female Genital System

Prefixes

Cervico	Cervix
Colpo	Vagina
Culdo	Rectouterine pouch
Episio	Vulva
Feto	Fetus
Gravido	Pregnancy
Gyneco	Female
Hystero	Uterus
Mammo, masto	Breast
Meno	Menses, menstruation
Metrio/metro	Lining of the uterus
Nato	Born
Omphalo	Umbilicus
Oophoro	Ovary
Para	Labor, delivery
Primi	First
Salpingo	Fallopian tube(s)
Utero	Uterus
Vagino	Vagina
Vulvo	Vulva

Terms

Abortion	Termination of pregnancy before fetus is viable
Amenorrhea	Lack of menstrual flow
Amniocentesis	Aspiration of amniotic fluid by a needle to diagnose for fetal abnormalities
Antepartum	First portion of pregnancy (before birth)
Cephalopelvic	Disproportion; infant's head larger than pelvic outlet
Dysplasia	Abnormal formation of cervical cells
Dysmenorrhea	Painful menstrual flow
Eclampsia	Serious form of hypertension in pregnancy
Ectopic pregnancy	Embryo outside the uterus
Endometriosis	Tissue making up lining of uterus is found outside the uterus
Episiotomy	Incision to widen vaginal orifice to avoid tearing during delivery
Gestation	Length of time from conception until birth
Hysterectomy	Excision or removal of uterus
Leiomyoma	Fibroids
Mastectomy	Excision or removal of breast
Menometrorrhagia	Excessive uterine bleeding other than from menstrual flow
Metrorrhagia	Uterine bleeding other than from menstrual flow
Multigravida	More than one pregnancy
Multipara	More than one delivery
Oophorectomy	Excision or removal of ovary
Placenta previa	Placenta malpositioned in uterus, covering the cervical opening
Postpartum	Period immediately after birth
Preeclampsia	Abnormal pregnancy condition characterized by edema, hypertension, proteinuria; also known as *toxemia*
Puerperium	Period immediately after birth
Salpingectomy	Excision or removal of fallopian tube(s)
Tubal ligation	Sterilization in which fallopian tubes are cut, ligated, and cauterized to prevent pregnancy

Abbreviations

CS	Cesarean section
D&C	Dilation and curettage
DUB	Dysfunctional uterine bleeding
ERT	Estrogen replacement therapy
FHR	Fetal heart rate
GPA	Number of pregnancies (G)/gravida, number of deliveries (P)/para, number of abortions/miscarriages (A)/abortion
HRT	Hormone replacement therapy
IUD	Intrauterine device
LMP	Last menstrual period
NST	Nonstress test
PID	Pelvic inflammatory disease
TAH BSO	Total abdominal hysterectomy with bilateral salpingo-oophorectomy
VBAC	Vaginal birth after cesarean section

STOP AND PRACTICE

Answer the following questions regarding the procedure described.

OPERATIVE REPORT

Patient information:

Patient name:
DOB:
MR#:

Preoperative diagnosis:

Urinary retention

Postoperative diagnosis:

Urinary retention

Procedure(s) performed:

Cystoscopy and **percutaneous** placement of **suprapubic** catheter

Anesthesia:

Assistant surgeon:

Description of procedure:

Patient was placed on operating table in the **lithotomy** position. Perineum was prepped and draped sterilely. 10cc Xylocaine jelly was injected into the urethra. The cystoscope was inserted. Urethra was unremarkable. Prostate was very large with **trilobar hypertrophy**.

Bladder shows catheter cystitis and a lot of **trabeculation**, diffusely inflamed.
Bladder was filled under vision with the cystoscope. Made a stab incision and using the dilator suprapublically dilated to 28 French leaving the catheter in place. The cystoscope was then removed. Patient tolerated the procedure without difficulty.

Rachel Perez MD

GODFREY REGIONAL HOSPITAL
123 Main Street • Aldon, FL 77714 • (407) 555-1234

STOP AND PRACTICE—cont'd

1. What procedure(s) were performed? Cystoscopy + percutaneous placement of suprapubic catheter
2. What technique was used to place the suprapubic catheter? stab incision
   What does this term mean? incision using a dialator for fluid removal
3. What were the findings through the cystoscope? Bladder showed catheter cystitis + trabeculation
4. In what position was the patient placed? lithotomy
5. How was the prostate described by the surgeon? very large with trilobar hypertrophy
6. Define the bolded terms.

percutaneous = incision/puncture
suprapubic = above pubis
lithotomy = stone removal
trilobar hypertrophy = abnormal growth
trabeculation = partician that divides

Nervous System and Sense Organs (Eyes and Ears)

GENERAL OVERVIEW

The nervous system is composed of the central nervous system and the peripheral nervous system.

The central nervous system consists of the brain and spinal cord (Figs. 1-24 and 1-25), which are protected by membranes known as the *meninges*. The brain is composed of four major structures: the cerebrum (Fig. 1-26), the cerebellum, brainstem, and diencephalons. The spinal cord transmits impulses from the body to the brain while the brain transmits muscle impulses to muscles and organs throughout the body.

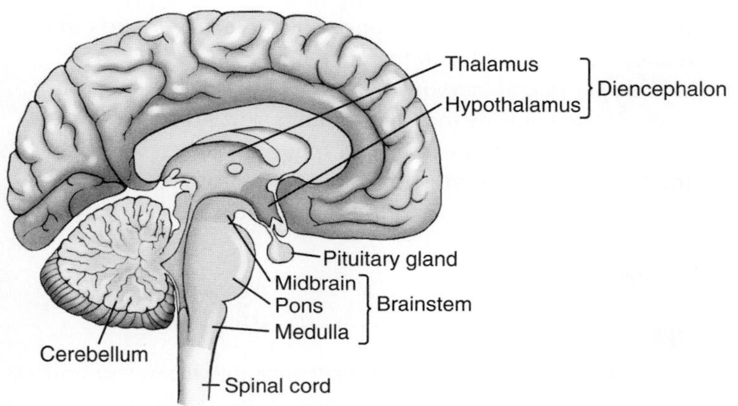

FIGURE 1-24. The brain.

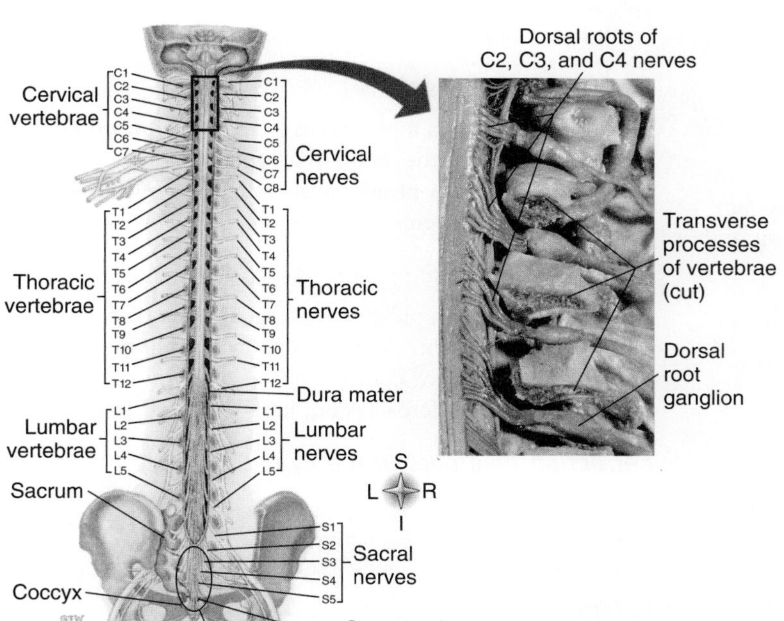

FIGURE 1-25. The spinal cord.

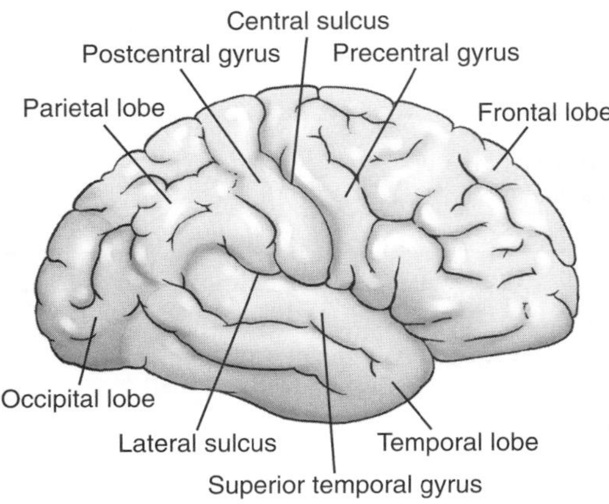

FIGURE 1-26. The cerebrum.

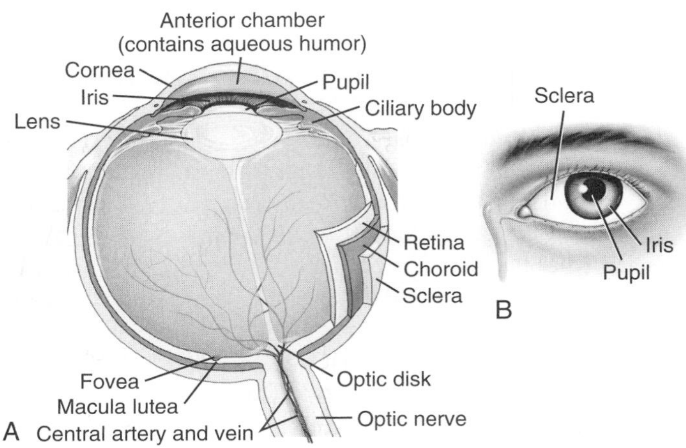

FIGURE 1-27. A, The eyeball viewed from above. **B,** The anterior view of the eyeball.

Both the brain and spinal cord receive limited protection from the meninges, which consist of three layers: the dura mater, the arachnoid, and the pia mater.

The peripheral nervous system consists of all nervous tissue located outside the spinal column and skull, composed of 12 pairs of cranial nerves carrying impulses to and from the brain. It is also composed of 31 pairs of spinal nerves carrying impulses to and from the spinal cord.

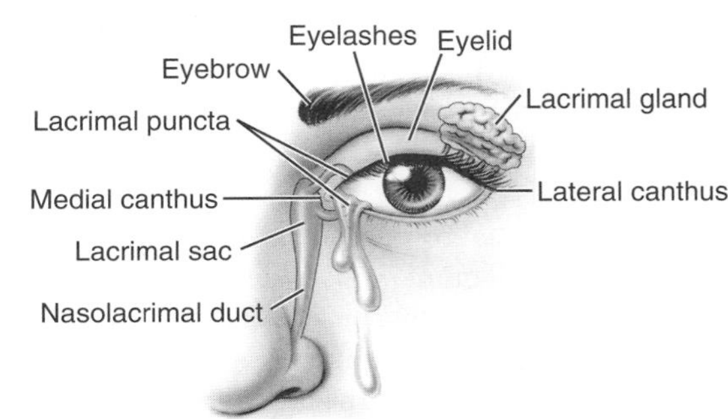

FIGURE 1-28. Ocular adnexa.

SENSE ORGANS

Eye

The outermost layer of the eyeball includes the sclera and cornea (Fig. 1-27). The cornea is one of the only body structures that does not contain capillaries and therefore relies on fluids from the eye for nourishment (Fig. 1-28). The conjunctiva covers the outer surface of the eye and lines the eyelids. The inner eye is composed of the choroids, iris, and ciliary body.

Ear

The ear consists of three sections: the external ear, middle ear (or tympanic cavity), and inner ear, referred to as the *labyrinth* (Fig. 1-29). The ears are responsible for hearing and body equilibrium.

COMMON NERVOUS SYSTEM AND SENSE ORGAN DISORDERS

Cerebrovascular Disease

Any disorders of blood vessels of the brain are referred to as *cerebrovascular disease.* These may be minor, with stroke symptoms such as brief blackout, dizziness, or blurred vision that resolve in 24 hours, known as a *transient ischemic attack,* or a cerebrovascular accident, which is more severe and frequently has more significant symptoms such as weakness or paralysis on one or more sides of the body. Impaired speech, lack of coordination, coma, and death may result from a cerebrovascular accident.

Seizure Disorders

Electrical disturbances to the brain result in seizures, which result in temporary loss of consciousness.

Parkinson's Disease

Parkinson's disease is a progressive neurologic disorder that affects the part of the brain that controls movement. As neurons of the brain progressively deteriorate, tremors and other abnormal movements result.

Multiple Sclerosis

Multiple sclerosis is a progressive, degenerative disease of the central nervous system. An individual with multiple sclerosis usually loses all motor control and becomes an invalid. The origin of multiple sclerosis is not known at this time.

Refraction Disorders of the Eye

Myopia	Nearsightedness
Hyperopia	Farsightedness
Presbyopia	Farsightedness characterized by aging

Cataracts

Cloudiness that occurs on the lens of the eye, impairing vision, is referred to as *cataracts.* Cataract extraction is a very

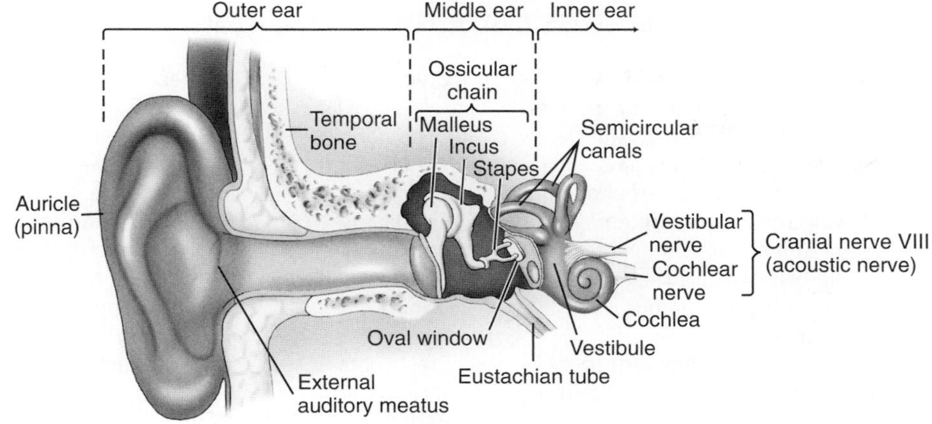

FIGURE 1-29. The ear.

common procedure for removing the defective lens, usually by phacoemulsification, and implanting an intraocular lens to replace it.

Glaucoma

Increased intraocular pressure, or glaucoma, creates increased pressure on the optic nerve and, if not controlled, may destroy the optic nerve and sight.

Strabismus

When one eye is misaligned with the other, resulting in the eyes not focusing in unison, the condition is referred to as *strabismus.* This is usually treated soon after birth and normal vision is restored at an early age. If not corrected early, vision may be lost in the affected eye.

Otitis Media

An inflammation of the middle ear is known as *otitis media.* Most common in children because of the inability of the body to drain fluids from the eustachian tube, a myringotomy or tympanostomy may be performed to make an incision into the eardrum, place a pressure-equalizing tube, or both, to assist in draining fluid from the ear.

Several figures in this chapter show the various components of the nervous system and sense organs. Review these illustrations to make certain you are familiar with the various components that comprise these systems. Table 1-7 contains key terms, suffixes, prefixes, and abbreviations for the nervous system and sense organs.

TABLE 1-7 NERVOUS SYSTEM AND SENSE ORGANS WORD LIST

Nervous System	
Prefixes	
Cerebello	Cerebellum
Encephalo	Brain
Meningo	Meninges
Myelo	Spinal cord
Radiculo	Nerve root
Rhizo	Nerve root
Spondylo	Vertebra
Terms	
Aphasia	Impairment of ability to form or understand speech
Concussion	Head injury characterized by loss of consciousness, amnesia, seizures, change in mental status
Dementia	Chronic, progressive organic mental disorder
Dysphagia	Difficulty swallowing
Encephalitis	Inflammation of brain
Epilepsy	Characterized by seizures, sensory disturbances, abnormal behavior, and/or loss of consciousness
Hemiparesis	Muscular weakness or slight paralysis on one side of body
Hemiplegia	Paralysis on one side of body
Hydrocephalus	Abnormal accumulation of fluid in ventricles of brain
Multiple sclerosis	Neurodegenerative disease characterized by destruction of myelin sheaths or central nervous system neurons
Neurorrhaphy	Suturing of severed nerve
Paraplegic	Paralysis of lower limbs and trunk
Paresthesia	Prickling, burning, numbness

Continued

TABLE 1-7 NERVOUS SYSTEM AND SENSE ORGANS WORD LIST—cont'd

Parkinson's disease	Progressive neurodegenerative diseases characterized by tremors, slow shuffling gait, hypokinesia, dysphasia, and dysphagia
Spina bifida	Spinal column has abnormal opening, allowing protrusion of meninges and/or spinal cord
Stroke/CVA	Ischemia of cerebral tissue caused by occlusion from thrombus
Syncope	Fainting or near fainting
Tay-Sachs	Inherited disease characterized by enzyme disorder that results in central nervous system deterioration
Tourette's syndrome	Condition characterized by facial grimaces, tics, involuntary arm or shoulder movements, involuntary vocalizations
Transient ischemic attack	Same characteristics of stroke except resolves or disappears within 24 hours
Vertigo	Dizziness
Abbreviations	
ALS	Amyotrophic lateral sclerosis
C1-C8	Cervical nerves
CNS	Central nervous system
CSF	Cerebrospinal fluid
CVA	Cerebrovascular accident
L1-L5	Lumbar nerves
LP	Lumbar puncture
MS	Multiple sclerosis
T1-T12	Thoracic nerves
TIA	Transient ischemic attack
SENSE SYSTEM: EYE AND EAR	
Eye	
Prefixes	
Blepharo	Eyelid
Conjunctivo	Conjunctiva
Irido	Iris
Kerato	Cornea
Lacrimo	Tear
Opto	Vision
Ophthalmo	Eye
Papillo	Optic disk
Phaco	Lens
Pupillo	Pupil
Retino	Retina
Sclero	Sclera
Vitreo	Vitreous
Terms	
Aphakia	Condition of no lens
Astigmatism	Malcurvature of cornea leading to blurred vision
Blepharitis	Inflammation of eyelid
Blepharoptosis	Drooping of upper eyelid
Cataract	Loss of transparency of lens
Chalazion	Hardened swelling of meibomian gland from blockage
Conjunctivitis	Inflammation of conjunctiva; also called *pinkeye*
Diplopia	Double vision
Ectropion	Turning outward of eyelid
Entropion	Turning inward of eyelid
Glaucoma	Abnormal intraocular pressure
Myopia	Nearsightedness
Nystagmus	Involuntary movement of eye
Presbyopia	Loss of elasticity of lens, usually from age
Radial keratotomy	Corneal incision that treats myopia by incising cornea in spokeline pattern
Strasbimus	Lack of coordination between eyes
Trabeculotomy	External excision of eye to promote intraocular circulation
Abbreviations	
EOM	Extraocular movements
IOL	Intraocular lens
IOP	Intraocular pressure
OD	Right eye
OS	Left eye
OU	Both eyes
Ear	
Prefixes	
Acousto	Hearing
Auro	Ear
Myringo	Eardrum
Ossiculo	Ossicles
Oto	Ear
Labyrintho	Inner
Salpingo	Eustachian tube
Stapedo	Stapes
Temporo	Temporal bone
Tympano	Eardrum
Terms	
Labyrinthitis	Inflammation of inner ear
Menière's disease	Chronic condition characterized by vertigo, hearing loss, tinnitus
Myringotomy	Incision of eardrum
Otitis externa	Inflammation of outer ear
Otitis media	Inflammation of middle ear
Tympanoplasty	Repair of middle ear, eardrum
Tympanostomy	Creating of opening through eardrum to promote drainage; commonly referred to as *myringtomy with tube placement*
Abbreviations	
AD	Right ear
AS	Left ear
AU	Both ears
ENT	Ears, nose, throat
OM	Otitis media

STOP AND PRACTICE

Answer the following questions regarding the procedure below.

OPERATIVE REPORT

Patient information:

Patient name:
DOB:
MR#:

Preoperative diagnosis:

Bilateral carpal tunnel syndrome

Postoperative diagnosis:

Left carpal tunnel release

Procedure(s) performed:

Anesthesia:

Assistant surgeon:

Description of procedure:

Patient was brought to the OR and placed under IV regional anesthetic. Left upper extremity was thoroughly prepped and draped in the usual sterile fashion. Curvilinear incision was carried across the **volar** aspect of the left wrist. Blunt **dissection** was carried down exposing the transverse carpal ligament. The **median** nerve was identified and protected while the transverse carpal ligament was divided completely. Hemostasis was achieved by **electrocautery**. Skin was closed utilizing interrupted simple sutures of 4-0 Nylon. Patient returned to Same Day Surgery in good condition having tolerated the procedure.

GODFREY REGIONAL HOSPITAL
123 Main Street • Aldon, FL 77714 • (407) 555-1234

STOP AND PRACTICE—cont'd

1. How was the procedure performed? open
2. Why was the procedure performed? Bilateral carpal tunnel syndrome
3. Where was the incision made? across the volar aspect of (L) wrist
4. What type of anesthetic was used? IV regional anesthetic
5. What does the abbreviation IV indicate? intravenous
6. Define the bolded terms.

Bilateral = both sides
volar = across
dissection = cut or divide
median = middle
electrocautery = burning of vessels to stop bleeding

Chapter in Review

Certification Review

- Identify key terms in the medical documentation for coding purposes.
- Understand the appropriate use and meaning of medical abbreviations.
- Define prefixes, suffixes, and word roots necessary to form medical terms.

Student Assignments

- Study Chapter 1.
- Review the Learning Objectives in Chapter 1.
- Review the Certification Review for Chapter 1.
- Complete the Stop and Practice exercise contained in Chapter 1.
- Complete the Chapter Review exercise to reinforce concepts learned in Chapter 1.
- Complete the practice exercises on the companion Evolve site for reinforcement of the concepts contained in Chapter 1.
- Complete the Workbook exercises for Chapter 1 as assigned by your instructor.

Chapter Review Exercise

Define the following terms or spell out the acronyms, then identify the appropriate system for each:

	Definition	System
1. FTSG	______	______
2. Lipoma	______	______
3. Cyanosis	______	______
4. Tracheotomy	______	______
5. SOB	______	______
6. Arthrocentesis	______	______
7. Rhinorrhea	______	______
8. Cardiomegaly	______	______
9. CAD	______	______
10. CHF	______	______
11. VAD	______	______
12. Dysphagia	______	______
13. Autograft	______	______
14. Gastritis	______	______
15. IUD	______	______
16. Blepharoplasty	______	______
17. Cataract	______	______
18. OU	______	______
19. Otitis media	______	______
20. Tympanoplasty	______	______

Practical Application

For the following coding scenarios, define the bolded terms.

1. Right total hip arthroplasty

The right lower extremity was prepped and draped in the usual sterile fashion. A curvilinear incision centered about the greater trochanter was made, and tissue and fascia were dissected. The piriformis and external rotator were taken off the **posterior femur**, exposing the underlying capsule. The hip was dislocated and the femoral head and neck **osteotomized** for preoperative templating. The acetabulum was dissected and reamed. After these procedures, a 52-mm prosthesis was implanted with proper abduction angle. Two cancellous screws were placed for fixation. Our attention was redirected to the **femur,** where the proximal femur was fashioned to accept a **prosthesis.** A size 12 femoral head was placed and the hip was reduced. The **fascia** was closed with interrupted sutures. Running 3-0 Vicryl was placed in the **subcuticular layer** and Steri-Strips placed across the skin.

Term	Definitions
______________	______________
______________	______________
______________	______________
______________	______________
______________	______________
______________	______________

2. *Therapeutic* ***bronchoscopy***

Acute bronchitis with exacerbation of chronic obstructive pulmonary disease.

Patient admitted for **dyspnea.** Bronchoscope was introduced through the right nostril. The **nasopharyngeal** mucosa, vocal cords, and trachea appear normal.

Washings from the **right lower lobe** bronchus were obtained and sent for **cytology.**

Term	Definitions
______________	______________
______________	______________
______________	______________
______________	______________
______________	______________

3. *Laparoscopic cholecystectomy*

Patient with classic **right upper quadrant** pain. A **periumbilical** incision was made and a port placed. The abdomen was insufflated with carbon dioxide gas. The gallbladder revealed **chronic cholecystitis** with **cholelithiasis.** The gallbladder was grasped and removed through the upper port.

Term	Definitions
______________	______________
______________	______________
______________	______________
______________	______________

4. ***Computerized tomographic angiography*** *of the brain and neck*

CTA of the brain and neck were performed, both with **intravenous** enhancement. No **stenosis** or occlusions were found. No saccular **aneurysms** were identified. **Atherosclerotic** formation at the right carotid bifurcation was identified. There were diffuse degenerative changes in the spine with posterior **spondylosis.**

Term	Definitions
______________	______________
______________	______________
______________	______________
______________	______________
______________	______________
______________	______________

5. *Modified radical* ***mastectomy***

Adenocarcinoma of the right breast

Breast was infiltrated and **superior** and **inferior** flaps were developed. Breast was taken off the chest and axillary **dissection** was also performed. **Hemostasis** was good.

Term	Definitions
______________	______________
______________	______________
______________	______________

2

Crucial Role of Documentation

LEARNING OBJECTIVES

After completing this chapter, the student will be able to:

- Comprehend the importance of physician documentation in the coding process.
- Understand that signature requirements are a vital component of the documentation process.
- Identify the various components of the medical chart needed for documentation in both office and hospital settings.
- Identify the various providers of service and locations of service where documentation occurs.
- Realize the importance of identifying documentation deficiencies.
- Understand the need for implementing documentation tools within the practice or facility to overcome documentation deficiencies.
- Develop specific tools and monitoring processes to correct and prevent documentation deficiencies identified in the practice setting.
- Apply documentation concepts to practice medical documents.

CODING REFERENCE TOOLS

Tool 2-1
Dictation Note Guide

Tool 2-2
History Check-off Guide

Tool 2-3
Examination Check-off Guide

Tool 2-4
Emergency Department Chart Documentation Requirements

Tool 2-5
ED Record of Treatment

Tool 2-6
History and Physical Examination Sample Dictation Model

Tool 2-7
Basic Documentation Do's and Don'ts

KEY TERMS

Assessment
Consultation
Discharge Summary
Examination
Fraud
History
The Joint Commission
Medical Decision Making
Medical Necessity
Medication Record
Objective
Patient History
Patient Quality Reporting Initiative (PQRI)
Pertinent Negative
Plan
Problem List
Qui Tam Action
Signature List
SOAP Format
Subjective

Documentation Drives the Coding Process

The first and perhaps most important aspect of medical coding is the documentation itself. Without appropriate documentation, coding is difficult, if not impossible. This chapter deals with physician documentation and its importance and role in both selecting correct coding for reimbursement and establishing medical necessity.

The first and foremost rule of coding and documentation is:

IF IT IS NOT DOCUMENTED, IT DID NOT HAPPEN.

If it did not happen, the provider may not code or collect payment for services. Billing for services that "did not happen" is the basic definition of **fraud**, an attempt to collect for services not furnished or to receive payment for services that would not otherwise be reimbursed. The specific definitions of fraud and abuse are discussed in Chapter 22.

In the same regard, if documentation is not *signed*, it does not exist. The provider of the service or the provider supervising the delivery of service must indicate that the work was performed or supervised by the provider for documentation to be complete. Carriers and other regulatory agencies differ regarding whether this documentation needs to be confirmed with a signature, initials, or other kind of identifying mark. The use of signature stamps in medical practice should be strongly discouraged; for most third-party carriers the signature stamp does not constitute the physician's authentication of services. Electronic signatures generated by computerized billing or medical records systems are becoming acceptable alternatives to original signatures. These electronic signatures should be verified as acceptable to federal, state, and other regulatory agencies before they are used. It is also prudent to maintain a signature log when more than one provider is represented so that all staff members are familiar with each provider's signature. This aspect is discussed later in the chapter.

The following examples may shed some light on the importance of documentation in the coding process.

Real Case Scenario

The gynecologic oncologist bills for an abdominal hysterectomy and an appendectomy. Diagnostic codes include malignant neoplasm of the cervix and malignant neoplasm of the appendix. The claim is sent to the insurance carrier, who reimburses for both services on the basis of medical necessity of the diagnoses listed.

Later medical review of the chart indicates no documented medical necessity because there was no diagnostic statement regarding malignancy to the appendix. The insurance carrier has reimbursed for services that are not "medically necessary" and thus are not covered.

Problem

Because the physician's documentation did not substantiate the appendectomy as other than incidental, payment was made inappropriately. If the carrier conducts a medical chart review, the provider will be liable for refunding the amount reimbursed for the appendectomy (the law now allows for up to three times the amount reimbursed). There may also be fines and penalties as well as a review of additional charts to identify other potentially fraudulent coding or billing. A representative sampling of similar charts may be made, and a percentage of the charges billed in error calculated, according to the results of that representative sampling. The percentage of all such procedures billed erroneously will be calculated as the error percentage, and that amount will be requested by the carrier for refund as overpayment.

In addition, the provider may be liable for fraud if services were billed and not provided or if services were deemed not medically necessary because of the lack of medical documentation. Fraud is penalized by the line item; therefore the number of cases calculated to be in error may be charged an average of $5000 per line item, with additional penalties and interest from the date of billing to the date of discovery by the carrier.

Although the amount reimbursed for the appendectomy represented may be only $400, the penalties will include triple the reimbursement (which equals $1200) plus a minimum $5000 line item fraud charge, plus interest. Therefore the single appendectomy refund to the carrier will easily exceed $6200, plus costs of the investigation into additional billing practices. The average gynecology/oncology office performs many of these services, and the amount assessed could easily run into many thousands of dollars.

In the real world of medical coding and billing, the coder attempts to impress upon the provider and documenter the importance of medical necessity in documentation. The provider may not comprehend such importance from a billing perspective but may fully understand the repercussions from a medical malpractice standpoint.

Until the last few decades, medical record documentation served solely as the mechanism for tracking patient visits and was used primarily by the physician in the office and by the medical staff. The physician or provider could document clearly and concisely, making review of documentation straightforward at the time of a future visit, or could handwrite charts illegibly because no one outside the office had to deal with the documentation.

More recently, the role of documentation in the coding and billing process has changed dramatically. These changes have become necessary in light of medical malpractice suits arising from poor documentation of medical care and an increase in fraud and abuse investigation by the federal government and third-party carriers (insurance companies). Increased emphasis on providing only medically necessary services requires that providers pay attention to which services will be paid or denied and submit properly documented claims.

MEDICAL MALPRACTICE AND DOCUMENTATION OF MEDICAL CARE

Because of the necessity of supporting documentation, the medical record serves as the best and perhaps the only line of defense against medical malpractice. The best protection from liability is well-documented patient care. Although many physicians may not comprehend the importance of good documentation from a coding and reimbursement perspective, they understand the necessity from a medical and legal standpoint. Take, for example, the following real-life scenario in which documentation was the determining factor for whether prudent medical care was, in fact, performed by the physician.

Real Case Scenario

Two years after a patient's death from myocardial infarction, the emergency department (ED) physician is sued for wrongful death. The patient's wife indicates in her suit that the ED physician failed to provide prudent medical care by not reading the electrocardiogram (ECG) performed on her husband during his last ED visit for chest pain before his death. As a result, the physician did not diagnose the myocardial infarction that caused the patient's death.

The physician's counsel argues that the physician did review the ECG, which showed no indication of an impending myocardial infarction. The plaintiff's attorney asks the physician to present evidence that the ECG was reviewed and yielded no significant findings. The ECG is present in the medical record; unfortunately, no evidence exists to support the claim that the physician had appropriately reviewed the ECG at the time of the patient's last visit.

Because of this lack of documentation, the ED physician was held accountable in part for the death of this patient. The outcome was that the plaintiff received a significant monetary award.

MEDICAL NECESSITY

Medical malpractice has not been the only factor that has increased the importance of medical documentation. Title XVIII of the Social Security Act of 1966 mandated that the Medicare program (for elderly and disabled Americans) pay only for those services that were deemed "medically necessary." To ensure that the standard of **medical necessity** was being met for all services paid by the Medicare program, the Centers for Medicare and Medicaid Services (CMS) began performing medical reviews. These reviews are performed based on analysis of computerized claims submitted to Medicare as well as postpayment reviews. Computerized claims submission also allows physician and practice profiling, including determination of physicians who might be submitting fraudulent claims, claims for procedures deemed not medically necessary, or claims for services either not provided or not documented. This process is responsible for saving the Medicare program billions of dollars annually.

With the implementation of the 1995 Evaluation and Management CPT (Current Procedural Terminology, fourth edition) code specifications, Medicare began conducting random claim audits to verify that the new codes were being used appropriately. To this day, the review of evaluation and management services remains a top priority of the federal government and other third-party carriers because the error rate remains significantly high for these services.

The federal government also implemented **qui tam action,** which allows individuals who are aware of potential fraudulent activity to report providers and be awarded a significant amount of the funds recouped from the resulting investigation. Commercial carriers also began to see the cost benefits of implementing claims review processes such as those implemented by Medicare, and they followed suit. Thus the coder needs to be aware that all entities may review charts for potential fraud and abuse and medical necessity; when appropriate, such entities may request refunds, interest, and perhaps penalties.

During the same time these review processes were being implemented, the cost of health care continued to soar. Third-party carriers recognized that these review processes identified overpayments and also assisted in containing health care costs. As a result, third-party carriers have invested significant time and resources to identify potential fraud, abuse, and overpayment for undocumented or inappropriately documented services.

REIMBURSEMENT

From the provider's perspective, medical record documentation also serves as the means for requesting correct reimbursement for services. The record is the primary source for identifying the appropriate procedures and services performed as well as the diagnostic documentation to support medical necessity. This information is then reviewed, interpreted, and translated into diagnostic and procedural codes, then billed for possible reimbursement. This is the primary role of the medical coder.

QUALITY ASSURANCE

The Tax Relief and Health Care Act of 2006 authorized the establishment of a physician quality reporting system by CMS, known as the **Physician Quality Reporting Initiative (PQRI)**. Under this program Medicare provided the possibility of a financial incentive to providers who report a set of designated quality measures in providing medical care to their patients. Providers who successfully provide these quality measures and report them appropriately are eligible for a financial incentive. In 2007 the bonus payment was designated at 1.5% of total allowed charges for billed services. This incentive has been offered in an attempt to ensure quality services to Medicare recipients. Obviously, medical documentation solely drives this process because the incentive bonus is available only with the submission of the documentation that specific quality measures for specific medical conditions have been met. This program is further described in Chapter 22.

The Medical Chart as a Whole

The patient medical record is a compilation of information gathered during the patient encounter and recorded to document the care provided and the medical necessity of those services. The record contains information regarding the patient's medical, social, and family history as well as information supplied by the patient regarding presenting complaints, examination findings by the physician, and medical decisions regarding the patient's care. Because much of the data secured during the patient encounter are recorded in the patient medical record and later used for requesting reimbursement or statistical analysis, the records must contain legible, accurate, and specific information regarding each encounter.

The information contained in the medical record is used to determine whether reimbursement is received for services. In addition, medical records are useful for vital statistics, utilization review, case management, quality assurance, and research.

There are several organizations, such as the American Hospital Association and The Joint Commission, which have developed minimum documentation requirements, such as the following:

- Medical record should be complete and legible.
- Relevant risk factors should be identified.
- All entries should be dated and authenticated.
- The medical necessity for all services should be apparent and documented.
- All diagnoses, past and present, should be accessible to the provider.
- A written plan of treatment should be included in the record.
- Patient's progress or any noncompliance should be reported.
- Each page of documentation should include the patient's name, date, and identification number.

One of the most common difficulties encountered by the medical biller or coder is the difference between medical terminology used in medical records and the descriptors found in CPT and ICD-9-CM (the International Classification, Ninth Revision, Clinical Modification) references. An understanding of medical terms, abbreviations, and acronyms is imperative in establishing the appropriate diagnostic and procedural codes of the services performed. A review of these terms, prefixes, and suffixes is included in the medical terminology review in Chapter 1.

The medical record document(s) may be electronic, handwritten, dictated, or typed notes or in the form of preprinted check-off forms.

Forms of Documentation

HANDWRITTEN DOCUMENTATION

Physicians are known for handwriting that is sometimes barely legible. Not only does handwritten documentation create ambiguities, it is lengthy and time consuming to read. The average handwritten chart is one and a half times longer than a dictated report. Dictated reports tend to be more organized, easier to read, and easier to defend in the event of a medical malpractice charge.

DICTATED OR TYPED DOCUMENTATION

Dictated notes tend to be more efficient, allowing quicker documentation in a more organized form. Many practices use macros with prewritten blocks of dictation to streamline the dictation process further.

CHECK-OFF SHEETS AND PREPRINTED FORMS

Although some physicians have abandoned the use of handwritten documentation, dictation may not provide a viable solution for their practices. A check-off style form may be used for documenting the data gathered during the encounter. Although this mechanism saves time and requires less space than handwritten documentation, it becomes almost too easy for the physician to "check off" items regardless of whether they are pertinent. Such a form may discourage documentation of more complete information by limiting space for findings. An alternative format would be a checklist that contains anatomic headings followed by multiple blank lines, thereby providing adequate space for documentation of significant observations.

ELECTRONIC MEDICAL RECORDS

Electronic medical records have become common in the medical office and facilities as well. There are a number of advantages to storing medical records electronically rather than in paper format, the most obvious being the reduction of costs associated with paper and record storage. However, the biggest advantage may be the ability of all personnel to access records simultaneously, coordinate care, and have immediate access to records. No longer does the provider need to wait for the transcription of the dictation or filing to be performed to access lab results or other urgent medical information. It also eliminates the illegible or undecipherable handwriting dilemma that faces the medical office staff. Unfortunately, electronic medical record systems can be cost prohibitive for a small practice; however, over time, they can actually represent a cost savings in the form of reduced copying, paper, computer supplies, dictation costs, and other costs associated with the paper record.

STANDARD ACRONYMS AND ABBREVIATIONS

No matter the format, documentation will almost certainly contain a number of abbreviations and acronyms. Specialty-specific abbreviations and any adopted by the individual physician should be avoided.

A list of standard abbreviations and acronyms used in a practice is helpful for the new transcriptionist, biller, or coder as well as during a third-party audit, utilization review, or other review of documentation. Unfortunately, many abbreviations can be interpreted more than one way. The following abbreviations are only a few examples:

"HS" could be interpreted as:
- at bedtime
- half strength
- hamstring
- heavy smoker
- heel spur
- high school

"CP" could be interpreted as:
- chest pain
- cleft palate
- chronic pain
- clinical pathway
- cor pulmonale

"LBP" could be:
- low back pain
- low blood pressure

A number of standardized abbreviations and acronyms are included in the system-specific reviews of medical terminology in Chapter 1.

SIGNATURE LISTS

A practice containing multiple providers should be capable of identifying each individual's signature in both the office and hospital setting. In the event of an audit, office personnel will be relied on to identify signatures that validate whether services coded and billed were documented appropriately. Practices with more than one provider should maintain a provider **signature list** in their files, with names and appropriate marks or signatures of each provider for signature authentication purposes (see Table 2-1).

Forms for Documentation Purposes

Myriad forms and formats may be used in gathering and recording the vital information stored in medical records; a few of the most common forms are reviewed in this chapter. Specific documentation guidelines for each type of service are addressed in more depth in specific chapters.

Because services may be provided in the office, outpatient or inpatient setting, or another facility, a number of documents are generated for record keeping, liability, and reimbursement.

OFFICE PROGRESS NOTE/HISTORY AND PHYSICAL

This document is one of the primary source documents for the physician's office. It may be conveyed in many formats and is usually typed or handwritten. Because of the variety of documents used for office notes, the coder must be familiar with a number of formats and be able to decipher both physicians' and patients' handwritten notes.

PATIENT HISTORY

In many instances the documentation process begins with the patient. Once the patient has registered, many medical practices ask the patient to complete a history and physical form that contains a multitude of questions regarding current complaint(s) and medical, family, and social history. If information from the patient's history form is used to determine the services provided, the physician must indicate he or she has reviewed the information by affixing a signature or acceptable authentication, date, and proof in the form of documentation. The physician may choose to incorporate relevant information from the history form into the patient progress note, in which case the review of the history form would not need to be documented.

In the event the **patient history** form is reviewed in subsequent visits for needed medical data, the physician will need to document each time that information from the form was used in medical decision making.

An example of the patient history and physical form is illustrated in Figure 2-1. Note the physician designation of "abnormals" and physician authentication by signature, date, and information reviewed on this document as appropriate.

PROGRESS NOTE/VISIT NOTE

The clinical staff, including nurses and medical assistants, may conduct the next part of the documentation process. The patient typically is directed to the clinical area after complet-

HISTORY AND PHYSICAL EXAMINATION

Godfrey Regional Hospital History & Physical
Admission: 12/01/00

The patient came from a nursing home and felt weak on the right side. Workers there thought she was alert, but confused. When seen in the ER, she was able to answer questions appropriately and to follow commands but was unable to lift her right leg. She had some motion in her right arm but was unable to squeeze her right hand. When evaluated by the ER physician, she was determined to be confused, and was difficult to understand. CT was obtained, with initial impression of a large, left hemispheric bleed.

Past medical history:

Remarkable for polymyalgia, GERD, hyperthyroid, DJD of the knees. Hospitalizations for pneumonia, gout, situational depression.
CURRENT MEDICATION: Prilosec 20 mg qd, Synthroid .125 mg daily, Propulsid 10 mg bid, Prednisone 20 mg daily, Cardizem CD 120 mg daily.

Family and social history

Unobtainable from patient.

Review of systems:

Unobtainable from patient.

Physical exam

Patient is alert but confused. She is not dysarthric. PERRL. Extraocular movements are normal. Sclera is clear. TMs normal. No skull lacerations noted. Slight right VII nerve weakness. Lungs clear. Abdomen is soft, nontender, without guarding or rebound. Neuro/MS: Full ROM except right arm and leg. Unable to raise her left leg or to move it at all with positive Babinski's on right. Normal labs.

Laboratory/radiology:

X-ray:

Assessment:

Intracranial bleed.

Plan:

GODFREY REGIONAL HOSPITAL
123 Main Street • Aldon, FL 77714 • (407) 555-1234

FIGURE 2-1. Patient history and physical form.

ing registration paperwork for "workup" documentation. The following information may be included:

Patient's reason for encounter (chief complaint)
Vital signs
Other pertinent medical data (laboratory results, other services performed that relate to the chief complaint)

These notes, made by clinical staff other than the physician, may be incorporated into the diagnostic statement and procedures only if the notes are also mentioned in the provider's report (similar to the patient history described above). The provider of service must document review of this information by signature/authentication and date or by incorporation in the provider's progress note.

Care should be taken that services provided by the clinical staff under the auspices of the health care professional are documented as ordered and performed to the provider's satisfaction. For instance, the patient arrives for an injection of vitamin K given by the nurse. An order for that service must exist in the record as well as the documentation that the service occurred, with review by the provider or billing entity that the provider supervised, reviewed, and approved both the service and its provision in the manner described in the notes.

An example of the staff note is illustrated in Figure 2-2. Note that this information may be incorporated in the physician's encounter documentation as in Figure 2-5, which is discussed below.

PROBLEM LIST

Some provider offices use a **problem list** similar to Figure 2-3 to record each time a patient presents with a new problem. This form serves as a medical summary of problems, medications, illnesses, and injuries. The provider should review this form at the time of each encounter for consideration in evaluating and managing the current problem. Again, this document must be reviewed and authenticated if information contained in the problem list will be used to determine diagnostic or procedural services or information incorporated in the physician progress note.

MEDICATION RECORD

Medications administered may be recorded on a separate document known as a **medication record** contained in the medical records. To be considered part of the diagnostic and procedural information used in the coding and billing process, these records must be documented as reviewed and approved, including orders for the medications and their appropriate administration as ordered by the physician. A minimum of the provider's signature or authentication; the date; and the name, dosage, strength, and administration route of the medication should be recorded. It will become apparent later why all this information is needed for billing and coding purposes. Figure 2-4 is an example of a medication record that may be present in the physician's office or health care provider's facility.

Documentation Formats

The provider or physician must document the examination of the patient and any relevant findings as well as the thought process in evaluating the patient and decision making regarding possible diagnosis and management options. This documentation should include positive findings and **pertinent negatives.** By indicating negative findings, the physician documents the thought processes required to arrive at final diagnosis(es) and the procedure(s) or service(s) that should be performed. Thus pertinent negatives, positive findings, and information regarding the history of the patient's chief complaint all play a part in the evaluation and management of the patient's condition.

Physician documentation usually is presented in one of two formats: SOAP or History, Exam, Medical Decision Making.

The **SOAP format** has been a nationally recognized method of recording patient visits for decades. The word SOAP is an acronym for ***s***ubjective ***o***bjective ***a***ssessment ***p***lan. However, this format has undergone major changes over the past few years because of documentation necessary for the assignment of evaluation and management procedure codes.

The **subjective** portion of the encounter takes into account all the information gathered from the patient, including information regarding the chief complaint, history of the patient, signs and symptoms, and a patient inventory of other system signs and symptoms.

The **objective** part of the visit consists of observed objective findings, including any pertinent negatives. For example, an observation of the patient by the provider might be recorded as "The patient, an elderly 56-year-old female, appears to be in no acute distress." Other objective findings may include observations from the physical examination.

The **assessment** portion consists of the patient's diagnosis or problem appropriately documented in the chart. It may also consist of a differential diagnosis or a list of possible diagnoses considered in the evaluation and management process.

The **plan** portion of the SOAP note is documentation of further workup or planned treatment. A plan for further treatment, workup, and follow-up is usually included in this portion of the record.

With the inception of the 1995 and 1997 evaluation and management guidelines from CMS came the need for more specific documentation guidelines. In some cases, the SOAP format was simply expanded to include these elements. In other instances, another format that encompassed the needed elements was devised.

As is discussed in Chapter 11, the patient record is composed of documentation regarding history, examination, and medical decision-making components of the encounter.

STAFF NOTES Patient name ______________________________

Date	Time	Staff notations

GODFREY MEDICAL ASSOCIATES
1532 Third Avenue, Suite 120 • Aldon, FL 77713 • (407) 555-4000

FIGURE 2-2. Staff/visit note.

Problem list	
Date	Problem

Date	Hospitalizations

Date	Surgeries

Date	Immunizations

Name ______________________

Phone #: ______________________

Allergies	

Current medications

Screening tests	Date	Date	Date
Mammogram			
Pap smear			
DRE/PSA			
12 Lead ECG			
ECG stress test			
Colonoscopy			

Last update:

GODFREY MEDICAL ASSOCIATES
1532 Third Avenue, Suite 120 • Aldon, FL 77713 • (407) 555-4000

FIGURE 2-3. Problem list.

MEDICATION FLOW SHEET

Name: ______________________ Pharmacy: ______________________

Phone: ______________________ Phone: ______________________

Allergies: ______________________

Medical HX: ______________________

Medication	Date	Date	Date	Date	Date

GODFREY MEDICAL ASSOCIATES

1532 Third Avenue, Suite 120 • Aldon, FL 77713 • (407) 555-4000

FIGURE 2-4. Medication flow sheet.

The **history** portion of the record includes the chief complaint and information provided by the patient for the reason for the visit as well as medical, social, and family history that may contribute to the current problem. Such information may include a review of systems gathered by the provider from patient statements or answers to questions.

The **examination** part of the record consists of the provider's findings. As with the history component, pertinent negatives or findings that rule out possible diagnoses are as important to the documentation process as positive findings.

The **medical decision-making** component of the record contains information regarding data, management and diagnostic options, risk, and morbidity or mortality. Clinical information such as x-ray findings, laboratory and other diagnostic tests, previous medical documentation, and discussion of the patient's condition or results with other medical providers is included in the review of data. Management and diagnostic options include whether the problem is new, established, stable, or worsening. The risk of morbidity or mortality refers to the effects the patient may experience if the condition is not treated appropriately. (These components are discussed in greater depth during review of the evaluation and management process in Chapter 11.)

Although the actual forms and formats differ significantly from practice to practice, Figures 2-5, 2-6, and 2-7 are representative samples of physician progress notes in the provider office setting. Variations in hospital and facility progress notes are highlighted later in this chapter.

Ancillary Reports

Ancillary records such as x-ray, laboratory, and other diagnostic tests are typically recorded on separate documents in the medical record. Two physicians are usually involved in this process: one ordering the procedure and one performing it and interpreting results. When two physicians are involved, only the physician responsible for the final interpretation can bill for the interpretative services. If one physician requires input or collaboration with the other physician (often known as an *overread*), then only the physician ultimately responsible for the interpretation may code and bill for the service. Documentation and billing for these services will differ on the basis of the providers involved. These documents may be found in both the physician chart and in the facility chart, depending on where services were performed and which provider was involved in treatment and interpretation.

For illustration, samples of a radiology report (Fig. 2-8), laboratory test results (Fig. 2-9), a surgical pathology report (Fig. 2-10), an ECG (Fig. 2-11), respiratory test outcomes (Fig. 2-12), and an electromyography report (Fig. 2-13) are provided. Specific documentation, signature requirements, and document contents are discussed in detail in the chapters on radiology, laboratory, and medicine services.

Hospital or Facility Records

The hospital record creates another complication in the documentation process. In many instances, either a practice does not have access to the documentation or access is extremely difficult. In addition, the provider typically does not dictate these hospital visit notes, except perhaps for the admission history and physical. As a result, the documentation is typically short, is sometimes marginally legible, and may not be accessible for every encounter so that level of service for coding and billing purposes may be determined.

In some instances the facility is treated as a "teaching facility," which requires additional guidelines for documentation purposes. When residents, interns, and medical students are involved in the care of patients, specific guidelines outline what services may be performed by which entities and what documentation is required for consideration for reimbursement.

In addition, requirements for hospital records often are above and beyond those of office records. **The Joint Commission,** a national organization that accredits hospitals, has developed additional guidelines for inpatient medical records that include the following:

- Patient's medical history
- Any known allergies
- Medical history completed within the first 24 hours of admission for inpatient
- Physical examination completed within the first 24 hours of admission for inpatient
- Conclusion drawn from the admitting history and physical examination
- Course of action statement planned for the stay
- Diagnostic and therapeutic orders
- Progress notes by all providers
- Consultation reports
- Nursing notes
- Ancillary procedure reports
- Conclusions or discharge summary at the end of the hospital stay

Keep in mind that facility documentation, in the form of nursing notes and notes by other facility employees, may not be considered as part of the provider's record unless the notes are documented as reviewed or are incorporated in the provider's medical record.

A number of documents, such as the following, may be included in hospital records:

- Admission history and physical
- Progress note
- Discharge summary
- Consultations
- Operative or surgical report
- Ancillary reports

Text continued on p. 52

PROGRESS NOTE

Chief complaint: ____________________

Date: ____________

Vital signs: BP______P______R______

History:

Exam:

Diagnosis/assessment:

Patient name: ____________________

Date of service: ____________

GODFREY MEDICAL ASSOCIATES

1532 Third Avenue, Suite 120 • Aldon, FL 77713 • (407) 555-4000

FIGURE 2-5. Physician progress note.

PROGRESS NOTE

Date: 02/05/XX	**Vital signs:** T	R
Chief complaint: Sore throat, difficulty swallowing	P	BP

02/05/XX This is a 7-year-old who has had a sore throat with some difficulty swallowing and a headache for the past two days. Not improving.

Examination:

She is afebrile. She has retro TM fluid on the left which is asymptomatic. The right side is normal. She has considerable amount of oropharyngeal inflammation, small tender anterior cervical node. Lungs are clear to auscultation. Heart, sinus without murmur.

Impression:

Strep tonsillitis

Plan:

She is placed on Amoxil 250 suspension tid for 10 days

Willen Obst MD

Patient name: Anne Novitz
DOB: 2/26/19XX
MR/Chart #: 63223

GODFREY REGIONAL OUTPATIENT CLINIC
3122 Shannon Avenue • Aldon, FL 77712 • (407) 555-7654

FIGURE 2-6. Physician progress note.

PROGRESS NOTE

Date: 01/18/XX	Vital signs: T	R
Chief complaint: Fever, nasal drainage	P	BP

01/18/XX

This 9-month-old child with Down's syndrome brought in today by mother with onset of fever and thick greenish drainage from his nose. Also developed a cough again. No history of ear infections and has had a history of pneumonia.

Physical examination:

General appearance of well-developed child in no acute distress

Head: Flat anterior fontanel

Ears: Canals small, cleared of cerumen

Neck: No adenopathy

Lungs: Clear, no wheezing but has noisy inspiratory respiration for which he had a recent bronchoscopy

Nose: He does have thick greenish drainage from his nose

Assessment:

Upper respiratory infection with symptoms of pulmonary infection

Plan:

Continue with Ibuprofen and decongestants
Placed on Augmentin 200 mg twice daily

Willem Obst MD

Patient name: Thomas Derringer
DOB: 4/16/20XX
MR/Chart #: 24481

GODFREY REGIONAL OUTPATIENT CLINIC
3122 Shannon Avenue • Aldon, FL 77712 • (407) 555-7654

FIGURE 2-7. Physician progress note.

RADIOLOGY REPORT

MR#:
DOB:
Dr.

Clinical summary:

Abdomen:

Conclusion:

Ddt/mm

D:
T:

, M.D. Date

GODFREY REGIONAL HOSPITAL
123 Main Street • Aldon, FL 77714 • (407) 555-1234

FIGURE 2-8. Radiology report.

Patient name: ______ Room #: ______
Age: ______ Sex: ______ Accession #: ______
Collected: ______ Received: ______
Reported: ______ Req. #/Med. Rec. #: ______
Requesting Phys: ______ Pt. ID #: ______

Test name	Results		Reference range	TL
	Out of range	In range		

Testing location (see reverse side)

GODFREY CLINICAL LABORATORIES
465 Dogwood Court • Aldon, FL 77712 • (407) 555-9876

FIGURE 2-9. Laboratory report.

SURGICAL PATHOLOGY REPORT

Name:__________ Hosp. No.:__________ Path. No.:__________

Date:______ Room:______ Age:_____ Sex:_____ Surgeon:__________ M.D.

Operation:__________

Material submitted:__________

Pre-op diagnosis:__________

Post-op diagnosis:__________

Previous material:__________ Pertinent history:__________

Diagnosis:

__________ M.D.
Pathologist

Gross description:

Micro description:

GODFREY CLINICAL LABORATORIES
465 Dogwood Court • Aldon, FL 77712 • (407) 555-9876

FIGURE 2-10. Surgical pathology report.

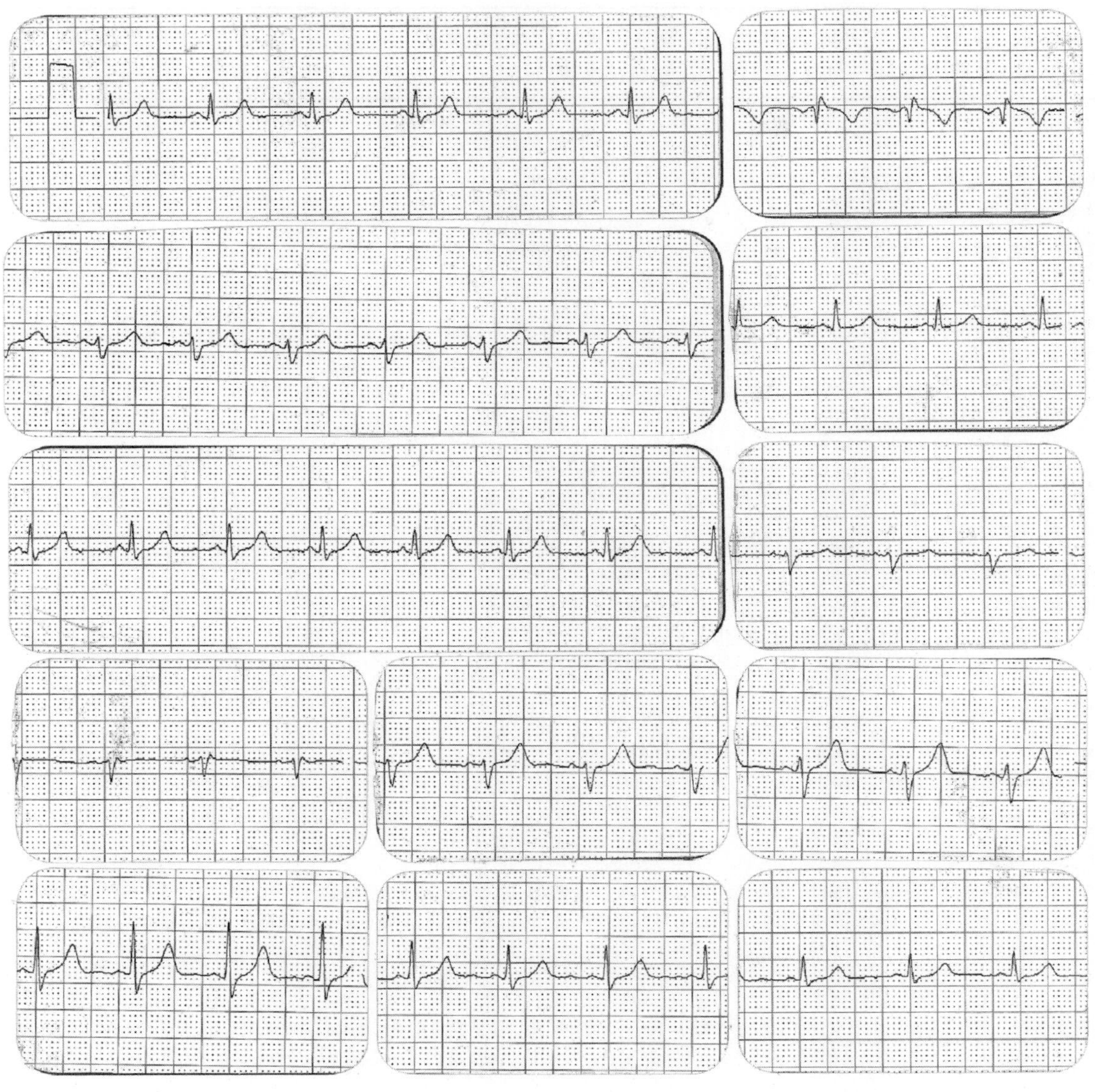

CLIN. DIAG.: Chest Pain

ECG DESCRIPTION: Stat 12 Lead

INTERPRETATION:

PATIENT: Jane Doe

DIG ( ) QUIN. ( ) AGE 29 SEX F B.P. 120/80

ECG REQUEST BY Dr. Hope U. Arewell

ATR. RATE 90 VENTR. RATE 90

INTERVALS: P-R .12 QRS .08 QTc

AXIS: Left Axis shift

RHYTHM: Normal Sinus Rhythm

INTERPRETED BY: H. Arewell MD

DATE:

FIGURE 2-11. Electrocardiogram.

Place top of report No. 3 here

PULMONARY FUNCTION REPORT

Name:____
ID #: ______________
Age: ________Ht:______Wt:_____
Reason for test: ______________
Smoker? ______________
Dyspnea: ______________
Lung surgery: ______________
Frequent cough: ______________
Pain breathing? ______________
Heart disease? ______________
Wheeze/asthma? ______________
Abnormal X-ray? ______________

Test	PRED	ACTL	%PRED
FVC	4.76		81%
FEV1	3.77		88%
FEV1/FVC	81%		107%
FEF 25%–75%	4.64		124%
MMET (sec.)	0.68		49%
FEF max	9.14		127%
FEF 25%	8.43		126%
FEF 50%	6.26		118%
FEF 75%	3.17		56%
ET (sec.)	—		—
Maximal FVC	4.76		81%
Maximal FEV1	3.77		88%
MVV (L/min.)	154.7		100%

BTPS factor:______________Last cal:______________
Primary normals source: Knudson.

Base:____________________
T____________________

Operator:____________________

Physician:____________________

GODFREY CLINICAL LABORATORIES
465 Dogwood Court • Aldon, FL 77712 • (407) 555-9876

FIGURE 2-12. Respiratory testing report.

ELECTROMYOGRAPHY LABORATORY REPORT

Nerve conduction studies

NR = No response
M = Motor
S = Sensory
Mx = Mixed
• = no increment after 10 sec. exercise
† = no decrement to 2/sec x3
X = Forearm median to ulnar crossover

Name:__________
Clinic number:__________ Age:_____
Birthdate:_______ Date:_______
Referring physician:__________

Nerve stimulated	(Recording site)	**Amplitude** (Sensory = uV; Meter = mV) Distal			Proximal		**Distal/peak latency** (mSec)			**Conduction velocity** (M/sec)			**F-wave latency** (mSec)		
		Right	Left	Normal	Rt	Lt	Rt	Lt	Normal	Rt	Lt	Normal	Rt	Lt	Normal
Lower right															
Sural (S) Pt.B	ankle						NH								
Peroneal (M) knee	EDB	3.0					14.8			45					
Peroneal (M) ankle	EDB	3.0					4.8								
Posterior tibia (M) knee	AH	1.0					14.8			41					
Posterior tibia (M) ankle	AH	1.5					4.2								
H-reflex							NR	NR							
Med (s) wrist	1st	9.0					3.6								
Med (m) elbow	thenar	2.8					9.6			58					
Med (m) wrist	thenar	2.8					4.4								
Ulnar (s) wrist	5th	1440					2.8								

Needle examination:

Summary:

Impression:

____________________, M.D.

GODFREY CLINICAL LABORATORIES
465 Dogwood Court • Aldon, FL 77712 • (407) 555-9876

FIGURE 2-13. Electromyography report.

ADMISSION HISTORY AND PHYSICAL

A hospital or facility requires that a history be taken and a physical examination be performed on all patients to assess their condition, needs, and plan for treatment. Because this is usually a comprehensive service that takes place during admission, the documentation is typically dictated and includes in-depth information regarding history, present illnesses, examination, and management options. In many facilities, such as hospitals that are governed by The Joint Commission accreditation standards, this admission history and physical examination, also known as an *HEP,* must be performed within 24 hours of admission. Figure 2-14 is an example of a hospital history and physical examination. Although the service may initially be performed by an intern or resident under the governance of the physician, the physician must see and evaluate the patient as well. Legal documentation requirements for residents and providers other than physicians are discussed in later chapters.

PROGRESS NOTE

The biggest problems with hospital daily visit notes are that they are often brief, handwritten, and sometimes illegible—or they may not be present at all. Some of the most significant fraud cases have involved services performed in the hospital setting that were not properly documented. When the provider sees the patient in the hospital, the evaluation of the patient and the provider's assessment and plan should be documented in the daily progress note. Because more than one provider may see the patient daily, each document should bear the provider's name, authentication, and date for specific services. Figure 2-15 is an example of a hospital or facility progress note.

DISCHARGE SUMMARY

The **discharge summary** should document the various services provided that prepare the patient for discharge from the inpatient facility. Discharge visits are based on the amount of time required to prepare the patient for discharge, including any services performed on the patient's floor. Services provided; the patient's progress during hospitalization; and discharge instructions, follow-up, and diagnoses are all included in the discharge summary, which is usually dictated because it tends to be lengthy and contains significant data. Figure 2-16 represents a typical discharge note for a hospital or facility. Again, format may differ from one facility to another, but the information contained in this document is typically the same.

CONSULTATIONS

A **consultation** involves one physician sending the patient to another physician for an expert medical opinion. Documentation must contain a written request and a written report (with findings) that was sent back to the requesting physician. Consultations are perhaps the most misunderstood medical documents and are often incorrectly coded and billed. For services to remain consultative in nature, the physician rendering an opinion may provide therapy but cannot assume primary care of the patient. Consultations may occur in many settings, including the hospital or facility, physician's office, or any setting where the criteria have been met. Figure 2-17 is an example of a dictated consultation report.

OPERATIVE OR PROCEDURE REPORT

A surgical procedure report, regardless of whether the procedure was performed in the hospital or in the office, would be documented in the same manner. The following elements should be included in all such documents:

- Patient identification (name, medical record number, date of birth, room number)
- Preoperative diagnosis
- Postoperative diagnosis
- Name of procedure
- Surgeon(s)
- Anesthesia/anesthesiologist(s)
- Indications
- Procedure detail
- Findings summary
- Complications or unusual service
- Postoperative condition

One of the most common mistakes made on the interpretation of operative reports is being misled by the word *summary* under "procedure performed." Because this summary is abbreviated, it often does not contain all the information necessary to assign diagnostic and procedural codes as appropriate. To code and bill for every service that was provided, the coder must review the entire operative record, sometimes multiple pages, abstract the key elements, and assign codes for all services provided. Chapter 13 illustrates how involved this process can be.

An example of an operative report form is given in Figure 2-18. In addition, the anesthesiologist would also generate a report of the preanesthesia services, administration of anesthesia, and patient monitoring (Fig. 2-19).

HEALTH CARE STAFF NOTES (NURSING NOTES)/PHYSICIAN EXTENDERS

Notes made by health care staff may be incorporated into the diagnostic statement only if these notes are mentioned in the provider's progress notes. If such documents are to be used in this manner, they must be referenced by the provider's own documentation (date, signature or authentication, and approval of actions taken or treatments provided). These nursing notes are similar to the visit note represented in Figure 2-2 except that the headings will reflect the hospital or facility's information rather than the physician's.

Text continued on p. 61

HISTORY AND PHYSICAL EXAMINATION

WHITE, Blanche
Admitted: 04/26/XXXX

John Parker, M.D.

Medical record number: 2253546

Patient is an 89-year-old female who presents with abdominal pain, nausea, vomiting and weakness. She has also had a fairly substantial weight loss over the last year or so. Symptoms started getting worse yesterday. She denies fever or chills. Bowels have moved, although not substantially. She says she really has not eaten enough to have a bowel movement at this time. She denied any blood in her emesis. No blood in her stool. The pain seems to be in the epigastric area, although it seems to radiate a little bit to the right side. Denies pain into the back at all. She also denies chest pain or SOB. She had become weak, enough that she has fallen. This had been a problem for her in the past, where she had fallen, but she has not had a fall for quite some time.

Past medical history:

Hypertension, cholelithiasis, depression, osteoarthritis and CHF. She also has cholelithiasis but no cholecystitis. She reports the recent onset of Type 2 diabetes mellitus. She reports an allergy to Penicillin and Amoxicillin.

Family and social history:

Noncontributory except she does smoke

Review of systems:

Denies dysuria or any difficulty urinating. She denies fever, chills or any swelling in her upper or lower extremities. No difficulties reported in breathing, joint pain, specifically knee pain she has reported in the past.

Physical exam

General: Alert, oriented, in no obvious distress
Vital signs: Temperature 98.4, respiration 20, BP 117/43
HEENT: Negative
Neck: Supple, no thyromegaly
Chest: Clear
Heart: Regular rate and rhythm, normal S1, S2, no gallops, rubs or murmurs
Abdomen: Soft, epigastric tenderness. No mass or organomegaly. No guarding, rebound or rigidity if noted
Back: No pain or spinal tenderness is noted on exam
Extremities: No swelling or edema noted
Neuro: She appears a little less alert and oriented than she has in the past

Laboratory/radiology:

Lab tests include WBC of 13,200, hemoglobin 11.8, platelet count 220,000. The differential appears within normal range. Panel 20 shows a decreased sodium of 133, Potassium 3.3, BUN and creatinine are 34 and 1.4. Calcium is 8.1, Bilirubin 1.1. Proteins normal, liver functions normal and TSH is 2.2. Urinalysis is normal.

X-ray:

Flat and upright of her abdomen are pending at this time.

Assessment:

Patient with abdominal pain, nausea, and weakness. This would be recurrent cholelithiasis or gastroenteritis.

Plan:

Admit to hospital, and will give her medications for her nausea. IV fluids for rehydration and watch for fever, chills. If things do not improve, will order ultrasound or CT.

John Parker MD

GODFREY REGIONAL HOSPITAL
123 Main Street • Aldon, FL 77714 • (407) 555-1234

FIGURE 2-14. Hospital admission and history.

PROGRESS NOTE

Date/time

04/27/XX

S:

Patient is feeling a little better, and she is not having as much abdominal pain.
She is still experiencing some trouble with confusion and loose stools. She appears to have lapsing periods of confusion, and even seeing people that are actually not there.
Otherwise she indicates she feels somewhat better. Denies chest pain, SOB, but reports she still feels a little weak.

O:

Afebrile, vital signs normal. Chest clear, heart regular rhythm, extremities show no appearance of edema.

A:

Abdominal pain with diarrhea, improved.
Confusion that may be related to infection.

P:

Will get blood cultures and start her on IV medications. If her confusion continues, may determine CT scan or ultrasound would be appropriate.

John Palermo

Patient ID

WHITE, Blanche
Admit: 04/26/XX
MR# 2253546

PROGRESS NOTES

GODFREY REGIONAL HOSPITAL
123 Main Street • Aldon, FL 77714 • (407) 555-1234

FIGURE 2-15. Hospital progress note.

DISCHARGE SUMMARY

WHITE, Blanche #2253546
DOB: 05/17/XX

Admitted: 04/26/XX
Discharged: 04/30/XX

Discharge diagnoses:

1. Diverticulosis
2. Abdominal pain with fever
3. Cholelithiasis
4. Confusion
5. Hypertension
6. Depression
7. Osteoarthritis
8. Congestive heart failure
9. Diabetes mellitus type 2

History:

Patient is an 89-year-old female who presented with abdominal pain, nausea, and vomiting. She was also weak. She had lost some weight, mostly I think because of dietary measures to control her newly diagnosed diabetes. She had no fever or chills. Her BMs had been fairly regular although not substantial. I do not feel that she is eating enough because of her recent symptoms to make bowel movements. There was no diarrhea. There has been no blood in the stool. She did have an emesis earlier that had no blood in it. Pain seemed to be over the epigastrium and left side, sometimes would radiate to the right side.

On exam, temperature was 98.4°, respiratory rate 20, blood pressure 117/43. HEENT examination was negative. Chest was clear. Heart had a regular rhythm, normal S1, S2, no gallops, rubs or murmurs. The abdomen was soft, there was epigastric tenderness. No mass or organomegaly. There was no guarding, rebound or rigidity. Extremities had no edema.

Laboratory and radiology studies:

Lab tests include a CBC showing a white count of 15,200, hemoglobin 11.8, platelet count 220,000. Follow-ups remained stable with an improving white count of 7,600. Hemoglobin had dropped to 10.8 with hydration.

On admission her sodium was 133, Potassium 3.3, BUN was elevated at 34, blood sugar 193. Calcium was low at 8.1. Bilirubin was up to 1.1 and her TSH was 2.2. Her sugars were followed in the hospital and they ranged fairly stable with a high being noted at 195, low of 75. Her potassium did respond to supplementation and was 3.9 on discharge. Her sodium also improved to 137 by discharge. BUN was back to normal as was the creatinine. Liver function testing was normal by discharge.

Urinalysis was remarkable for 2–3 WBCs per hpf. Blood cultures were negative.

Flat and upright of abdomen showed degenerative changes and a probable gallstone.

Abdominal ultrasound showed cholelithiasis.

Hospital course:

Patient was admitted to the hospital because of her abdominal symptoms. She was started on Protonix 40 mg IV as well as Demerol for pain. Her pre-hospital medications were continued. Blood cultures were obtained and she was placed on Levaquin 500 mg every 24 hours. Amaryl was also started for her blood sugars, which remained stable except for a low of 56. She was a little symptomatic with this and so sugar was given. Her potassium was supplemented with cocktails in addition to the IV fluids. Over the course of her hospitalization she did feel better with her stomach. She did have some trouble with confusion on occasion, but mostly with the initial episode of her illness and during the time she had a fever. Over the course of her stay however, she was still weak and we needed to watch her blood sugars closely. She was switched to oral Levaquin, told to monitor her blood sugars closely, and continue the Amaryl. She will be started on OT and PT to help in strengthening her gait.

John Palermo MD

D: 04/30/XX
T: 05/02/XX

GODFREY REGIONAL HOSPITAL
123 Main Street • Aldon, FL 77714 • (407) 555-1234

FIGURE 2-16. Discharge summary.

CONSULTATIONS

Indication for consultation:

Ventricular tachycardia

History:

54-year-old with known history of cardiac disease who was undergoing outpatient arthroscopy of the knee. Patient's cardiac rhythm was noted to have multiple runs of non-sustained ventricular tachycardia. Patient remained asymptomatic stable.
Status post MI 15 years ago.

FAMILY/SOCIAL HISTORY:
Non-contributory

Exam:

PHYSICAL EXAM:
Head: Normocephalic, atraumatic
Neck: Supple, w/o evidence of JVP, mass or bruit
Chest: Clear to auscultation
Cardiac: Normal carotid upstroke with normal contour
Abdomen: Soft, nontender, no evidence of mass
Extremities: Showed no evidence of clubbing, cyanosis, or edema
Neurologic: Grossly intact, nonfocal
EKG: Ectopic atrial rhythm with delayed precordial transmission

Diagnosis/assessment:

IMPRESSION:
Known history of coronary atherosclerotic heart disease and atrial fibrillation, now presents with run of nonsustained V tach per report. It would be prudent to continue patient on his current medications and allow him to follow-up with his primary cardiologist.

We appreciate the opportunity to participate in the overall evaluation and management of this patient.

Patient name: ____________________

Date of service: ____________________

GODFREY MEDICAL ASSOCIATES
1532 Third Avenue, Suite 120 • Aldon, FL 77713 • (407) 555-4000

FIGURE 2-17. Dictated consultation report.

OPERATIVE REPORT

Patient information:
Patient name: DOB: MR#:
Preoperative diagnosis:
Postoperative diagnosis:
Procedure(s) performed:
Anesthesia:
Assistant surgeon:
Description of procedure:

GODFREY REGIONAL HOSPITAL
123 Main Street • Aldon, FL 77714 • (407) 555-1234

FIGURE 2-18. Operative report.

PRE-ANESTHESIA EVALUATION

Age	Sex	Height	Weight	Pre-procedure vital signs
	☐ M ☐ F	in./cm.	lb./kg.	B/P P R T

Proposed procedure

Previous anesthesia/operations *(if none, check here☐)*

Current medications *(if none, check here☐)*

Family history of anesthesia complications *(if none, check here☐)*

Allergies *(if NKDA, check here☐)*

Airway/teeth/head and neck

History from
☐ **Parent/guardian** ☐ **Poor historian** ☐ **Chart**
☐ **Significant other** ☐ **Patient**

System	WNL	Comments	Pertinent study results
Respiratory Asthma, Pneumonia Bronchitis, Productive cough COPD, Recent cold Dyspnea, SOB Orthopnea, Tuberculosis	☐	Tobacco use: ☐ No ☐ Yes ____ Pack/Day for ____ Years	Chest X-ray Pulmonary studies
Cardiovascular Angina, MI Arrhythmia, Murmur CHF, MVP Exercise tolerance, Pacemaker Hypertension, Rheumatic fever	☐		ECG
Hepato/gastrointestinal Bowel obstruction, Jaundice Cirrhosis, N&V Hepatitis, Reflux/heartburn Hiatal hernia, Ulcers	☐	Ethanol use: ☐ No ☐ Yes Frequency________	
Neuro/musculoskeletal Arthritis, Paresthesia Back problems, Syncope CVA/stroke, Seizures DJD, TIAs Headaches, Weakness Loss of consciousness Neuromuscular disease Paralysis	☐		
Renal/endocrine Diabetes Renal failure/dialysis Thyroid disease Urinary retention Urinary tract infection Weight loss/gain	☐		
Other Anemia Bleeding tendencies Hemophilia Pregnancy Sickle cell trait Transfusion history			

Problem list/diagnoses / Planned anesthesia/special monitors	ASA PS	Lab studies
Problem list/diagnoses	1 2	**Lab studies** Hgb/HcT/CBC Electrolytes Urinalysis
Planned anesthesia/special monitors	3 4 5 E	Other

Post-anesthesia note

Pre-anesthesia medications ordered

Signature of evaluator(s)

Signed Date Time

Optional form 517 back

GODFREY REGIONAL HOSPITAL
123 Main Street • Aldon, FL 77714 • (407) 555-1234

FIGURE 2-19. Anesthesia report.

History from: ☐ Patient ☐ Parent/guardian ☐ Significant other ☐ Chart ☐ Poor historian ☐ Language barrier

PRE-ANESTHESIA EVALUATION

☐ See previous anesthesia record dated ________ for information

Proposed procedure | **Age** | **Sex** ☐ M ☐ F | **Height** in/cm | **Weight** lb/kg

***Pre-procedure* vital signs**
B/P: P: R: T: O_2 SAT %:

Current medications ☐ None

Previous anesthesia/operations ☐ None

Airway
☐ MP1 ☐ MP2 ☐ MP3 ☐ MP4
☐ Unrestricted neck ROM ☐ T-M distance = ________ ☐ Obesity ☐ ↓ neck ROM:
☐ ↓ mouth opening/TMJ ☐ Hx difficult airway ☐ Teeth poor repair ☐ Teeth chipped/loose:
☐ Edentulous ☐ Facial hair ☐ Short muscular neck

Family HX anes. problems

Allergies ☐ None

System | **Comments** | **Diagnostic studies**

☐ WNL Respiratory
Asthma/RAD, Bronchiolitis, COPD, Emphysema, Bronchitis, Respiratory failure, Pleural effusion, Pulmonary embolism, Sinusitis/rhinitis, Environ. allergies, Chronic tonsillitis, Chronic OM, Recent URI, TB/+PPD, Pneumonia, Productive cough, SOB/dyspnea, OSA, Orthopnea, Wheezing

Tobacco use: ☐ Yes ☐ No ☐ Quit _____ Packs/Day for _____ Years

***Pre-procedure* pulmonary assessment:**

☐ WNL Cardiovascular
Hypertension, Hyperlipoproteinemia, CAD/cardiomyopathy, Angina, Stable/unstable, Myocardial infarction, CHF DOE PND, Peripheral vascular Dz, Exercise tolerance, Excellent/fair/poor, Abnormal ECG, Dysrhythmia, Hypovolemia, Chronic fatigue, Pacemaker/AICD, Murmur, Valvular Dz/MVP, Rheumatic fever, Endocarditis, Aneurysm

***Pre-procedure* cardiac assessment:**

☐ WNL Hepato/gastrointestinal
Obesity, Cirrhosis, Hepatitis/jaundice, Bowel obstruction, Ulcers, Hiatal hernia, GERD, N & V, Diarrhea, IBS, Pancreatitis, Gallbladder Dz, Diverticulum, Colon polyps

Ethanol use: ☐ Yes ☐ No ☐ Quit Frequency________ ☐ Hx ETOH abuse

☐ WNL Neuro/musculoskeletal
Arthritis/DJD, Back problems (LBP), CVA/TIA, Psychiatric disorder, Headaches, ↑ ICP/head injury, Loss of consciousness, Muscle weakness, Neuromuscular Dz, Paralysis, Paresthesia(s), Syncope, Seizures, Epilepsy

☐ WNL Renal/endocrine
Thyroid disease, Cushing's syndrome, Renal failure/dialysis, Renal insufficiency, Renal stones, Adrenocortical insuff., Prostate, BPH/CA, Diabetes mellitus, Type I/II/Gest., UTI, Pituitary disorder

☐ WNL Other
Anemia, Bleeding disorder, Cancer, Chemotherapy, Radiation Tx, Dehydration, HIV/AIDS, Immunosuppressed, Sickle cell Dz/trait, Recent steroids, Transfusion Hx, Weight loss/gain, Herbal/OTC drug use, Illicit drug use

☐ WNL Pregnancy
TIUP, Pre-eclampsia, HELLP, SGA, LGA, PROM, Multiple gestation, VBAC, IUGR

☐ AROM ☐ SROM ☐ Pitocin drip ☐ Induction ☐ Mg drip ________ gm/hr G: P: Weeks gest: EDC:

ECG

Chest X-ray

Pulmonary studies

Laboratory studies

PT/PTT/INR: T&S/T&C:

HCG: LMP: U/A:

Other diagnostic tests

Surgical diagnosis/problem list

Planned anesthesia/special monitors

Pre-anesthesia medications ordered

Evaluator signature | **Date**

Physical status 1 2 3 4 5 E

Post-anesthesia care notes

Location | Time
B/P | O_2 Sat %
Pulse | Resp | Temp

☐ Awake ☐ Stable ☐ Mask O_2
☐ Somnolent ☐ Unstable ☐ NC O_2
☐ Unarousable ☐ Oral/nasal airway
Intubated - ☐ T-piece ☐ Ventilator
Regional - dermatome level:
☐ Continuous epidural analgesia
☐ Direct admit to hospital ward (PACU recovery not required)
☐ Recovery recorded on anes. form

Controlled medications			
Medication	Used	Destroyed	Returned

Provider | **Witness**

☐ No anesthesia related complications noted
☐ Satisfactory post anesthesia/analgesia recovery
☐ See progress notes for anesthesia related concerns

Provider | Date | Time

GODFREY REGIONAL HOSPITAL
123 Main Street • Aldon, FL 77714 • (407) 555-1234

FIGURE 2-19, cont'd.

Continued

ANESTHESIA RECORD

Date | OR# | Page of | Procedure(s) | Surgeon(s)

	Start	Stop
Anesthesia		
Procedure		
Room time **in:**		**out:**

Pre-procedure

☐ Identified ☐ ID band ☐ Questioned
☐ Chart reviewed ☐ Permit signed
☐ NPO since
☐ Patient reassessed prior to anesthesia & surgery - Ready to proceed
☐ Peri-operative pain management discussed with patient/guardian, plan of care completed
Pre-anesthetic state:
☐ Awake ☐ Anxious ☐ Uncooperative
☐ Calm ☐ Lethargic ☐ Unresponsive
Other:

Patient safety

☐ Anesthesia machine# ______ checked
☐ Secured with safety belt
☐ Arm(s) secured on armboards: L R
☐ Arm(s) tucked: L R ☐ Axillary roll
☐ Pressure points checked, padded, monitored
☐ Eye care: ☐ Taped closed ☐ Ointment ☐ Saline ☐ Pads ☐ Goggles
☐ No pressure on orbits when prone

Monitors and equipment

☐ Steth: ☐ Esoph ☐ Precordial ☐ Suprasternal
☐ Non-invasive B/P ☐ V lead ECG
☐ Continuous ECG ☐ ST/Dysrhy. analysis
☐ Pulse oximeter ☐ Nerve stimulator:
☐ End tidal CO_2 ☐ Ulnar ☐ Tibial
☐ Oxygen monitor ☐ Facial ☐ ______
☐ ET agent analyzer ☐ Fluid/blood warmer
☐ Temp: ______ ☐ Cell saver ☐ BIS
☐ Body warmer ☐ TEE ☐ ICP
☐ Airway humidifier: ☐ FHT monitor ☐ EEG
☐ Evoked potential:
☐ NG/OG tube ☐ SSEP ☐ BAEP ☐ MEP
☐ Foley catheter ☐ Doppler: ______
☐ Arterial line
☐ CVP
☐ PA line
☐ IV(s)

Anesthetic technique

GA induction: ☐ Intravenous ☐ Pre-O_2 ☐ RSI
☐ Cricoid pressure ☐ Inhalation ☐ IM ☐ PR
GA maintenance: ☐ Inhalation ☐ Inhalation/IV
☐ GA/regional combination ☐ TIVA
Regional: Epidural- ☐ Thoracic ☐ Lumbar ☐ Caudal
☐ SAB ☐ Ankle ☐ Femoral ☐ Axillary ☐ Interscalene
☐ CSE ☐ Bier ☐ Continuous spinal ☐ Cervical plexus
☐ Other:
Regional technique: ☐ Position
☐ See remarks ☐ Prep
☐ Local ☐ Site
☐ Needle
☐ LA
☐ Narcotic
☐ Additive
☐ Test dose Rx
☐ Attempts x ______ ☐ Level
☐ Catheter ☐ Test dose response: + −
Space ______ cm Skin ______ cm ☐ Secured
☐ Sedation & analgesia/monitored anesthesia care

Airway management

☐ Oral ETT ☐ RAE ☐ L.T.A. ☐ Magill forceps
☐ Nasal ETT ☐ LMA # ______
☐ Stylet ☐ LMA fastrach # ______
☐ DVL ☐ LMA ProSeal # ______
☐ Tube size: ______ ☐ FOI ☐ Awake
☐ Blade: ______ ☐ Laser ETT ☐ LIS
☐ Attempts x ______ ☐ EMG ETT ☐ Bougie
☐ Grade: I II III IV ☐ Armored ETT ☐ Blind
☐ Secured at ______ cm ☐ DLT ______
☐ ET CO_2 present ☐ Univent ______
☐ Breath sounds = bilateral ☐ ______
☐ Cuffed-min. occ. pres. with: ☐ Air ☐ NS ☐ ______
☐ Uncuffed-leaks at ______ cm H_2O
☐ Oral airway ☐ Nasal airway ☐ Bite block
Circuit: ☐ Circle system ☐ NRB ☐ Bain
☐ Mask case ☐ Via tracheotomy/stoma
☐ Nasal cannula ☐ Simple O_2 mask ☐ ______
Nebulizer:
Topicalization:
Nerve block(s):

Time:

Agents
☐ Des ☐ Iso ☐ Sevo ☐ Halo (%)
☐ N_2O ☐ Air (L/min)
Oxygen (L/min)
( ) ( ) ( ) ( ) ( ) ( ) ( ) ( ) ( )

Totals

Fluids

Monitors
Urine (ml)
EBL (ml)
Gastric (ml)
ECG
% Oxygen inspired (FiO_2)
O_2 saturation (SaO_2)
End Tidal CO_2
Temp: ☐ C ☐ F
PNS/TOF

Peri-op meds

200 180 160 140 120 100 80 60 40 20
150 120 100 80 50

Symbols
V Λ B/P cuff pressure
⊥ T Arterial line pressure
X Mean arterial pressure
• Pulse
O Spontaneous respiration
Ø Assisted respiration
⊠ Controlled respiration
T Tourniquet

Vent
Tidal volume (ml)
Respiratory rate
Peak pressure (cm H_2O)
☐ PEEP ☐ CPAP (cm H_2O)
Symbols for remarks
Position

Time of delivery:
Sex: M F
Apgars: /

Provider(s)

Remarks:

Patient identification

GODFREY REGIONAL HOSPITAL
123 Main Street • Aldon, FL 77714 • (407) 555-1234

FIGURE 2-19, cont'd.

ANCILLARY TEST FINDINGS

Other tests may be considered part of the history, examination, and medical decision-making components used for diagnostic and procedural coding if the physician provides written interpretation. This interpretation may be recorded on the order slip along with the date and signature or authentication of the provider, or it may be incorporated in the progress note signed and dated by the provider. Reports regarding provider documentation have been previously discussed. Keep in mind that facility tests are performed by employees of the facility or hospital; a qualified provider must perform the interpretations.

For certain ancillary services to be considered for coding, billing, and reimbursement, a minimal amount of information must be provided in the interpretive statement. For example, to consider reimbursement for an ECG, most third-party insurance carriers require a minimum of heart rate, rhythm, and ectopy notation. If physicians provide various ancillary services, the coder must determine the minimal documentation requirements for reimbursement specified by each carrier so that requests for reimbursement may be submitted in the proper format.

Specific guidelines exist regarding what services may be provided by physician extenders, such as physician assistants and nurse practitioners. In addition, signature requirements and billing guidelines for these providers differ greatly by carrier. More information on this topic can be found in Chapter 21.

Other Documentation Needs

In addition to the requirements for specific services previously discussed, some general guidelines exist for documenting services. Certain terms are acceptable in some services but may be disallowed in others. For example, the notation "patient doing well" is not acceptable for complete documentation of a patient visit. As has already been described, history, physical examination, and medical decision-making documentation should be recorded for all such visits. The conclusion or impression of "doing well," however, might be acceptable for an outpatient office visit, with the inclusion of a diagnosis or diagnostic impression. The documentary note "doing well" would NOT be acceptable, however, for a critical care visit, which requires constant attendance to the care of a critically ill or injured unstable patient. In fact, the note "doing well" would be contradictory to the billing of a critical care visit; it would imply that the patient was, in fact, not critically ill but rather "doing well." Thus the provider should be careful in the choice of words when recording services.

Descriptors for visits should be chosen carefully. The type of service to be billed should be aligned carefully with the content of the visit documentation. This is described at length in Chapter 11.

Determining Medical Documentation Needed for Coding and Billing Purposes

One of the most important aspects of coding and billing is extracting the key elements from the documentation provided for coding and billing purposes. Although the documentation may be present on one or more of the forms or in different formats, the coder must read the records and identify key words that will be necessary to assign the appropriate ICD-9-CM diagnostic codes, CPT procedure codes, or both. At first the coder may select more codes than necessary; however, the goal is to read through the documentation once only and list the key words that may be necessary. As we begin our review of ICD-9-CM coding and CPT coding, we will identify words that can be eliminated.

In reading through the documentation, the coder looks for two key components: WHAT services were provided and WHY those services were provided and were medically necessary. Any additional detail for these two key elements should be captured and unnecessary elements eliminated when ICD-9-CM and CPT codes are assigned.

Look at the following sample operative report (Fig. 2-20) and determine the WHAT and WHY:

WHAT was performed:	Colonoscopy
Additional details:	Advanced to the cecum
WHY it was performed:	Dysphagia
	Rectal bleeding due to hemorrhoids
	GERD
	Gastritis

This is the information we will use to assign ICD-9-CM diagnostic codes for the WHY and CPT procedures codes for WHAT was performed during this encounter. Do not concern yourself whether all these terms will be necessary; this is discussed in depth throughout the following chapters.

OPERATIVE REPORT

Patient information:

Patient name:
DOB:
MR#:

Preoperative diagnosis:

Dysphagia, rectal bleeding

Postoperative diagnosis:

GERD, Gastritis, Rectal Bleeding due to Hemorrhoids

Procedure(s) performed:

Colonoscopy

Anesthesia:

Assistant surgeon:

Description of procedure:

The patient was placed in the left lateral decubitus position. After conscious sedation, the colonoscope was passed through anal verge and advanced to the cecum. Colonic mucosa was normal, and the scope was retroflexed and showed the cause of the rectal bleeding was Grade II internal hemorrhoids.

Patrick Adam MD

GODFREY REGIONAL HOSPITAL
123 Main Street • Aldon, FL 77714 • (407) 555-1234

FIGURE 2-20. Sample operative report.

STOP AND PRACTICE

Read the following reports and determine the WHAT and WHY.

1. Chart #1

CT localization was obtained showing good visualization of the liver lesions. The right upper abdomen was prepped and a 20-gauge percutaneous needle biopsy was performed of the right lobe of the liver. Because of the patient's right shoulder pain, a chest x-ray was obtained to rule out any pneumothorax.

Service #1: ______________________
WHAT performed: ______________________
WHY performed: ______________________
Service #2: ______________________
WHAT performed: ______________________
WHY performed: ______________________

2. Chart #2

Preoperative diagnosis: Suspect chronic cholecystitis
Postoperative diagnosis: Chronic cholecystitis

A supraumbilical incision was made, trocar introduced, and pneumoperitoneum insufflated. Ports were placed where we found chronic cholecystitis. Fluoroscopic cholangiogram was performed and the gallbladder dissected from the liver and removed through the umbilical port site. Released the pneumoperitoneum and closed the area with sutures and staples.

Service #1: ______________________
WHAT performed: ______________________
WHY performed: ______________________
Service #2: ______________________
WHAT performed: ______________________
WHY performed: ______________________

3. Chart #3

Diagnosis: Carpal tunnel syndrome
Procedure: Release of carpal tunnel of the wrist

The left arm was scrubbed and draped in the usual sterile manner. Incision was started on the flexor surface of the left wrist just proximal to the wrist crease. This was carried down through the subcutaneous tissue. The proximal end of the transverse carpal ligament was then incised and a groove director was inserted underneath the transverse carpal ligament, after which the whole extent of the transverse carpal ligament was then released from the proximal to the distal end.

Service #1: ______________________
WHAT performed: ______________________
WHY performed: ______________________

4. Chart #4

Presenting complaint: Left shoulder pain

53-year-old patient who has been having pain in the left shoulder for years. No reported trauma.

Past medical history: Negative
Review of systems: Joint pain in shoulder
Medications: Flonase
Allergies: Augmentin

Exam reveals a 53-year-old patient, appropriate height and weight, well oriented to time, place, and person. Exam of shoulder revealed full range of motion. No acromioclavicular joint tenderness. Full power of rotator cuff including supraspinatus, rotators, and subscapularis. No signs of instability are noted. Shoulder x-ray was negative.

Diagnosis: Mild subacromial bursitis

Service #1: ______________________
WHAT performed: ______________________
WHY performed: ______________________
Service #2: ______________________
WHAT performed: ______________________
WHY performed: ______________________

5. Chart #5

History: Abdominal cramping, uterine bleeding

Transabdominal pelvic ultrasound was performed. The uterus is midline. The echotexture is homogeneous. A small amount of free cul-de-sac fluid was appreciated. Both ovaries demonstrate normal echotexture and normal color flow.

Impression: Normal pelvic ultrasound

Service #1: ______________________
WHAT performed: ______________________
WHY performed: ______________________

Developing Documentation Tools for the Practice

One of the coder's responsibilities is to identify problem areas in the documentation process and educate the staff in rectifying these problems. A number of steps can be taken in this process. The coder must determine effective methods and means for successfully correcting documentation problems within the practice.

The coder enters the coding profession as a career choice. The physician has usually entered the medical profession for the primary purpose of diagnosing and treating patients—not to appropriately document the patient chart for coding and billing. With this in mind, the coder must develop strategies to ensure the collection of proper documentation for coding. Some suggestions for optimizing data collection in patient records are offered below.

STANDARDIZED DICTATION NOTE GUIDES

Make certain that the physician, provider, or transcriber has available a list of the elements that must be assessed and noted in the medical documentation during the patient encounter. Develop a guide for these elements presented in a format that is usable by the person responsible for dictating or documenting the record. This may take the form of an outline posted in the dictation area or a "pocket card" that can be carried by the provider at all times for reference. A copy of a sample "History and Physical" dictation pocket card is shown in Tool 2-1.

Other useful tools for making certain that patient records include all the vital elements of documentation are illustrated in Tools 2-2, 2-3, and 2-4.

STANDARDIZED PROGRESS NOTE FORMS

Another way to ensure proper documentation is to incorporate specific guidelines into the medical practice's standardized forms. For instance, column notations that outline needed documentation such as social history, family history, and differential diagnosis can be used. Stress to those documenting the need to record "noncontributory" and "not applicable" when appropriate. Emphasize the importance of following a set format so that third-party carriers and staff can locate specific information at a particular place on the form.

In the event the documenter handwrites the documentation, a standardized form can incorporate time-saving mechanisms such as descriptive words that can be circled when appropriate. Even if the documenter dictates at a later time, the circled information will assist in providing a complete record.

An example of a standardized progress note or record of treatment for the emergency department setting is illustrated in Tool 2-5.

In addition, a number of excellent tools are available that allow the documenter to check off normal and abnormal elements without the need for much writing. These serve as excellent alternatives for the physician who uses handwritten progress notes as documentation. Figures 2-21 through 2-26 are excellent representative selections of these documentation tools.

STANDARDIZED LANGUAGE FOR DICTATION

If providers dictate documentation, coders can assist them by developing "macros" for specific conditions. Software word-processing packages provide the capability of programming a set paragraph and labeling it as a macro (such as "PHYSICAL"). When the transcriptionist enters the macro command, the body of the text appears, and the health care provider must dictate only the information needed to fill in the blanks. A macro titled PHYSICAL might appear as follows:

This ( )-year-old (female, male) presents with the complaint(s) of ( ). Family history and social history are noncontributory to the patient's complaints. Review of systems reveals no significant findings. Vital signs are BP ( ) and pulse ( ); respirations are ( ).

An example of a history and physical template as described is included in Tool 2-6.

"GOOD WORDS/BAD WORDS" LIST

Provide a list of descriptive words considered acceptable in certain medical documentation and a list of terms that are not acceptable. Post it prominently wherever dictation or documentation is performed. These terms will vary by specialty. "Doing well" may be acceptable documentation (although not preferred) in a family physician's chart, but it would not be appropriate for documenting service provided to a critical care patient.

DOCUMENTATION DO'S AND DON'TS LIST

After a thorough review of the habits and practices of dictating or documenting information, develop a list of words and phrases that should be included and a list of those that should be excluded in documentation, as illustrated in Tool 2-7.

REVIEWING SIGNATURE REQUIREMENTS

Documentation is crucial to the provider from a reimbursement standpoint as well as from a legal one. When appropriate signature requirements are not met, the documentation is of no value in regard to reimbursement and may leave the practice vulnerable to legal difficulties.

Records are often filed after a visit and subsequent dictation has been concluded. Develop a procedure for reviewing each medical record to ensure that signatures have been provided. Put into writing whether such a procedure is to be

Text continued on p. 72

TOOL 2-1

DICTATION NOTE GUIDE

ADMISSION HISTORY AND PHYSICAL EXAMINATION

Date
Patient's name
Attending

HISTORY

Chief complaint
History of present illness
Past medical history
Past surgical history
Medications
Allergies
Social history (ETOH, tobacco)
Family history
Immunizations

Review of Systems:

Constitutional
Eyes
Cardiovascular
Respiratory
Musculoskeletal
Integumentary
Neurologic
Psychological
GI
GU
Ears, nose, mouth, throat
Allergic/immunologic
Endocrine
Hematologic/lymphatic

PHYSICAL EXAMINATION

Body Areas:

General appearance (AO, WDWN, NAD)
Head/face
Neck
Abdomen
Back
Each extremity
Chest/breasts
Genitalia/groin/buttocks

Organ Systems:

Eyes
Cardiovascular
Respiratory
GI
GU
Psychological
Ears, nose, mouth, throat
Musculoskeletal
Skin
Neurologic
Hematologic/lymphatic/immunologic

HISTORY AND PHYSICAL PROGRESS NOTE FORMATS

SOAP FORMAT

S: Subjective

Major events (ROS, FH, SH, HPI)
Better or worse
Patient's complaints

O: Objective

Vital signs
Physical examination
Labs/ancillaries

A: Assessment

Review of data
Diagnosis

P: Plan

Treatment
Discharge plan

SNOCAMP FORMAT

S: Subjective

Major events (ROS, FH, SH, HPI)
Better or worse
Patient's complaints

N: Nature of Presenting Problem

O: Objective

Vital signs
Physical examination
Lab values/ancillaries

C: Counseling/Coordination of Care

Document time
Document issue(s)

A: Assessment

Review of data
Diagnosis

M: Medical Decision Making

Differential diagnosis
Review of data
Risk of morbidity/mortality

P: Plan

Treatment
Discharge plan

TOOL 2-1

DICTATION NOTE GUIDE—cont'd

ADMISSION HISTORY AND PHYSICAL EXAMINATION

MEDICAL DECISION MAKING

Ancillary services ordered/interpret
Medical data review
Risk of morbidity/mortality

ASSESSMENT/PLAN

Diagnosis
Treatment plan
Discharge instructions

OP NOTE

Date
Patient's name
Medical record #
Preoperative diagnosis
Postoperative diagnosis
Operative procedures
Surgeon
Assistants
Anesthesia
Surgical procedures in detail
Findings
Estimated blood loss
Drains/tubes
Pathology, specimens, cultures
Complications
Disposition/condition

POSTOPERATIVE CHECK/NOTE

Subjective
Objective
Vital signs
Inputs/outputs
Fluids: volume, blood products, urine output, drains, bowel movements, blood loss
Lab values
CBC, SMAC, CXR, ABG
Physical examination: lungs, dressings, incisions, pulses
Assessment plan

HISTORY AND PHYSICAL PROGRESS NOTE FORMATS

ADMIT/TRANSFER ORDERS/NOTE (ACDAVANDIML)

A: Admit (floor, ICU, unit, etc.), attending/consulting MDs
C: Condition (stable, fair, guarded)
D: Diagnosis
A: Activities (ad lib, bed rest)
V: Vital signs monitoring (check BP hourly)
A: Allergies
N: Nursing (dressing changes, IV care)
D: Diet (clear liquids, NPO)
I: IV (access site)
M: Medications: preadmission, antibiotics, pain meds
L: Labs and ancillary services

DISCHARGE SUMMARY

Patient's name
Medical record #
Attending MD
Admit date/discharge date
Primary/associated diagnoses
Surgical procedures
Hospital course
Consults
Complications
Discharge condition
Discharge instructions (follow-up)
Copies to:

ETOH, Alcohol; *AO,* alert and oriented; *GI,* gastrointestinal; *GU,* genitourinary; *WDWN,* well developed, well nourished; *NAD,* no apparent distress; *CBC,* complete blood count; *SMAC,* Sequential Multiple Analyzer Computer (blood test); *CXR,* chest x-ray; *ABG,* arterial blood gases; *ROS,* review of systems; *FH,* family history; *SH,* social history; *HPI,* history of present illness; *ICU,* intensive care unit; *BP,* blood pressure; *IV,* intravenous; *NPO,* nothing by mouth.

TOOL 2-2

HISTORY CHECK-OFF GUIDE (Indicate [+] or [–] in Applicable Boxes)

FAMILY HISTORY/SOCIAL HISTORY

FAMILY HISTORY	☐ Marital status	☐ Parents	☐ Siblings					
	FAMILY HISTORY OF:	☐ Genetic disease	☐ Diabetes	☐ Hypertension	☐ Arteriosclerotic heart disease (ASHD)	☐ Cancer	☐ Hyperlipidemia	☐ Cerebrovascular accident (CVA)
		☐ Kidney disease	☐ Psychiatric illness	☐ Tuberculosis	☐ Arthritis	☐ Sickle cell		
SOCIAL HISTORY	☐ Smoker	☐ Alcohol	☐ IV drug use	***SEXUAL PREFERENCE***	Place of birth: ____________			
	☐ Packs/day	☐ Caffeine	☐ PCP	☐ Heterosexual	Occupation: ____________			
	☐ Years	☐ Diet	☐ Crack	☐ Homosexual	Education: ____________			
	☐ Cigarettes/pipe	☐ Exercise	☐ Cocaine	☐ Bisexual	Religion: ____________			
	☐ Cigar		☐ Other					
REVIEW OF SYSTEMS								
GENERAL	☐ Weight change	☐ Appetite	☐ Sleeping habits					
HEENT								
HEAD	☐ Cephalgia	☐ Head injury	☐ Migraines					
EYES	☐ Blurriness	☐ Cataracts	☐ Diplopia	☐ Photophobia	☐ Vision changes			
EARS	☐ Discharge	☐ Hearing changes	☐ Tinnitus					
NOSE	☐ Sinusitis	☐ Rhinorrhea	☐ Epistaxis	☐ Fracture				
MOUTH	☐ Tenderness	☐ Lesions						
THROAT	☐ Sore throat	☐ Dysphagia	☐ Hoarseness					
NECK	☐ Injury	☐ Masses	☐ Pain	☐ Stiffness				
RESPIRATORY	☐ Asthma	☐ Bronchitis	☐ Chronic obstructive pulmonary disease (COPD)	☐ Chronic cough	☐ Hemoptysis	☐ Shortness of breath (SOB)	☐ Tuberculosis	☐ Tachypnea
CARDIOVASCULAR	☐ Angina	☐ Congestive heart failure (CHF)	☐ Claudication	☐ CVA	☐ Cyanosis	☐ Dizziness	☐ Dyspnea	☐ Hypertension
	☐ Orthopnea	☐ Palpitations	☐ Phlebitis	☐ Precordial pain	☐ Stroke (TIA)			
GASTROINTESTINAL	☐ Constipation	☐ Diarrhea	☐ Dysphagia	☐ Gallbladder disease	☐ Hematemesis	☐ Hematochezia	☐ Hemorrhoids	☐ Hepatitis
	☐ Hernia	☐ Indigestion	☐ Jaundice	☐ Melena	☐ Nausea/vomiting	☐ Pancreatitis		☐ Rectal bleeding
GENITOURINARY	☐ Anuria	☐ Dysuria	☐ Hematuria	☐ Nocturia	☐ Discharge			
	☐ Frequency	☐ Hesitancy	☐ Incontinence	☐ Chronic urinary tract infection (UTI)	☐ Sexually transmitted disease (STD)	☐ Prostatitis		
OB/GYN	☐ Pregnancy							
	☐ Contraceptive use							
BREASTS	☐ Discharge	☐ Enlargement	☐ Pain	☐ Tenderness	☐ Prior surgery	☐ +Mammogram		
NEUROMUSCULAR	☐ Anesthesias	☐ Paresthesias	☐ Arthralgias	☐ Myalgias	☐ Nervousness	☐ Syncope	☐ Vertigo	☐ Weakness
ENDOCRINE	☐ Hot/cold intolerance	☐ Paresthesias	☐ Polydipsia	☐ Polyphagia	☐ Polyuria			
	☐ Anemia	☐ Excess bruising/bleeding	☐ Diabetes	☐ Thyroid problems				
NEUROLOGIC	☐ Dizziness	☐ Syncope	☐ Seizures	☐ Vertigo	☐ Paresthesias	☐ Weakness	☐ Tremor	
RHEUMATOLOGY	☐ Arthritis	☐ Joint stiffness/swelling	☐ Myalgias	☐ Gout	☐ Lyme's disease	☐ Back pain		
VASCULAR	☐ Phlebitis	☐ Varicose veins	☐ Claudication	☐ Cramping	☐ Raynaud's disease			
HEMATOLOGY	☐ Anemia	☐ Easy bruising/bleeding	☐ Transfusions	☐ Blood type	☐ Pain	☐ Fever	☐ Chills	☐ Night sweats
DERMATOLOGY	☐ Rashes	☐ Moles (recent changes)	☐ Birthmarks	☐ Dryness	☐ Pruritus	☐ Lumps	Pigmentation change: ____________	
PSYCHOLOGICAL	☐ Depression	☐ Agitation	☐ Panic/anxiety	☐ Memory	☐ Hallucinations	☐ Personality changes		

TOOL 2-3

EXAMINATION CHECK-OFF GUIDE (Indicate [+] or [–] in Applicable Boxes)

PHYSICAL EXAMINATION							
GENERAL:	☐ Alert	☐ Oriented	☐ Well developed	☐ Nourished	☐ NAD	Race: ______	Sex: ______
HEAD/SCALP:	☐ Normocephalic	☐ Condition scalp					
EYES:	☐ PERRLA	☐ EOMI	☐ Discs	☐ Retinal vessels	☐ Lids	☐ Conjunctiva	
	☐ Sclera	☐ Visual fields	☐ Visual acuity				
EARS:	☐ Pinnae	☐ External auditory canal	☐ Eardrum	☐ Rinne test	☐ Weber's test	☐ Acuity	
NOSE:	☐ Mucosa	☐ Septum	☐ Polyps				
THROAT/ORAL:	☐ Lips	☐ Buccal mucosa	☐ Palate	☐ Tongue	☐ Tonsils		
	☐ Gingiva	☐ Teeth/dentures	☐ Gag reflex				
NECK:	☐ Trachea-larynx	*THYROID:*	☐ Goiter	☐ Nodules	☐ Bruits		
		CAROTID ARTERY:	☐ Contour	☐ Bruit	☐ Jugular venous pressure with waveforms		
RESPIRATORY:	☐ Contour	*BREATH SOUNDS:*	☐ Wheezes	☐ Rales	☐ Rhonchi	☐ Rub	
		☐ Resonance	☐ Diaphragm movement		☐ Intercostal muscle retraction		
CARDIAC:	☐ Heart sounds: S1, S2, S3, S4		☐ Systolic click	☐ Opening snap	☐ Mid-diastolic murmur		
MURMUR:	☐ Systolic	☐ Diastolic	☐ Continuous	☐ Radiation			
	Location: ______	Location: ______	☐ Loudness	☐ Pitch	☐ Quality		
ABDOMEN:	☐ Appearance	☐ Bowel sounds	☐ Scars	☐ Distention	☐ Bruits	☐ Liver	
	☐ Spleen	☐ Guarding	☐ Rebound	☐ Kidneys	☐ Costovertebral tenderness		
	☐ Ventral hernia	☐ Bladder	☐ Masses				
GU (male):	☐ Penis	☐ Scrotum	☐ Testicles	☐ Varicocele	☐ Hydrocele	☐ Hernia (inguinal/femoral)	
GU (female):	☐ External genitalia	☐ Bartholin gland	☐ Urethra				
	INTERNAL EXAM:	☐ Cervix	☐ Uterus	☐ Adnexa	☐ Rectovaginal area		
RECTAL:	☐ External lesions	☐ Hemorrhoids	☐ Fissures	☐ Sphincter tone	☐ Sphincter tenderness		
MUSCULOSKELETAL:	*APPEARANCE:*	☐ Muscle swelling	☐ Deformity	☐ Tenderness	☐ Range of motion		
		☐ Bone	☐ Deformity	☐ Tenderness			
		☐ Joint swelling	☐ Deformity	☐ Tenderness	☐ Range of motion		
	☐ Hypertrophy	☐ Spasm	☐ Muscle group atrophy				
	☐ Spinal kyphosis	☐ Spinal scoliosis					
BREAST:	☐ Symmetry	☐ Skin changes	☐ Retraction	☐ Nipple-areola	☐ Masses		
	☐ Tenderness	☐ Nipple discharge					
VASCULAR:	*ARTERIAL PULSE CONTOUR/BRUITS:*		☐ Radial ulnar	☐ Brachial	☐ Carotid		
			☐ Abdominal aorta	☐ Femoral	☐ Popliteal	☐ Post tibial	☐ Dorsalis
EXTREMITIES:	☐ Clubbing	☐ Cyanosis	☐ Edema	☐ Color	☐ Pigmentation		
	☐ Turgor	☐ Texture	☐ Temperature	☐ Lesions	☐ Nailbeds		
NEUROLOGIC:	☐ Mental status	☐ Orientation	☐ Memory	☐ Arithmetic	☐ Abstract concepts		
	☐ Speech	☐ Cortical integration	☐ Cranial nerves	☐ Motor	☐ Sensory	☐ Reflexes	

NAD, No acute distress; *PERRLA*, pupils equal, round, and reactive to light and accommodation; *EOMI*, extraocular movements intact; *GU*, genitourinary.

TOOL 2-4

ED CHART DOCUMENTATION REQUIREMENTS

	Chart Documentation Requirements	Chart Content (examples)	Levels of Documentation
HISTORY **Chief Complaint**	Document in patient's own words	"Pt states"	Req All Levels
Hx Present Illness	Must be documented by ED phy	Location, Timing, Assoc S/S Quality, Context, Mod Factors Severity, Duration	Brief 1–3 elements Extended >4 elements
Past FH/SH/PMH	May be documented by staff and **confirmed** by ED phy Review pertinent –/+	"Reviewed and agree with nurse/ resident's notes"	Req Levels 4/5
Review of Systems	May be documented by staff and **confirmed** by ED phy "All other systems negative" acceptable after pert problems	*ROS Identified:* Constitutional, Musculoskel, Eyes, Integumen, Neuro Ears,Throat, Nose, Mouth, Cardiovasc, Psych, Endocrine Gastro, Hema/Lymph, GU, All/Immun	Prob Foc Prob Pert Only Extend 2–9 rel systems Complete all systems
PHYSICAL EXAM	All abnormal findings of affected areas must be documented "Negative" or "normal" OK for findings of unaffected areas Must be able to identify system(s) from negatives listed	*Organ Systems Identified:* Constitutional, Eyes, Ears, Nose, Mouth, throat, Cardiovasc Respiratory, GI, GU, Musculoskel, Skin Neurologic, Psych, Hema/ Lymph/Imm *Body Areas Identified:* Ea Extremity, Neck, Abdomen Genitalia, Groin, Buttocks, Chest, incl breasts, Head, incl face, Back, incl spine	Prob Foc 1 element Exp Prob Foc 2–4 elements Detailed 5–7 elements Complete 8 or more
MED DECISION **Dx/Mgt Options**	Minimal "improving, resolved(ing)" Limited "self-limited" Multiple "inadequately controlled" Extensive "worsening" "failing to respond"	Differential Diagnosis Final Diagnosis Drug Therapy(ies) Procedure(s) Disposition of Patient/Consultations	Minimal 1 Limited 2 Multiple 3 Extensive 4
Amt /Complexity of Data Reviewed	Path/Lab 1>test =1 Rad 1>test =1 Dx Test 1>test =1 Comp Test Results Ea 1 test =2 Old Records Eval Need =1 OR Old Records Obtain/Review =2 Discuss with Physician =1	Physician Documentation of: Medical Necessity of Tests/Orders Test Results Independent Interpretation Eval of Need for Records Eval/Review of Old Records Repeat Procedures Repeat Evaluations/Treatments	Minimal/None 1 Limited 2 Moderate 3 Extensive 4 or more
Risk /Morbidity/ Mortality	Presenting Prob Severity Diagnostic Proc Ordered Management Options Selected Discharge Status Discharge Instructions	Mild, moderate, progressive X-Rays, Labs, Procedures Home/Admit/Resolution or Non-Resolution of symptoms Rest, Gargle, Bandages Non-Rx drugs Drug Therapy(ies) IV fluids w/ or w/o additives Minor procedures	Straightforward Minimal Self-Lmtd/Minor Problem Low >2 Self-Lmtd/Minor 1 Stable Chronic Illness Acute Uncompl Illness/Inj Moderate >1 chronic ill/mild exac >2 stable chronic ill/inj undiag new problem acute complicated injury Extensive >1 chronic ill/severe exac acute/chronic illnesses poses threat life/limb abrupt chg in neuro status

TOOL 2-5

EMERGENCY DEPARTMENT RECORD OF TREATMENT

Admit#:	Date:	Time:	Age:	Sex:	Race:
Name:		Address:			
SSN:	DOB:		Phone:		
Chief Complaint:			Medications:		
Vitals:			Allergies:		

HISTORY

CHIEF COMPLAINT

HX PRESENT ILLNESS

PAST MED HX/FAMILY HX

(P=Pt F=Family)	P F	Other Hx Information:
HTN/Card/Stroke/Chol		
Cancer/Bleed		
Seizures/Headaches		
Weakness/Coordination		
DM/Kidney/Abdominal		
Surgical Procedures		
Other:		

SOCIAL HX

Occupation/Living Arrangement

Alcohol/Smoking/Drugs

REVIEW OF SYSTEMS	NL if WNL	Noted System Abnormalities:
Constitutional		
Allergic/Immun		
Integumentary		
Eyes		
Ears, Nose, Mouth, Throat		
Cardiovasc		
Hematologic		
Endocrine		
Respiratory		
GI		
GU		
Musculoskeletal		
Neurologic		

MEDICAL DECISION MAKING

Procedures/Treatments/Re-Evaluation:

Prescriptions:

	NL if WNL	Finding Abnormalities
Lab Results:		
CBC		
UA		
ABG		
Cultures		
ECG		
Enzymes		
Pulse Ox		
X-Ray: Specify________		
Other: _______________		
Other: _______________		

Consults:

Resident Signature/Date:

EXAM	NL if WNL	Noted Exam Abnormalities:
Constitutional		
Skin		
Eyes		
Ears, Nose, Mouth, Throat		
Neck		
Respiratory		
Cardiovascular		
Chest		
GI		
GU		
Musculoskeletal		
Neurological		
Lymph/Immun		
Psych		

Other Exam Abnormalities:

FINDINGS:

Differential Dx(s):

Final Dx(s):

DISPOSITION:
Discharge:
Admit:
Transfer to:
CONDITION:
Improved/Stable
Worse/Expired
INSTRUCTIONS:

I hereby attest that I have reviewed and concurred with Resident Findings/Treatment:
Physician Signature/Date:

Name: ____________ DoB __/__/__ Cht.# ____________ Seen with: ☐ Mth. ☐ Fth. ☐ Other ________

History

Nutrition: ☐ Breast ☐ Formula ________ ☐ WIC

Present ____________

Past ____________

Family/social ____________

Drug allergies? ☐ yes ☐ no ____________

Physical Exam ☑ Nl ☒ Abn

Temp ______ Head Cir./% ___/___ Wt %/Ht % ___/___

Constitutional ☐	Head, fontanels ☐	Gastrointestinal ☐
Alertness ☐	Eyes ☐	Genitourinary ☐
Hearing ☐	ENMT ☐	Back ☐
Language ☐	Lymphatics ☐	Extremities, hips ☐
Nutrition ☐	Respiratory ☐	Muscle tone ☐
Growth ☐	Cardiovascular ☐	Skin ☐
Motor develop. ☐	Femoral pulses ☐	Neuromuscular ☐

Procedures ☐ Hep B ____________

Immun. current? ☐ yes ☐ no ____________

Plan ____________

Next visit:

Anticipatory Guidance ☐ Immunization (risks/benefits) ☐ Growth ☐ Development ☐ Nutrition (solids) ☐ Fluoride ☐ Sleep (night crying) ☐ Safety (shaking, no walkers, poisons, Ipecac) ☐ Fear of strangers ☐ Educational handouts ________

Provider's sig. ►

9 mo.	Date/Time	Age	Weight	Height	Assessment: ☐ Referral

FIGURE 2-21. Forms for regularly scheduled interval examinations are used to record the information needed for medical and documentation purposes.

Name: ____________ DoB __/__/__ Cht.# ____________ Seen with: ☐ Mth. ☐ Fth. ☐ Other ________

History

Date of injury __/__/__ Time of injury ________ Time of visit ________ Location ________

Description of injury/complications

Date of last tetanus: __/__/__

Physical Findings ____________

Treatment/Plan

Referral? ☐ yes ☐ no Dr. ____________ Findings/recommendations: ________

Anticipatory Guidance ☐ Discussed signs of possible complications and appropriate intervention. ________

Provider's sig. ► ☐ Follow up: ☐ phone call ________ ☐ return visit ________

Injury	Date/time	Description: ☐ Referral

FIGURE 2-22. Forms designed to ask injury-specific information are separated from the usual physical examination and illness documentation forms.

Name: ____________ DOB __/__/__ Cht.# ____________ Seen with: ☐ Mth. ☐ Fth. ☐ Other ____________

Physical Exam ☑ Nl ☒ Abn (Circle Abn)

Temp ____ P ____ R ____ BP ____ Peak Fl ____

Constitutional ☐ looks ill 1^+, 2^+, 3^+ Hydration ☐ ____
Fontanel ☐
Eyes ☐ red, drainage (clear, pur.), Fundi ☐ ____
Ears: . Rtm ☐ red, dull, thick, ↓ mobility, retract., bulging fluid (ser, pur), perf, scarred, tube (in, out)
Ltm ☐ red, dull, thick, ↓ mobility, retract., bulging fluid (ser, pur), perf, scarred, tube (in, out)
Ext. canal ☐ cerumen, swollen, tender, pur. drainage
Nose ☐ drainage (watery, mucoid, pur.), Sinuses ☐
Mouth/throat ☐ ulcers, drainage (mucoid, pur.) inj. ____
Tonsils ☐ enlarged 1^+, 2^+, 3^+, 4^+, exudate, petechiae
Lymphatic ☐
Neck ☐
Cardiovascular ☐
Respiratory ☐ rhonchi, wheezes, rales, ↓ br. sounds, retract.
R ___ L ___ resp. distress 0, 1^+, 2^+, 3^+ ____
Gastrointestinal ☐
Genitourinary ☐
Musculoskeletal ☐
Skin ☐
Neurological ☐

CPT: PF / EPF / D / C

History ☒ Positive ☑ Negative ☐ Follow-up visit

Chief complaint/duration: ____________

restless ☐	fussy ☐	awake at night ☐	↓ appetite ☐

Fever ☐	Earache ☐	Back pain ☐	Vomiting ☐
Congestion ☐	Sw. glands ☐	Musc/jnt pain ☐	Diarrhea ☐
Cough ☐	Red eyes ☐	Abd. pain ☐	Urinary sx. ☐
Sore throat ☐	Headache ☐	Constipation ☐	Skin rash ☐

Over ☐

Systems reviewed ☐ Family/Social Hx reviewed ☐
Past Hx reviewed ☐ Immunizations current? Yes ☐ No ☐
Current meds: ____________
Drug allergies? Yes ☐ No ☐

CPT: PF / EPF / D / C

Treatment ____________

Provider's sig. ► Over ☐

CPT: SF / LC / MC / HC

☐ Report back in 24 hrs. ☐ Call in 48 hrs., prn ☐ Re-examine

Sick	Date/Time	Age	Weight	Height	Diagnosis:	☐ After hrs. ☐ Referral

FIGURE 2-23. Forms designed specifically for "sick" visits are used to record information regarding presenting complaint, history of present illness, physical examination, and medical decision making for both medical and documentation purposes.

implemented just before the next visit or the next time the chart is pulled. As part of the office policy, this procedure should be clearly outlined and distributed to all employees. In addition to the established procedures for optimizing documentation, a monitoring process must also be included. The components of a successful compliance and monitoring program for a medical practice are discussed in Chapter 22.

MONITORING PROCESS FOR DOCUMENTATION SUCCESS

After providing input and devising tools for effective documentation, monitor their implementation and success. If documenters still are not providing acceptable documentation, continue to educate and identify alternative tools and techniques that may be more successful. In a large medical practice, monitoring techniques must be incorporated into the company compliance program as well.

After the coder has developed effective tools and techniques to optimize the documentation process, the first skill to be developed for successful diagnostic and procedural coding is selecting appropriate information from the medical documentation. Some primary rules exist for this selection process and are specific to physician coding for services. In Chapters 19 and 20, the differences in physician and hospital coding, and the rationale for those differences, are discussed.

Godfrey Regional Hospital Providers and Facilities

As previously discussed, a number of forms and formats may be used for record keeping and reimbursement purposes. These forms and formats may also occur in different locations. As mentioned in the Preface, this text has adapted a real-life scenario approach to help students understand the coding process. Toward this end, providers from various locations are represented throughout the textbook and its ancillaries. Some charts are dictated and typed and others are handwritten, sometimes bordering on illegible. Other charts lack some of the appropriate medical record documentation to code appropriately. A list of these providers and facilities is included in Table 2-2.

Providers and locations have been established so that students may practice the multiple skills required in medical coding. A signature log is required so that office personnel may identify signatures of individual physicians providing the various services. Table 2-1 contains the signature log for the medical groups.

Text continued on p. 83

Name: ______________ DoB __/__/__ Age ________ Chart No. [ ]

Assessment

Plan

Provider's signature ______________ Return visit ________

Physical Exam

Ht. ____ Wt. ____ Temp. ____ Resp. ____
B.P. sit. or stand. ___/___ Supine ___/___
Pulse rate and regularity ______________

Circle abnormal and pertinent normal findings.
Describe abnormalities above.

☑ Normal ☒ Abnormal

1. Constitutional
- a. ☐ gen. appear., development, body shape, nutrition, deformities, grooming

2. Eyes
- a. ☐ conjunctivae, lids
- b. ☐ pupils, irises
- c. ☐ fundi (optic discs, vessels, exudate, hemorr.)

3. Ears, nose, throat, and mouth
- a. ☐ appearance of ears, appearance of nose
- b. ☐ auditory canals, tympanic membranes
- c. ☐ hearing (whis. voice, finger rub, tun. fork)
- d. ☐ nasal mucosa, septum, turbinates
- e. ☐ lips, teeth, gums
- f. ☐ oropharynx (mucosa, saliv. glands, hard and soft palates, tongue, tonsils, post. pharynx)

4. Neck
- a. ☐ appearance, masses, symmetry, tracheal position, crepitus
- b. ☐ thyroid (enlargement, tenderness, mass)

5. Respiratory
- a. ☐ respiratory effort (intercostal retractions), use of accessory muscles, diaphragm move.
- b. ☐ percussion (dullness, flatness, hyper-reson.)
- c. ☐ palpation (tactile fremitus)
- d. ☐ auscultation (breath sounds, rhonchi, wheezes, rales, rubs)

6. Cardiovascular
- a. ☐ palpation (location of p.m.i., size, thrill)
- b. ☐ auscultation (abnormal sounds, murmurs)
- c. ☐ carotid arteries (pulse amplitude, bruits)
- d. ☐ abdominal aorta (size, bruits)
- e. ☐ femoral arteries (pulse amplitude, bruits)
- f. ☐ pedal pulses (pulse amplitude)
- g. ☐ extremities (edema, varicosities)

7. Chest (breasts)
- a. ☐ inspection (size, symmetry, nipple discharge)
- b. ☐ palpation of breasts and axillae (masses, lumps, tenderness)

8. Gastrointestinal (abdomen)
- a. ☐ examination for masses, tenderness
- b. ☐ examination of liver, spleen
- c. ☐ examination for presence or absence of hernia
- d. ☐ examination of (when indicated) anus, perineum, rectum: (sphincter tone, hemorrhoids, masses)
- e. ☐ stool for occult blood when indicated

9. Genitourinary
- a. ☐ scrotum (hydrocele, spermatocele), tenderness of cord, testicular mass)
- b. ☐ examination of penis
- c. ☐ digital exam of prostate (size, symmetry, nodularity, tenderness)

10. Lymphatic
- a. ☐ palpation of lymph nodes in 2 or more areas: (Circle: neck, axillae, groin, other)

11. Musculoskeletal
- a. ☐ examination of gait and station
- b. ☐ inspection and/or palpation of digits and nails (clubbing, cyanosis, inflammatory conditions, petechiae, ischemia, infections, nodes)
- c. ☐ assessment of range of motion (pain, crepitation, contracture)
- d. ☐ Examination of joint, bone, and muscle of 1 or more of the following 6 areas (circle)
  - head/neck
  - rt. upper extremities
  - spine, ribs, and pelvis
  - lt. upper extremities
  - rt. lower extremities
  - lt. lower extremities
- e. ☐ inspection and/or palpation (misalignment, asymmetry, crepitation, defects, tenderness, masses, effusion)
- f. ☐ assessment of stability: dislocation (luxation), subluxation or laxity
- g. ☐ muscle strength and tone (flaccid, cogwheel, spastic), atrophy or abnormal movement

12. Skin
- a. ☐ inspection of skin and sub-Q tissue (rashes, lesion, ulcers)
- b. ☐ palpation of skin and sub-Q tissue (induration, sub-Q nodules, tightening)

13. Neurology
- a. ☐ test cranial nerves: notation of deficits
- b. ☐ examination of DTRs with notation of pathological reflexes (e.g., Babinski)
- c. ☐ examination of sensation (touch, pain, vibration, proprioception)

14. Psychiatric
- a. ☐ description of patient's judgment and insight

Brief assessment of mental status:
- b. ☐ orientation to time, place, and person
- c. ☐ recent and remote memory
- d. ☐ mood and affect (depression, anxiety, agitation)
- e. ☐ other

Procedures and Immunizations

☐ Hearing ☐ Glucose ☐ Cholesterol ☐ CXR
☐ Vision ☐ PT ☐ HDL/LDL ☐ ECG
☐ CBC ☐ Urine ☐ TSH

Are immunizations current? ☐ yes ☐ no

☐ dT ☐ Hep B ☐ Influenza

Drug Allergies

Male 19-39	Date/Time	Summary	☐ Referral

FIGURE 2-24. Forms designed specifically for complete physical examinations, which are also specific to age and sex, are used to detail the information specific to the particular patient groups.

Name: ______________________ Date ___/___/___

HPI Chief Complaint:

Current Meds.:

Past/Family History

THIS SECTION TO BE COMPLETED BY PATIENT.

Personal/Social History

Are you ... ☐ single ☐ married
☐ live-in partner ☐ divorced ☐ widowed

Do you have children? ☐ yes ☐ no
Age(s) of child(ren) ______________

Occupation ______________

	YES	NO
a. Are your immunizations up to date?	☐	☐
Date of last tetanus shot: ______________		
b. Do you have any pain or blood on urination?	☐	☐
c. Do you have lesions, sores or drainage from penis?	☐	☐
d. Do you have any lumps, swelling, tenderness or pain in groin, scrotum, or testicles?	☐	☐
e. Are you sexually active now?	☐	☐
☐ same sex ☐ opposite sex ☐ single partner ☐ multiple partners		
Have you had more than 4 lifetime partners?	☐	☐
f. Do you use condoms?	☐	☐
g. Do you have concerns about sexual orientation, sexually transmitted diseases, or exposure to HIV or other sexual concerns?	☐	☐
h. Do you feel safe/comfortable in your home, with your family, and/or your partner relationship?	☐	☐
i. Do you smoke or use tobacco products now?	☐	☐
j. Do you use recreational drugs?	☐	☐
k. Do you drink alcohol?	☐	☐
☐ daily ☐ weekly ☐ rarely		
# of drinks ______________		
If yes, do you drink: ☐ beer ☐ wine ☐ liquor		

Review of Systems

Are you concerned about? (circle concerns)

	YES	NO
1. Recent changes in health status	☐	☐
2. Eye problems: vision, pain, tearing	☐	☐
3. Ear, nose, mouth, throat problems	☐	☐
4. Heart problems: chest pain, blood pressure	☐	☐
5. Lung problems: coughing, wheezing, infections	☐	☐
6. Abdominal pain, stomach, bowel problems	☐	☐
7. Kidney or bladder problems	☐	☐
8. Muscle, bone, joint or back problems	☐	☐
9. Skin, hair or nail problems	☐	☐
10. Neurologic problems: headaches, dizziness, numbness	☐	☐
11. Nervousness, anxiety, depression, suicidal thoughts	☐	☐
12. Excessive thirst and urine output, recent weight changes	☐	☐
13. Anemia, bruising, blood clots, swollen glands	☐	☐
14. Food allergies, hay fever, eczema, asthma, decreased immunity	☐	☐
Do you have any other concerns?	☐	☐

____
____
____
____

______________ ______
Patient's signature Date

Provider Comments:

☐ PFSH and ROS have been reviewed. ☐ Unresolved problems from previous visit have been addressed.

______________ ______
Provider's signature Date

Anticipatory Guidance

☐ Nutrition
☐ Exercise
☐ Dental care
☐ Cardiovascular risks
☐ Sun exposure
☐ Smoking cessation
☐ Alcohol/drugs
☐ Sexual issues
☐ STD prevention
☐ Self-exam: testes, skin, oral cavity
☐ School/work
☐ Family
☐ Recreation/hobbies
☐ Safety/injury/gun safety
☐ Auto seat belts
☐ Smoke detectors
☐ Domestic violence
☐ Stress
☐ Educational handouts

FIGURE 2-24, cont'd.

New Patient Record (Adults)

Date ________ DoB __/ /__ Chart No. [ ]

Name: ______________________ Sex ☐ M ☐ F Referred By ______________

Current Medical Problems *List all medical problems and approximate time they began.*

Problems Onset date

____

____

____

____

Current Medications *List all medications you take (including nonprescription medication).*

1 ________ 5 ________
2 ________ 6 ________
3 ________ 7 ________
4 ________ 8 ________

Current Allergies or Sensitivities *List anything you are allergic to and describe how it affects you.*

____

____

____

____

Work History

Are you currently employed? ☐ Yes ☐ No
☐ Homemaker ☐ Retired ☐ Disabled
Present type of work ______________
In your work are you exposed to:
☐ Harmful toxins ☐ Extremes in temperatures
☐ Heavy lifting ☐ Undue stress, pressure
☐ Other ______________

Health Care Providers *What other health care providers have cared for you in the past five years?*

Year	Doctor/provider	City and state

Do you have other concerns or problems? ☐ Yes ☐ No

____

____

____

Signed ______________________ Date ________

Family Medical History

Relative	Age(s)	Health is: Good	Poor	Deceased
Father	____	☐	☐	☐
Mother	____	☐	☐	☐
Brothers	____	☐	☐	☐
Sisters	____	☐	☐	☐
Spouse	____	☐	☐	☐
Children	____	☐	☐	☐

Illness(es) ______________________

____

____

Cause(s) of Death ______________________

____

Check if you or a member of your family have had the following illnesses or problems. List which family member.

☐ Allergies ________
☐ Asthma ________
☐ Eczema, rashes ________
☐ Eye problems ________
☐ Thyroid problems ________
☐ Lung problems ________
☐ Heart diseases ________
☐ Cholesterol problems ________
☐ High blood pressure ________
☐ Phlebitis ________
☐ Stomach or intestinal problems ________
☐ Liver diseases ________
☐ Kidney problems ________

☐ Diabetes ________
☐ Hereditary diseases ________
☐ Cancer ________
☐ Anemia or blood diseases ________
☐ Epilepsy ________
☐ Nervous breakdown or mental illnesses ________
☐ Depression ________
☐ Suicide attempt ________
☐ Alcohol or drug problem ________
☐ Other ________

____

History updated (date)

500-50

FIGURE 2-25. New patient records should include specific medical information for the new patient so that all the pertinent history and medical information is included both for the physician and for documentation purposes.

Name: ______________________ DoB __/__/__ Age ________ Chart No. [ ]

Assessment

Plan

Provider's signature ____________ Return visit ____________

Physical Exam

Ht. ____ Wt. ____ Temp. ____ Resp. ________
B.P. sit. or stand. ___/___ Supine ___/___
Pulse rate and regularity ______________

Circle abnormal and pertinent normal findings.
Describe abnormalities.
☑ Normal ☒ Abnormal

1. **Constitutional**
   a. ☐ gen. appear. (e.g., development, nutrition, body habitus, deformities, attention to grooming)

2. **Head and face**

3. **Eyes**
   a. ☐ inspection of conjunctivae and lids (e.g., xanthelasma)

4. **Ears, nose, throat and mouth**
   a. ☐ inspection of teeth, gums and palate
   b. ☐ inspection of oral mucosa with notation of presence of pallor or cyanosis

5. **Neck**
   a. ☐ examination jugular veins (e.g., distention; a, v or cannon a waves)
   b. ☐ examination of thyroid (e.g., enlargement, tenderness, mass)

6. **Respiratory**
   a. ☐ assessment of respiratory effort (e.g., intercostal retractions, use of accessory muscles, diaphragmatic movement)
   b. ☐ auscultation of lungs (e.g., breath sounds, adventitious sounds, rubs)

7. **Cardiovascular**
   a. ☐ palpation of heart (e.g., location, size and forcefulness of the point of maximal impact; thrills; lifts; palpable S3 or S4)
   b. ☐ auscultation of heart, including normal sounds, abnormal sounds and murmurs
   c. ☐ measurement of blood pressure in two or more extremities when indicated (e.g., aortic dissection, coarctation)

   Examination of:

   d. ☐ carotid arteries (e.g., waveform, pulse amplitude, bruits, apical-carotid delay)
   e. ☐ abdominal aorta (e.g., size, bruits)
   f. ☐ femoral arteries (e.g., pulse, amplitude, bruits)
   g. ☐ pedal pulses (e.g., pulse, amplitude)
   h. ☐ extremities for peripheral edema and/or varicosities

8. **Chest (breasts)**

9. **Gastrointestinal (abdomen)**
   a. ☐ examination of abdomen with notation of presence of masses or tenderness
   b. ☐ examination of liver and spleen
   c. ☐ obtain stool sample for occult blood from patients who are being considered for thrombolytic or anticoagulant therapy

10. **Genitourinary (abdomen)**

11. **Lymphatic**

12. **Musculoskeletal**
    a. ☐ examination of the back with notation of kyphosis or scoliosis
    b. ☐ examination of gait with notation of ability to undergo exercise testing and/or participation in exercise program
    c. ☐ assessment of muscle strength and tone (e.g., flaccid, cogwheel, spastic) with notation of any atrophy and abnormal movements

13. **Extremities**
    a. ☐ inspection and palpation of digits and nails (e.g., clubbing, cyanosis, inflammation, petechiae, ischemia, infections, Osler's nodes)

14. **Skin**
    a. ☐ inspection and/or palpation of skin and subcutaneous tissue (e.g., stasis dermatitis, ulcers, scars, xanthomas)

15. **Neurological/psychiatric**
    Brief assessment of mental status:
    a. ☐ orientation to time, place, and person
    b. ☐ mood and affect (e.g., depression, anxiety, agitation)

Comments:

Procedures

☐ CBC
☐ Urine
☐ Glucose
☐ BUN
☐ Creatinine
☐ Electrolytes
☐ Liver funct. tests
☐ Cholesterol
☐ HDL/LDL
☐ Triglycerides
☐ Serum enzymes
☐ PT time
☐ Digitalis level
☐ CXR
☐ ECG
☐ Ambulatory ECG
☐ Echocardiogram
☐ Stress test
☐ Other

Drug Allergies:

Cardiology	Date/Time	Summary	☐ Referral ☐ Consultation

FIGURE 2-26. Patient records that are specialty specific detail the information needed for evaluating, treating, and managing specific specialty problems, such as those in cardiology.

Name: ______________________________ Date ___/___/___

HPI Chief Complaint:

Current Meds.:

Past, Family/Social History

THIS SECTION TO BE COMPLETED BY PATIENT.

Review of Systems

Are you concerned about? (circle concerns)

YES NO

1. Have you had recent health concerns (circle): changes in the way you feel, weight loss or gain, ↓ appetite, ↓ energy, ↑ tiredness or weakness, problems with sleep? ☐ ☐
2. Eye problems: vision, pain, tearing ☐ ☐
3. Ear, nose, mouth, throat problems ☐ ☐
4. Heart problems:
   a. Have you had any heart problems? ☐ ☐
   b. Have you ever had high blood pressure? ☐ ☐
   c. Do you take any heart, blood pressure, or cholesterol medications? ☐ ☐
   d. Do you have any chest pain? If yes, (circle) does it occur with rest, after exercise, after eating, during stress or emotional strain, associated with shortness of breath, nausea or vomiting? ☐ ☐
   e. Do you have any shortness of breath? ☐ ☐
   f. Do you sleep on more than one pillow? ☐ ☐
   g. Have you noticed any fluttering, skipped beats, pounding or heart irregularity? If yes, is this worse after drinking tea, coffee or colas? ☐ ☐
   h. Have you had any fainting or passing out episodes? ☐ ☐
   i. Have you been tiring more easily? ☐ ☐
   j. Have you noticed ankle or leg swelling? If yes, does the swelling decrease after resting and elevation of legs? ☐ ☐
   k. Do you have pain in the calves of your legs after walking? ☐ ☐
   l. Have you been coughing up blood? ☐ ☐
   m. Have you noticed any bluish discoloration or paleness to your skin? ☐ ☐
   n. Do you smoke? ☐ ☐
   o. Do you drink alcoholic beverages? ☐ ☐
5. Lung problems: coughing, wheezing, infections ☐ ☐
6. Abdominal pain, stomach or bowel problems ☐ ☐
7. Kidney or bladder problems ☐ ☐
8. Muscle, bone, joint or back problems ☐ ☐
9. Skin, hair or nail problems ☐ ☐
10. Neurologic problems: headaches, dizziness, numbness ☐ ☐
11. Nervousness, anxiety, depression, suicidal thoughts ☐ ☐
12. Excessive thirst and urine output, recent weight changes ☐ ☐
13. Anemia, bruising, blood clots, swollen glands ☐ ☐
14. Food allergies, hay fever, eczema, asthma, decreased immunity ☐ ☐

Do you have any other concerns?

____

____

______________________ ________
Patient's signature Date

Provider Comments:

☐ PFSH and ROS have been reviewed. ☐ Unresolved problems from previous visit have been addressed.

______________________ ________
Provider's signature Date

Anticipatory Guidance

☐ Nutrition
☐ Low-salt diet
☐ Weight reduction
☐ Exercise
☐ Aspirin
☐ Smoking cessation
☐ Caffeine
☐ Alcohol
☐ Work
☐ Stress
☐ Oral contraceptive risks
☐ Postmenopausal hormones

FIGURE 2-26, cont'd.

Name: ______________________ DoB __/__/__ Age __________ Chart No. [ ]

Assessment

Plan

______________________ ____________
Provider's signature Return visit

Physical Exam

Ht. ____ Wt. ____ Temp. ____ Resp. ________
B.P. sit. or stand. ___/___ Supine ___/___
Pulse rate and regularity ________________

Circle abnormal and pertinent normal findings. Describe abnormalities.

☐ Normal ☐ Abnormal

1. **Constitutional**
   a. ☐ gen. appear., development, body habitus, nutrition, deformities, grooming
2. **Head and face**
3. **Eyes**
4. **Ears, nose, throat and mouth**
5. **Neck**
   a. ☐ appearance, masses, symmetry, tracheal position, crepitus
   b. ☐ thyroid (enlargement, tenderness, mass)
6. **Respiratory**
   a. ☐ respiratory effort (intercostal retractions) use of accessory muscles, diaphragm move
   b. ☐ auscultation (breath sounds, rhonchi, wheezes, rales, rubs)
7. **Cardiovascular**
   a. ☐ femoral arteries (pulse amplitude, bruits)
   b. ☐ pedal pulses (pulse amplitude)
   c. ☐ extremities (edema, varicosities)
8. **Chest (breasts)**
   a. ☐ inspection and palpation of breasts (e.g., masses or lumps, tenderness, symmetry, nipple discharge)
9. **Gastrointestinal (abdomen)**
   a. ☐ examination for masses, tenderness
   b. ☐ examination of liver and spleen
   c. ☐ examination for presence or absence of hernia
   d. ☐ stool for occult blood when indicated
   e. ☐ digital rectal examination including sphincter tone, presence of hemorrhoids, rectal masses
10. **Genitourinary**
    Pelvic exam. (with or without specimen collection for smears or cultures), including:
    a. ☐ external genitalia (e.g., gen. appearance, hair distribution, lesions)
    b. ☐ urethral meatus (e.g., size, location, lesions, prolapse)
    c. ☐ urethra (e.g., masses, tenderness, scarring)
    d. ☐ bladder (e.g., fullness, masses, tenderness)
    e. ☐ vagina (e.g., gen. appearance, estrogen effect, discharge, lesions, pelvic support, cystocele, rectocele)
    f. ☐ cervix (e.g., gen. appearance, lesions, discharge)
    g. ☐ uterus (e.g., size, contour, position, mobility, tenderness, consistency, descent or support)
    h. ☐ adnexa/parametria (e.g., masses, tenderness, organomegaly, nodularity)
    i. ☐ anus and perineum
11. **Lymphatic**
    a. ☐ palpation of lymph nodes in neck, axillae, groin, other locations _____
12. **Musculoskeletal**
13. **Extremities**
14. **Skin**
    a. ☐ inspection and/or palpation of skin and sub-Q tissue (e.g., rashes, lesions, ulcers)
15. **Neurological/psychiatric**
    Brief assessment of mental status:
    a. ☐ orientation to time, place, and person
    b. ☐ mood and affect (depression, anxiety, agitation)

Comments:

Procedures and Immunizations Are immunizations current? ☐ yes ☐ no

	☐ Cholesterol	☐ PAP test	☐ Other
	☐ HDL/LDL	☐ Mammogram	☐ dT
☐ CBC	☐ FSH	☐ Stool guaiac	☐ Hep B
☐ Glucose	☐ Prolactin	☐ Chlamydia screen	☐ Influenza
☐ TSH	☐ Estradiol	☐ Rubella screen	☐ Rubella
☐ Urine	☐ VDRL	☐ GC screen	

Drug Allergies:

GYN	Date/Time	Summary	☐ Referral

FIGURE 2-27. Another example of specialty-specific history, examination, and medical decision-making form that helps the physician properly document patient information for charting purposes and fulfill documentation requirements.

Name: ______________________ Date ___/___/___

HPI Chief Complaint:

Current Meds.:

Past/Family History

THIS SECTION TO BE COMPLETED BY PATIENT.

Personal/Social History

Are you ... ☐ single ☐ married ☐ live-in partner ☐ divorced ☐ widowed

Do you have children? ☐ yes ☐ no
Age(s) of child(ren) ______
No. of pregnancies ____ Miscarriages ____
Occupation ______

YES NO

a. Do you have concerns about your breasts? (circle): changes in size or shape, changes in skin color, lumps, tenderness, ulcerations, discharge or blood from nipple, inverted nipple ☐ ☐
b. Do you have concerns about your menstruation (circle): frequency of periods, amount of flow, cramping, premenstrual tension, menopausal symptoms, postmenopausal bleeding? ☐ ☐
c. Do you take hormones (estrogen)? ☐ ☐
d. Do you have concerns about (circle): vaginal itching, dryness or discharge; pain or bleeding with intercourse; fertility problems; lack of enjoyment of sex? ☐ ☐
e. Concerns about lesions, lumps or swelling on your vulva or vagina? ☐ ☐
f. Do you have (circle) pain on urination, blood in urine, repeated urinary infections, awakening at night to urinate, urine leakage or incontinence? ☐ ☐
g. Do you have concerns about abdominal pain or swelling, constipation or diarrhea, laxative or antacid use, rectal pain or bleeding, hemorrhoids? ☐ ☐
h. Approximate date of last menstruation ______
i. Approximate date of last pelvic exam ______
j. Approximate date of last Pap test ______
k. Approximate date of last mammogram ______
l. Are you sexually active now? ☐ ☐
☐ same sex ☐ opposite sex
☐ single partner ☐ multiple partners
Have you had more than 4 lifetime partners? ☐ ☐
m. Birth control method ______
n. Do you have concerns about sexual orientation, sexually transmitted diseases, exposure to AIDS or other sexual concerns? ☐ ☐
o. Do you feel safe/comfortable in your home, with your family, and/or your partner relationship? ☐ ☐
p. Do you smoke or use tobacco products now? ☐ ☐
q. Do you use recreational drugs? ☐ ☐
r. Do you drink alcohol? ☐ ☐
☐ daily ☐ weekly ☐ rarely
# of drinks ______
If yes, do you drink: ☐ beer ☐ wine ☐ liquor

Review of Systems

Are you concerned about? (circle concerns)

YES NO

1. Recent changes in health status ☐ ☐
2. Eye problems: vision, pain, tearing ☐ ☐
3. Ear, nose, mouth, throat problems ☐ ☐
4. Heart problems: chest pain, blood pressure ☐ ☐
5. Lung problems: coughing, wheezing, infections ☐ ☐
6. Abdominal pain, stomach or bowel problems ☐ ☐
7. Kidney or bladder problems ☐ ☐
8. Muscle, bone, joint or back problems ☐ ☐
9. Skin, hair or nail problems ☐ ☐
10. Neurologic problems: headaches, dizziness, numbness ☐ ☐
11. Nervousness, anxiety, depression, suicidal thoughts ☐ ☐
12. Excessive thirst and urine output, recent weight changes ☐ ☐
13. Anemia, bruising, blood clots, swollen glands ☐ ☐
14. Food allergies, hay fever, eczema, asthma, decreased immunity ☐ ☐

Do you have any other concerns? ☐ ☐

______

______

Patient's signature ______ Date ______

Provider Comments:

☐ PFSH and ROS have been reviewed. ☐ Unresolved problems from previous visit have been addressed.

Provider's signature ______ Date ______

Anticipatory Guidance

☐ Nutrition
☐ Exercise
☐ Calcium
☐ Multivit. with folate
☐ Cardiovascular risks
☐ Osteoporosis risks
☐ Estrogen
☐ Sun exposure
☐ Smoking cessation
☐ Alcohol/drugs
☐ Sexual issues
☐ Family planning/contraception
☐ STD prevention
☐ Menopause
☐ Self-exam: breasts, skin, oral cavity
☐ Family
☐ Recreation/hobbies
☐ Safety/injury/gun safety
☐ Auto seat belts
☐ Domestic violence
☐ Stress
☐ Educational handouts

FIGURE 2-27, cont'd.

TOOL 2-6

HISTORY AND PHYSICAL EXAMINATION SAMPLE DICTATION MODEL

Patient:
Age:
Gender:
Date of physical:

If applicable:
Attending physician:
Date of admission:
Room #:

Chief Complaint

As related to provider by patient
Character, location, onset, radiation, intensity, duration, intermittency, events associated with, palliative, provocative factors

Past Medical History:

Patient denies/positive for:

Arthritis	Diabetes	Hepatitis	Rheumatic fever
Asthma	Emphysema	Heart disease	Seizure
Blood disease	Epilepsy	Hypertension	Thyroid disease
Bronchitis	Flu	Liver disease	Tuberculosis
Cancer	Gout	Pneumonia	Ulcers
			UTI

Past Surgical History:

Injuries:

Chronic Diseases/Disabilities:

Family History:

Social History:

Patient presently lives with:
Occupation:
Patient denies/positive for history of:
- Cigarettes/smoking (# of years/packs per day)
- ETOH (frequency, # of years)
- Substance abuse (# of years/substance)

Medications:

Allergies:

Review of systems:

General:	Recent change in weight, appetite, sleeping habits
HEENT:	Head: Cephalgia, head injury, migraines Eyes: Blurring, cataracts, diplopia, photophobia, vision changes Ears: Discharge, hearing changes, tinnitus Nose: Chronic sinusitis, decreased smell, rhinorrhea, epistaxis, nasal fractures Mouth/throat: Tenderness/lesions oral cavity, frequent sore throats, dysphagia, persistent hoarseness Neck: History of injury, masses, pain, stiffness
Respiratory:	Asthma, bronchitis, COPD, chronic cough, hemoptysis, SOB, tuberculosis, tachypnea
Cardiovascular:	Angina, CHF, claudication, CVA, cyanosis, dizziness, exertional dyspnea, hypertension, orthopnea, palpitations, phlebitis, precordial pain, TIA
Gastrointestinal:	Constipation, diarrhea, dysphagia, gallbladder disease, hematemesis, hematochezia, hemorrhoids, hepatitis, hernia, indigestion, jaundice, melena, nausea, vomiting, pancreatitis, rectal bleeding

Continued

TOOL 2-6

HISTORY AND PHYSICAL EXAMINATION SAMPLE DICTATION MODEL—cont'd

Genitourinary:	Dysuria, hematuria, nocturia, discharge, frequency, hesitancy, incontinence, chronic UTI, STD, prostatitis
Ob/GYN:	Pregnancy history, past Pap/breast exam, contraceptive use, menstrual history
Breasts:	Discharge, enlargement, pain, tenderness, prior surgery/biopsy, +mammogram
Neuromuscular:	Anesthsias, paresthesias, arthralgias, myalgias, nervousness, syncope, vertigo, weakness
Endocrine:	Hot/cold intolerance, paresthesias, polydipsia, polyphagia, polyuria, anemia, excessive bruising/ bleeding, diabetes, thyroid enlargement/problems

Physical Examination

Vital signs:	BP, P, T, R
General:	This is a ___ year old ____ who appears well hydrated and properly nourished and whose appearance is appropriate with the stated age. The patient is alert, cooperative, and in no acute distress at this time.
Skin:	Skin texture, turgor, and pigmentation appear normal. No rashes, cyanosis. Normal hair pattern for sex and age.
Head:	Atraumatic, normocephalic, symmetrical, and without deformities. Eyes: PERRLA EOMI bilaterally. No conjunctival injection, ptosis, or sclera icterus. Funduscopic examination reveals no AV nicking, retinal hemorrhages, or retinopathy seen. Ears: External ear exam reveals no abnormalities seen. External ear canals are patent, TM intact with normal light reflex, and without injection. Nose: No deviated septum, turbinates normal appearing. Moist mucosa without discharge noted. Mouth: Pink gums without bleeding. Mucosa moist. Teeth appear in good condition. Throat: Trachea midline and mobile. No JVD, thyroid not palpable or enlarged. No cervical lymphadenopathy or rigidity present.
Lungs/thorax:	Lungs clear to auscultation, no rales, rhonchi, or wheezes. Breath sounds normal without prolonged expiratory phase. Respirations normal with good chest motion. No lymphadenopathy noted. Active bowel sounds noted in all quadrants. No pulsations, bruits, or flank pain.
Extremities:	No clubbing, cyanosis, edema, or varicosities noted. Pulses equal and adequate.
Neurologic:	Patient oriented ×3. DTRs equal and adequate in upper and lower extremities. Good grip strength noted bilaterally. Sensation intact.

UTI, Urinary tract infection; *ETOH,* ethyl alcohol; *HEENT,* head, ears, eyes, nose, throat; *COPD,* chronic obstructive pulmonary disease; *SOB,* shortness of breath; *CHF,* congestive heart failure; *CVA,* cerebrovascular accident; *TIA,* transient ischemic attack; *STD,* sexually transmitted disease; *BP,* blood pressure; *P,* pulse; *T,* temperature; *R,* respirations; *PERRLA,* pupils equal, round, and reactive to light and accommodation; *EOMI*, extraocular muscles intact; *AV,* atrioventricular; *TM,* tympanic membrane; *JVD,* jugular venous distension; *DTRs*, deep tendon reflexes.

TOOL 2-7

BASIC DOCUMENTATION DO'S AND DON'TS

	Do's	Don'ts
HISTORY		
Present	Vital signs review Duration/severity of symptoms	Allow other personnel to document history, presenting illness
Past	Pertinent negative history Pertinent positive history	
Systems review	Document all systems history review; include "WNL" notations	
Family/social	Include notations such as not available/ noncontributory; unable to obtain due to_____	
PHYSICAL EXAM	Include body areas/organ systems, abnormal findings notated, pertinent negatives notated	
MEDICAL DECISION MAKING		
Diagnostic tests	Document orders Document interpretations INTERPRETATIONS NOT DOCUMENTED CANNOT BE CHARGED	Document diagnosis interpretations as "WNL" or "Abn"—document specifics that make them normal/abnormal
Clinical impression	Record primary/secondary diagnoses Record contributory diagnoses that may have resulted in increased level of care Include differential diagnoses	Use "rule out,""probable,""suspect," as part of the diagnostic statement
Treatment plan	Record all medications/orders and sign Record all discharge instructions, including preprinted handouts Resolution/nonresolution of symptoms Documentation of risks	Allow nurse documentation of medications unless signed off by the physician
Signature Requirements	Sign all charts Countersign all academic residents Include notation "examined and concur" CHARTS NOT SIGNED ARE CONSIDERED NOT DOCUMENTED—NO CHARGE	Allow signature stamps Allow "dictated but not read"
Special Notations	Document additional time spent for: Excessive data review/counseling due to: lengthy past medical history, lengthy review of records, patient inability to comprehend Procedures documented separately	Forget to document time for these elements

WNL, Within normal limits; *Abn,* abnormal.

TABLE 2-1 GODFREY REGIONAL MEDICAL SIGNATURE LOG

Provider	Signature	Provider	Signature
Maurice Doates, MD	Maurice Doates, MD	John Parker, MD	John Parker MD
Robert Rais, MD	Robert Rais MD	Nathan Brady, MD	Nath Brady MD
Stanley Krosette, MD	Stanley Krosette, MD	Luis Perez, MD	Luis Perez MD
William Obert, MD	William Obert MD	Steven Speller, MD	Steven Speller MD
Felix Washington, MD	Felix Washington MD	Maria Callaway, MD	Maria Callaway MD
Jay Corman, MD	Jay Corman MD	Patrick Adams, MD	Patrick Adams MD
Nancy Connelly, MD	Nancy Connelly MD	James Ellicott, MD	James Ellicott MD
Adam Westgate, MD	Adam Westgate MD	Linda Patrick, MD	Linda Patrick MD
Patrick Chung, MD	Patrick Chung MD	Vincent DiMarco, MD	Vincent DiMarco MD
Rachel Perez, MD	Rachel Perez MD		
Lisa Valhas, MD	Lisa Valhas MD		

Keep in mind that physicians may provide services in a number of facilities at different locations. As an exercise, put together one medical chart and review the documents contained in that chart. Typically, the physician chart will be tabbed on the basis of like services and like locations, such as the following:

Office visit/progress notes
Laboratory/x-ray tests
Other ancillaries
Hospital services
Correspondence/patient records

Typically, the following would be included in the record, starting from front to back:

Tab 1: Office Visits/Progress Notes (chronologic order, current first)
Figure 2-3 Problem list
Figure 2-4 Medication flow sheet
Figure 2-2 Staff/visit note (chronologic order, current first)
Figure 2-5 Progress note (most current)
Figure 2-6 Progress note (oldest)

Tab 2: Lab/X-Ray
Figure 2-8 Radiology report (chronologic order, current first)
Figure 2-9 Laboratory report (chronologic order, current first)

Tab 3: Other Ancillaries
Figure 2-11 Respiratory report (chronologic order, current first)
Figure 2-13 Electromyography report (chronologic order, current first)

Tab 4: Hospital Services
Figure 2-16 Discharge summary (chronologic order, current first)
Figure 2-15 Hospital progress note (chronologic order, current first)
Figure 2-14 Admission and history (chronologic order, current first)
Figure 2-18 Operative report (chronologic order, current first)
Figure 2-19 Anesthesia report

Tab 5: Correspondence/Patient Records
Figure 2-17 Consultation report (chronologic order, current first)
Figure 2-1 Patient history

TABLE 2-2 GODFREY REGIONAL HEALTH FACILITIES AND PROVIDERS

Facility Names and Addresses

Facility	Address	Facility	Address
Godfrey Regional Outpatient Clinic	3122 Shannon Ave. Aldon, FL 77712 (407) 555-7654	Godfrey Clinical Laboratories	465 Dogwood Court Aldon, FL 77712 (407) 555-9876
Godfrey Regional Hospital	123 Main Street Aldon, FL 77714 (407) 555-1234	Godfrey Medical Associates	1532 Third Ave. Suite 120 Aldon, FL 77713 (407) 555-4000

Provider Names

PROVIDER	SPECIALTY	LOCATION(S) OF SERVICE
Patrick Adams, MD	Gastroenterologist	Godfrey Regional Hospital Godfrey Medical Associates
Nathan Brady, MD	Internal Medicine/Cardiology	Godfrey Regional Hospital Godfrey Regional Outpatient Clinic Godfrey Medical Associates
Maria Callaway, MD	Surgical Pathologist	Godfrey Regional Hospital Godfrey Regional Outpatient Clinic
Patrick Chung, MD	Surgeon/Orthopedics	Godfrey Regional Hospital Godfrey Regional Outpatient Clinic Godfrey Medical Associates
Nancy Connelly, MD	Emergency Department	Godfrey Regional Hospital
Jay Corman, MD	Internal Medicine	Godfrey Regional Hospital Godfrey Medical Associates
Vincent DiMarco, MD	Neurologist	Godfrey Regional Hospital Godfrey Regional Outpatient Clinic
Maurice Doates, MD	Internal Medicine	Godfrey Regional Hospital Godfrey Regional Outpatient Clinic Godfrey Medical Associates
James Ellicott, MD	Otolaryngologist	Godfrey Regional Hospital Godfrey Regional Outpatient Clinic
Stanley Krosette, MD	Internal Medicine	Godfrey Regional Hospital Godfrey Regional Outpatient Clinic Godfrey Medical Associates
William Obert, MD	Family Medicine	Godfrey Regional Hospital Godfrey Medical Associates
John Parker, MD	Internal Medicine	Godfrey Regional Hospital Godfrey Regional Outpatient Clinic Godfrey Medical Associates
Linda Patrick, MD	Ophthalmologist	Godfrey Regional Hospital Godfrey Medical Associates
Luis Perez, MD	Anesthesiologist	Godfrey Regional Hospital Godfrey Regional Outpatient Clinic
Rachel Perez, MD	Surgeon/General	Godfrey Regional Hospital Godfrey Regional Outpatient Clinic Godfrey Medical Associates
Robert Rais, MD	Emergency Department	Godfrey Regional Hospital
Steven Speller, MD	Pathologist	Godfrey Clinical Laboratories
Lisa Valhas, MD	Radiologist	Godfrey Regional Hospital Godfrey Regional Outpatient Clinic
Felix Washington, MD	Family Medicine	Godfrey Regional Hospital Godfrey Medical Associates
Adam Westgate, MD	Surgeon/General	Godfrey Regional Hospital Godfrey Regional Outpatient Clinic Godfrey Medical Associates

Chapter in Review

Certification Review

At this point, it is assumed that you have not completed your studies and are not prepared to take the certification examination. Therefore certification exercises are included in the coding chapters that occur later in the text.

Coding Concepts

- The cardinal rule of coding is: If it is not documented, it did not happen.
- All documentation used for coding must be appropriately signed to be considered complete.
- Documentation is important from both coding and medical liability standpoints.
- Identify the key words that identify WHAT was performed and WHY the services were medically necessary for coding purposes.
- Complete ancillary records include medication records, health care staff notes, operative notes, and laboratory and other ancillary test results.
- Documentation requirements for hospital records include history and physical examination, admission records, hospital progress notes, and consultations.
- Documentation tools can help in the development of adequate medical documentation for medical coding and compliance.

Student Assignments

- Study Chapter 2.
- Review the Learning Objectives for Chapter 2.
- Complete the Chapter Review exercise to reinforce the concepts learned in this chapter.
- Complete and discuss the Practical Application exercise.
- Complete practice exercises on the companion Evolve site for reinforcement of the concepts contained in Chapter 2.
- Complete the Workbook exercises for Chapter 2 as assigned by your instructor.

Chapter Review Exercise

Identify where the following services might be performed and, on the basis of that location, identify the appropriate form(s) that would be used.

	Location	Type of Form(s)
1. Patient visit Godfrey Regional Hospital	________	________
2. Patient visit Godfrey Medical Associates	________	________
3. Patient visit Godfrey Regional Outpatient Clinic	________	________
4. Patient visit Emergency Department, Godfrey Regional Hospital	________	________
5. Laboratory report	________	________
6. Radiology report	________	________
7. Admission history and physical	________	________
8. Staff documentation of office visit	________	________
9. Patient history	________	________
10. Patient problem list	________	________
11. Anesthesia record	________	________
12. Operative report	________	________
13. Discharge summary	________	________
14. Consultation	________	________

Practical Application

Review the following reports and discuss what type of report they represent and in what setting these forms might be used. Also identify WHAT services were performed and WHY they were medically necessary.

1. Chart #1

This is a 12-year-old male who presents with a sore left shoulder after a fall at school today. He says he was tackled at school and landed on his shoulder in the region of the collar bone. His father states they have been using ice on his shoulder; however, this seems not to have provided him any relief. He indicates he can move his shoulder, but it is painful to do so.

He is on no medications. No known drug allergies.

Vital signs are stable. Patient is alert and oriented. He is in a fair amount of distress. He is quite tearful, but he answers questions appropriately. Regarding appearance of the left shoulder, there is no step-off deformity noted on exam. There is no swelling noted of the shoulder, but there is some bruising over the top aspect of the shoulder in the region of the collar bone and shoulder blade.

X-ray of the shoulder did not demonstrate any dislocation or acute bony abnormality.

Patient will be discharged at this time to follow up with his private physician in the office or return to the emergency department if needed.

Report type: ____________________
Service #1: ____________________
WHAT performed: ____________________
WHY performed: ____________________
Service #2: ____________________
WHAT performed: ____________________
WHY performed: ____________________

2. *Chart #2*

Progress Note

Sputum specimen obtained from last evening showed numerous gram-positive diplococci. This may be early streptococcal pneumonia developing. Her white count has actually increased since admission, so we will start her on IV Levaquin for presumed early pneumonia. Lungs are still clear to auscultation. Trace wheezing. Will continue updraft treatments and check white count tomorrow to determine whether she will need further treatment or may be discharged.

Report type: ____________________
Service #1: ____________________
WHAT performed: ____________________
WHY performed: ____________________
Service #2: ____________________
WHAT performed: ____________________
WHY performed: ____________________

3. *Chart #3*

Preoperative diagnosis: Left pleural effusion
Postoperative diagnosis: Same
Procedure: Thoracentesis

The patient was brought into the operating room and positioned on the table. The left back was prepped and draped over a marker that had been placed on the left posterior chest prior to x-ray to mark the level of the pleural effusion.

The patient had approximately 35 cc of pleural effusion over the eighth mid-scapular line in the left posterior chest. Using a 22-gauge needle, the pleural space was infiltrated and approximately 100 to 200 cc of straw-colored pleural fluid was extracted. The needle was removed with a small dressing placed over the left back puncture site.

Report type: ____________________
Service #1: ____________________
WHAT performed: ____________________
WHY performed: ____________________
Service #2: ____________________
WHAT performed: ____________________
WHY performed: ____________________

4. *Chart #4*

Follow-up Visit

Two months status postoperative low anterior resection, multiple positive lymph nodes, vascular invasion liver metastases complicated by rupture of the gastroduodenal artery after an attempted dissection for catheter placement.

Physical examination is unremarkable. Rectal examination reveals a very well-healed anastomosis. Her colostomy has no edema. I will discuss with her surgeon the timing of her colostomy closure.

Report type: ____________________
Service #1: ____________________
WHAT performed: ____________________
WHY performed: ____________________
Service #2: ____________________
WHAT performed: ____________________
WHY performed: ____________________

5. *Chart #5*

88-year-old brought in by a friend for evaluation of low back pain as well as pain in the right hip and pelvis. She fell 3 weeks ago, tripping on a branch at home. Pain has been present but tolerable. She has not used any analgesics. She also has some pain in the right leg. No numbness or weakness.

Physical Examination

She had no difficulty lying down. There is some paraspinal spasm in the T12-L1 area. No pain on percussion of the entire spine. No pain on compression of pelvis, mild pain on palpation on the right greater trochanter. Lumbosacral spine x-rays show compression fracture of L1. No other abnormalities except for marked degenerative joint disease of the spine.

Impression

Compression fracture of L1

Plan

Discussed admission with the patient; however, she feels she is capable of getting along at home. She does not want to be hospitalized. Will give her Celebrex, 100 mg a day. She should follow up with her primary care physician in the next week, but sooner if pain increases or numbness or weakness of extremities develop.

Report type: ____________________
Service #1: ____________________
WHAT performed: ____________________
WHY performed: ____________________
Service #2: ____________________
WHAT performed: ____________________
WHY performed: ____________________

SECTION 2

ICD-9-CM Diagnostic Coding

In Section 1 of this text, many documents and techniques used in the documentation process were identified. This section contains diagnostic coding guidelines applicable to physicians and providers and provides an explanation of how to apply these rules to actual physician documents. The format of the ICD-9-CM diagnostic code book and its use for correct diagnostic code assignment are covered. Hospital and facility diagnostic coding is discussed in depth later in this text.

A brief review of the steps in the process of correctly identifying and coding diagnostic components of the medical documentation, or WHY services were performed, follows. This outline is intended to provide a simple approach to the complicated process covered in depth by this part of the text.

Many think that diagnostic coding involves only the selection of the correct numeric ICD-9-CM diagnostic code; however, the process also involves many rules and considerations. As mentioned in Chapter 2, documentation plays a key role in determining which diagnostic statements are the correct ones to use. The steps for identifying correct diagnostic codes include the following:

Step 1: Identify key elements and words for possible use in the diagnosis.

Step 2: Determine which diagnostic statements are necessary for proper diagnosis coding purposes.

Step 3: Determine the appropriate diagnostic code order.

Step 4: Assign diagnostic codes to diagnoses selected from the ICD-9-CM code book.

After thoroughly reading the discussion of each step, use the Diagnostic Documentation Worksheet to evaluate the information contained in the coding example. This form appears on the companion Evolve site.

The current version of diagnostic coding, the International Classification of Diseases, 9th Revision, Clinical Modification (ICD-9-CM), will soon be replaced by a new version, the International Classification of Diseases, 10th Revision, Clinical Modification (ICD-10-CM), which will be discussed throughout Section 2.

In anticipation of the implementation of ICD-10-CM in the near future, implementation impact comments have been included where significant changes will occur between the current ICD-9-CM code and the ICD-10-CM code to come. ■

3

Determining Physician Diagnosis

LEARNING OBJECTIVES

After completing this chapter, the student will be able to:

- Identify key elements and words in physician documentation.
- Identify which key elements and words should be used for coding and documentation purposes.
- Recognize the differences between signs, symptoms, and diagnoses.
- Determine correct diagnostic code order.
- Apply diagnostic coding concepts to practical coding scenarios.

CODING REFERENCE TOOLS

Tool 3-1
Rules for Selecting Appropriate Diagnoses for Physician Coding

Tool 3-2
Signs and Symptoms Rules

Tool 3-3
Diagnosis Do's and Don'ts

Tool 3-4
Diagnostic Order Rules

ICD-9-CM Physician Diagnostic Coding

The rules for diagnostic coding for outpatient facility and physician coding differ greatly from inpatient facility diagnostic coding. Keep in mind that ALL the discussions in the following chapters relate specifically to physician coding only.

It is also important to mention that additional diagnostic statements, signs, or symptoms should NOT be added if the intent is solely to enhance reimbursement. Coding guidelines must be followed, and additional diagnostic statements should be added only when appropriate.

Keeping the above in mind, let's take a detailed look at the steps for determining what diagnosis or diagnostic statements would be appropriate for inclusion.

STEP 1: IDENTIFY KEY ELEMENTS AND WORDS FOR POSSIBLE USE IN THE DIAGNOSIS

Some primary rules exist for selecting appropriate diagnoses from medical documentation. These rules are specific to physician coding for services. The differences between physician and hospital coding, and the rationale for those differences, are described later in the chapter. Keep in mind when reviewing the medical documentation that one must identify WHY the services are being provided. Although only interested in assigning diagnoses at this point, the student must also identify services for the purpose of making certain all services have an appropriate diagnosis assigned.

Some basic guidelines for diagnostic selection are included in Tool 3-1. We have already discussed in Chapter 2 the cardinal rule of coding: If it is not documented, it did not happen.

Let's take a look at the additional rules contained in Tool 3-1 in detail:

—The condition, problem, or other circumstance chiefly responsible for the health encounter, visit, or problem is reported. This will be referred to as the "chief reason for the encounter."

The patient may present for a number of complaints or problems; however, the chief reason for the encounter will be the condition, sign, or symptom that prompted the visit. For instance, if the patient presents with rhinorrhea (nasal discharge) and cough but fever is what prompted the visit to the physician, fever would be assigned as the chief reason for the encounter.

If the patient presented for rhinorrhea, cough, and fever, and, before the conclusion of the visit, the physician diagnosed sinusitis as the diagnosis, the sinusitis would be the primary diagnosis because the other phrases are signs or symptoms of the sinusitis. (This will be covered further during the discussion of Tool 3-2.)

—Unconfirmed diagnoses described as "possible," "probable," "questionable," "rule out," "ruled out," and "suspect(ed)" cannot be used for physician diagnoses or physician coding.

Only conditions that are confirmed by the physician may be used for coding purposes. Therefore if the physician, at the conclusion of the encounter, has not made a definitive diagnosis, signs and symptoms may need to be used for that visit.

For example, if the patient presents with the complaint of cough and fever and the physician suspects an upper respiratory infection, the diagnosis for that encounter would be cough and fever. Only if the physician makes a definitive diagnosis of upper respiratory infection before the conclusion of that visit may that diagnostic statement be used. In many of these circumstances, the physician requires additional workup such as laboratory or x-ray findings to make a definitive diagnosis.

—Code the condition to the highest level of specificity.

When a definitive diagnosis has been made before the conclusion of the encounter and signs and symptoms of that condition are also available, the diagnosis would be assigned first. An example would be the diagnosis of bronchitis with presenting signs or symptoms of cough. Because the diagnosis of bronchitis was made before the conclusion of the encounter, it would be considered more specific, or the highest level of specificity. Therefore bronchitis would be the primary, or first, diagnosis. In some cases, when only signs and symptoms are available at the conclusion of the encounter, they may be the condition coded to the highest level of specificity.

—If the physician does not identify a definite condition or problem at the conclusion of the patient visit, the coder should select the documented chief complaint or chief reason for the encounter.

This is similar to the previously mentioned guidelines, in that when the physician does not make a specific diagnosis at the conclusion of the visit, the coder will need to use the presenting complaints of the patient for the primary diagnosis.

—Never code a diagnosis not listed by the physician.

It is important that the coder recognize that he or she may not code for any conditions not listed by the physician. The coder may not make any conclusions regarding diagnosis that may have been omitted or not clearly identified in the record. For instance, the recording of a blood pressure of 200/120 mm Hg probably means that the patient has hypertension; however, the coder may not make that conclusion. Without a definitive diagnosis made by the physician, the coder may only assign a diagnosis of "elevated blood pressure without a diagnosis of hypertension."

Using the basic coding documentation rules discussed in Tool 3-1, look at the progress note in Figure 3-1, and identify items that would or would not be selected as key elements or phrases.

In the example in Figure 3-1, identify components that might be used for diagnostic and procedural coding. Look for elements that identify WHY (diagnosis, signs, or symptoms) the encounter took place, as well as WHAT (procedures, services) was provided to help the patient. Later chapters on ICD-9-CM diagnostic coding and CPT (Current Procedural

TOOL 3-1

RULES FOR SELECTING APPROPRIATE DIAGNOSES FOR PHYSICIAN CODING

1. **If it is not documented, it did not happen.**
2. The condition, problem, or other circumstance chiefly responsible for the health encounter, visit, or problem is reported. This will be referred to as **chief reason for encounter.**
3. Unconfirmed diagnoses described as "possible," "probable," "questionable," "rule out," "ruled out," and "suspect(ed)" CANNOT be used for physician diagnoses or physician coding.
4. Code the condition to the **highest level of specificity.** In some cases this may be the sign, symptom, abnormal test, or reason for visit or encounter.
5. If the physician does not identify a definite condition or problem at the conclusion of the patient encounter, the coder should select the documented chief complaint or chief reason for the encounter.
6. Never code a diagnosis not listed by the physician. In the event the coder believes the physician has not listed an appropriate diagnosis, the coder must check with the physician.

   If the physician believes the information has been omitted in error, the provider may add an addendum to the original medical record and, at that time, the coder may code accordingly.

TOOL 3-2

SIGNS AND SYMPTOMS RULES

Signs and symptoms should be used **ONLY** when:

1. Principal diagnosis has not been established at the conclusion of the encounter.
2. No more specific diagnosis for the specific condition can be made at the end of the encounter.
3. Presenting signs and symptoms are transient and no definitive diagnosis is made.
4. The symptom is treated in an outpatient setting without the additional workup necessary to arrive at a more definitive diagnosis at the conclusion of the visit or encounter.

   Signs and symptoms need NOT be used when they are an integral part of the underlying diagnosis or condition already coded.

Terminology, 4th edition) procedural coding examine which elements should be retained for coding purposes. Because all documentation will not be the same, it is important to keep in mind that the medical record should be reviewed for more than "impression." In some instances, additional information is contained in the body of the documentation. A complete review will be necessary to select the correct diagnostic statements for coding purposes.

Look at the key words identified in the sample documentation that are needed for diagnostic and procedural coding purposes.

WHAT (Service Elements)	WHY (Diagnostic Elements)
Physician office visit	Cough, fever, cold symptoms Upper respiratory infection Urinary frequency, urinary tract infection
Chest x-ray	Cough, fever, cold symptoms Upper respiratory infection
Complete blood cell count (CBC)	Cough, fever, cold symptoms Upper respiratory infection
Urinalysis	Urinary frequency, urinary tract infection

Note the necessity of matching WHAT service was provided with WHY that particular service was necessary. Refer to Figure 3-2 for completing Step 1 (identifying key elements for possible use in coding) of the Diagnostic Documentation Worksheet.

PROGRESS NOTE

Date:	Vital signs: T	R
Chief complaint:	P	BP

This is a 65-year-old female who presents due to ongoing problem with cough, fever, and cold symptoms.

Examination:

Chest x-ray and CBC are ordered, which indicate the presence of an upper respiratory infection. Patient also complains of urinary frequency; therefore, a urinalysis is performed that confirms the diagnosis of urinary tract infection.

Impression:

Upper respiratory infection
Urinary tract infection

Plan:

The patient will be treated with antibiotics and should follow-up in approximately 7–10 days.

Patient name:
DOB:
MR/Chart #:

GODFREY REGIONAL OUTPATIENT CLINIC
3122 Shannon Avenue • Aldon, FL 77712 • (407) 555-7654

FIGURE 3-1. Progress note.

DIAGNOSTIC DOCUMENTATION WORKSHEET

Chart#/Patient Name:

	WHAT (Service/Procedure)	**WHY (MEDICAL NECESSITY)** (Diagnostic Information)
Step 1 Select all words for possible use as diagnosis/diagnostic statement from the document	Office Visit	Cough, Fever, Cold Symptoms, Upper Respiratory Infection
		Urinary Frequency, Urinary Tract Infection
	Chest X-Ray	Cough, Fever, Cold Symptoms, Upper Respiratory Infection
	CBC	Cough, Fever, Cold Symptoms, Upper Respiratory Infection
	Urinalysis	Urinary Frequency, Urinary Tract Infection
Step 2 Determine which words are appropriate for inclusion: (Carry these forward) Diagnosis vs. signs/symptoms		
Step 3 Based on each service performed, determine the appropriate order of diagnosis for each service performed		
Step 4 Look up/assign the proper dx codes		

FIGURE 3-2. Step 1 of the diagnostic coding process.

STOP AND PRACTICE

Review the following diagnostic information and identify the key words that would be appropriate for determining diagnostic statements that may be considered for diagnostic purposes.

Use for diagnostic purposes?

		Yes	No
1.	Rule out pneumonia	______	______
	Cough	______	______
2.	Dysuria	______	______
	Probably urinary tract infection	______	______
3.	Leg pain	______	______
	Tibia fracture	______	______
4.	Femur fracture	______	______
	Closed femur fracture	______	______
5.	Tonsillitis	______	______
	Strep tonsillitis	______	______
6.	Bronchitis	______	______
	Acute bronchitis	______	______
7.	Abdominal pain	______	______
	Rule out appendicitis	______	______
8.	Shortness of breath	______	______
	Asthma	______	______
	Asthma, status asthmaticus	______	______
9.	Abdominal pain	______	______
	Right upper quadrant	______	______
	Abdominal pain	______	______
	Possible cholecystitis	______	______
10.	Upper respiratory illness	______	______
	Upper respiratory infection	______	______

STEP 2: DETERMINE WHICH DIAGNOSTIC STATEMENTS ARE NECESSARY FOR PROPER DIAGNOSIS CODING PURPOSES

Step 2 involves determining which of the elements selected will be used for diagnostic coding. This requires elimination of unneeded signs and symptoms and determination of those that are necessary for coding. In an actual medical document, a number of statements can be found regarding why the patient is being seen or why the services are being performed. Some of these statements are diagnoses—statements after the patient's evaluation have taken place. Signs and symptoms are information gathered throughout the course of the evaluation. In some instances the physician may be unable to make a final diagnosis, in which case the final diagnostic statement may be nothing more than signs and symptoms. The physician may make a final diagnostic statement after the conclusion of the encounter. Therefore these statements may not be used for that encounter.

For instance, the patient has symptoms of cough and fever. At the conclusion of the encounter, the physician orders a chest x-ray and makes a diagnosis of cough, ruling out pneumonia. The final diagnostic statement encompassing "rule out" cannot be used; the cough and fever may be coded as signs and symptoms because the pneumonia diagnosis has not been definitively established at the conclusion of the encounter.

When the patient arrives at the radiology center to undergo a chest x-ray, and the diagnosis of pneumonia is determined before the chest x-ray visit has ended, pneumonia may be used as a diagnosis for the chest x-ray services but not for the physician office visit.

In the event that it is necessary to use signs, symptoms, or other conditions that do not qualify as a true diagnosis, the additional rules found in Tool 3-2 also apply.

Signs and symptoms, or complaints that are not a specific diagnosis, are used only when:

—Principal diagnosis has not been established at the conclusion of the visit or encounter.

When signs and symptoms are the only definitive statements in the documentation, they will be used as the diagnosis statement.

—No more specific diagnosis for the specific condition can be made at the end of the encounter.

As mentioned previously, when the physician is unable to make a definitive diagnosis, such as upper respiratory infection, the signs and symptoms such as cough and fever would be used in these instances.

—Presenting signs and symptoms are transient and no definitive diagnosis is made.

An example would be the patient who presents with elevated blood pressure, but the physician cannot made a definitive diagnosis of hypertension until further review or testing concludes that the patient indeed has hypertension instead of elevated blood pressure.

—The symptom is treated in an outpatient setting without the additional workup necessary to arrive at a more definitive diagnosis at the conclusion of the encounter.

When additional testing is necessary to make a definitive diagnosis, signs or symptoms may need to be used for that encounter. If the testing is completed before the visit has ended and the physician makes a more conclusive diagnosis, it may be used.

STOP AND PRACTICE

Look at the following diagnostic statements. Identify whether the statements are "signs and/or symptoms" (SS) or "diagnosis" (D).

	SS	D
1. Upper respiratory infection	______	______
2. Nausea	______	______
3. Vomiting	______	______
4. Headache	______	______
5. Angina	______	______
6. Abdominal pain	______	______
7. Ovarian cyst	______	______
8. Shoulder strain	______	______
9. Ankle fracture	______	______
10. Shortness of breath	______	______
11. High blood pressure	______	______
12. Ankle contusion	______	______
13. Viral illness	______	______
14. Nasal congestion	______	______
15. Fatigue	______	______
16. Sore throat	______	______

In questions 17 to 26, try to eliminate (cross out) the diagnoses, signs, or symptoms that are an integral part of the final diagnosis for each case. This will leave only statements that should be used for coding purposes.

17. Upper respiratory infection
    Cough
    Acute bronchitis
18. Nausea
    Vomiting
    Gastroenteritis
19. Shortness of breath
    Chronic obstructive pulmonary disease
20. Angina
    Coronary artery disease
    Status post bypass graft
21. Otitis media
    Acute bronchitis
    Diaper rash
    Cough
22. Urinary retention
    Urinary frequency
    Urinary tract infection
23. Urinary tract infection
    Kidney stone
24. Abdominal pain
    Appendicitis
25. Fever
    Influenza
26. Fever
    Urinary tract infection

In accordance with the rules, the signs and symptoms that are an integral part of the diagnostic statement can be eliminated in the sample. The procedure (service) elements are addressed in the CPT procedural section of the textbook.

WHY (Diagnostic Elements)
Cough, fever, cold symptoms
Upper respiratory infection
Urinary frequency, urinary tract infection

Several of the key elements and phrases previously identified in the sample chart as diagnostic elements to be considered for diagnosis coding can now be eliminated based on these additional guidelines.

COUGH, FEVER, COLD SYMPTOMS These are signs and symptoms that are part of the actual diagnosis of upper respiratory infection. This is referred to as "coding to the highest level of specificity." Be as specific as possible. Obviously, an upper respiratory infection has the symptoms of cough, fever, and cold as an integral part of the upper respiratory infection diagnosis. Therefore the diagnosis of upper respiratory infection is coded to the highest specific level possible.

As long as the coder is confident that the signs and symptoms listed are integral to that disease or diagnostic process, they need not be coded.

URINARY FREQUENCY This is considered a sign or symptom of the more specific diagnosis of urinary tract infection. Because urinary frequency signs and symptoms are an integral part of the urinary tract infection diagnosis, it is not necessary to code this sign or symptom.

Refer to Figure 3-3 for completion of Step 2 in determining the diagnostic statements to eliminate or include in this coding exercise and then proceed to the Stop and Practice exercise.

Key elements have been identified for diagnostic statements; signs and symptoms not necessary to list and code have been determined. Next are additional diagnostic statements that may be found in the documentation.

ADDITIONAL DIAGNOSTIC DO'S AND DON'TS

Physician documentation frequently includes statements regarding previous conditions, chronic conditions, and abnormal findings. Tool 3-3 provides additional rules entitled for determining which of the diagnoses selected thus far should be coded.

Do code:

—*Chronic conditions that require continued clinical evaluation and monitoring during each visit, such as hypertension, Parkinson's disease, chronic obstructive pulmonary disease, and other systemic diseases.*

Because patients with these diseases require continual monitoring, and other conditions and medications interact

DIAGNOSTIC DOCUMENTATION WORKSHEET

Chart#/Patient Name:

	WHAT (Service/Procedure)	**WHY (MEDICAL NECESSITY)** (Diagnostic Information)
Step 1 Select all words for possible use as diagnosis/diagnostic statement from the document	Office Visit	Cough, Fever, Cold Symptoms, Upper Respiratory Infection
		Urinary Frequency, Urinary Tract Infection
	Chest X-Ray	Cough, Fever, Cold Symptoms, Upper Respiratory Infection
	CBC	Cough, Fever, Cold Symptoms, Upper Respiratory Infection
	Urinalysis	Urinary Frequency, Urinary Tract Infection
Step 2 Determine which words are appropriate for inclusion: (Carry these forward) Diagnosis vs. signs/symptoms	Office Visit	Upper Respiratory Infection
		Urinary Tract Infection
	Chest X-Ray	Upper Respiratory Infection
	CBC	Upper Respiratory Infection
	Urinalysis	Urinary Tract Infection
Step 3 Based on each service performed, determine the appropriate order of diagnosis for each service performed		
Step 4 Look up/assign the proper dx codes		

FIGURE 3-3. Step 2 of the diagnostic coding process.

TOOL 3-3

DIAGNOSIS DO'S AND DON'TS

1 For previous conditions stated as diagnosis when previous condition has no bearing on current visit—**DO NOT CODE**

Coder may use a "V" code (history of) if significant

2 Chronic conditions not the thrust of treatment—**DO CODE**

Certain diseases such as hypertension, Parkinson's disease, diabetes, and COPD are examples of systemic diseases that require continued clinical evaluation and monitoring during each visit.
If visit does not involve evaluation of condition—**DO NOT CODE**

3 Conditions that ARE an integral part of the disease—**DO NOT CODE**

Example: Patient with nausea and vomiting caused by infectious gastroenteritis. Nausea and vomiting are common symptoms of this disease process and need not be coded.
Conditions that are NOT an integral part of the disease—**DO CODE**
Example: 5-year-old with 104° F fever associated with pneumonia also experienced convulsions. Pneumonia is coded (fever usually associated with pneumonia need not be coded) and convulsions are coded (not always associated with pneumonia or fever).

4 Diagnosis not listed in final diagnostic statement—**CHECK WITH PHYSICIAN**

If integral to correct coding, ask the physician to incorporate this information into the final diagnostic statement.

5 Abnormal findings—**CODE WHEN NECESSARY**

Should be assigned only when physician is unable to arrive at a diagnosis before the conclusion of the encounter. If abnormal findings is the only diagnostic information available, the coder should check with the physician to make certain a codeable diagnosis is not available.

COPD, Chronic obstructive pulmonary disease.

with or exacerbate their conditions, these systemic chronic diseases usually would be coded in addition to the reason for the encounter. However, if they are not the chief reason for the encounter, that would not be assigned as the primary diagnosis.

—Conditions that are not an integral part of a diagnosis or disease.

When a definitive diagnosis has been made before the conclusion of the visit, but that diagnosis does not involve signs or symptoms also documented, those signs and symptoms should also be incorporated in the diagnosis statement.

—Abnormal findings when necessary.

In some instances diagnosis tests will not be conclusive. They may indicate only an abnormality. In these instances a diagnosis such as "abnormal chest x-ray" may be appropriate.

Don't code:

—Conditions that have no bearing on the current condition or treatment.

When previous conditions that are no longer present have no bearing on the current complaint or diagnosis, they should not be coded. For instance, if the patient is presenting because of an upper respiratory infection and he or she has a history of a fractured femur, the fracture would not be relevant to evaluating the patient's current condition. Therefore the fractured femur, or, as correctly coded, history of fracture, would not be assigned. If, however, the patient has a past history of lung cancer, which is considered in the diagnostic options of the patient presenting with an upper respiratory infection, "history of" lung cancer would be relevant.

—Conditions that are an integral part of the diagnosis or disease.

Signs and symptoms are usually presenting complaints or physician observations made during the encounter that are not a diagnostic conclusion. For instance, the physician or patient may state that the patient has rhinorrhea (nasal discharge); however, a diagnosis regarding why the patient has nasal discharge is not made. However, in instances when a specific diagnosis is made, signs and symptoms that encompass that condition do NOT need to be assigned additional codes.

Differentiating signs and symptoms used as the diagnosis from those that are an integral part of a stated disease or condition is a cornerstone of the basic guidelines for reviewing documentation and identifying key elements.

Reevaluate the choice of diagnostic statements presented in Figure 3-3 to make certain these diagnostic statements are still appropriate according to the coding guidelines discussed thus far. All the key elements can be identified by circling, marking, or highlighting the information within the physician documentation. Then the elements not necessary for coding purposes can be eliminated.

STEP 3: DETERMINE THE APPROPRIATE DIAGNOSTIC CODE ORDER

Order is significant in coding and reimbursement. Keep in mind that some third-party carriers allow only one diagnostic code per service billed. In those instances the first diagnosis for each service billed is the ONLY diagnosis code considered. Also, it is assumed that the most acute or severe diagnoses typically would be the chief reason for the encounter. Each service billed should include the appropriate "matching" reason WHY that service was medically necessary. Although the diagnosis code is indicative of the medical necessity for the service, it will justify only services billed in the correct combination.

Additional rules for diagnostic order are found in Tool 3-4:

—Signs and symptoms should be assigned after definitive diagnosis and only when they are not an integral part of a diagnostic statement.

—Acute conditions are coded as primary diagnosis in most instances.

Based on ICD-9-CM coding guidelines, the word *acute* implies that the condition is the chief reason for the encounter. Therefore acute bronchitis would be assigned as a primary diagnosis as opposed to impetigo when both conditions are evaluated or treated during the same encounter.

—Chronic conditions are coded secondary.

When chronic conditions are evaluated secondary to the presenting complaint or diagnosis, they should be assign secondary codes.

Take another look at the medical chart in Figure 3-1. Each listed service should specifically include the primary reason that the service was provided (medical necessity), followed by any contributing diagnoses that support the intensity or complexity of that particular service. For instance, a patient in the physician's office with multiple complaints typically would have multiple diagnoses for the office visit. These additional diagnoses add to the complexity of the physician's office visit. In the case of laboratory services, blood specimens or urine specimens, for example, would include specific diagnostic statements for results identified from these tests.

Revisit the previous example and look at the order of diagnosis for each of the services identified.

WHAT (Service Elements)	WHY (Diagnostic Elements)
Physician office visit	Upper respiratory infection, urinary tract infection
Chest x-ray	Upper respiratory infection
CBC	Upper respiratory infection
Urinalysis	Urinary tract infection

Physician Office Visit

On the basis of the rules already discussed, several of the elements identified as signs or symptoms of a stated condition or disease have been eliminated. Therefore the remaining diagnostic statements for the physician office visit are the following:

TOOL 3-4

DIAGNOSTIC ORDER RULES

1. Signs and symptoms are assigned only after diagnoses and only when NOT an integral part of the diagnostic statement.

2. Acute conditions are coded as the primary diagnosis in most instances because they are assumed to be the primary reason for the encounter. The exception would be the case of a significantly more serious condition.

   EXCEPTION: Myocardial infarction not listed as acute otitis media.
   (Note that many serious conditions are "automatically" assumed as acute.)

3. Chronic conditions (when coded by previous rules) are coded secondary to any acute conditions or primary reasons for encounter. Make sure to use chronic codes when applicable.

4. Physician diagnosis allows for only four diagnoses per service (line item) billed on the physician claim form. Choose them wisely, keeping in mind that some insurance carriers consider only the first diagnosis per service in determining medical necessity for the service and whether reimbursement is made.

   Select more than four diagnoses in total for all services if necessary; however, only four may be used per service.

Urinary tract infection
Upper respiratory infection

Several factors would be considered in determining which diagnosis would best justify the medical necessity of the office visit. Because neither condition listed is acute or chronic, those considerations are not involved. Certainly, the fact that the patient reports ongoing problems with the signs and symptoms now diagnosed as upper respiratory infection (probably prompting the visit to the physician in the first place) would be a consideration.

The other consideration would be the complexity of each diagnosis. The upper respiratory infection necessitated both a chest x-ray and a CBC, both more significant than the urinalysis ordered for the urinary tract infection. Thus the upper respiratory infection would be coded as the primary diagnosis for the physician visit. This does NOT mean it necessarily will be the primary diagnosis for each of the other services provided.

Certainly, a urinalysis would not be necessary for the primary diagnosis of upper respiratory infection, nor would the urinalysis be justified from a medical necessity standpoint.

Chest X-Ray

This radiologic test allowed the provider to render unequivocally the diagnosis of upper respiratory infection. Symptoms of cough, fever, and cold were eliminated as integral parts of the upper respiratory infection diagnosis. The urinary tract infection has no bearing on a radiologic test; therefore it is not used at all to justify this service.

Complete Blood Cell Count

The CBC would not be considered medically necessary for the diagnosis of urinary tract infection. This test was performed only for the medical necessity of establishing the diagnosis of upper respiratory infection.

Urinalysis

Urinalysis is performed on a specimen for the symptom of urinary frequency, diagnosed to the higher level of specificity of urinary tract infection. The other diagnosis of upper respiratory infection has no bearing on the medical necessity of a urinalysis; therefore it is not used to justify this service.

The following is a recap of the services, the appropriate diagnoses, and the order of the diagnostic statements for these services.

Service/Encounter (WHAT)	Diagnosis (WHY)
Physician office visit	Upper respiratory infection, urinary tract infection
Chest x-ray	Upper respiratory infection
CBC	Upper respiratory infection
Urinalysis	Urinary tract infection

Note that each encounter or service may include a different diagnosis. Some encounters or services may have more than one diagnosis. Figure 3-4 is the correct diagnostic code order for this sample chart. Use this same technique in coding Step 3 in the Stop and Practice section.

STOP AND PRACTICE

Review the following diagnostic statements, signs, and symptoms. Eliminate unnecessary statements and place the remaining diagnostic statements in appropriate order for an office encounter. Place a numeric assignment next to each remaining statement.

1. Upper respiratory infection
   Rule out pneumonia
   Acute bronchitis
2. Cholecystitis
   Cholecystitis with cholelithiasis
3. Cough
   Fever
   Bronchitis
4. Seizures
   Epilepsy ruled out
5. Shortness of breath, cause undetermined
6. 2-year-old child with fever, rhinorrhea
   Diagnosis: acute sinusitis and acute otitis media
7. Bronchitis with cough
8. Congestive heart failure with shortness of breath
9. Headache
   Probably migraine
10. Abdominal mass with jaundice
    Consider hepatitis

Because all the required steps have been completed before the assignment of the proper ICD-9-CM code, code selection for the diagnosis can now proceed. These steps may seem of little consequence for the simple physician charts discussed here, but the same guidelines are used to determine the assignment of diagnostic codes in even the most complex situations.

So far, the steps discussed have helped accomplish the following:

- Identify the key elements and phrases used in diagnostic coding.
- Distinguish signs or symptoms from actual diagnoses and determine when their use is appropriate.
- Identify the rules for coding.
- Determine the appropriate order of diagnoses for services rendered.

The last step of the diagnostic coding process is to open the ICD-9-CM coding books and begin assigning appropriate codes.

DIAGNOSTIC DOCUMENTATION WORKSHEET

Chart#/Patient Name:

	WHAT (Service/Procedure)	**WHY (MEDICAL NECESSITY)** (Diagnostic Information)
Step 1 Select all words for possible use as diagnosis/diagnostic statement from the document	Office Visit	Cough, Fever, Cold Symptoms, Upper Respiratory Infection
		Urinary Frequency, Urinary Tract Infection
	Chest X-Ray	Cough, Fever, Cold Symptoms, Upper Respiratory Infection
	CBC	Cough, Fever, Cold Symptoms, Upper Respiratory Infection
	Urinalysis	Urinary Frequency, Urinary Tract Infection
Step 2 Determine which words are appropriate for inclusion: (Carry these forward) Diagnosis vs. signs/symptoms	Office Visit	Upper Respiratory Infection
		Urinary Tract Infection
	Chest X-Ray	Upper Respiratory Infection
	CBC	Upper Respiratory Infection
	Urinalysis	Urinary Tract Infection
Step 3 Based on each service performed, determine the appropriate order of diagnosis for each service performed	Office Visit	1) Upper Respiratory Infection (addtl services performed)
		2) Urinary Tract Infection (1 addtl service performed)
	Chest X-Ray	1) Upper Respiratory Infection
	CBC	1) Upper Respiratory Infection
	Urinalysis	1) Urinary Tract Infection
Step 4 Look up/assign the proper dx codes		

FIGURE 3-4. Step 3 of the diagnostic coding process.

STEP 4: ASSIGN DIAGNOSTIC CODES TO DIAGNOSES SELECTED FROM THE ICD-9-CM CODE BOOK

Keep in mind that the universal insurance claim form (CMS-1500) or inpatient billing form (UB-04) that is used for coding, billing, and reimbursement to insurance carriers gives the coder the opportunity to assign code numbers only to WHAT services are rendered (CPT procedural codes) and WHY those services are medically necessary (ICD-9-CM diagnostic codes). There is insufficient room on the claim form to add descriptions or further describe services and diagnoses. In addition, most health insurance claim forms are now read by optical scanners that are unable to decipher descriptors other than code numbers. Therefore a justification exists for the ICD-9-CM, a standardized coding method for reporting diagnosis information with numeric codes only.

ICD-10-CM Implementation Impact

Although the process for determining physician diagnosis will not change with the implementation of ICD-10-CM, the information gathered perhaps will need to be more detailed than currently necessary to assign the appropriate diagnosis code(s). In general, the tenth revision, known as ICD-10-CM, resulted in a significant increase in the clinical detail of diagnostic information. This will make it necessary to gather all diagnostic information on an encounter.

For example, under ICD-9-CM:

Code 451.0	Phlebitis and thrombophlebitis of superficial vessels of lower extremities

Under ICD-10-CM:

Code 180.03	Phlebitis and thrombophlebitis of superficial vessel of lower extremities, bilateral

Therefore it would be necessary to gather additional information from the documentation, such as bilateral, unilateral, complications, and other details that may not have been necessary under the ICD-9-CM system.

Chapter in Review

Certification Review

- Always code the chief reason for the encounter or service as the primary diagnosis.
- Always code to the highest level of specificity.
- Always select appropriate diagnoses that tie to the services performed.
- Every chart should have a WHY (diagnostic code) and WHAT (CPT code) in completely describing the services performed and the medical necessity for those services.
- Conditions stated with words such as "rule out," "probable," and "possible" may NOT be selected for physician diagnostic coding.
- Acute conditions or those with the word "acute" included in the diagnostic statement should be coded as primary because they are assumed to be the chief reason for the encounter.
- Chronic systemic conditions should be coded in addition to the primary reason(s) for encounter when such conditions influence the physician's decision making and final diagnostic statement.
- Signs and symptoms may be used for diagnostic statements; however, they should be used only when a more specific diagnosis is not available.

Student Assignments

- Study Chapter 3.
- Review the Learning Objectives for Chapter 3.
- Review the Certification Review for Chapter 3.
- Complete the Stop and Practice exercises contained in Chapter 3.
- Complete the Chapter Review exercise to reinforce concepts learned in Chapter 3.
- Complete the Practical Application exercises for Chapter 3.
- Complete the practice exercises on the companion Evolve site for reinforcement of the concepts in Chapter 3.
- Complete the Workbook exercises for Chapter 3 as assigned by your instructor.

Chapter Review Exercise

Determine which of the following diagnoses would be used in the final diagnostic statement as well as the appropriate order for the diagnoses selected.

Diagnostic Statement(s)	Selected in Appropriate Order
1. Otitis media	________
Dehydration	________
Nausea/vomiting	________
2. Strep throat	________
Acute pharyngitis	________
Sore throat	________
3. Unstable angina	________
Hypertension (previously diagnosed)	________
Coronary artery disease (previously diagnosed)	________
4. Gastroenteritis, probably viral	________
Nausea and vomiting	________
5. Chickenpox	________
Dehydration	________
6. Acute sinusitis	________
Bronchitis	________
7. Viral hepatitis	________
Viral illness	________
8. Abdominal pain, right upper quadrant, caused by pancreatitis or cholecystitis	________
9. Chest pain, probably angina	________
10. Syncope with a fever in a 6-year-old child	
Rule out meningitis	________

Practical Application

Using the concepts presented in Chapter 3, identify the key elements or statements used for diagnostic purposes and place them in appropriate diagnostic order in the charts on the following pages. The Diagnostic Coding Worksheet for assigning diagnoses found on the companion Evolve site may be used.

1. Borderline hypercholesterolemia

PROGRESS NOTE

Chief complaint: ____________

Date: ____________

Vital signs: BP_____ P_____ R_____

History:

This 45-year-old patient came to the physician for evaluation of her borderline hypercholesterolemia for which she takes niacin in doses of 1500 mg daily. Her cholesterol initially was 345, and it has now dropped to 252. She has a history of hypoglycemia, which has improved with diet and supplements. She also has an approximately 6-month history of insomnia. Allergy to codeine. Has had some bloating after meals and extremely cold extremities for which she wears gloves in the house during the winter months.
Family history—mother with valvular heart disease, father with heart attack.

SOCIAL/FAMILY HISTORY:
Drinks coffee and rarely alcohol.

Exam:

Diagnosis/assessment:

Borderline hypercholesterolemia
Hypoglycemia
Insomnia
Cold extremities/intolerance to cold

Stacy Kroll MD

Patient name: ____________

Date of service: ____________

GODFREY MEDICAL ASSOCIATES
1532 Third Avenue, Suite 120 • Aldon, FL 77713 • (407) 555-4000

Service provided: office visit only

Diagnostic statement #1: ____________

Diagnostic statement #2: ____________

Diagnostic statement #3: ____________

2. Shortness of breath versus angina

PROGRESS NOTE

Date:	Vital signs: T	R
Chief complaint:	P	BP

This 58-year-old female noted a sensation of shortness of breath in the high substernal region of her chest. She also describes a feeling of heaviness or pressure. I believe that this sensation is more consistent with angina than true air hunger. This sensation reportedly lasted about 20 minutes. There was no radiation with discomfort and no associated symptoms.

Physical examination:

EXAM: Neck supple without masses. Thyroid gland not enlarged. Carotid arterial pulses equal and full. Prominent normal jugular venous pulsations with patient in supine position. Chest is symmetrical with equal respiratory sounds. No thoracic deformity or tenderness. Breast normal, free of masses or tenderness. No visible or palpable precordial activity. There is a grade III/VI systolic ejection murmur. Lungs clear to auscultation and percussion. Extremities free of cyanosis, clubbing, and peripheral edema. Femoral and distal pulses are present and normal. EKG reveals T-wave inversions that are symmetrical in leads V1 and V3; lead V4 reveals very flat T wave, consistent with anterior myocardial ischemia.

Assessment:

Angina

Plan:

Will order stress test and possible cardiac catheterization as ECG already shows ischemic heart disease.

Maurice Doater, MD

Patient name:
DOB:
MR/Chart #:

GODFREY REGIONAL OUTPATIENT CLINIC
3122 Shannon Avenue • Aldon, FL 77712 • (407) 555-7654

Service provided: ____________________
Diagnostic statement #1: ____________________
Diagnostic statement #2: ____________________
Diagnostic statement #3: ____________________

Service provided: ____________________
Diagnostic statement #1: ____________________
Diagnostic statement #2: ____________________
Diagnostic statement #3: ____________________

3. Pain in chest

PROGRESS NOTE
Chief complaint: ______________________
Date: ____________

Vital signs: BP_____ P_____ R_____

History:

This 40-year-old gentleman presents to this office because of pain in the chest that has been noted for some time. The pain is radiating in nature, and the patient has become concerned.

Medical history reveals no diabetes or history of rheumatic fever. Social history is one-pack-a-day cigarette smoker, no ETOH intake. Family—both parents died as the result of strokes.

Exam:

Neck is supple, no carotid bruit. Lungs clear to percussion and auscultation. Heart reveals regular rate and rhythm with no gallop, rub, or murmur. ECG is within normal limits. Treadmill stress test using the Bruce protocol was normal; no abnormalities were noted.

Diagnosis/assessment:

Chest pain, noncardiac in nature; probably musculoskeletal in nature

John Parkermo

Patient name: ______________________
Date of service: ____________

GODFREY MEDICAL ASSOCIATES
1532 Third Avenue, Suite 120 • Aldon, FL 77713 • (407) 555-4000

Service provided: ______________________
Diagnostic statement #1: ______________________
Diagnostic statement #2: ______________________
Diagnostic statement #3: ______________________

Service provided: ______________________
Diagnostic statement #1: ______________________
Diagnostic statement #2: ______________________
Diagnostic statement #3: ______________________

4. Slow heartbeat

EMERGENCY ROOM RECORD

Name:	Age:	ER physician:
	DOB:	
Allergies/type of reaction:	**Usual medications/dosages:**	

Triage/presenting complaint: This 65-year-old patient presents to the emergency room complaining of an irregular heart beat and shortness of breath. The patient has a history of COPD.

Initial assessment:

Time	T	P	R	BP	Other:					

Medication orders:

Lab work:

X-Ray:

Physician's report:

Following the administration of O_2, ABG, ECG, and chest x-ray, the final diagnosis is bradycardia and severe exacerbation of COPD. The patient will be admitted for further study and treatment.

Diagnosis:	**Physician sign/date**
	Nancy Connolly MD
Discharge Transfer Admit Good Satisfactory Other:	

GODFREY REGIONAL HOSPITAL
123 Main Street • Aldon, FL 77714 • (407) 555-1234

Service provided: ____________________
Diagnostic statement #1: ____________________
Diagnostic statement #2: ____________________

Service provided: ____________________
Diagnostic statement #1: ____________________
Diagnostic statement #2: ____________________

Service provided: ____________________
Diagnostic statement #1: ____________________
Diagnostic statement #2: ____________________

Service provided: ____________________
Diagnostic statement #1: ____________________
Diagnostic statement #2: ____________________

5. Motor vehicle accident

EMERGENCY ROOM RECORD

Name:	Age:	ER physician:
	DOB:	
Allergies/type of reaction:	**Usual medications/dosages:**	

Triage/presenting complaint: This 46-year-old male presents to the emergency room via ambulance following a motor vehicle accident where he lost control of his car and hit a tree off the side of the road. Upon presentation, the patient complains of pain to the lower right extremity, especially when the leg is moved. It appears to have obvious deformity.

Initial assessment:

Time	T	P	R	BP	Other:

Medication orders:

Lab work:

X-Ray:

Physician's report:

An x-ray of the femur and hip reveal a right comminuted intertrochanteric fracture as well as a distal transverse femur fracture. The patient also complains of abdominal pain, and bruising and contusions appear throughout the abdominal area. Urinalysis reveals frank hematuria. The patient's lower extremity is splinted for mobility and the patient is transferred for evaluation of the above-listed problems.

Diagnosis:	Physician sign/date
	Robert Rai MD
Discharge Transfer Admit Good Satisfactory Other:	

GODFREY REGIONAL HOSPITAL
123 Main Street • Aldon, FL 77714 • (407) 555-1234

Service provided: ______________________
Diagnostic statement #1: ______________________
Diagnostic statement #2: ______________________

Service provided: ______________________
Diagnostic statement #1: ______________________
Diagnostic statement #2: ______________________

Service provided: ______________________
Diagnostic statement #1: ______________________
Diagnostic statement #2: ______________________

Service provided: ______________________
Diagnostic statement #1: ______________________
Diagnostic statement #2: ______________________

6. Chest pain in elderly patient

PROGRESS NOTE

Date:	**Vital signs:** T R
Chief complaint:	P BP

A 92-year-old female presents with recurrent chest pain along with dizziness and weakness. The patient has been in the office on numerous occasions with similar complaints.

Examination:

Following examination, a chest x-ray, ECG, and cardiac enzymes are performed.

Impression:

The patient is diagnosed with chest pain, probably anxiety-related.

Plan:

Willen Obst MD

Patient name:
DOB:
MR/Chart #:

GODFREY REGIONAL OUTPATIENT CLINIC
3122 Shannon Avenue • Aldon, FL 77712 • (407) 555-7654

Service provided: ______________________________
Diagnostic statement #1: ______________________________
Diagnostic statement #2: ______________________________
Service provided: ______________________________
Diagnostic statement #1: ______________________________
Diagnostic statement #2: ______________________________

Service provided: ______________________________
Diagnostic statement #1: ______________________________
Diagnostic statement #2: ______________________________
Service provided: ______________________________
Diagnostic statement #1: ______________________________
Diagnostic statement #2: ______________________________

7. Upper abdominal pain

EMERGENCY ROOM RECORD

Name:	Age:	ER physician:
	DOB:	
Allergies/type of reaction:	Usual medications/dosages:	

Triage/presenting complaint: This 47-year-old male presents to the emergency room with abdominal pain, especially in the right upper abdomen. The patient has had these symptoms for the past 4–5 days, more at night while sleeping. Nothing has improved the symptoms, and they have steadily increased over the last 24 hours.

Initial assessment:

Time	T	P	R	BP	Other:				

Medication orders:

Lab work:

X-Ray:

Physician's report:

Exam of the abdomen, chest, HEENT, and labs (liver enzymes) are performed. Liver enzymes are significantly elevated. The patient will be watched for probable cholelithiasis in the observation unit.

Diagnosis: | **Physician sign/date**

Discharge Transfer Admit Good Satisfactory Other:

GODFREY REGIONAL HOSPITAL
123 Main Street • Aldon, FL 77714 • (407) 555-1234

Service provided: ______________________
Diagnostic statement #1: ______________________
Diagnostic statement #2: ______________________
Service provided: ______________________
Diagnostic statement #1: ______________________
Diagnostic statement #2: ______________________

Service provided: ______________________
Diagnostic statement #1: ______________________
Diagnostic statement #2: ______________________
Service provided: ______________________
Diagnostic statement #1: ______________________
Diagnostic statement #2: ______________________

8. Severe headache

PROGRESS NOTE

Date:	**Vital signs:** T	R
Chief complaint:	P	BP

This 7-year-old presents with a 2–3 hour history of severe headaches, including intermittent nausea and vomiting. The patient refused vehemently any diagnostic testing including labs, CT scans, etc.

Physical examination:

Assessment:

Plan:

The patient will be seen by the pediatric neurologist and admitted to rule out seizures and migraine headaches.

Felix Washington MD

Patient name:
DOB:
MR/Chart #:

GODFREY REGIONAL OUTPATIENT CLINIC
3122 Shannon Avenue • Aldon, FL 77712 • (407) 555-7654

Service provided: ______________________
Diagnostic statement #1: ______________________
Diagnostic statement #2: ______________________

Service provided: ______________________
Diagnostic statement #1: ______________________
Diagnostic statement #2: ______________________

9. Finger laceration

PROGRESS NOTE

Date: **Chief complaint:**	**Vital signs:** T R P BP

A 25-year-old male presents with a laceration of finger which resulted from a knife cut while working at the bakery where he is currently employed.

Examination:

Laceration appears deep, almost down to the bone. It is examined for vessel and tendon involvement, which appears to be negative. An x-ray of the finger reveals no other damage other than the laceration. The wound is irrigated and sutured appropriately.

Impression:

Plan:

Jay Corman MD

Patient name:
DOB:
MR/Chart #:

GODFREY REGIONAL OUTPATIENT CLINIC
3122 Shannon Avenue • Aldon, FL 77712 • (407) 555-7654

Service provided: ____________________
Diagnostic statement #1: ____________________
Diagnostic statement #2: ____________________

Service provided: ____________________
Diagnostic statement #1: ____________________
Diagnostic statement #2: ____________________

10. Shortness of breath

EMERGENCY ROOM RECORD

Name:	Age: / DOB:	ER physician:
Allergies/type of reaction:	**Usual medications/dosages:**	

Triage/presenting complaint: A patient is brought in with shortness of breath and history of COPD. The patient appears diaphoretic, in obvious distress.

Initial assessment:

Time	T	P	R	BP	Other:				

Medication orders:

Lab work:

X-Ray:

Physician's report:

A chest x-ray and ABG are performed. The patient will be admitted for acute exacerbation of COPD, with impending ARDS.

Diagnosis:	**Physician sign/date**
	Robert Rai MD
Discharge Transfer Admit Good Satisfactory Other:	

GODFREY REGIONAL HOSPITAL
123 Main Street • Aldon, FL 77714 • (407) 555-1234

Service provided: ____________________
Diagnostic statement #1: ____________________
Diagnostic statement #2: ____________________

Service provided: ____________________
Diagnostic statement #1: ____________________
Diagnostic statement #2: ____________________

Service provided: ____________________
Diagnostic statement #1: ____________________
Diagnostic statement #2: ____________________

11. Chest discomfort

PROGRESS NOTE

Date:	Vital signs: T	R
Chief complaint:	P	BP

A 26-year-old patient presents to the office with complaints of chest discomfort. He presents with history that he fell while taking out the trash approximately two weeks ago, and experienced some chest discomfort following the fall. Today, he fell while walking down the steps to his home and the pain afterward appeared to become worse.

Examination:

A chest x-ray and rib x-ray were performed which revealed multiple rib fractures, probably the 5th and 6th ribs.

Impression:

Plan:

He was advised on the treatment for this injury and tape was applied to the rib cage.

Willem Obst MD

Patient name:
DOB:
MR/Chart #:

GODFREY REGIONAL OUTPATIENT CLINIC
3122 Shannon Avenue • Aldon, FL 77712 • (407) 555-7654

Service provided: ______________________
Diagnostic statement #1: ______________________
Diagnostic statement #2: ______________________

Service provided: ______________________
Diagnostic statement #1: ______________________
Diagnostic statement #2: ______________________

Service provided: ______________________
Diagnostic statement #1: ______________________
Diagnostic statement #2: ______________________

12. Injury trauma

EMERGENCY ROOM RECORD

Name:	Age:	ER physician:
	DOB:	

Allergies/type of reaction:	Usual medications/dosages:

Triage/presenting complaint: This 28-year-old male presents with complaints of pain to the lower back area following an accident where he lost control of his car, hitting a nearby tree.

Initial assessment:

Time	T	P	R	BP	Other:					

Medication orders:

Lab work:

X-Ray:

Physician's report:

Back x-rays were performed which were negative. However, a urinalysis revealed hematuria and kidney trauma is suspected. A kidney ultrasound was also negative. The patient will be admitted for further evaluation and treatment.

Diagnosis:	Physician sign/date
	Nancy Connolly, MD
Discharge Transfer Admit Good Satisfactory Other:	

GODFREY REGIONAL HOSPITAL
123 Main Street • Aldon, FL 77714 • (407) 555-1234

Service provided: ____________________
Diagnostic statement #1: ____________________
Diagnostic statement #2: ____________________

Service provided: ____________________
Diagnostic statement #1: ____________________
Diagnostic statement #2: ____________________

Service provided: ____________________
Diagnostic statement #1: ____________________
Diagnostic statement #2: ____________________

13. History of bipolar disorder

PROGRESS NOTE

Date:	**Vital signs:** T	R
Chief complaint:	P	BP

This 42-year-old male presents with shortness of breath and history of bipolar disorder.

Examination:

Upon the patient's insistence, an ECG, chest x-ray, and cardiac enzymes were ordered, all of which were negative.

Impression:

Plan:

The patient was discharged with a diagnosis of shortness-of-breath episode due to anxiety.

Robert Rai MD

Patient name:
DOB:
MR/Chart #:

GODFREY REGIONAL OUTPATIENT CLINIC
3122 Shannon Avenue • Aldon, FL 77712 • (407) 555-7654

Service provided: ______________________
Diagnostic statement #1: ______________________
Diagnostic statement #2: ______________________

Service provided: ______________________
Diagnostic statement #1: ______________________
Diagnostic statement #2: ______________________

Service provided: ______________________
Diagnostic statement #1: ______________________
Diagnostic statement #2: ______________________

14. Admitted patient with chills

PROGRESS NOTE

Date/time

04/27/XX

S:

Pt states she feels tired, no more chills, denies cough denies N/V/D
C/o dysuria

O:

Lungs, clear, T 102. Abdomen, positive bowel sounds, soft untender
WBC: 16.7, 85.8% segs

A:

Fever of unknown origin, cultures pending

P:

Continue IVF and antibiotics. Will repeat UA for symptoms

Maurice Doater, MD

PROGRESS NOTES

GODFREY REGIONAL HOSPITAL
123 Main Street • Aldon, FL 77714 • (407) 555-1234

Service provided: ______________________
Diagnostic statement #1: ______________________
Diagnostic statement #2: ______________________

Service provided: ______________________
Diagnostic statement #1: ______________________
Diagnostic statement #2: ______________________

Service provided: ______________________
Diagnostic statement #1: ______________________
Diagnostic statement #2: ______________________

15. Shortness of breath this evening—emergency department visit

EMERGENCY ROOM RECORD

Name:	Age:	ER physician:
	DOB:	

Allergies/type of reaction:	Usual medications/dosages:
None	

Triage/presenting complaint:

Initial assessment:

Time	T	P	R	BP	Other:					

Medication orders:

Lab work:

X-Ray:

Physician's report:

Check-off form completed.

Diagnosis:	Physician sign/date
	Nancy Connolly MD 11/24/XX
Discharge Transfer Admit Good Satisfactory Other:	

GODFREY REGIONAL HOSPITAL
123 Main Street • Aldon, FL 77714 • (407) 555-1234

Service provided: ______________________
Diagnostic statement #1: ______________________
Diagnostic statement #2: ______________________

Service provided: ______________________
Diagnostic statement #1: ______________________
Diagnostic statement #2: ______________________

Service provided: ______________________
Diagnostic statement #1: ______________________
Diagnostic statement #2: ______________________

16. Episode of dyspnea

HISTORY AND PHYSICAL EXAMINATION

Stanley Krosette, MD

This 67-year-old female noticed trembling and restlessness in her left leg, eventually had shortness of breath and presented to the ER. Her chest x-ray, ECG and basic labs were normal. Her venous Doppler study of the LLE revealed no evidence of deep vein thrombosis. She will be admitted for possible DVT.

Past medical history:

Recently hospitalized for perforated appendix. Patient has had multiple admissions for other health problems.
CURRENT MEDICATIONS:
These include Synthroid 0.3 mg 4 X weekly, Digoxin 0.25 daily, Reglan 10 mg qid and prn Tylenol.

Family and social history

The patient and her spouse have been able to maintain with the help of family members. The patient does not drink or smoke.

Review of systems:

Musculoskeletal, patient has had numerous and gradually increasing musculoskeletal symptoms and reports many years of trembling or restless leg syndrome.

Physical exam

General: Patient's temperature was 98.6, pulse 54 and regular, respiratory rate of 18
Patient's BP 127/51, patient is very hard of hearing
HEENT: Pupils equal and reactive to light and accommodation. EOM intact
CHEST: Mild degree of kyphosis and breath sounds relatively distant. No dullness to percussion of the thorax. No rales.
CV: Normal first and second heart sounds, no jugular venous distention
ABDOMEN: Soft, flat, nontender. Well healed surgical scars present on the central abdomen.

Laboratory/radiology:

X-ray:

CXR and Doppler normal

Assessment:

Episode of Dyspnea, LLE Restlessness, Severe hearing loss, Recent perforated appendix with peritonitis

Plan:

Stanley Krosette, MD

GODFREY REGIONAL HOSPITAL
123 Main Street • Aldon, FL 77714 • (407) 555-1234

Service provided: ______________________
Diagnostic statement #1: ______________________
Diagnostic statement #2: ______________________

Service provided: ______________________
Diagnostic statement #1: ______________________
Diagnostic statement #2: ______________________

Service provided: ______________________
Diagnostic statement #1: ______________________
Diagnostic statement #2: ______________________

17. Radiology report—venous Doppler ultrasound

RADIOLOGY REPORT

MR#:
DOB:
Ordered by: Dr.Stanley Krosette, MD

Clinical summary:

Shortness of breath

Abdomen:

CHEST BEDSIDE:
Single frontal view of the chest was obtained and compared with last chest x-ray performed 02/28/xxxx. The heart is normal in size, lungs clear. Diaphragm slightly flat raising the possibility of chronic obstructive pulmonary disease. Otherwise negative.

Conclusion:

IMPRESSION:
Hyperinflation of the lungs with possible COPD

Ddt/mm

D:
T:

_________________________, M.D. Date

GODFREY REGIONAL HOSPITAL
123 Main Street • Aldon, FL 77714 • (407) 555-1234

Service provided: ______________________
Diagnostic statement #1: ______________________
Diagnostic statement #2: ______________________

Service provided: ______________________
Diagnostic statement #1: ______________________
Diagnostic statement #2: ______________________

Service provided: ______________________
Diagnostic statement #1: ______________________
Diagnostic statement #2: ______________________

18. Note

PROGRESS NOTE

Date/time
03/01/xxxx

S:

"My leg has trembled off and on for years"

O:

Alert, great loss of hearing, lungs, clear, no dyspnea

A:

Restless leg syndrome
Dyspnea

P:

Chronic and progressive health problems
Will almost certainly need full nursing home care

Stacy Kravitz, MD

PROGRESS NOTES

GODFREY REGIONAL HOSPITAL
123 Main Street • Aldon, FL 77714 • (407) 555-1234

Service provided: ______________________
Diagnostic statement #1: ______________________
Diagnostic statement #2: ______________________

Service provided: ______________________
Diagnostic statement #1: ______________________
Diagnostic statement #2: ______________________

Service provided: ______________________
Diagnostic statement #1: ______________________
Diagnostic statement #2: ______________________

19. Fever of unknown origin

RADIOLOGY REPORT

MR#:
DOB:
Ordered by: Dr. Stanley Krosette, MD

Clinical summary:

Fever of unknown origin

Abdomen:

PA and lateral chest:
Pulmonary markings are prominent with definite infiltrate identified. No change. Heart size is normal.

Conclusion:

Normal chest

Ddt/mm

D:
T:

__________, M.D. Date

GODFREY REGIONAL HOSPITAL
123 Main Street • Aldon, FL 77714 • (407) 555-1234

Service provided: ____________________
Diagnostic statement #1: ____________________
Diagnostic statement #2: ____________________

Service provided: ____________________
Diagnostic statement #1: ____________________
Diagnostic statement #2: ____________________

Service provided: ____________________
Diagnostic statement #1: ____________________
Diagnostic statement #2: ____________________

20. Bilateral pedal edema

PROGRESS NOTE

Date:	Vital signs: T	R
Chief complaint:	P	BP

56-year-old male presents with bilateral pedal edema increasingly getting worse. Patient states he has a prior history of heart failure and recently discontinued all of his medications on his own accord.
PAST MEDICAL HISTORY: No known allergies, discontinued all meds on his own
Bilateral hernia repair, gallbladder removal 1995. CHF, cirrhosis of liver, COPD, ETOH. Abuse.

Examination:

Patient does not appear to be in discomfort. Vital Signs: T 98.3, P 92, R 22, BP 180/72. Chest normal, heart irregularity. Irregular rhythm, regular rate, no murmurs, rubs. Abdomen, flat, positive bowel sounds
MS: Good range of motions of all joints. No erythema, tenderness or swelling. Pedal edema 2+ bilaterally in lower extremities. Radial and dorsalis pedal pulses +2 out of 4 bilaterally.

Impression:

Pedal Edema
CHF

Plan:

Restart meds

Jay Corman MD

Patient name:
DOB:
MR/Chart #:

GODFREY REGIONAL OUTPATIENT CLINIC
3122 Shannon Avenue • Aldon, FL 77712 • (407) 555-7654

Service provided: ______________________
Diagnostic statement #1: ______________________
Diagnostic statement #2: ______________________

Service provided: ______________________
Diagnostic statement #1: ______________________
Diagnostic statement #2: ______________________

Service provided: ______________________
Diagnostic statement #1: ______________________
Diagnostic statement #2: ______________________

4

Using the ICD-9-CM Code Book

LEARNING OBJECTIVES

After completing this chapter, the student will be able to:

- Comprehend the reasons for the establishment of a uniform coding system.
- Use the ICD-9-CM code book conventions and format.
- Correctly locate diagnoses in the ICD-9-CM code book.
- Understand the use of the tabular and alphabetical sections of the ICD-9-CM code book.
- Know the terminology unique to ICD-9-CM.
- Recognize the signs and symbols unique to ICD-9-CM and their application in the diagnostic coding process.
- Apply the concepts for using the ICD-9-CM code book to practical coding scenarios.

CODING REFERENCE TOOLS

Tool 4-1
Helpful Hints in Locating Diagnoses in ICD-9-CM

Tool 4-2
Ten Steps to Accurate Coding from the ICD-9-CM Book

Tool 4-3
CMS Guidelines for ICD-9-CM Coding

Tool 4-4
Index to ICD-9-CM Tabular List (by Disease Process)

Introduction to ICD-9-CM

ICD

Two versions of the ICD (International Classification of Diseases) are available. The original version, known only as **ICD,** was developed by the World Health Organization (WHO) to facilitate standardized reporting of diseases throughout the world. It is still used today by that same organization. The medical profession in the United States has created an adaptation of this widely used reference book.

ICD-9-CM CODE BOOK

All ICD reference books use the revision number following the abbreviation *ICD.* Thus ICD-9 represents the ninth revision of the reference book. Medical professionals have adapted the ICD version developed by WHO for use in statistical reporting and medical services billing in the United States. This clinical modification is identified as ICD-9-CM for International Classification of Diseases, 9th Revision, Clinical Modifications.

ICD-10

WHO has already released the tenth revision of ICD; however, the ICD-10-CM version is not expected to be available until sometime after 2013. Proposed changes in ICD-10-CM are discussed in Chapter 8. The ICD-9-CM serves as a standardized means of reporting medical diagnostic information for the health care industry in the United States. Hospitals, physicians, and medical facilities, as well as the nation's health care insurance industry, all accept ICD-9-CM as the standard for reporting diagnostic information regarding services, medical necessity, and why services are performed.

USES OF ICD-9-CM

Hospitals use ICD-9-CM when billing for services and for maintaining a statistical database of admitting diagnoses, principal diagnoses, days of hospital stay, and required government statistics, such as tumor registries and medical indexes. Although hospitals report statistical data for billing and reimbursement on a different form than physicians do, they use the standard coding found in ICD-9-CM for reporting both medical necessity and the chief reason(s) for the encounter.

Physicians also use ICD-9-CM for reporting medical necessity for services performed and for including this information in statistical databanks. This same information is used for grant and research projects and for the determination of specific diagnostic protocols referred to as *standards of care.* Because the ICD-9-CM code is the only means of communicating medical necessity for services provided, the health care provider must ensure that coding is performed accurately to attain maximum reimbursement.

Third-party carriers, or insurance companies, use these diagnostic codes to evaluate the medical necessity for services billed by physicians, hospitals, and other health care entities. They also store these data for reference purposes in determining matters such as preexisting conditions. In addition, this statistical evidence is used to examine the incidences of certain diagnoses and to classify data according to age group, gender, and other categories. For example, statistical evidence that breast cancer is the number one disease in women ages 30 to 45 years is the result of coding from ICD-9 and ICD-9-CM.

Because these data are of considerable magnitude in the health care field, the importance of accurate coding and the negative impact of incorrect coding on reimbursement, statistics, and insurance rates can be understood. Following are a few real case scenarios that demonstrate the importance of correct (or incorrect) diagnosis coding.

REAL CASE SCENARIO 1

A 4-year-old girl was seen by the hematologist/oncologist for a suspicious cyst on her face. The cyst, which proved to be benign, was removed. Coding, however, indicated "malignant neoplasm of the brain." Many years later, when the child is now an adult who has not maintained insurance coverage over the previous few years, her application for life insurance is denied because of "preexisting conditions."

Problem

Several years after the cyst was removed, the patient was faced with attempting to determine who coded the service incorrectly, contacting that physician's office, having the error corrected, and making certain all sources were informed of the correction after needed changes were made. This process can take an excessive amount of time. In some instances the individual may never be able to determine at exactly what time and place the error occurred.

REAL CASE SCENARIO 2

A 34-year-old man presents to the physician's office with a laceration to the left hand after an accident. Health insurance claim forms filed to the carrier are denied, indicating "previous amputation of left hand in 1999," and a physician audit takes place because of the possibility of fraudulent billing.

Problem

The patient had a traumatic amputation of the right *hand in 1999—not the left as indicated at the time of amputation. Therefore claims for injuries would not be considered until the correction on the 1999 amputation claim was made.*

REAL CASE SCENARIO 3

A 45-year-old woman is involved in an automobile accident in which she is a passenger in a vehicle driven by another individual. Injuries are significant; the patient is seen in the emergency department and is subsequently admitted. Hospital charges are reported to the patient's auto insurance carrier. Charges are denied on the basis of "no accident report for this insured" because they are filed to her *insurance carrier.*

Problem

The patient was the passenger *in the vehicle, and the claim should be filed first to the driver's automobile insurance, where an accident report has been made. The diagnosis coded for the injuries, however, was "motor vehicle accident,* driver,*" which led the insurance carrier to believe incorrectly that the patient was indeed the driver of the accident vehicle.*

REAL CASE SCENARIO 4

According to the statistical data coded from several area hospitals in the Southeast, the average hospital stay for an appendectomy with perforation has dropped from 6 to 3 days. The Centers for Medicare and Medicaid Services (CMS) in the southeast office computes these data and attains a new average stay of 4 days for this hospital procedure in the southeast CMS region. Reimbursement for these hospital diagnosis-related groups is adjusted accordingly, and all hospitals in the Southeast have their reimbursements lowered.

Problem

After complaints from several hospitals in the Southeast, the data were investigated. It appeared that several hospitals were coding inappropriately. What had been coded as an appendectomy with perforation was, in fact, a simple appendectomy without perforation, for which the correct average stay is 3 days. Resubmission of corrected claims and reanalysis of statistical data were necessary at all hospitals involved as well as with the CMS data. The hospitals that had coded these data incorrectly were audited for the possibility of fraudulent billing practices because they did not perform the services as reported.

The previous examples demonstrate only a few of the many situations that can result from incorrect diagnostic coding and its effect on reimbursement, patients, and statistical data.

ICD-9-CM AND MEDICAL NECESSITY

The data integrity of ICD-9-CM depends on both coding to the highest level of specificity and correct coding compliance. Medical necessity has become a hot topic with the federal government, specifically with claims filed to the Medicare and Medicaid programs. Fraud and abuse occur daily in the United States, and millions of dollars in reimbursement are lost because of inadequate documentation for medical necessity. In addition to lost revenue, fraud and abuse fines are frequently charged. If found guilty, the provider is responsible for repayment of overpaid claims at three times the original payment amount, along with fines that vary from $2000 to $10,000 per service billed.

The medical record often does not accompany the medical claim for services, so the ICD-9-CM code is the only effective means of communicating medical necessity for services. In the event that the insurance carrier needs additional information regarding medical necessity, the medical chart documentation must substantiate the ICD-9-CM diagnostic codes used. The coder then must not only code for accurate reimbursement purposes but act as statistician as well.

DIFFERENCES IN HOSPITAL AND PHYSICIAN DIAGNOSTIC CODING

It is important to understand the basic principles underlying the diagnostic coding differences for inpatient and physician coding. Hospitals are reimbursed for resources used to provide medical care to the patient. They are reimbursed one set amount based on the principal or primary diagnosis. The theory behind this reimbursement method is that the hospital provides certain services to a patient as a result of procedures and workups for conditions or suspected conditions. Therefore the hospital has the ability to incorporate diagnosis codes with descriptions such as "rule out," "suspect," and "probable." An example of this can be seen in two patients entering the hospital with an admitting diagnosis of "chest pain, rule out MI" (myocardial infarction). Although MI was subsequently diagnosed in one patient, the other was later discharged with a diagnosis of "chest pain, rule out MI." The diagnosis-related group might remain the same for both patients because their workups included such services as electrocardiograms, chest x-rays, laboratory tests, and hospital days. Both received services and workups for a possible MI.

Physicians would be reimbursed only on the services performed and documented at the time of the encounter. The emergency department physician in the situation described previously would be paid for the documented history, physical examination, and medical decision making performed for chest pain. Therefore the physician's diagnostic statement based on the chief reason for the encounter would probably be "chest pain."

In the outpatient setting, hospitals code for facility charges associated with a procedure performed by a provider or physician. They use procedural coding from the Current Procedural Terminology (4th edition) manual as well as ICD-9-CM coding from Volume 3—Procedural Coding, to indicate the procedure performed rather than the medical necessity for that facility charge.

Hospital and outpatient coding is discussed in detail in Section 4. The rules discussed thus far are specific to physician or provider coding.

Before ICD-9-CM codes can be properly assigned, the correct use of the ICD-9-CM coding book must be learned.

ICD-9-CM Conventions and Formats

GENERAL FORMAT

First, a look at the format, abbreviations, and symbols used in the ICD-9-CM is appropriate. The ICD-9-CM coding book is divided into several sections. The three primary areas include the following:

1. Numeric (Tabular Listing of Diseases: Volume 1)
2. Alphabetical (Alphabetical Index to Diseases: Volume 2)
3. Procedural (Index to Procedures: Volume 3), if applicable

The coder must understand that many ICD-9-CM books incorporate multiple volumes in one book. Thus physician coders typically purchase only Volumes 1 and 2 together in one book because they do not need Volume 3. Hospital coders, however, must have all three volumes, usually purchased in one book. Despite the differences in selecting the correct key elements, diagnoses, signs, or symptoms for coding purposes, the methods for using the ICD-9-CM are universal across all types of coding—physician, hospital, and outpatient surgery alike.

A look at the ICD-9-CM book reveals that main terms are located flush with the left margin. Indentations indicate further information regarding the diagnosis listed. These indented terms are referred to as *subterms* or *essential modifiers*. These notations may add additional information to the selection of the appropriate diagnostic code. Nonessential modifiers, located directly after the main term in parentheses, clarify the code selection but do not change the code assignment selection process. An example of this follows:

Blepharitis (eyelid)	373.00
Angularis	373.01
Ciliaris	373.00
With ulcer	373.01
Marginal	373.00
With ulcer	373.01
Simple blepharitis of the eyelid, not otherwise specified	373.00
Angularis blepharitis	373.01
Ciliaris blepharitis with ulcer	373.01

One of the most common errors made in selecting the correct ICD-9-CM code from the key elements, diagnosis, signs, and symptoms is selecting a code without reviewing all available choices. Make certain, after locating the correct terms, to review all indented codes for possible higher specificity, which would include more diagnostic information than the key element alone.

ABBREVIATIONS

NOS

The designation of *not otherwise specified* (NOS) indicates a lack of sufficient detail to permit assignment to a more specific code. This abbreviation is used when the physician, provider, or documenter does not further specify the condition.

Physician documents "otitis media"
Code 382.9 otitis media NOS

A number of other otitis media codes that are more specific are listed in ICD-9-CM; however, the physician has not provided further information to allow coding to a higher level of specificity.

NOTE: These codes may not be reimbursed by some insurance carriers. In the case of specialists, insurance carriers expect a higher level of specificity.

NEC (Other Specified)

The abbreviation of *not elsewhere classifiable* (NEC) indicates that the physician has further classified the diagnosis to a higher level of specificity; however, ICD-9-CM does not contain a code to the same level of specificity stated. For example, consider the following diagnosis:

Physician documents "viral rickettsiosis fever"

Diagnosis given by the physician is more specific than the diagnoses listed in ICD-9-CM. Rickettsiosis is coded as 083 with the additional fourth digit of "8" for other specified, or NEC. Therefore the correct ICD-9-CM code is 083.8, other specified rickettsiosis.

PUNCTUATION

Parentheses

Parentheses ( ) enclose supplementary words that may be present or absent in a statement of diagnosis. *Parentheses do not affect the code number assigned.* Information in parentheses is provided to aid in selection of an ICD-9-CM code that is as close to the information provided by the physician as possible.

Physician documents "subacute bacterial endocarditis"
Code 421.0 Acute and subacute bacterial endocarditis
Endocarditis (acute) (chronic) (subacute)

NOTE: The information contained in ICD-9-CM in this example indicates that the words in parentheses may or may not be part of the physician's diagnostic statement.

Brackets

Brackets [ ] are used to enclose synonyms, alternate words, or explanatory phrases. Many physicians use a variety of phrases or abbreviations to describe one diagnosis or condition.

Physician documents "SBE"
Code 421.0 Acute and subacute bacterial endocarditis [SBE]

Colon

A colon (:) is used after an incomplete term that requires one or more modifiers.

Bronchitis: (need additional modifiers)
Asthmatic
Chronic

Braces

Braces { } are used to connect a series of terms to a common stem.

Endocarditis Myoendocarditis Periendocarditis	} Acute/subacute

TYPEFACES

Bold	All codes and titles in a tabular list are in bold.
Italic	All exclusion notes are in italics.

RELATED TERMS

AND	Interpreted for ICD-9-CM as "and/or."
WITH	Both parts of the title must be present in the diagnostic statement.

SYMBOLS

Several symbols are used in ICD-9-CM to provide instructional notes regarding the proper use of specific codes. Although the symbols vary from one code book to another, the concepts they represent remain the same. Reviewing the specific color and shape representation for each of these concepts in its respective ICD-9-CM code book may be helpful. Although the shapes and colors for these symbols will vary from one ICD-9-CM coding book to another, the legend for these symbols is typically located at the bottom of each page of the ICD-9-CM coding book.

Differing code symbol	Indicates that a code and its description are not the same in ICD-9-CM and ICD-9.
New code symbol	Indicates that a code is new to this revision.
Text revision symbol	Denotes a revision of an existing code in text or notes.
Additional digit symbol	Indicates that additional digits are required.
Nonspecific code symbol	Denotes a nonspecific code; a more specific code should be used if possible. These codes may not be reimbursed by some carriers.
Unspecified code symbol	Denotes an unspecified code; a more specific code should be used if possible. These codes may not be reimbursed by some carriers.
Manifestation code symbol	Indicates an unacceptable principal diagnosis, meaning that a given diagnosis is a manifestation of another disease process. The other primary diagnosis should be coded first (the code typically references the primary diagnosis needed).

INSTRUCTIONAL NOTATIONS

Includes	Indicates separate terms, modifying adjectives, sites, or conditions entered under a subdivision, such as category. Used to further define or give examples of content of category.
Excludes	Enclosed in a box and printed in italics to draw attention to presence. In other words, all terms after the word "excludes" are coded elsewhere. ICD-9-CM usually refers the coder to the correct codes.
Notes	Used to define terms and to give coding instructions.
See	Acts as a cross-reference and directs the coder elsewhere. Often found when the referenced term is not the appropriate medical term for the condition (e.g., Headache, See Cephalgia).
See category	Refers the coder to a specific category for assigning a correct code.
See also	Refers the coder to a reference elsewhere if the main term or subterms alone are not sufficient for coding.
Code also	Used when more than one code is required to fully describe a stated condition or diagnosis. Notation requires that the underlying disease be coded first and the particular manifestation coded second.
Use additional code	The coder may wish to add further information by using an additional code to give a more complete description of the diagnosis or the medical necessity.

ICD-10-CM Implementation Impact

Many of the coding conventions and formats remain relatively the same for ICD-10-CM as they are currently represented in ICD-9-CM.

The following are a few of the changes to the terminology used in ICD-10-CM.

UNSPECIFIED CONDITIONS

In ICD-9-CM, the main terms listed in bold all had to be met for that term and diagnosis code to be assigned. In ICD-10-CM, a term without an essential modifier is the unspecified form of the condition whether or not all the words in the main term in bold are met.

Example:

J40 Bronchitis, not specified as acute or chronic
Will include Bronchitis NOS

Example:

I05 Rheumatic mitral valve diseases
Will include mitral valve disorders whether specified as rheumatic or not

BRACES

Braces have been eliminated from ICD-10-CM. In ICD-9-CM a series of terms, each pertaining to the word, were followed by a bracket.

Example:

ICD-9-CM

560.9 Unspecified intestinal obstruction

Enterostenosis Obstruction Occlusion Stenosis Stricture	} of intestine or colon

ICD-10-CM

K56.6 Other and unspecified intestinal obstruction
Enterostenosis
Obstructive ileus NOS
Occlusion of colon or intestine
Stenosis of colon or intestine
Stricture or colon or intestine

Numeric (Tabular; Volume 1) and Alphabetical Index (Volume 2)

The ICD-9-CM book is NOT intended to be used with the numeric or the alphabetical section alone. These two indexes are intended to complement each other.

Codes should be located in the alphabetical volume, identified to the highest level of specificity, and cross-referenced in the numeric volume. Additional notes, such as fifth-digit classification information, "includes," "excludes," and other instructional notes, are included ONLY in the numeric volume when cross-referencing occurs. Take extreme caution to ALWAYS cross-reference these codes. Most coding errors can be avoided if coders make certain to perform this "cross-check" every time they select a code.

Take time to look at some entries in the ICD-9-CM code book and become familiar with the format, lookup, and abbreviations so that key elements, signs and symptoms, and diagnoses identified for coding purposes will be correctly coded. Complete the exercises on the following pages to develop those skills.

ICD-10-CM Implementation Impact

Unlike ICD-9-CM, in which each chapter represents an anatomic system, such as Endocrine, Neoplasms, Infectious/Parasitic Disease, Gastrointestinal, or Genitourinary, the ICD-10-CM system chapters may encompass more than one letter, and more than one chapter may share a letter.

Example:
Chapter 2—Neoplasms—encompasses C00-D48.
Chapter 3—Diseases of the Blood/Blood Forming Organs and Certain Disorders Involving the Immune System—encompasses D50-D89.

The tabular list of ICD-10-CM includes 21 chapters, whereas ICD-9-CM totals only 17 main chapters (Table 4-1). Also, in ICD-10-CM each chapter will start with an overview of the structure of the chapter. See the following example from Chapter 14 of ICD-10-CM.

CHAPTER 14: DISEASES OF THE GENITOURINARY SYSTEM

N00-N08	Glomerular diseases
N10-N16	Renal tubulo-interstitial diseases
N17-N19	Renal failure
N10-N23	Urolithiasis
N25-N29	Other disorders of the kidney and ureter
N30-N39	Other diseases of the urinary system
N40-N51	Diseases of the male genital organs
N50-N64	Disorders of the breast
N70-N77	Inflammatory diseases of female pelvic organs
N80-N98	Noninflammatory disorders of female genital tract
N99	Other disorders of the genitourinary system

TABLE 4-1 CHAPTER BREAKDOWN OF ICD-9-CM AND ICD-10-CM

ICD-9-CM CHAPTERS	ICD-10-CM CHAPTERS
Infectious and parasitic diseases	Certain infectious diseases
Neoplasms	Neoplasms
Endocrine, nutritional, and metabolic diseases and immunity disorders	Diseases of the blood and blood-forming organs and certain disorders involving the immune mechanism
Diseases of the blood and blood-forming organs	Endocrine, nutritional, and metabolic diseases
Mental disorders	Mental and behavioral disorders
Diseases of the nervous system	Diseases of the nervous system
Diseases of the sense organs	Diseases of the eye and adnexa
Diseases of the circulatory system	Diseases of the ear and mastoid process
Diseases of the respiratory system	Diseases of the circulatory system
Diseases of the digestive system	Diseases of the respiratory system
Diseases of the genitourinary system	Diseases of the digestive system
Complications of pregnancy, childbirth, and the puerperium	Diseases of the skin and subcutaneous tissue
Diseases of the skin and subcutaneous tissue	Diseases of the musculoskeletal system and connective tissue
Diseases of the musculoskeletal system and connective tissue	Diseases of the genitourinary system
Congenital anomalies	Pregnancy, childbirth and the puerperium
Certain conditions originating in the perinatal period	Certain conditions originating in the perinatal period
Symptoms, signs, and ill-defined conditions	Congenital malformations, deformations and chromosomal abnormalities
Injury and poisoning	Symptoms, signs, and abnormal clinical and laboratory findings, not elsewhere classified
E and V codes: External causes of injury and supplemental classification	Injury, poisoning, and certain other consequences of external causes
	External causes of morbidity and mortality
	Factors influencing health status and contact with health services
	Codes for special purposes

STOP AND PRACTICE

Take each diagnostic statement and indicate where the diagnosis will be located in the ICD-9-CM code book.

Diagnosis	Location (Where to Look Up)
Upper respiratory infection	INFECTION, Respiratory, Upper
Headache	CEPHALGIA

1. Acute myocardial infarction ______
2. Finger laceration ______
3. Otitis media ______
4. Gastrointestinal hemorrhage ______
5. Abdominal pain ______
6. Fractured femur ______
7. Bacterial pneumonia ______
8. Senile cataract ______
9. Incarcerated inguinal hernia ______
10. Sepsis ______
11. Renal insufficiency ______
12. Congestive heart failure ______
13. Upper respiratory infection (URI), possible pneumonia ______
14. Chronic obstructive pulmonary disease with acute bronchitis ______
15. Ingrown toenail ______
16. Acute bronchitis with URI ______
17. Femur fracture, closed ______
18. Cough, normal chest ______
19. Chronic pulmonary edema ______
20. Acute URI caused by pneumococcus ______

Additional Guidelines

Now that you are becoming more familiar with the specific format, standardized abbreviations, and symbols of the ICD-9-CM code book, use Tool 4-1 to gather additional hints for locating codes. These helpful hints will assist in locating the correct term or word for proper coding of diagnoses the **first** time.

—Cross-reference codes in alphabetical/numeric indexes.

Although time is an important factor in efficient coding, the coder should NEVER skip the step of cross-referencing. Once the coder has identified the appropriate key word for locating the diagnosis in ICD-9-CM and has found the category for the code, he or she must also reference the numeric index for the inclusions, exclusions, and other notations previously discussed. Only by performing these functions does the coder ensure correct selection of code(s).

—Code to the highest level of specificity.

Although this guideline has been previously discussed, it bears repeating. When identifying a diagnosis, it is important to gather all the specifics regarding that diagnosis. For instance, diabetes mellitus can be defined as type 1 or type 2, controlled or uncontrolled, with or without manifestations. All these additional data will change the diagnostic code(s) assignment(s).

—Do not assume chronic or acute unless specified by physician.

Make certain all key words are obtained from the documentation. If a diagnosis code requires the documentation of "acute" to assign that code, determine whether that documentation is present and, if necessary, query the physician.

—Determine the "root word" that all other words modify to look up the code correctly.

Because time is of the essence in assigning correct code(s) for the encounter, it is important to look up the key word first, not after multiple attempts that will take sufficiently more time. Keep in mind that when using ICD-9-CM you are looking for the disease, sign, or symptom, so the key word should describe that problem.

For instance, take upper respiratory infection. If one asks, what is the disease?

"Infection" would be the disease, sign, or symptom.
The type of infection would be respiratory.
The type of respiratory infection would be upper.
Therefore the correct order for looking up "upper respiratory infection" would be:
Infection
Respiratory
Upper

—Make sure to convert nonmedical terminology to medical terms.

Although there are cross-references for a number of common terms for conditions, additional time will be spent looking in multiple locations in the ICD-9-CM code book unless the non-medical terms are converted to medical terminology.

Correct coding is important; however, time is also valuable. Many facilities require a specified correct coding rate and a minimum chart load per day, per coder. Because time is an important element in successful coding, coders must make certain that they quickly identify the key elements and locate the correct codes in ICD-9-CM. In the exercises on the following pages, practice a few more diagnostic terms and determine how they will be identified for lookup in the ICD-9-CM book.

TOOL 4-1

HELPFUL HINTS IN LOCATING DIAGNOSES IN ICD-9-CM

1 Cross-reference codes in alphabetical/numeric indexes.

Always look up the code in the alphabetical section and cross-verify with the tabular section for correct code selection as well as highest level of specificity.

2 Code to highest level of specificity.

Make certain you have gathered all modifying words to the selected key elements, such as acute, chronic, open, closed.

3 Do not assume chronic or acute unless specified by the physician.

If diagnosis requires presence of chronic or acute to use the code selected, make certain the physician has indicated such. Remember that most acute conditions are identified as the chief reason for the encounter.

4 Determine the "root word" that all other words modify to look up the code correctly the first time.

EXAMPLE: Diagnosis as stated:
Stress fracture, tibia
ICD-9-CM: **Fracture, pathologic, tibia—733.16**
TIP: Think of identifying the proper "term" much like diagramming sentences in school. Identify the subject, the noun, and all other words and descriptive modifiers. In this way, diagnoses that appear to be complex are, in fact, just as simple as the one- or two-word diagnostic statements.

EXAMPLE: Cystic breast disease
Main subject—disease
Modifying factor—breast = disease, breast
Additional modifying factor—cystic
Look-up will be as follows:
Disease, breast, cystic—ICD-9-CM: 610.1

5 Make sure to convert nonmedical terminology to medical terms.

If the documentation does not use a medical term, the coder may need to convert nonmedical terms for coding purposes:
EXAMPLES: Headache = Cephalgia
Heart attack = Infarction, myocardial

STOP AND PRACTICE

For each diagnostic statement, indicate where the diagnosis will be located in the ICD-9-CM code book.

Diagnosis	Location (Where to Look Up)
Abdominal pain	Pain, abdominal

1. Chronic obstructive pulmonary disease ________
2. Closed wrist fracture ________
3. Laceration repair, thumb ________
   (This is WHAT service was provided; for the correct selection of diagnosis, think about WHY laceration repair was necessary.)
4. Abscess of right great toe ________
5. Infectious gastroenteritis ________
6. Streptococcal infection ________
7. Fibrocystic breast disease ________
8. Fracture of tibia/fibula ________
9. Coronary artery disease ________
10. Bilateral pedal edema ________
11. Postoperative wound infection ________
12. Right upper quadrant, left lower quadrant abdominal pain ________
13. Dupuytren's contracture ________
14. Rupture, head of biceps
    Chronic shoulder pain ________
15. Acute respiratory distress syndrome with shortness of breath ________
16. Abdominal pain
    Abdominal mass
    Rule out liver metastases (mets) ________
17. Obstructive sleep apnea with adenotonsillar hyperplasia ________
18. Acute appendicitis
    Appendicitis with peritonitis ________
19. Cholelithiasis with acute cholecystitis ________
20. Rule out endometriosis and uterine anomaly lesions, right utero ligament ________

Take the time to identify key elements and choose the correct lookup *before* locating the diagnosis in the ICD-9-CM; both are essential time-saving steps. A summary of the steps for accurate coding from ICD-9-CM is found in Tool 4-2.

—Locate the main term within the diagnostic statement.

Again, this will be the diagnosis, sign, or symptom, not the words that add additional information to that diagnostic statement.

—Locate the main term in the alphabetical index.

—Refer to all notes under the main term.

—Examine any modifications appearing in parentheses next to the main term.

These modifications or alternative words are intended to assist in the correct selection of diagnosis. Many times the physician will document other terms for the same diagnosis.

An example would be the diagnosis Pneumonia, 486. It may be referred to in such terms as *benign, bilateral, double, primary, progressive,* or *purulent* because these are all listed in parentheses as additional words that may be present; however, do not change the code assignment of 486 for the condition.

—Note subterms indented beneath the main term.

These are more specific conditions that may need to be assigned a different, more specific code. Again, for pneumonia, some of the subterms are as follows:

Allergic pneumonia	518.3
Aspiration pneumonia	507.0
Fetal pneumonia	770.18

Therefore the code assignment will differ if these additional specific key words are present in the documentation.

—Follow any cross-reference instructions.

If the coder looks up pulmonary disease correctly, he or she will look under:

Disease, pulmonary, which will direct to "See also disease, lung"

—Confirm your code selection in the numeric (tabular) Volume 1.

Often the code listed in the alphabetical index will not include required fourth and fifth digits, so this is another reason to always cross-reference from the alphabetical index to the numeric index.

—Follow the instructional terms in Volume 1.

"See also," for instance, directs the coder to look at other possibilities for consideration and should be researched before making a final code selection. For instance, code 595.89, other specified types of cystitis, may refer to any of the following:

Abscess of bladder
Bullous cystitis
Emphysematous cystitis
Glandularis cystitis

Another example would be code 484.8, pneumonia in other infectious diseases classified elsewhere. Instructions direct the coder to code the underlying disease first; specific examples such as the following are given:

Q fever (083.0)
Typhoid fever (002.0)

—Assign the code number you have determined to be correct.

—Place the diagnostic code(s) for each service in appropriate order.

TOOL 4-2

TEN STEPS TO ACCURATE CODING FROM THE ICD-9-CM BOOK

1 Locate the main term in the diagnostic statement.

2 Locate the main term in the Alphabetical Index (Volume 2).
Keep in mind that:
— Primary arrangement for main terms is by condition
— Main terms can be referred to in ill-defined lay terms

3 Refer to all notes under the main term. Check instructions in any notes appearing in the box immediately after the main term.

4 Examine any modifications appearing in parentheses next to the main term.
Check if any of these apply to the qualifying terms used in the diagnostic statement.

5 Note the subterms indented beneath the main term.

6 Follow any cross-reference instructions (terms such as "see" or "see also" must be followed to ensure correct codes).

7 Confirm your code selection in the Tabular List (Volume 1).

8 Follow instructional terms in the Tabular List (Volume 1). Watch for exclusion notes as well as fourth- or fifth-digit requirements. Be sure to check all the way back to the original heading for that section because the instructional information may be located on one or more pages preceding the actual page where the code is located.

9 Assign the code number you have determined to be correct. Repeat these steps for each diagnostic code selected, making certain those integral to another diagnosis are not coded.

10 Place the diagnostic code(s) for each service in the appropriate order.

The CMS has also provided additional guidelines for coding standardization. These are shown in Tool 4-3.

The first exercise is to identify the diagnosis needed to code and select the correct code from the ICD-9-CM book. Try the following examples and remember to locate the MAIN term first before attempting to locate the correct codes.

	Diagnostic Term	ICD-9-CM Code to Reference
1. Acute bronchitis	Bronchitis, acute	______
2. Cough	______	______
Fever	______	______
Upper respiratory infection	______	______

Hints:

1. Acute bronchitis.
   Bronchitis is the key term, with *acute* as a modifier (adjective) to the description. Therefore, bronchitis, acute, would be looked up.
2. Cough
   Fever
   Upper respiratory infection

Fever and cough are both signs and symptoms of a URI. Therefore neither of these must be coded. The only diagnosis for this chart is upper respiratory infection. The main term here is *infection*, modified by *respiratory*, which is further modified by *upper*. This diagnosis can be located under infection, respiratory, upper.

Helpful Coding Hints

To prevent selection of an incorrect code, consider the following in your selection of correct ICD-9-CM codes.

1. Always check the anatomic or system area selected. It may not be possible to memorize all the codes, but if the breakdowns within ICD-9-CM become familiar enough, confirmation that a selection is at least in the correct category is possible.

TOOL 4-3

CMS GUIDELINES FOR ICD-9-CM CODING

1 Identify each service, procedure, or supply with an ICD-9-CM code from 002.0 through V82.9 to describe the **diagnosis, symptom, complaint, condition, or problem.**

2 Identify services or visits for circumstances other that disease or injury, such as follow-up care for chemotherapy, with **V codes.**

3 **Code the principal diagnosis first,** followed by the secondary code, and so on. Code any coexisting conditions that may affect the treatment or outcome of treatment of the patient for that service as supplementary information.

4 **Do not code a diagnosis that is no longer applicable.**

5 **Code to the highest level of specificity.** Carry the numeric code to the appropriate fourth or fifth digit. There are only approximately 100 codes with three digits; therefore most of the codes should be four or five digits in length.

6 **Code chronic diseases when applicable** to the patient's treatment or service for that encounter.

7 When **ancillary services** are provided, **list the appropriate V code first** and the problem second. This follows the rule that the primary diagnosis should be the chief reason for the encounter or service being billed.

8 For surgical procedures, code the procedure that is most applicable to the principal diagnosis.

STOP AND PRACTICE

IN CLASS

Select the diagnoses that should be coded and locate the correct diagnosis codes. See Figure 4-1 to review the complete diagnostic coding selection process.

	Diagnostic Term	ICD-9-CM Code to Reference
1. Incomplete miscarriage	______	634.91
2. URI	______	465.9
3. Acute bronchitis with cough	______	466.0
4. Virus, varicella	______	______
5. Viral syndrome	______	______
6. Psychogenic ulcerative colitis	______	______
7. Diabetes mellitus	______	______
8. Benign hypertension	______	______
9. Acute lymphocytic leukemia	______	______
10. Blood loss anemia	______	______
11. Acute serous otitis media	______	______
12. Streptococcal pneumonia	______	______
13. Irritable bowel syndrome	______	______
14. Gastrointestinal bleed	______	______
15. Chronic obstructive pulmonary disease with bronchitis	______	______
16. Hepatitis C	______	______
17. Cholelithiasis with cholecystitis	______	______
18. Asthmatic dyspnea	______	______
19. URI with cough	______	______
20. Fever, cough, pneumonia	______	______

DIAGNOSTIC DOCUMENTATION WORKSHEET

Chart#/Patient Name:

	WHAT (Service/Procedure)	WHY (MEDICAL NECESSITY) (Diagnostic Information)
Step 1 Select all words for possible use as diagnosis/diagnostic statement from the document	Office Visit	Cough, Fever, Cold Symptoms, Upper Respiratory Infection
		Urinary Frequency, Urinary Tract Infection
	Chest X-Ray	Cough, Fever, Cold Symptoms, Upper Respiratory Infection
	CBC	Cough, Fever, Cold Symptoms, Upper Respiratory Infection
	Urinalysis	Urinary Frequency, Urinary Tract Infection
Step 2 Determine which words are appropriate for inclusion: (Carry these forward) Diagnosis vs. signs/symptoms	Office Visit	Upper Respiratory Infection
		Urinary Tract Infection
	Chest X-Ray	Upper Respiratory Infection
	CBC	Upper Respiratory Infection
	Urinalysis	Urinary Tract Infection
Step 3 Based on each service performed, determine the appropriate order of diagnosis for each service performed	Office Visit	1) Upper Respiratory Infection (addtl services performed)
		2) Urinary Tract Infection (1 addtl service performed)
	Chest X-Ray	1) Upper Respiratory Infection
	CBC	1) Upper Respiratory Infection
	Urinalysis	1) Urinary Tract Infection
Step 4 Look up/assign the proper dx codes	Office Visit	Upper Respiratory Infection = Infection, Respiratory, Upper 465.9
		Urinary Tract Infection = Infection, Urinary Tract 599.0
	Chest X-Ray	Upper Respiratory Infection = Infection, Respiratory, Upper 465.9
	CBC	Upper Respiratory Infection = Infection, Respiratory, Upper 465.9
	Urinalysis	Urinary Tract Infection = Infection, Urinary Tract 599.0

FIGURE 4-1. Step 4 of the diagnostic coding process.

EXAMPLE:
Diabetes mellitus
Code erroneously selected was 350.00
Because the 300 series of ICD-9-CM codes is psychiatric in nature, the code selected cannot be correct. The correct code series for diabetes is 250.XX.

CODING TIP: Develop an index for the tabular section of ICD-9-CM to cross-check selections easily. An example is shown in Tool 4-4. This may be incorporated directly into the ICD-9-CM book as a reference.

2. Always check fourth and fifth digits carefully. Only the third or fourth digit may have been selected correctly. Necessary additional digits may not have been selected, or incorrect additional digits may have been selected.

EXAMPLE:
Diabetes mellitus
Code selected was 250.0
The coder selected the correct first four digits; however, a fifth digit is necessary. Omitted additional digits result in denial from insurance carriers.

3. Make certain to read all notes regarding "excludes," "includes," and so forth. The correct code may seem to have been selected; however, there may be an exclusion listed for the specific condition or diagnosis coded. The ICD-9-CM book will direct the coder to the appropriate code.

EXAMPLE:
Congenital dentofacial deformities
Code selected was 754.0, congenital skull, face, jaw deformities
This code **excludes** dentofacial anomalies. ICD-9-CM directs the coder to code 524.0-524.9.

4. Remember to cross-reference all codes from the alphabetical to the numeric sections, reading all information from one indentation to the next, to ensure correct coding.

Additional Coding Resources

In addition to the ICD-9-CM guidelines discussed, the ICD-9-CM Official Guidelines for Coding and Reporting are developed to accompany and complement the instructions included in ICD-9-CM. These are extensive and are included as Appendix A in this text. These guidelines are updated yearly and are usually published before the October 1 ICD-9-CM implementation date.

In addition, *Coding Clinic for ICD-9-CM* is an official publication of the American Hospital Association and endorsed by CMS for ICD-9-CM coding guidelines, advice, and clarification. The *Coding Clinic* is published quarterly and offers additional guidelines and clarification to promote the most accurate coding possible.

As we advance into specific coding guidelines, you will see references to *Coding Clinic* guidelines frequently. Care should be taken by the coder to only use resources considered definitive sources, such as *Coding Clinic* and the *ICD-9-CM Official Guidelines for Coding and Reporting*.

TOOL 4-4

INDEX TO ICD-9-CM TABULAR LIST (BY DISEASE PROCESS)

Infectious and Parasitic Diseases	001-139
Neoplasms	140-239
Endocrine, Nutritional and Metabolic Diseases, Immunity Disorders	240-279
Diseases of Blood/Blood-Forming Organs	280-289
Mental Disorders	290-319
Inflammatory Diseases of Central Nervous System	320-326
Hereditary/Degenerative Diseases of Central Nervous System	330-337
Other Diseases of Central Nervous System	340-349
Disorders of Peripheral Nervous System	350-359
Disorders of Eye and Adnexa	360-379
Diseases of Ear and Mastoid Process	380-389
Diseases of Circulatory System	390-459
Diseases of Respiratory System	460-519
Diseases of Digestive System	520-579
Diseases of Genitourinary System	580-629
Complications of Pregnancy, Childbirth, and Puerperium	630-677
Diseases of Skin and Subcutaneous Tissue	680-709
Diseases of Musculoskeletal System and Connective Tissue	710-739
Congenital Anomalies	740-759
Certain Conditions Originating in the Perinatal Period	760-779
Symptoms, Signs, and Ill-Defined Conditions	780-799
Injury and Poisoning	800-999

Chapter in Review

Certification Review

- The ICD-9-CM code book is an offshoot of the ICD book published by WHO.
- The ICD-9-CM codebook is composed of three sections:
  1. Numeric (tabular, Volume 1)
  2. Alphabetical (Volume 2)
  3. Procedural (Volume 3)
- Volume 3 (procedures) is used primarily for coding hospital services.
- When using the ICD-9-CM code book, the coder should always cross-reference the selection in the numeric section of the code book.
- ICD-9-CM signifies the use of an incomplete code number with the use of a specific symbol.
- NEC (not elsewhere classifiable) defines diagnostic statements in which the physician has classified the diagnosis to a higher level than what is available in the ICD-9-CM code book.
- NOS (not otherwise specified) pertains to diagnostic statements in which the physician has not classified the diagnosis to the highest level available in ICD-9-CM.
- The term *and* is interpreted as "and/or" for the purpose of the ICD-9-CM code book.

Student Assignments

- Study Chapter 4.
- Review the Learning Objectives for Chapter 4.
- Review the Certification Review for Chapter 4.
- Complete the Stop and Practice exercises in Chapter 4.
- Complete the Chapter Review exercise to reinforce concepts learned in Chapter 4.
- Complete the practice exercises on the companion Evolve site for reinforcement of the concepts presented in Chapter 4.
- Complete the Practical Application exercise for Chapter 4.
- Complete the Workbook exercises for Chapter 4 as assigned by your instructor.

Chapter Review Exercise

Assign diagnostic codes as appropriate for the following:

Diagnosis	Code(s)
1. Osteomyelitis	730.20
2. Rheumatoid arthritis, hand	714.0
3. Infectious otitis media	382.9
4. Pelvic mass, rule out cervical neoplasm	789.30
5. Nonunion of fracture, tibia	733.82
6. Laceration of hand	882.0
7. Angina	413.9
8. Pendred's syndrome	243
9. Nontraumatic perforation of bowel	569.83
10. *Klebsiella* pneumonia	482.0
11. Abdominal distress	789.00
12. Athlete's foot	110.4
13. Epileptic attack	345.90
14. Low back pain	724.2
15. Barrett's syndrome	530.85
16. Bell's disease	296.00
17. Bell's palsy	351.0
18. Bennett's fracture	815.01
19. Premature infant birth	765.10
20. Birthmark	757.32
21. Centipede bite	989.5
22. Fever blister	054.9
23. Bright's disease	583.9
24. Bradycardia	427.89
25. Bronchospasm with acute bronchiolitis	466.19
26. Burkitt's tumor	200.20
27. Acquired limb deformity	736.9
28. Degenerative spinal cord	336.8
29. Single episodic depression	296.20
30. Allergic eyelid dermatitis	373.32
31. Bacterial diarrhea	008.5
32. Capsulitis, hip	726.5
33. Cervicalgia	723.1
? 34. Cervicitis during pregnancy	646.60
35. Acute cholecystitis	575.0
36. Ear canal cholesteatoma	385.30
37. Alcoholic cirrhosis	571.2
38. Charcot's cirrhosis	571.6
39. Eating compulsion	307.51
40. Abdominal cramps	789.00

Diagnosis	Code(s)
41. Fatty cirrhosis	571.8
42. Forearm contusion	923.10
43. Epigastric pain	789.06
44. Liver contusion	864.01
45. Smoker's cough	491.0
46. Muscle cramps	729.82
47. Congenital spine curvature	754.2
48. Baker's cyst	727.51
49. Ovarian cyst	620.2
50. High-frequency hearing loss	389.8
51. Amino acid deficiency	270.9
52. Clotting deficiency	286.9
53. Elbow dislocation	832.00
54. Difficulty breastfeeding	676.80
55. Rubber dermatitis	692.4
56. Mitral valve deficiency	424.0
57. Arterial dilation	447.8
58. Bouillaud's disease	391.9
59. Heart disease with acute pulmonary edema	428.1
60. Acute gastric dilation	536.1
61. Congenital heart disease	746.9
62. Osteofibrocystic disease	252.01
63. Paget's disease	731.0
64. Adult polycystic kidney disease	753.13
65. Dislocation anterior hip	835.03
66. Stress disorder	308.9
67. Dislocation, humerus, proximal end	831.00
68. Sympathetic reflux dystrophy	337.20
69. Elevated SGOT (serum glutamate oxaloacetate transaminase)	790.4
70. Distal end ulnar dislocation	833.09
71. Petit mal epilepsy	345.00
72. Exposure to cold	991.9
73. Parrot fever	073.9
74. Abnormal heart sounds	785.3
75. Rocky Mountain spotted fever	082.0
76. Anal fissure	565.0
77. Abnormal thyroid function	794.5
78. Ureterosigmoid abdominal fistula	593.82
79. Foreign body, anus	937
80. Toxic goiter	242.00
81. Liver hematoma	573.8
82. Traumatic liver hematoma	864.01
83. Hemophilia A	286.0
84. Obstructed Richter's hernia	552.9
85. Postoperative hematoma	998.12
86. Adrenal hypoplasia	759.1
87. Idiopathic hypotension	458.1
88. Hormonal imbalance	259.9
89. Eye infection	360.00
90. Bartholin's gland inflammation	616.89
91. Breast inflammation	611.0
92. Irritable bowel	564.1
93. Cold intolerance	780.99
94. Postpartum breast inflammation	675.24
95. Inflammation, lumbar disc	722.93
96. Intelligence quotient under 20	318.2
97. Krukenberg's tumor	3
98. Spinal cord lesion	336.9
99. Infective mastitis	611.0
100. Myocarditis with rheumatic fever	398.0
101. Breast mass	611.72
102. Nursemaid's elbow	832.2
103. Nystagmus	379.50
104. Phase of life problem	V62.89
105. Vasomotor phenomenon	780.2
106. Food aspiration pneumonia	507.0
107. Positive stool culture	792.1
108. Premature ventricular contractions	427.69
109. Premature labor	644.20
110. Rales	786.7
111. Diaper rash	691.0
112. Rasmussen's aneurysm	011.20
113. Radiculitis, arm	723.4
114. Rapid respirations	786.06
115. Fluid retention	276.6
116. Granulomatous rhinitis	472.0
117. Leg scar	709.2
118. Allergic reaction	995.3
119. Burning sensation	782.0
120. Seborrheic wart	702.19
121. Abnormal heart rhythm	427.9
122. Sleeping sickness	086.5
123. Sleep disorder	780.56
124. Convulsions	780.39
125. Splenic flexure syndrome	569.89
126. Spina bifida with hydrocephalus	741.00
127. Fertility testing	V26.21
128. Hemoptysis	786.3

Diagnosis	Code(s)
129. Sternoclavicular sprain	848.41
130. Cardiac bypass graft status	V45.81
131. Suture abscess	998.59
132. Thyroid storm	242.91
133. Rectal stricture from chemical burn	947.3
134. Drug-induced delusional syndrome	292.11
135. Shaken infant syndrome	995.55
136. Jet lag syndrome	327.35
137. Parkinsonism	332.0
138. Central nervous system syphilis	094.9
139. Congenital syphilis	090.9
140. Tay-Sachs disease	330.1
141. Articular cartilage tear	718.00
142. Grinding teeth	306.8

Diagnosis	Code(s)
143. Child temper tantrum	312.10
144. Saphenous vein thrombosis	453.6
145. Thrombocytopenia	287.5
146. Omental torsion	560.2
147. Shortness of breath	786.05
148. Congestive heart failure with mild pedal edema	428.0, 782.3
149. Abnormal electrocardiogram	794.31
150. Cough, normal chest	786.2

Practical Application

Now that all four steps of the ICD-9-CM diagnostic coding guidelines have been completed, follow the steps to assign the appropriate ICD-9-CM diagnostic code(s) for the charts on the following pages and place the codes in the correct order.

1. Acute onset of left-side chest pain

PROGRESS NOTE

Date:	Vital signs: T	R
Chief complaint:	P	BP

This 21-year-old presents with acute onset of left-sided-only chest pain. His ECG performed in the office today is entirely within normal limits, and is not suggestive of pericarditis.

Examination:

Examination shows no rub, gallop, or pathological heart sounds. I suspect he has no organic heart disease.

Impression:

Chest pain, musculoskeletal in nature.

Plan:

I recommended he take the rest of the week off work, rest, take analgesics for pain, and return to work after that time, if he is pain free.

Willem Obst MD

Patient name:
DOB:
MR/Chart #:

GODFREY REGIONAL OUTPATIENT CLINIC
3122 Shannon Avenue • Aldon, FL 77712 • (407) 555-7654

Diagnostic statement #1: ______________

ICD-9-CM code: ______________

Diagnostic statement #2: ______________

ICD-9-CM code: ______________

2. Postpartum with multiple complaints

PROGRESS NOTE

Date:	**Vital signs:** T	R
Chief complaint:	P	BP

This is a 32-year-old female who presents today with a cough of 2 weeks' duration, now producing yellow-colored mucus. She presents today because of these symptoms, as well as hemorrhoidal bleeding, which has increased over the past 2 to 3 days, and diarrhea, which began yesterday. Of note, the patient is 6 weeks postpartum vaginal delivery.

Examination:

Circumferential external hemorrhoids noted, nonthrombosed, very indurated, and tender. HEENT unremarkable except for slight nasal drainage. Chest—perhaps some faint wheezing present, consistent with bronchial involvement process.

Impression:

Diarrhea, acute bronchitis, external hemorrhoids

Plan:

Will treat with amoxicillin 500 mg bid x 10 days for acute bronchitis. Patient instructed on care of external hemorrhoids and given diet instructions for complaints of diarrhea, which is not considered to be severe at this time.

Jay Corman MD

Patient name:
DOB:
MR/Chart #:

GODFREY REGIONAL OUTPATIENT CLINIC
3122 Shannon Avenue • Aldon, FL 77712 • (407) 555-7654

Diagnostic statement #1: ______________

ICD-9-CM code: ______________

Diagnostic statement #2: ______________

ICD-9-CM code: ______________

Diagnostic statement #3: ______________

ICD-9-CM code: ______________

3. Leg pain/bacterial infection

PROGRESS NOTE

Date:	**Vital signs:** T	R
Chief complaint:	P	BP

This is a 66-year-old female who comes to the physician's office complaining that she has a bacterial infection in her legs. She has already been treated for this infection but states she is having severe pain and is unable to buy the bandages for dressing changes. Patient denies diabetes. Has had history of hypertension and myocardial infarction in 1993. Medications are Monoket, Cotrim, Lasix, and Altace. Family and social history are noncontributory. Patient is having no chest pain, no shortness of breath, and no abdominal pain, but feels nauseated.

Physical examination:

Vital signs are normal; patient is alert. HEENT is unremarkable. Abdomen–obese, soft, and nontender. She has marked edema of the lower extremities. She has erythema from the knees to the feet. Has a necrotic ulceration on the left tibial aspect of her left lower leg. She has marked oozing, crusting, and drainage from both legs consistent with venous stasis and cellulitis. Peripheral pulses are intact, and she has good capillary refill.

Assessment:

DIAGNOSIS: Venous stasis with cellulitis of lower extremities

Plan:

There is no way she can care for herself at home; therefore, we will admit her for care to include whirlpool treatments, dressing changes, and antibiotic therapy.

Maurice Doater, MD

Patient name:
DOB:
MR/Chart #:

GODFREY REGIONAL OUTPATIENT CLINIC
3122 Shannon Avenue • Aldon, FL 77712 • (407) 555-7654

Diagnostic statement #1: ______________

ICD-9-CM code: ______________

Diagnostic statement #2: ______________

ICD-9-CM code: ______________

Diagnostic statement #3: ______________

ICD-9-CM code: ______________

4. Abdominal pain

PROGRESS NOTE

Date/time

S:

Patient is feeling better and not having the same level of abdominal pain. She is still experiencing dysuria and incontinence. Otherwise she indicates she feels somewhat better. Denies chest pain, SOB, reports she still feels a little weak.

O:

Afebrile, vital signs normal. Chest clear. Extremities normal, Abdomen normal

A:

Abdominal pain, possible UTI

P:

Treat with IV medications

Felix Washington MD

PROGRESS NOTES

GODFREY REGIONAL HOSPITAL
123 Main Street • Aldon, FL 77714 • (407) 555-1234

Diagnostic statement #1: ______________

ICD-9-CM code: ______________

Diagnostic statement #2: ______________

ICD-9-CM code: ______________

Diagnostic statement #3: ______________

ICD-9-CM code: ______________

5. Possible hypertension

PROGRESS NOTE

Date:	**Vital signs:** T	R
Chief complaint:	P	BP

This is a 56-year-old male who presents with headaches and possible high blood pressure.

Examination:

Chest clear, Vital signs normal, Abdomen, soft, nontender. Repeated BP were all within normal range.

Impression:

Headaches with possible HTN

Plan:

Follow with BP History for next 30 days.

Willen Obert MD

Patient name:
DOB:
MR/Chart #:

GODFREY REGIONAL OUTPATIENT CLINIC
3122 Shannon Avenue • Aldon, FL 77712 • (407) 555-7654

Diagnostic statement #1: ______________

ICD-9-CM code: ______________

Diagnostic statement #2: ______________

ICD-9-CM code: ______________

Diagnostic statement #3: ______________

ICD-9-CM code: ______________

6. Severe epigastric cramping

EMERGENCY ROOM RECORD

Name:	Age:	ER physician:
	DOB:	
Allergies/type of reaction:	**Usual medications/dosages:**	

Triage/presenting complaint: 60-year-old male presents with severe epigastric cramping. He states that the pain started after eating dinner tonight. He has had continual cramping and severe abdominal discomfort. The patient has taken some Lorazepam and had 2 episodes of emesis but no fever and does not feel nauseated at the present time.

Initial assessment: Severe epigastric cramping

Time	T 98	P 70	R 16	BP182/98	Other:					

Medication orders:

Lab work:

X-Ray: Labs show WBC 4.5, Hgb 12, platelets 86, sodium 41, potassium 3.9, BUN 21. Reglan 10 mg IV given.

Physician's report:

Patient unable to lie on bed, walking back and forth with distress. Lungs clear, heart regular, abdomen minimally distended but soft. He has hyperactive but non-tympanitic bowel symptoms.

Diagnosis:	Physician sign/date
Abdominal pain unclear etiology Anxiety	Nancy Connolly MD
Discharge Transfer Admit Good Satisfactory Other:	

GODFREY REGIONAL HOSPITAL
123 Main Street • Aldon, FL 77714 • (407) 555-1234

Diagnostic statement #1: ______________

ICD-9-CM code: ______________

Diagnostic statement #2: ______________

ICD-9-CM code: ______________

Diagnostic statement #3: ______________

ICD-9-CM code: ______________

7. Radiology report, abdominal pain

RADIOLOGY REPORT

MR#:
DOB:
Ordered by: Maurice Doates, MD

Clinical summary:

Abdominal pain since 11 AM

Abdomen:

ABDOMEN, 1 VIEW:
One view of the abdomen was obtained. Non-obstructive bowel gas pattern. No calcification overlying kidneys or ureters.

Conclusion:

IMPRESSION:
No abnormality on one view of abdomen

Ddt/mm

D:
T:

, M.D. Date

GODFREY REGIONAL HOSPITAL
123 Main Street • Aldon, FL 77714 • (407) 555-1234

Diagnostic statement #1: ______________

ICD-9-CM code: ______________

Diagnostic statement #2: ______________

ICD-9-CM code: ______________

Diagnostic statement #3: ______________

ICD-9-CM code: ______________

8. Garbled speech, gait instability

HISTORY AND PHYSICAL EXAMINATION

William Obert, MD

82-year-old with episode of shortness of breath, some vague chest pain. Said he got confused, had some slurred speech and could not walk. His wife indicates they were coming home and she noticed he was more mixed up and confused and having some garbled speech. She says that he has had two previous episodes of this in the past. Denies any cough, fever, chills, nausea or vomiting. Evidence of some COPD, is an ex-smoker. No history of CAD.

Past medical history:

Systolic hypertension, DJD, hyperlipidemia, COPD, has had left cataract extraction.

Family and social history

Review of systems:

Denies any weight changes, appetite changes, fever or chills. Denies any problems with tinnitus, hearing loss. Denies sore throat, dysphagia. No history of CAD. Denies cough or hemoptysis. Lot of arthritis, denies dysuria, urgency, frequency. Denies any anemia.

Physical exam

General:	Alert, oriented male resting comfortably. No acute distress.
VITAL SIGNS:	BP 132/78, Pulse 97, Respirations 20
HEENT:	Normocephalic and atraumatic
NECK:	Supple without adenopathy
CARDIAC:	Regular rate and rhythm
LUNGS:	Decreased lung exchange throughout with some fine crackles
NEUROLOGICAL:	Alert, oriented to person, place and time. Somewhat vague in his history. Finger-to-toe able to complete.

Laboratory/radiology:

CBC shows WBC 14,000, Hgb 12.4, 84 neutrophils, 4 bands. BMP sodium 137, potassium 3.8, chloride 106. Troponin 0.1. ECG shows normal sinus rhythm. Chest x-ray is normal.

X-ray:

Assessment:

Plan:

Episode of garbled speech with gait instability, possible cerebrovascular accident versus transient ischemic attack. We will check neuros and vital signs every two hours. Repeat his ECG and enzymes in four hours. Needs a CT scan of his head.

William Obert MD

GODFREY REGIONAL HOSPITAL
123 Main Street • Aldon, FL 77714 • (407) 555-1234

Diagnostic statement #1: ______________

ICD-9-CM code: ______________

Diagnostic statement #2: ______________

ICD-9-CM code: ______________

Diagnostic statement #3: ______________

ICD-9-CM code: ______________

9. Consultation

CONSULTATION

Indication for consultation:

Ventricular tachycardia

History:

54-year-old with known history of cardiac disease who was undergoing outpatient arthroscopy of the knee. Patient's cardiac rhythm was noted to have multiple runs of non-sustained ventricular tachycardia. Patient remained asymptomatic stable.
Status post MI 15 years ago.
FAMILY/SOCIAL HISTORY:
Non-contributory

Exam:

PHYSICAL EXAM:
Head: Normocephalic, atraumatic
Neck: Supple, w/o evidence of JVP, mass or bruit
Chest: Clear to auscultation
Cardiac: Normal carotid upstroke with normal contour
Abdomen: Soft, nontender, no evidence of mass
Extremities: Showed no evidence of clubbing, cyanosis, or edema
Neurologic: Grossly intact, nonfocal
ECG: Ectopic atrial rhythm with delayed precordial transmission

Diagnosis/assessment:

IMPRESSION:
Known history of coronary atherosclerotic heart disease and atrial fibrillation, now presents with run of nonsustained V tach per report. It would be prudent to continue patient on his current medications and allow him to follow-up with his primary cardiologist.

We appreciate the opportunity to participate in the overall evaluation and management of this patient.

Patient name: ____________________

Date of service: __________

GODFREY MEDICAL ASSOCIATES
1532 Third Avenue, Suite 120 • Aldon, FL 77713 • (407) 555-4000

Diagnostic statement #1: __________

ICD-9-CM code: __________

Diagnostic statement #2: __________

ICD-9-CM code: __________

Diagnostic statement #3: __________

ICD-9-CM code: __________

10. Knee arthroscopy

OPERATIVE REPORT

Patient information:

Patient name:
DOB:
MR#:

Preoperative diagnosis:

Torn medial meniscus, left knee

Postoperative diagnosis:

Torn medial meniscus, left knee

Procedure(s) performed:

Arthroscopy of left knee with partial medial Meniscectomy, medial femoral condyle chondroplasty

Anesthesia:

General

Assistant surgeon:

Description of procedure:

Patient placed supine on table and satisfactory general anesthetic was given. Left leg was prepped and draped in the usual sterile fashion. Arthroscope cannula was introduced via anterolateral port at the joint line. Knee was distended with normal saline, there was no pathology or loose body in the suprapatellar area. The medial plica showed no evidence of pathology or damage. The cartilaginous surface of the medial femoral condyle showed extensive changes of chondromalacia. The posterior horn of the medial meniscus was torn of its free edge. A combination of hand-held cutters and rotary shavers were used to trim back to the tear of the posterior horn of the medial meniscus.

The knee was irrigated throughout the procedure via normal saline delivered by the arthroscopy pump. All instruments were removed.

GODFREY REGIONAL HOSPITAL
123 Main Street • Aldon, FL 77714 • (407) 555-1234

Diagnostic statement #1: ______________

ICD-9-CM code: ______________

Diagnostic statement #2: ______________

ICD-9-CM code: ______________

Diagnostic statement #3: ______________

ICD-9-CM code: ______________

5

V Codes and E Codes

LEARNING OBJECTIVES

After completing this chapter, the student will be able to:

- Understand the proper use of V codes.
- Understand the proper use of E codes.
- Understand that primary guidelines for assigning the chief reason for encounter apply, even with the assignment of E codes as primary when appropriate.
- Use an index for V code and E code sections of the ICD-9-CM code book for inclusion as tools with the coding book.
- Apply V and E coding concepts to practical coding scenarios.

CODING REFERENCE TOOLS

Tool 5-1
V Code Index

Tool 5-2
E Code Index

KEY TERMS

External Causes (E Codes)

V Codes

In addition to the numeric codes used for diagnostic coding, ICD-9-CM has a series of special codes that are applied in specific circumstances. For the most part, these codes are NOT used as primary diagnostic codes; however, there are always exceptions to the rules.

V Codes

APPROPRIATE USE

This section of the ICD-9-CM book deals with instances when events other than disease or injury classifiable to the numeric section are recorded as the diagnosis, problem, condition, or chief reason for the encounter. A section on V codes in the ICD-9-CM book ("Supplementary Classification of Factors Influencing Health Status and Contact with Health Services") covers codes V01 through V82. V codes are typically used for the following reasons:

- Patient does not present with a problem or condition, yet a physician encounter takes place for a specific purpose, such as organ donation or vaccination. In most instances these events probably would not occur in the hospital setting but rather in the outpatient or physician office setting.
- Patient with a specific disease or problem has an encounter for the purpose of specific treatment of that disease or problem (e.g., chemotherapy for malignancy). Remember that under the basic rules for coding the chief reason for an encounter or service, the primary diagnosis in the previous instance would require a V code for chemotherapy, followed by the supplemental malignancy diagnosis.
- Patient with a circumstance or problem that influences health status but currently is not an illness or injury (e.g., exposure of a pregnant patient to a communicable disease).

Identify the subsection within the V code section in which the appropriate code is located. This saves time in the coding process because the coder avoids thumbing through the entire V code section, and it helps in cross-checking whether the code selected is from the correct chapter.

V CODE INDEX

V codes are indexed in the alphabetical index of ICD-9-CM along with the other diseases, signs, and symptoms. Unlike other ICD-9-CM descriptors located under the condition, illness, injury, sign, or symptom, V codes are located under the terms that describe the reason for the encounter or visit. The following terms categorize services that have assigned V codes:

Admission
Aftercare
Attention (to)
Care
Carrier (suspected)
Contact
Contraception, contraceptive
Convalescence
Counseling
Dependence
Dialysis
Donor
Examination
Exposure
Fitting (of)
Follow-up
Health
History (personal)
Maintenance
Newborn
Observation
Outcome of delivery
Pregnancy
Problem
Prophylactic
Replacement artificial/mechanical device
Resistance, resistant
Screening
Status
Supervision
Test
Therapy
Transplant
Unavailability of medical facilities
Vaccination

Most ICD-9-CM code books do not include a general classification range of V codes. Tool 5-1 is provided as a valuable aid that can be included in the coder's ICD-9-CM code book.

V01-V06: Persons with Potential Health Hazards Related to Communicable Diseases

These codes are used for encounters with patients who are exposed to, who are in contact with, or who need prophylactic treatment for a disease. Codes from this subsection are identified by the following key word(s):

Contact
Exposure
Prophylactic
Vaccination

EXAMPLES:

V01.6 Contact/exposure to venereal disease
V02.1 Carrier or suspected carrier of typhoid
V03.7 Need for prophylactic vaccination tetanus toxoid
V06.4 Need for prophylactic multiple vaccination, mumps, measles, rubella

V07-V09: Persons with Need for Isolation, Other Potential Health Hazards, and Prophylactic Measures

Codes from this category are typically used when medical documentation indicates resistance to specific medications or

TOOL 5-1

V CODE INDEX

Persons with Potential Health Hazards Related to Communicable Disease(s)	V01-V06
Persons with Need for Isolation, Other Potential Health Hazards, and Prophylactic Measures	V07-V09
Persons with Potential Health Hazards Related to Personal and Family History	V10-V19
Persons Encountering Health Services in Circumstances Related to Reproduction and Development	V20-V28
Observation and Evaluation of Newborns and Infants for Suspected Conditions Not Found	V29
Liveborn Infants According to Type of Birth	V30-V39
Persons with Conditions Influencing Their Health Status	V40-V49
Persons Encountering Health Services for Specific Procedures and Aftercare	V50-V59
Persons Encountering Health Services in Other Circumstances	V60-V69
Persons Without Reported Diagnosis Encountered During Examination and Investigation of Individuals and Populations	V70-V82

health hazards or potential health hazards. Codes from this subsection are identified by the following key words:

Resistance (resistant)
Replacement

EXAMPLES:

V07.4 Postmenopausal hormone replacement therapy
V09.0 Infection with microorganisms resistant to penicillin

V10-V19: Persons with Potential Health Hazards Related to Personal and Family History

When personal history or family history of certain diseases influences the health status of the patient or is a pertinent contribution to the health status of the patient, a code from this section will be used. Care should be taken to differentiate between family history and personal history by assigning codes from the following categories:

V10-V15 Personal history
V16-V19 Family history

Codes from this section are located under the alphabetical heading History.

EXAMPLES:

V10.3 Personal history, malignant breast neoplasm
V16.3 Family history, malignant breast neoplasm
V10.11 Personal history, malignant lung neoplasm
V16.1 Family history, malignant lung neoplasm

V20-V29: Persons Encountering Health Services in Circumstances Related to Reproduction and Development

Codes from this range are used to describe supervision of pregnancy, care of infant, postpartum care, contraceptive management, sterilization, outcome of delivery, and antenatal screening. Codes from the V22 category are typically used in the outpatient setting because the supervision of a normal pregnancy most often does not require inpatient services. Code V22.2 is assigned either to indicate the primary reason for the encounter or to indicate a pregnant patient who is seen for an unrelated condition that is not complicated or related to the pregnancy. Codes from the V24 series are indicative of uncomplicated follow-up during the postpartum period. V27 codes are used as an additional diagnostic code on the mother's medical record to indicate the outcome of delivery. Codes from this category will be identified with the following key word(s):

Pregnancy
Observation
Postpartum
Contraception
Outcome of delivery

EXAMPLES:

V20.2 Routine child health care
V22.2 Supervision of first normal pregnancy
V23.0 Pregnancy with history of infertility
V24.2 Routine postpartum follow-up
V25.2 Sterilization
V27.0 Single liveborn
V28.0 Screening for chromosomal anomalies by amniocentesis
V29.2 Observation for suspected respiratory condition

V30-V39: Liveborn Infants According to Type of Birth

Recorded as the first diagnosis on the newborn hospital record, codes from the V30 range describe the number of live and stillborn births as well as the location of birth and type of delivery (e.g., cesarean). Fourth (and in some instances fifth) digits are required for this section as follows:

Fourth digit identifies location of birth:

.0 Born in hospital (also requires fifth digit)
.1 Born before hospital admission
.2 Born outside hospital and not hospitalized

Fifth digit (required when fourth digit is "0"):

0 Delivered without mention of cesarean delivery
1 Delivered by cesarean delivery

EXAMPLES:

V30.00 Single liveborn, born in hospital without mention of cesarean delivery
V32.01 Twin, mate stillborn, born in a hospital, delivered by cesarean delivery

V40-V49: Persons with Conditions Influencing Health Status

This subcategory of codes is used for conditions that influence the patient's health and increase the complexity of the patient's chief reason for the encounter. Conditions including transplant status, the presence of an artificial opening such as a tracheostomy, and status postoperative (S/P) conditions—such as S/P coronary artery bypass grafting—are all included in this category. Key words for this category are the following:

Status
Dependence

EXAMPLES:

V42.1 Transplant, heart, S/P
V44.0 Tracheostomy

V50-V59: Persons Encountering Health Services for Specific Procedures and Aftercare

This range of codes covers encounters that take place for the purpose of dealing with residual states or to prevent recurrence of diseases or injuries that are no longer present. These codes may be assigned for the fitting and adjustment of prosthetic devices, orthopedic aftercare (e.g., removal of an internal fixation device), attention to artificial openings, encounters for dialysis, physical therapy, speech therapy, and other therapies. Key words for this subcategory would include the following:

Admission
Aftercare
Attention to

EXAMPLES:

V54.81 Aftercare following joint replacement
V58.11 Encounter for chemotherapy

V60-V69: Persons Encountering Health Services in Other Circumstances

When encounters are for purposes other than disease, illness, injury, signs, or symptoms, codes from this category would be appropriate. Examples would be convalescent and palliative care and visits for the purpose of follow-up examinations. Key words for this category would be the following:

Admission
Follow-up

EXAMPLES:

V67.00 Postoperative examination unspecified
V68.2 Request expert evidence

V70-V72: Persons without Reported Diagnosis Encountered During Examination and Investigation of Individuals and Populations

General medical examinations, observation for suspected conditions that are not found, and special examinations are included in this category. There are a number of medical examinations, and they are subcategorized within this section as follows:

V70.0 Routine general medical examination
V70.1 General psychiatric examination, requested by authority
V70.2 General psychiatric examination, other/unspecified
V70.3 Other examinations for administrative purposes
V70.4 Examinations for medicolegal reasons
V70.5 Examinations for defined population
V70.6 Examinations for population surveys
V70.7 Examinations for clinical trial participant
V70.8 Other specified medical examinations
V70.9 Unspecified medical examinations

Key words would include such terms as the following:

Admission
Observation

EXAMPLES:

V70.0 Routine general medical examination
V71.4 Observation following accident

V73-V83: Screening Examinations for Specified Conditions

When patient encounters are screening examinations for conditions that are currently inactive, codes from this subcategory would be appropriate. A key word to identify services from within this section is the following:

Screening

EXAMPLES:

V76.1 Screening for malignant neoplasm
V79.2 Screening for mental retardation

STOP AND PRACTICE

Assign the appropriate V codes to the following:

		Section Where Located	V Code
1.	Pregnancy examination	______	______
2.	Preoperative examination	______	______
3.	Exposure to rubella	______	______
4.	Visit for tetanus immunization	______	______
5.	Donation of bone marrow	______	______
6.	Personal history of malignant liver neoplasm	______	______
7.	Visit for normal pregnancy	______	______
8.	Visit for routine child care	______	______
9.	Contraceptive counseling	______	______
10.	General medical examination	______	______
11.	Removal of surgical rods	______	______
12.	Dressing changes	______	______
13.	Peritoneal dialysis	______	______
14.	Chemotherapy administration	______	______
15.	Physical therapy	______	______
16.	Single liveborn birth	______	______
17.	Supervision of high-risk pregnancy, multiple births	______	______
18.	Family history of malignant neoplasm of gastrointestinal (GI) tract	______	______
19.	Observation following automobile accident	______	______
20.	Visits to the laboratory for routine blood work	______	______

E Codes

APPROPRIATE USE

The **External Causes (E code)** section of the ICD-9-CM coding book is included to provide a mechanism for coding "external" causes of injury and poisoning. This section is used to code environmental events, circumstances, and conditions that cause injury, poisoning, or other adverse effects.

The E code is NEVER used as the primary diagnostic code for services because this event typically is not the chief reason for the encounter or service. The illness, injury, poisoning, or condition resulting from the external cause is usually the primary diagnosis and the primary reason for the encounter.

The E code is important from a reimbursement perspective. This code typically clarifies how, where, and why an accident happened. It is therefore used to help assign liability and responsibility of the appropriate insurance carrier.

EXAMPLE:
Open wound of the arm
Occurred during a worksite fire

The appropriate numeric code for the chief reason for the encounter, "Wound, open, arm," should be assigned. The E code for "Worksite fire" should also be coded because this indicates that workers' compensation should be billed rather than private health insurance.

Omission of appropriate E codes results in either inappropriate or delayed payment until this information is provided on request from the carrier. Requests from the carrier for information typically result in a much longer time for payment than required if the information is provided initially. The health insurance carrier typically has an average of 30 days to process a claim. After processing the claim and determining the need for additional information about an injury, the carrier sends a request letter to the provider. The average response time for the provider adds another 7 to 10 days to the process. The additional claim information is now mailed to the carrier, adding 7 to 10 more days for mailing and receipt.

Unlike the laws passed by most states that specify a certain amount of time that insurance carriers have to initially process a claim, there typically are no rules on how quickly they must respond when additional information is needed. Coding must be complete so that payment may be demanded and received within a reasonable period.

General coding guidelines for the assignment of E codes include the following:

- E codes may be used in conjunction with codes from the 001-999 and V01-V83 ranges to indicate an injury, illness, or adverse effect from an external cause.
- E codes should be assigned for all initial treatments of injuries, illnesses, or adverse effects; however, if the encounter is not for the initial treatment, it would not be appropriate to assign an E code.
- As many E codes as necessary should be assigned to fully explain how, why, and where the injury occurred.
- E codes can never be used as a primary diagnosis.

E800-E848: Vehicle/Transport Accidents

Vehicle accidents are classified by the type of vehicle as well as the designated person; that is, driver, passenger, or unspecified. The majority of vehicle accident E codes require five digits, including a fifth digit that designates the person.

For example, the category Motor Vehicle Traffic Accidents (E810-E819) indicates that the fifth digit should be assigned as follows:

0 Driver other than motorcycle
1 Passenger other than motorcycle
2 Motorcyclist
3 Passenger on motorcycle
4 Occupant of streetcar
5 Rider of animal, occupant of animal-drawn vehicle
6 Pedal cyclist
7 Pedestrian
8 Other specified person
9 Unspecified person

E849.0-E849.9: Place of Occurrence Codes

Place of occurrence codes are intended to specify where a specific accident or injury occurred. Care should be taken NOT to routinely assign "E849.9 unspecified place" when the place of occurrence is not known.

E850-E869: Accident Poisoning Codes

These codes are discussed at length in the discussion on ICD-9-CM tables in Chapter 6.

E870-E879: Misadventures or Abnormal Reaction to Surgical or Medical Care

When complications arise from a surgical procedure, whether through an accidental "misadventure" or without complication but resulting in an abnormal reaction, these incidents are assigned codes from the E870-E879 range.

E880-E888: Accidental Falls

Falls that resulted in injuries or suspected injuries are assigned code(s) for the complaints or injuries as well as an E code from the range E880 to E888. All codes from this category require a total of five digits, including instances when an accidental fall occurs but no additional information is available, in which case E888.9 would be assigned.

E890-E899: Accidents by Fire or Flame

Injuries that result from fire or flame are assigned to this category. The fire or flame may be controlled or uncontrolled (the latter termed *conflagration*).

E900-E909: Accidents from Natural and Environmental Factors

Conditions such as excessive heat or cold, changes in air pressure, neglect, and lack of food or housing are included in this section. Excessive exposure to weather conditions such as hail and humidity are also included in this section.

E910-E915: Accidents by Submersion, Suffocation, and Foreign Bodies

Accidental drowning or submersion is included in this section. Drowning or submersion when NOT intentional appears in the Homicide or Purposefully Inflicted Injury of Others section.

E916-E928: Other Accidents

Accidents not included in any of the above categories are included in this section. Examples of "other accidents" included in this category are the following:

- Struck accidentally by falling object
- Striking against or struck accidentally by objects or persons
- Caught accidentally in or between objects
- Machinery accidents
- Cutting or piercing instruments
- Electric current

E929: Late Effects of Accidents

This category is intended to be used as the cause of death or disability from an accidental injury previously received.

E930-E949: Drugs and Medicinal and Biologic Substances Causing Adverse Effects in Therapeutic Use

This section is discussed in depth in Chapter 6.

E950-E959: Suicide and Self-Inflicted Injury

This category would be used for suicide or attempted suicide, or injuries that are specified in documentation as being intentional.

E960-E969: Homicide and Injury Purposefully Inflicted by Others

This category is used for injuries inflicted by other persons intentionally for the purpose of attempting to kill or injure another person. Documentation must specify that the injuries inflicted were intentional, not accidental.

E970-E978: Legal Intervention

These codes are used for injuries inflicted by law enforcement in the act of arresting or attempting to detain, suppressing disturbances, maintaining order, or engaging in other legal actions.

E979: Terrorism

Added in recent years, this category is intended when injuries occur in the act of unlawful use of force or violence against a government or civilian population.

E980-E989: Injury Undetermined Whether Accidental or Purposefully Inflicted

Codes from this category should be assigned when injuries occur and whether they were accidental or intentional has not been determined. In many instances this results from the lack of documentation or the inability of the provider to make a specific determination.

E990-E999: Injury Resulting from Operations of War

This category is used for injuries to both military personnel and civilians caused by war or civil insurrections.

E Code Index

The alphabetical index to External Causes is a separate index in ICD-9-CM. It is found in different locations according to the publisher and edition of ICD-9-CM used in the practice. It is organized by main terms that identify an accident, event, or specific cause of injury or adverse effect. In some instances these external causes are environmental, such as an earthquake, or are caused by other sources, such as dog bites or broken glass. In addition to providing information regarding how the accident or injury occurred, an additional E code assignment may be made for the place of occurrence (i.e., the location where the injury or accident occurred). As with the V codes, most ICD-9-CM books do not include a general index for the E code section, so such an index has been provided in Tool 5-2.

The External Cause codes provide a break from some of the more difficult exercises completed thus far. Remember, the chief encounter for each service is the primary diagnosis; therefore E codes are NOT primary. Identifying where the code is located in the E code section prevents the coder from looking through the entire E code section.

TOOL 5-2

E CODE INDEX

Railway Accidents	E800-E807
Motor Vehicle Traffic Accidents	E810-E819
Motor Vehicle Nontraffic Accidents	E820-E825
Other Road Vehicle Nontraffic Accidents	E826-E829
Water Transport Accidents	E830-E838
Air and Space Accidents	E840-E845
Vehicle Accidents Not Classified Elsewhere	E846-E848
Place of Occurrence	E849
Accidental Poisoning by Drugs, Medicinal Substances, Biologics	E850-E858
Accidental Poisoning by Other Solid and Liquid Substances, Gases, Vapors	E860-E869
Misadventure to Patients During Surgical/Medical Care	E870-E876
Surgical/Medical Procedures Cause of Abnormal Reaction of Patient or Later Complication, Without Mention of Misadventure at Time of Procedure	E878-E879
Accidental Falls	E880-E888
Accidents by Fire and Flames	E890-E898
Accidents Due to Natural/Environmental Factors	E900-E909
Accidents Caused by Submersion, Suffocation, and Foreign Bodies	E910-E915
Other Accidents	E916-E928
Late Effects of Accidental Injury	E929
Drugs, Medicinal and Biologic Substances Causing Adverse Effects in Therapeutic Use	E930-E949
Suicide and Self-Inflicted Injury	E950-E959
Homicide and Injury Purposely Inflicted by Other Persons	E960-E969
Legal Intervention	E970-E978
Injury Undetermined Whether Accidentally or Purposely Inflicted	E980-E989
Injury Resulting from Operations of War	E990-E999

STOP AND PRACTICE

Assign the appropriate E codes to the following:

	Section Where Located	E Code
Boiling water	Other Accidents	E924.0
1. Cut from electric can opener	________	E910.2
2. Auto accident, driver	________	E819.0
3. Burns from fire, warehouse	________	E891.9
4. Scuba diving accident	________	E910.3
5. Contusion from fall	________	E888.9
6. Struck by fellow soccer player	________	E917.0
7. Rape	________	E960.1
8. Stabbing	________	E966
9. Gunshot wound	________	E922.9

	Section Where Located	E Code
10. Tripped and fell on stairs	________	E880.9
11. Fell from bed	________	E884.4
12. Cut finger with piece of glass	________	E920.8
13. Scuba accident	________	E910.1
14. Accidental drowning	________	E910.9
15. Accident from farm cultivator	________	E919.0
16. Struck by furniture	________	E917.3
17. Fell into well	________	E883.1
18. Fall from ladder	________	E881.0
19. Lightning exposure	________	E907
20. Dog bite	________	E906.0

ICD-10-CM Implementation Impact

Although the concept of V codes and E codes does not change significantly in ICD-10-CM, they have been reassigned code numbers or new code families as defined in ICD-10-CM.

The codes currently assigned E codes in ICD-9-CM will be assigned codes in the V00-Y97 range, which comprise Chapter 20, External Causes of Morbidity, in ICD-10-CM. In ICD-9-CM, the last digit of the external cause code signifies the person injured, for example:

0—Driver
1—Passenger
2—Motorcyclist
7—Pedestrian

In ICD-10-CM the second digit will indicate the identity of the person injured, for example:

V00-V09—Pedestrian Injured in Transport Accident
V10-V19—Pedal Cycle Rider Injured in Transport Accident
V20-V29—Motorcycle Rider Injured in Transport Accident

Codes currently assigned V codes in ICD-9-CM will be reassigned to the Z code family in ICD-10-CM. For example:

Z00—Encounter for general exam without complaint, suspected or reported diagnosis
Z01—Encounter for other special examination without complaint, suspected or reported diagnosis

A number of V codes and E codes have been moved and incorporated in other areas, such as the T code family for Poisoning and Adverse Affects of Drugs, Medicaments, and Biological Substances.

Chapter in Review

Certification Review

- V codes constitute the Supplemental Classification of Factors Influencing Health Status and Contact with Health Services section in the ICD-9-CM code book.
- V codes are used when a patient does not present with any diagnoses, signs, or symptoms, yet an encounter takes place.
- V codes may be the primary diagnosis when the chief reason for encounter is best described by the use of a V code (e.g., encounter for chemotherapy).
- E codes are NOT applied for primary diagnoses because they provide additional information for coding the cause of the injury or poisoning.
- E codes are important from a reimbursement perspective because they assign liability and the appropriate insurance carrier responsibility.
- Clean claims are those received and processed without the need for additional information, correction, or research.
- Clean claims ensure prompt payment because they are processed on the initial submission.
- Many states have laws specifying time limits within which carriers must adjudicate (provide payment or response for) clean claims submitted.

Student Assignments

- Study Chapter 5.
- Review the Learning Objectives for Chapter 5.
- Complete the Certification Review for Chapter 5.
- Complete the Stop and Practice exercises contained in Chapter 5.
- Complete the Chapter Review exercise to reinforce concepts learned in Chapter 5.
- Complete the practice exercises on the companion Evolve site for reinforcement of the concepts contained in Chapter 5.
- Complete the Practical Application exercises.
- Complete the Workbook exercises for Chapter 5 as assigned by your instructor.

Chapter Review Exercise

Assign V codes, E codes, and ICD-9-CM codes as appropriate.

Code/V Code/Other

1. Exposure to human immunodeficiency virus (HIV) ______
2. History of hypertension ______
3. Malignant neoplasm of cervix, treated successfully 10 years ago ______
4. Fracture of tibia, removal of screws and pins ______
5. Dialysis treatment for end-stage renal disease ______
6. Coronary artery bypass grafting status ______
7. Pregnancy ______
8. Well-child examination ______
9. Worried well (examination for which there is no diagnosis) ______
10. Viral illness with exposure to strep throat ______
11. Family history ovarian cancer ______
12. Exposure to sexually transmitted disease ______
13. History of colon carcinoma ______
14. Single delivery, liveborn ______
15. Status post (S/P) tracheostomy ______
16. HIV counseling ______
17. Postmenopausal state ______
18. History of malaria ______
19. History of alcoholism ______
20. Removal of orthopedic pin ______
21. Substance abuse counseling ______
22. Family history of mental illness ______
23. S/P percutaneous transluminal coronary angioplasty ______
24. Newborn, suspicion of brain damage ______

25. Supervision of first pregnancy V22.0
26. Infant, single liveborn V30.00
27. Screening sickle cell V78.2
28. Adjustment of arm prosthetic V52.0
29. Evaluation following rape V71.5
30. Glaucoma screening V80.1
31. History of renal stones V13.01
32. History of myocardial infarction 412
33. Insertion of intrauterine device V25.1
34. Sterilization V25.2
35. Supervision of high-risk pregnancy V23.89
36. S/P pacemaker V45.01
37. S/P heart transplant V42.1
38. S/P aortic valve replacement V42.2
39. Amniocentesis screening chromosome abnormalities V28.0
40. History of allergy to penicillin V14.0
41. History of colon polyps V12.72
42. History of malignant melanoma V10.82
43. History of cigarette smoking V15.82
44. Family history of mental retardation V18.4
45. Need for DTP immunization V06.1
46. Renal dialysis status V45.1
47. Breast augmentation V50.1
48. Screening mammogram V76.12
49. Preemployment physical V70.5
50. Replacement gastrostomy tube V55.1
51. High-risk screening mammogram V76.11
52. HIV-positive status V08
53. Fall on steps of bus E817.1
54. Bicycle accident E826.1
55. Fall off steps of airplane, passenger E843.3
56. Traffic accident E819.0
57. Auto accident involving tree E823.1
58. Fall from ladder on boat E833.9
59. Injury in private driveway E849.0
60. Accidental fall E888.9
61. Fall from bed E884.4
62. Injury on football field E849.4
63. Injury at beach E849.8
64. Lead poisoning, lead-based paint at home E861.5
65. Barbiturate poisoning, accidental E851
66. Fall into storm drain E833.2
67. Fall on stairs E880.9
68. Fall out of tree E884.9
69. Drowning/submersion in bathtub E910.4
70. Injury from colliding with another person E917.9
71. Fall on pitchfork E920.4
72. Adverse reaction, chlorine fumes 987.6, E869.8
73. Crushed by crowd E917.1
74. Injury from foreign body, ear E915
75. Suicide by hanging E953.0
76. Suicide by jumping from window of home E957.0
77. Adverse reaction to bee sting 989.5, E905.3
78. Injury from lifting heavy objects E927.9
79. Injury from can opener E920.4
80. Accidental overdose, acetaminophen 965.4, E866.8
81. Inhalation of asbestos 989.81, E866.8
82. Family history of congenital defects V19.5
83. Need for flu vaccine V04.81
84. Need for rabies immunization V04.5
85. Fall on escalator E880.0
86. Fall from tripping E885.9
87. Sprain/strains from strenuous activity E927.9
88. Injury occurring at industrial site E849.3
89. Adverse effects, digoxin taken correctly 972.1, E858.3
90. Adverse effects, hormones taken correctly 962.9, E932.9
91. Injury from electric can opener E920.2
92. Intentional self-inflicted knife wound E956
93. Gunshot wound, homicide attempt E965.4
94. Injured by object dropped on patient E916
95. Fall in bathtub E884.9
96. School physical V70.3
97. Sports physical V70.3
98. Car versus car highway accident E812.9
99. Family history of breast cancer V16.3
100. S/P loss of limb, below knee V49.75

Practical Application

Review the following case scenarios and assign ICD-9-CM codes as appropriate. Assign both numeric and V codes and E codes as appropriate, listing them in the correct order for each service.

1. Progress note

PROGRESS NOTE

Chief complaint: ______________________

Date: ______________

Vital signs: BP_____ P_____ R_____

History:

Patient arrives for visit relating her brother recently underwent colon resection for colon cancer and would like to discuss need for colonoscopy screening.

The patient is a 48-year-old female who presents with no symptoms, no dysuria, no change in bowel habits, no recent weight loss, concerned about the history of colon cancer in her family.

She relates that her brother was recently diagnosed with colon cancer, and in 2002, her mother was diagnosed with colon cancer as well as two other siblings in the past ten years.

She is on no medications, no chronic problems, past surgical history is cesarean section times two with two normal healthy children, now age 28, and 26. She indicates she does not smoke or drink, and is currently unemployed.

Exam:

On exam, the patient is alert and oriented. HEENT exam reveals PERRLA, EOM. Neck supply, no carotid bruits, no thyroidmegaly noted. Heart sounds are regular, no murmurs, rubs or gallops. Lungs clear to auscultation. Neurologically intact.

Diagnosis/assessment:

Discussed with patient the need for screening colonoscopy for over age 40 adults as well as with her significant family history of colon cancer. We will get her scheduled for a screening colonoscopy in the near future. She presents with no signs or symptoms indicative of colon disease; however, would recommend screening colonoscopy due to age and family history.

Stacy Kraft, MD

Godfrey Regional Outpatient Clinic

Patient name: ______________________

Date of service: ______________

GODFREY MEDICAL ASSOCIATES

1532 Third Avenue, Suite 120 • Aldon, FL 77713 • (407) 555-4000

Codes: ______________________

2. Progress note

PROGRESS NOTE

Date:	**Vital signs:** T	R
Chief complaint:	P	BP

2-year-old returns for MMR and Oral Polio immunization series. At her last visit, she was diagnosed with otitis media. Due to the fact she was running a low grade fever, we opted to hold off on her immunizations.

Examination:

Vital signs, including temperature, are normal.

Impression:

Plan:

We will proceed with her MMR immunization and Oral Polio today.

Mom understands the benefits and risks of these immunizations, and warning signs, and wishes to proceed.

Willen Obst MD

Patient name:
DOB:
MR/Chart #:

GODFREY MEDICAL ASSOCIATES
1532 Third Avenue, Suite 120 • Aldon, FL 77713 • (407) 555-4000

Codes: ______________________

3. Progress note

PROGRESS NOTE

Chief complaint: ______________________

Date: ______________

Vital signs: BP_____ P_____ R_____

History:

22-year-old patient presents today with complaints of abdominal pain, and amenorrhea for approximately 6–8 weeks. She is currently not on any birth control, married, and suspects she may be pregnant.

Exam:

On exam, the patient presents as a normal, healthy 22-year-old female who wishes to determine whether she is pregnant. Patient is alert and oriented, HEENT is normal, neck supple, abdomen, soft, no masses, heart normal rate and rhythm.

Diagnosis/assessment:

Laboratory pregnancy test was performed which was positive. We will refer patient to an Ob/Gyn for care during her pregnancy, and she will return to our office for any non-pregnancy related problems.

Godfrey Regional Hospital

Patient name: ______________________

Date of service: ______________

GODFREY MEDICAL ASSOCIATES
1532 Third Avenue, Suite 120 • Aldon, FL 77713 • (407) 555-4000

Codes: ______________________

4. Progress note

PROGRESS NOTE

Date:	**Vital signs:** T	R
Chief complaint:	P	BP

SUBJECTIVE:
22-year-old complains that she fell and injured her right ankle in the parking lot of her office building yesterday. Of note, the patient is approximately 22 weeks pregnant, G1 P1 A 0. She is being followed by Dr. Smith for her pregnancy.
PAST MEDICAL HISTORY:
Allergies, None
Medications, None

Physical examination:

OBJECTIVE:
Alert, oriented pregnant female. BP 120/80, respirations 20, pulse 70. She appears in no distress. She has moderate swelling of the right ankle, tender over the lateral malleolar area. Good range of motion, good pulses. We will not x-ray at this time due to her pregnancy.

Assessment:

Right ankle sprain, elevate the leg, immobilze with Swede-O splint.

Plan:

Take Tylenol only (no narcotics) on a PRN basis. Avoid walking any more than is necessary during the next 2–3 days.

Jay Corman MD

Patient name:
DOB:
MR/Chart #:

GODFREY REGIONAL OUTPATIENT CLINIC
3122 Shannon Avenue • Aldon, FL 77712 • (407) 555-7654

Codes: ______________________

5. Progress note

PROGRESS NOTE

Date:	**Vital signs:** T	R
Chief complaint:	P	BP

Patient presents for follow-up exam for breast cancer. She was seen approximately one year ago, following mastectomy, chemotherapy and radiation therapy for infiltrating ductal carcinoma of the left breast. She has had no recurrence, and was instructed to follow-up on a yearly basis.

Examination:

Alert, female, in no acute distress. Weight 170, pulse 90, temperature 98.6. Examination of the breasts reveals no masses, no abnormalities. Left breast reveals well healed surgical scar. She indicates she is doing well, without complaints. Has continued to perform monthly breast self exams and has felt no lumps or masses. There is no lymphadenopathy. Neck is supple, no thyroidmegaly.

Impression:

Plan:

We will order a mammogram and CA-125 and await the test results, however, appears to be a resolved infiltrating ductal carcinoma without reoccurrence.

Adam Westgate MD

Patient name:
DOB:
MR/Chart #:

GODFREY REGIONAL OUTPATIENT CLINIC
3122 Shannon Avenue • Aldon, FL 77712 • (407) 555-7654

Codes: ______________________________

6. Progress note

PROGRESS NOTE

Date:	Vital signs: T	R
Chief complaint:	P	BP

Patient presents having been injured at home while walking across the lawn. He apparently was pushing a lawnmower, tripped and hit his head on the curb along the sidwalk. Complains of headache, nausea and nasal pain caused by impact. Also complaints of skin laceration to nose. No previous hospitalizations, surgeries or major illnesses. He is up-to-date on his immunizations, including tetanus toxoid.

Examination:

25-year-old male who was working in his yard on this date and apparently tripped, hit his head and presents with a 2.0 cm laceration of the nose. Examination reveals a 2.0 cm gaping laceration along the septal edge, and apparently a deviated septum which resulted from his fall. He indicates the septal defect was not present prior to the accident. This may need reconstructive surgery in the future. He reports no loss of consciousness or other symptoms other than some nausea and headache from the impact. Head, normal symmetry, no motor or sensory deficits noted. Normal gait. He reports no dizziness or light-headedness. Eyes, PERRLA, EOM, neck supple, full ROM without any limitation. Lungs clear to auscultation, heart regular rate and rhythm, abdomen, nondistended, non-tender. Back and extremities appear normal, no contusions, abrasions, lacerations, full ROM.

Impression:

Laceration to the nose was approximated and closed with 2 sutures, bandaged and taped.

Plan:

Patient to return in 7–10 days for suture removal and re-evaluation of septal defect. Patient should clean wound daily with hydrogen peroxide and water, change bandage as needed and avoid extensive nose blowing for the next 24 hours.

John Parker MD

Patient name:
DOB:
MR/Chart #:

GODFREY REGIONAL OUTPATIENT CLINIC
3122 Shannon Avenue • Aldon, FL 77712 • (407) 555-7654

Codes: ______________________

7. Progress note

PROGRESS NOTE

Date:	**Vital signs:** T	R
Chief complaint:	P	BP

19-year-old male was playing soccer and was accidentally kicked by another player instead of the soccer ball. Patient experiencing pain in the calf area and unable to bear full weight on right leg.

Examination:

X-ray was negative for fracture or other injury.

Impression:

Leg pain from leg contusion due to kick

Plan:

Will treat conservatively with NSAIDS and Tylenol for pain.

Felix Washington MD

Patient name:
DOB:
MR/Chart #:

GODFREY REGIONAL OUTPATIENT CLINIC
3122 Shannon Avenue • Aldon, FL 77712 • (407) 555-7654

Codes: ______________________________

6

ICD-9-CM Tables

LEARNING OBJECTIVES

After completing this chapter, the student will be able to:

- Understand the proper use of the drugs and chemicals table located in the ICD-9-CM code book.
- Understand the proper use of the decision tree (Tool 6-1) for determining the appropriate ICD-9-CM codes for assigning the adverse effects of drugs or poisonings.
- Determine whether ingestion of drugs and chemicals is the result of:
  Accidental poisoning
  Therapeutic use of drugs
  Suicide or assault
  Undetermined causes
- Properly use the hypertension table located in the ICD-9-CM code book.
- Comprehend the relations of other medical conditions that complicate hypertension with assumptions made in coding these conditions.
- Understand the proper rules and guidelines for assigning codes to neoplasms.
- Identify the differences among the categories of neoplasms identified in ICD-9-CM.
- Know the proper use of the neoplasm table contained in the ICD-9-CM code book.
- Know the correct assignment order of primary and secondary neoplasms.
- Perceive the proper use of V codes for neoplastic diagnoses.
- Apply concepts from the ICD-9-CM tables to practical coding scenarios.

CODING REFERENCE TOOLS

Tool 6-1

Adverse Effects of Drugs and Poisonings

Tool 6-2

Neoplastic Diagnostic Coding Rules

KEY TERMS

Accidental Overdose
Assault
Benign
Carcinoma in Situ
Malignant
Metastatic from
Metastatic to
Neoplasm
Poisoning
Primary
Secondary
Suicide Attempt
Therapeutic Use
Uncertain Behavior
Unspecified Behavior

In the alphabetical section of ICD-9-CM are diagnoses that are so extensive that the codes are arranged in a table format. For these tables to be used correctly, there are specific guidelines for coding and selecting the appropriate code(s). The hypertension and neoplasm tables are contained in the alphabetical section, whereas the drugs and chemicals table is frequently independent of the alphabetical section.

Drugs and Chemicals Table

APPROPRIATE USE

The drugs and chemicals table found in the ICD-9-CM book provides a concise guide to **poisoning** and external causes for adverse effects of drugs and other chemical and biologic substances. Each of the listed drugs, chemical substances, and biologic substances is assigned a code on the basis of the diagnostic statement regarding whether the cause is the result of the following:

- Poisoning
- Overdose
- Wrong substance given or taken
- Intoxication

Codes from the drugs and chemicals table are used only when the chief reason for the encounter is the result of exposure to a drug or chemical. Codes in the drugs and chemicals table are arranged by the drug or chemical name in alphabetical order.

The categories in the drugs and chemicals table are as follows (Fig. 6-1):

- Poisoning
- Accident
- Therapeutic Use
- Suicide Attempt
- Assault
- Undetermined

960-979: Poisoning

Codes from this category are used ONLY when the substance involved was not taken according to physician instructions. Examples of the appropriate use of the poisoning codes would include scenarios such as the following:

- Wrong dosage of medication given in error
- Medication given to wrong person

Substance		External Case (E-Code)				
	Poisoning	Accident	Therapeutic Use	Suicide Attempt	Assault	Undetermined
Adalin (acteyl)	967.3	E852.2	E937.3	E950.2	E962.0	E980.2
Adenosine (phosphate)	977.8	E858.8	E947.8	E950.4	E962.0	E980.4
Adhesives	989.89	E866.8	—	E950.9	E960.1	E980.9
ADH	962.5	E858.0	E932.5	E950.4	E962.0	E980.4
Adicillin	960.0	E856	E930.0	E950.4	E962.0	E980.4
Adiphenine	975.1	E855.6	E945.1	E950.4	E962.0	E980.4
Adjunct, pharmaceutical	977.4	E858.8	E947.4	E950.4	E962.0	E980.4
Adrenal (extract, cortex, or medulla) (glucocorticoids) (hormones) (mineralocorticoids)	962.0	E858.0	E932.0	E950.4	E962.0	E980.4
ENT agent	976.6	E858.7	E946.6	E950.4	E962.0	E980.4
ophthalmic preparation	976.5	E858.7	E946.5	E950.4	E962.0	E980.4
topical NEC	976.0	E858.7	E946.0	E950.4	E962.0	E980.4

FIGURE 6-1. Excerpt from drugs and chemicals table in the ICD-9-CM.

- Medication taken by wrong person
- Patient takes wrong medication
- Intoxication (other than that resulting from cumulative ingestion)
- Overdose
- The combination of medications with other substances (e.g., other medications, alcohol, over-the-counter medications), which creates an adverse effect

In addition to the assignment of a poisoning code when appropriate, the external cause for the condition should also be assigned an appropriate external code (E code).

E850-E869: Accident

These codes include **accidental overdose** of drug, wrong substance, drug taken in error, accidents in the use of drugs or biologicals during medical or surgical procedures, and external causes of poisoning classifiable to 980-989.

E930-E949: Therapeutic Use

These codes include the correct substance administered properly and as prescribed in therapeutic or prophylactic dosage.

E950-E952: Suicide Attempt

These codes are used when self-inflicted injuries or poisonings are involved. Make certain that the diagnostic statement confirms that injuries or poisonings are self-inflicted. Many times the physician or provider is unable or unwilling to make the diagnosis of **suicide attempt** because he or she may be unable to ascertain, especially in the case of drug overdose, whether the injury or poisoning was intentional or accidental.

E961-E962: Assault

The codes for **assault** indicate injury or poisoning that has been inflicted by another person, with the intent to do bodily harm, injure, or kill. This information must be documented and included in the diagnostic information used for coding.

E980-E981: Undetermined

Undetermined codes are used when the intent of the poisoning or injury is similar to that mentioned in the suicide attempt or assault section and the provider cannot or will not make a definite diagnostic statement regarding whether the injury was accidental or intentional.

DOCUMENTATION REQUIREMENTS

As with all the other ICD-9-CM diagnosis codes that have been discussed so far, the drug and chemical codes depend on documentation. In some instances documentation will be unclear about the circumstances under which the drug or chemical was ingested. Consider the following example:

A 30-year-old woman presents to the emergency department by ambulance because of seizures from an overdose of acetaminophen (Tylenol). Physician documentation does not specify whether the overdose was intentional, for the purpose of suicide, or accidental.

In this instance the coder must assign an undetermined external cause code. Even when intent seems apparent and is likely the cause of the adverse effect, caution must be taken to make certain the information is documented appropriately. See the following example:

A 35-year-old man presents to the emergency department for abdominal bleeding caused by an ingestion of rat poison.

Without further information the coder cannot assume that the ingestion is the result of an accident. The ingestion could have been accidental (self-inflicted or inflicted accidentally or intentionally by another individual) or self-inflicted in a suicide attempt. Take extreme caution to consider all possibilities before assigning the E code for drug and chemical codes. The undetermined code will often be assigned because of insufficient or unclear documentation. In some cases the physician may be unable to determine the cause, as in the example of the patient who ingested acetaminophen.

In addition to the appropriate code(s) for poisoning as well as the E code that indicates accidental, therapeutic, suicide, assault, or undetermined, the chief reason for the encounter will remain the presenting problem, such as headache, seizures, or abdominal bleeding, followed by the codes that indicate the poisoning code (when applicable) and external cause (E code).

DRUGS AND CHEMICALS FLOWCHART

The most complex part of coding arises from the inability to determine from the documentation provided whether poisoning is the result of an accident, proper therapeutic use, a suicide attempt, or assault. Because of the complexity of this decision-making process, a diagnosis flowchart can be helpful in this determination (Tool 6-1). Keep in mind that code assignment will typically require a minimum of two codes for any scenario. In some situations three codes will be assigned to code these appropriately.

As discussed in the introductory chapters on ICD-9-CM coding, the condition would be assigned as the chief reason for the encounter, followed by the poisoning codes and the external cause code when applicable. In most instances this would be the presenting condition, such as coma, seizures, or abdominal pain caused by the drugs and other substances, followed by the cause of the adverse effect.

Following are a few examples; assign code(s) appropriate for them using the decision tree. Use the section of the drugs and chemicals table illustrated in Figure 6-1.

CONDITION: Poisoning due to antidiuretic hormone prescribed 5 months prior to mother of patient

TOOL 6-1

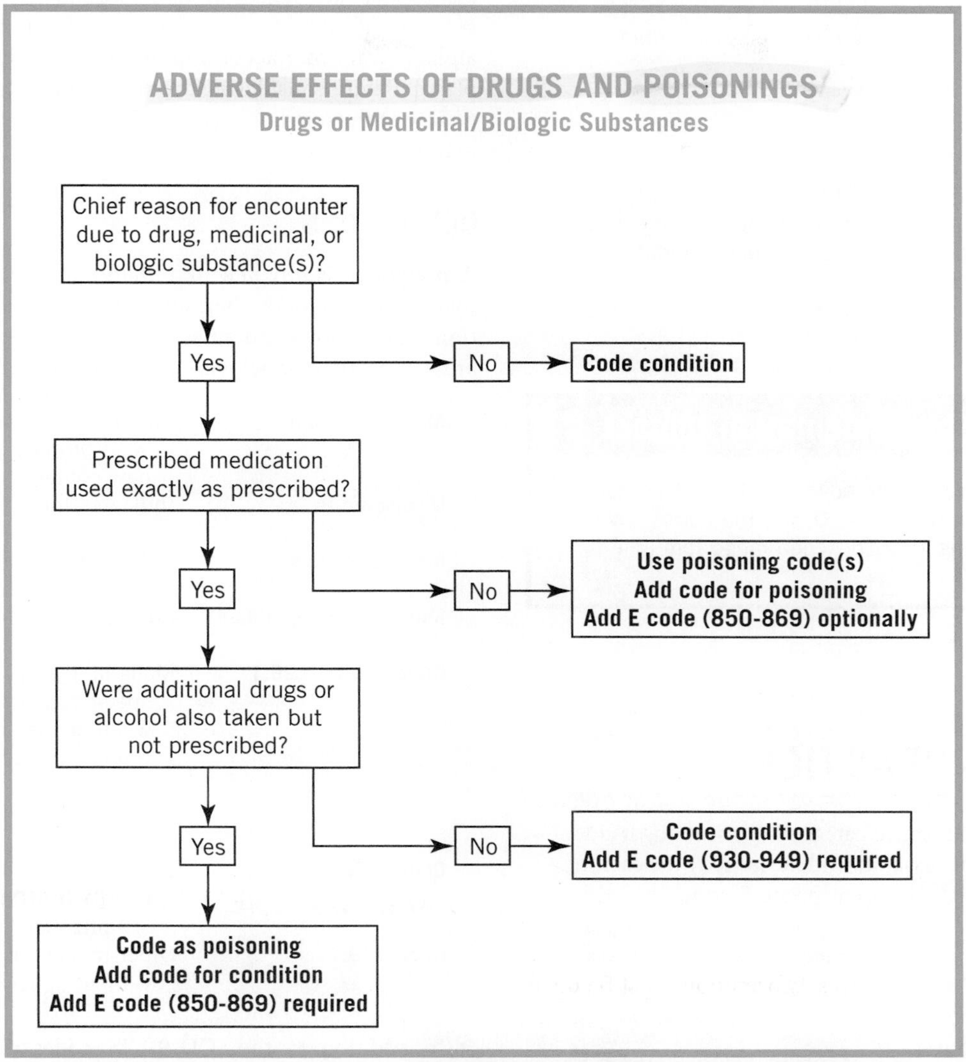

ADVERSE EFFECTS OF DRUGS AND POISONINGS
Drugs or Medicinal/Biologic Substances

Chief reason for encounter due to drug, medicinal, or biologic substance(s)?
- Yes → Prescribed medication used exactly as prescribed?
  - Yes → Were additional drugs or alcohol also taken but not prescribed?
    - Yes → **Code as poisoning / Add code for condition / Add E code (850-869) required**
    - No → **Code condition / Add E code (930-949) required**
  - No → **Use poisoning code(s) / Add code for poisoning / Add E code (850-869) optionally**
- No → **Code condition**

Starting at the top of the decision tree, answer the first question:

Chief reason for encounter due to drug, medicinal, or biologic substance? YES

Continue DOWN to the next question:

Prescribed medication used exactly as prescribed? NO. The medication was old and not prescribed for the patient.

Continue ACROSS:

Use poisoning code	962.5
Add external cause code	E858.0 for accidental

Therefore the correct answer would be the condition that prompted the encounter, such as rash, headache followed by:

962.5	Poisoning ADH
E858.0	Accidental

Take another example that uses the ICD-9-CM code book:

CONDITION: Patient presents with seizures from intentional ingestion of rat poison

Starting at the top of the decision tree, answer the first question:

Chief reason for encounter due to drug, medicinal, or biologic substance? YES

Continue DOWN to the next question:

Prescribed medication used exactly as prescribed? NO. Rat poison is not a prescribed medication.

Continue ACROSS:

Use poisoning code: 989.4

Add external cause code: E980.7 for undetermined

Therefore the correct answer would be:

780.39	Seizures
989.4	Poisoning ADH
E980.7	Undetermined poisoning, documentation does not state whether suicidal, accident, or assault

ICD-10-CM Implementation Impact

Although the logic for the adverse effects does not change significantly in ICD-10-CM, the codes have been moved to the T36-T50 code range family in ICD-10-CM.

STOP AND PRACTICE

Identify the external cause category (poisoning, accident, therapeutic, suicide, assault, undetermined) for each of the following. Assign the appropriate E code.

	External Cause	E Code Category
1. Overdose of fluoxetine		
2. Digoxin toxicity		
3. Accidental ingestion of diphenhydramine		
4. Suicidal ingestion of acetaminophen		
5. Ingestion of antifreeze		
6. Rattlesnake bite		
7. Intentional poisoning of another individual, rat poison		
8. Ingestion of smelter fumes		
9. Ingestion of poisonous plant, not classified		
10. Vitamin B_{12} toxicity		

Neoplasms

Neoplasms are listed in table format in the alphabetical section of ICD-9-CM. These codes are arranged in alphabetical order according to the anatomic site of the neoplasm. Before considering the neoplasm table, however, some review of the terminology associated with neoplasms may be helpful.

DEFINITIONS

A **neoplasm** is *any new and abnormal growth.* That growth may be **malignant** or **benign** or as yet undetermined. Additional definitions and rules for coding neoplastic diagnoses are necessary to assist with correct coding.

Metastatic from	Spread to a distant site of the solid primary neoplasm with a new center of malignancy.
Metastatic to	Indicates the site mentioned is secondary or metastatic.
Metastatic from	Site mentioned is the primary site.
Metastatic (unqualified)	Code as unspecified site for that type.
Codes 199.0-199.1	Malignant neoplasms without specification regarding whether the site used is primary or secondary. These codes should be used when no further information is documented.
Code 199.0	Disseminated malignant neoplasm without specification of site.
Code 199.1	Other malignant neoplasm without specification of site.

In addition to the ICD-9-CM codes discussed in this chapter, the ICD-9-CM code book includes morphology codes, which are prefixed by an M. Hospital coders specifically use these codes, usually for the purpose of identifying tumor locations for tumor registries. Although these are used solely by the inpatient/outpatient facility coder, an understanding of the code breakdown is necessary. The first four digits identify the type of neoplasm and the fifth digit identifies the behavior, such as in the following:

/0	Benign
/1	Uncertain or borderline malignancy
/2	Carcinoma in situ Intraepithelial Noninfiltrating Noninvasive
/3	Malignant, primary site
/6	Malignant, metastatic site Secondary site
/9	Malignant, uncertain whether primary or secondary

GUIDELINES FOR USE

In addition to the guidelines already discussed, those found in Tool 6-2 should be used for the coding of neoplastic diseases. Although they are used to cover specific coding complexities, many of the rules are simply delineations of the rules already learned. For instance, because the primary diagnosis for each encounter or service will always be the chief reason for that encounter or service, most of the specific neoplasm guidelines are no different than those guidelines already presented.

The ICD-9-CM Official Guidelines for Coding and Reporting offers some additional direction regarding the assignment of neoplastic codes:

- The neoplasm table in the alphabetical index should be referenced first.
- If the histologic term is documented, that term should be referenced first to determine which column of the neoplasm table should be used.
- Anemia associated with malignancy should be assigned anemia as the primary diagnosis using code 285.22, Anemia in neoplastic disease.
- Anemia associated with chemotherapy or other neoplastic treatment should be coded with anemia as the primary diagnosis and E933.1 as an additional code, followed by the malignancy code.
- Primary malignancy previously excised. If the primary malignancy has been previously eradicated or excised and no further treatment is directed at the site, a "History of" code for the site should be assigned.

DOCUMENTATION GUIDELINES

As with the other service codes in the ICD-9-CM book, appropriate neoplastic diagnostic codes rely on good documentation. Basic coding guidelines apply to neoplasm codes as well. When the neoplasm is not specified as primary or secondary malignancy, it will be assigned as primary. As with the other ICD-9-CM codes, the chief reason for the encounter is assigned as the primary diagnostic code. Consider the following example:

> A 42-year-old woman presents for chemotherapy for metastatic cervical cancer originating in the breast. The breast cancer was treated approximately 5 years ago and is no longer present.

The primary code is assigned to the encounter for chemotherapy, the second code is given to the secondary neoplasm of the uterus, and a V code is added for history of breast carcinoma as the third code.

V58.1	Encounter for chemotherapy
198.82	Secondary malignant neoplasm, uterus
V10.3	Personal history of breast carcinoma

TOOL 6-2

NEOPLASTIC DIAGNOSTIC CODING RULES

1. When treatment is directed at the primary site, the malignancy is designated as the principal site. (Chief reason for encounter still applies.)

2. When treatment is directed at the secondary or metastatic site, the secondary site would be designated as the principal diagnosis, followed by the primary site listed as a secondary diagnosis. (Again, the chief reason for this encounter is the secondary site; therefore the chief reason for the encounter rule applies here as well.)

3. Care for ancillary services such as chemotherapy or radiotherapy—chief reason for these encounters would be coded with V58.0-V58.1 because these are the chief reasons for this service or encounter. The neoplastic disease being treated with the radiotherapy or chemotherapy may be listed as additional diagnosis(es).

4. When the primary neoplasm is no longer under treatment, it is not appropriate to code the encounter with a neoplasm code. The V codes, or personal history, would be used as the chief reason for encounter. An example of the use of personal history V codes would be patients who return annually for a re-examination to their hematologist or oncologist who are not being and have not been treated for the disease for some time because the neoplasm is no longer present.

5. Admissions for complications associated with a malignant neoplasm would be coded with that complication listed first. Again, the chief reason for this encounter or service would be the chief complaint or condition rather than the malignant neoplasm. The primary or secondary diagnosis could be the primary and/or secondary neoplasm, whichever is still present.

In those instances in which neoplasms are not specified as benign or malignant, codes from the uncertain or unspecified behavior categories are applicable.

CATEGORIZATION OF NEOPLASMS

The following are the main categories for the neoplasm table.

140-208: Malignant Neoplasms

Malignant or cancerous neoplasms are further defined as tumor cells that extend or attach themselves to an adjacent structure and spread to distant sites. Two types of malignant neoplasms are coded as the following:

Solid malignant neoplasms (140-199)	Single localized point of origin. These neoplasms tend to metastasize to adjacent or remote sites.
Hematopoietic/ lymphatic neoplasms (200-208)	Reticuloendothelial and lymphatic system and blood-forming tissue neoplasms: Primary neoplasms of lymph nodes or glands (200-202) Lymphoma—can be malignant or benign Hodgkin's disease Multiple myeloma/leukemia (203-208)

Malignant neoplasms are further subdivided in the neoplasm table as **primary,** the site where the neoplasm originated, and **secondary,** the site where the neoplasm has spread. When a malignant neoplasm is not specified as primary or secondary, it is assumed to be primary in nature.

230-234: Carcinoma in Situ

Carcinoma in situ codes refer to malignant neoplasms undergoing malignant changes; however, they remain confined at the point of origin without any invasion of surrounding normal tissue.

210-229: Benign

When neoplasms, or new growths, do not invade or spread and are noncancerous, they are designated benign neoplasms. Use codes from the benign column of the neoplasm table. These neoplasms are not invasive; they do not spread to other sites.

235-238: Uncertain Behavior

When neoplasms have the behavior of both benign and malignant neoplasms and the pathologist has been unable to determine the specific nature, they will be coded to the category of **uncertain behavior**. These codes might also be used for an initial visit to the physician when a neoplasm is identified during an examination. The behavior of the neoplasm is unknown and cannot be ascertained until a biopsy or an excision is performed.

239: Unspecified Behavior

In some instances the nature of the neoplasm has not been specified in the medical documentation. A code would be used from this column of the neoplasm table. This designation should not be confused with behavior that cannot be determined. In the case of **unspecified behavior,** the diagnostic information has not specified the nature of behavior that may be known.

A look at the layout of the neoplasm table shows how these codes are further divided (Fig. 6-2).

ICD-10-CM Implementation Impact

Neoplasms in ICD-10-CM will be represented within 17 code families with the first character of either C or D. A table will still be present with the same headings as currently included in ICD-9-CM. The code families for neoplasms in ICD-10-CM are proposed as follows:

MALIGNANT NEOPLASMS

C00-C75	Stated or presumed primary, specified sites, except lymphoid, hematopoietic, related tissue
C00-C14	Lip, oral cavity, pharynx
C15-C26	Digestive organs
C30-C39	Respiratory and intrathoracic organs
C40-C41	Bone and articular cartilage
C43-C44	Skin
C45-C49	Mesothelial and soft tissue
C50	Breast
C51-C58	Female genital organs
C60-C63	Male genital organs
C64-C68	Urinary tract
C69-C72	Eye, brain, other parts of central nervous system
C73-C75	Thyroid and other endocrine glands
C76-C80	Malignant neoplasms, ill-defined, secondary, and unspecified sites
C81-C96	Malignant neoplasms, stated or presumed primary, lymphoid, hematopoietic, and related tissue
D00-D09	In situ neoplasms
D10-D36	Benign neoplasms
D37-D48	Neoplasms of uncertain behavior
D49	Neoplasms of unspecified behavior

STOP AND PRACTICE

For the following neoplasms, determine to which coding category they should be assigned. The categories are malignant (primary, secondary, in situ), benign, uncertain behavior, and unspecified behavior.

Neoplasm	Behavior/Category
1. Metastatic neoplasm of the spine	198.5
2. Breast cancer	174.9
3. Breast cancer, in situ	233.0
4. Breast neoplasm	238.3
5. Breast lipoma	214.1
6. Adenocarcinoma of the thyroid	193
7. Adrenal adenoma	227.0
8. Acute myeloid leukemia	205.00
9. Carcinoma of the brain from the lung	162.9, 198.3
10. Acute lymphatic leukemia	204.00

Table 6-1 delineates the proper assignment of ICD-9-CM diagnostic code(s) based on the reason for encounter.

MEDICAL TERMINOLOGY

Medical terminology is important in the proper assignment of diagnostic codes. Following are a few additional terms related to neoplasms:

Mass Not regarded as a neoplasm, not determined to be a new growth

Carcinoma Cancerous tumor

Sarcoma Malignant neoplasm of connective tissue

Lymphosarcoma Form of non-Hodgkin's lymphoma

Burkitt's tumor Form of non-Hodgkin's lymphoma

Dysplasia Precursor condition to carcinoma

	Malignant					
Neoplasm *(continued)*	Primary	Secondary	Ca in situ	Benign	Uncertain Behavior	Unspecified
bone (periosteum)	170.9	198.5	—	213.9	238.0	239.2
Note—Carcinomas and adenocarcinomas, of any type other than intraosseous or odontogenic, of the sites listed under "Neoplasm, bone," should be considered as constituting metastatic spread from an unspecified primary site and coded to 198.5 for morbidity coding and to 199.1 for underlying cause of death coding.						
acetabulum	170.6	198.5	—	213.6	238.0	239.2
acromion (process)	170.4	198.5	—	213.4	238.0	239.2
ankle	170.8	198.5	—	213.8	238.0	239.2
arm NEC	170.4	198.5	—	213.4	238.0	239.2
astragalus	170.8	198.5	—	213.8	238.0	239.2
atlas	170.2	198.5	—	213.2	238.0	239.2
axis	170.2	198.5	—	213.2	238.0	239.2
back NEC	170.2	198.5	—	213.2	238.0	239.2
calcaneus	170.8	198.5	—	213.8	238.0	239.2

FIGURE 6-2. Excerpt from table of neoplasms in the ICD-9-CM.

STOP AND PRACTICE

Assign the appropriate ICD-9-CM diagnostic code(s) in the correct order to the following conditions.

	ICD-9-CM Code(s)
1. Right renal mass	______
2. Severe dysplasia, cervix; chronic cervicitis	______
3. Bronchial adenoma	______
4. Neurofibromatosis, type 2	______
5. Carcinoma in situ, skin of anus	______
6. Metastatic carcinoma from lung	______
7. Metastatic carcinoma to brain	______
8. Metastatic carcinoma of brain	______
9. Acute myeloblastic leukemia	______
10. Benign lymphoma of axillary nodes	______

TABLE 6-1 NEOPLASM CODING ORDER GUIDELINES

REASON FOR ENCOUNTER	CODE(S) TO ASSIGN
Primary neoplasm	Primary neoplasm
Chemotherapy/radiation	V code chemotherapy V code radiation Malignant site being treated Other site(s) if appropriate
Complications from chemotherapy/ treatment	Complications V code for treatment modality Malignant site being treated Other site(s) if appropriate
Admission for removal of malignancy with treatment during admission	Primary neoplasm V code for treatment modality
Malignant neoplasm with signs/symptoms	Malignant neoplasm only
Encounter for follow-up for previous malignancy	History of code only
Encounter for condition related to malignancy	Condition Malignant neoplasm

Hypertension

APPROPRIATE USE

Hypertension is coded from the table in the alphabetical index of ICD-9-CM. All hypertensive disorders and diseases, and those associated with hypertension, are listed in the hypertension table. There are four columns in the table, which are outlined as follows:

Column 1 Hypertensive condition (e.g., antepartum, cardiovascular).

Column 2 Malignant hypertension.
Accelerated severe form of hypertension.
Symptoms may include headaches, blurred vision, dyspnea, or uremia.

Column 3 Benign hypertension.
Relatively stable hypertension (usually mild, continuous blood pressure elevation) that with proper treatment does not threaten the life span of the patient. It is considered a risk factor for heart disease and cerebrovascular disease.

Column 4 Unspecified hypertension.
Hypertensive heart disease refers to secondary effects of prolonged hypertension on the heart.
Hypertensive disorders should be coded as in Figure 6-3.

Hypertension, hypertension, essential, or NOS Hypertension defined as essential, primary, systemic, or not otherwise specified would be coded as category 401. Do not use malignant or benign hypertension designations unless the documentation supports this diagnosis.

Hypertension, controlled This category of codes 401 through 405 is usually assigned to hypertension that is controlled with therapy.

Hypertension, uncontrolled This designation refers to either untreated hypertension or hypertension that is not responding to medical treatment or therapy. Codes 401 through 405 are used for coding this type of hypertension.

Hypertension, transient When elevated blood pressure is documented without a diagnosis of hypertension (code 796.2), transient hypertension should be assigned unless there is a documented, established diagnosis of hypertension for the patient.

HYPERTENSION DOCUMENTATION GUIDELINES

Often the documentation of hypertension lacks specificity. As a result, the diagnosis code 401.9 (hypertension, unspecified) must be assigned when documentation lacks information regarding the nature of the hypertension (benign compared

	Malignant	Benign	Unspecified
Hypertension, hypertensive (arterial) (arteriolar) (disease) (essential) (fluctuating) (idiopathic) (intermittent) (labile) (low rennin) (orthostatic) (paroxysmal) (primary) (systemic) (uncontrolled) (vascular)	401.0	401.1	401.9
with			
heart involvement (conditions classifiable to 428, 429.0-429.3, 429.8, 429.9 due to hypertension) (*see also* Hypertension, heart)	402.00	402.10	401.90
with kidney involvement – *see* Hypertension, cardiorenal			
renal involvement (only conditions classifiable to 585, 586, 587) (excludes conditions classifiable as 584) (*see also* Hypertension, kidney)	403.00	403.10	403.90
with heart involvement – *see* Hypertension, cardiorenal			
failure (and sclerosis) (*see also* Hypertension, kidney)	403.01	403.11	403.91
sclerosis without failure (*see also* Hypertension, kidney)	403.00	403.10	403.90
accelerated (*see also* Hypertension, by type, malignant)	401.0	—	—
antepartum – *see* Hypertension, complicating pregnancy, childbirth, or the puerperium			

FIGURE 6-3. Excerpt from the hypertension table in the ICD-9-CM.

with malignant). Other descriptive words may accompany the diagnosis of hypertension, including hypertensive crisis, orthostatic hypertension, uncontrolled hypertension, essential hypertension, intermittent hypertension, primary hypertension, or systemic hypertension. These terms do not specify the nature of the hypertension, though. Therefore these diagnostic statements will also be assigned a diagnosis code of 401.9, hypertension, unspecified. The use of malignant or benign hypertension codes is not appropriate without supporting medical documentation.

OTHER CODING GUIDELINES

When another condition complicates the treatment of hypertension, typically both conditions are coded. The primary reason for the encounter, which may be the complicating condition, is coded as the primary diagnosis and the hypertension is coded as the secondary diagnosis. Complicating conditions of hypertension, clarified in the *ICD-9-CM Official Guidelines for Coding and Reporting,* include the following.

Hypertension in Pregnancy

As indicated in Chapter 7, complications that arise during or after pregnancy are assigned codes from the 600 series of ICD-9-CM. This guideline also applies to hypertension in pregnancy. Regardless of whether the condition occurred during pregnancy or was present before pregnancy, a code from the 600 series would be assigned. If the condition of hypertension still exists after the postpartum period, a diagnostic code from the 400 series would again be assigned.

Hypertension with Heart Disease

Certain heart conditions (codes 425.8, 428, and 429) are assigned a code from category 402 when the stated condition is the result of hypertension or the statement implies that such is the case (use of the word *hypertensive* in the documentation). The coder must use only the code from category 402 in these instances. When this relation is not stated, each condition is coded separately.

Hypertensive Renal Disease with Chronic Renal Failure

When conditions coded in categories 585 through 587 occur with hypertension, codes from category 403 are appropriate. ICD-9-CM assumes a relation between chronic renal failure and hypertension. Acute renal failure is not included in this assumption.

Hypertensive Heart and Renal Disease

Combination codes from category 404 are used for coding these two diseases. The coder may assign a relation between hypertension and renal disease when both are stated in the diagnosis, whether or not they are connected.

Other Associated Complications of Hypertension Requiring Two Codes

Hypertensive cerebrovascular disease
Hypertensive retinopathy
Secondary hypertension

These complications of hypertension must be assigned two diagnostic codes for the conditions stated. One code is assigned for the underlying condition and the other for the hypertension.

Hypertension Coding as a Chronic Condition

Because many patients will have hypertension in addition to other illnesses, injuries, signs, and symptoms, it is important to keep in mind that only conditions chiefly responsible for the encounter would be appropriate. If the patient presents for the evaluation and treatment of hypertension or if the condition of hypertension is involved in evaluation and management during the encounter, the assignment of hypertension is appropriate. Only when the chief reason for the encounter is hypertension would this condition be listed first. When hypertension is a contributing illness, it is listed as a secondary diagnostic code. Keep in mind that the coding guidelines are relative to physician coding and that facility coders may use the hypertension diagnosis in other circumstances (discussed in the brief overview of hospital/facility coding in Chapters 1 and 2).

ICD-10-CM Implementation Impact

Hypertensive diseases will be included in ICD-10-CM in the code family I10-I15. In addition, hypertension no longer uses the type of hypertension as an axis for classification.

STOP AND PRACTICE

Code the following hypertension-related conditions.

	ICD-9-CM Code(s)
1. Hypertension	________
2. Postoperative hypertension	________
3. Elevated blood pressure	________
4. Postpartum hypertension	________
5. Pulmonary hypertension	________
6. Myocarditis from hypertension	________
7. Hypertension with chronic renal failure	________
8. Hypertension from brain tumor	________
9. Gestational hypertension	________
10. Hypertension, possibly malignant	________

Chapter in Review

Certification Review

- The table of drugs and chemicals located in ICD-9-CM is intended to simplify the assignment of adverse effects.
- Each drug or chemical is assigned a code based on the diagnostic statement regarding whether the injury is the result of poisoning, overdose, wrong substance given or taken, or intoxication.
- Some adverse effects require two ICD-9-CM codes: one for the poisoning and an additional E code for the external cause.
- When the cause of adverse effects is not stated by the physician, the coder must use the Undetermined category. This is particularly important in potential suicide cases in which the physician does not or will not state that the adverse effects were intentionally inflicted.
- Adverse effects from therapeutic use occur only when the correct substance is administered correctly as prescribed.
- Accidental poisoning codes are used only when accidental overdose of a drug, wrong substance, drug taken in error, or accidents in the use of drugs or biologic substances are identified.
- Drugs and chemicals listed in the drugs and chemicals table in the ICD-9-CM code book are listed alphabetically; generic names are used for prescription drugs.
- A neoplasm is defined as any new and abnormal growth. That growth may be malignant, benign, or undetermined.
- Masses are not coded or classified as neoplasms unless the physician states "neoplasm" or "neoplastic" in the diagnostic statement.

- When secondary or metastatic neoplasms are coded, the primary site should always be coded. If the site is known, use the appropriate code. If the site is not known but is known to exist, use 199.0 or 199.1. If the site no longer exists, use history of malignant neoplasm codes.
- Carcinoma in situ refers to malignant neoplasms that stay confined to the point of origin without invading surrounding areas.

Student Assignments

- Study Chapter 6.
- Review the Learning Objectives for Chapter 6.
- Complete the Stop and Practice exercises for Chapter 6.
- Complete the Certification Review for Chapter 6.
- Complete the Chapter Review exercises to reinforce concepts learned in this chapter.
- Complete the practice exercises on the companion Evolve site for reinforcement of the concepts contained in Chapter 6.
- Complete the Practical Application exercise for Chapter 6.
- Complete the Workbook exercises for Chapter 6 as assigned by your instructor.

Chapter Review Exercise

Code the following:

	Code(s) Assigned
1. Essential hypertension	________
2. Suicide attempt by cocaine	________
3. Open wound of abdomen from shotgun blast to abdomen	________
4. Overdose of phenobarbital, prescribed by physician, taken as directed	________
5. Hypertensive heart and renal disease	________
6. Attempted homicide by rat poison	________
7. Hypertension in pregnancy, antepartum	________
8. Secondary hypertension from pulmonary edema	________
9. Allergic reaction to spider bite	________
10. Asbestos poisoning	________
11. Secondary hypertension	________
12. Pulmonary hypertension	________
13. Transient hypertension of pregnancy	________
14. Accidental overdose, doxycycline	________
15. Accidental ingestion, gas fumes/vapors	________
16. Benign hypertension	________
17. Preexisting hypertension in pregnancy with preeclampsia	________
18. Adverse effects of bupivacaine hydrochloride (Marcaine), administered subcutaneously	________
19. Renovascular hypertension	________
20. Suicide attempt by ingestion of gas	________
21. Overdose of diazepam, accidental	________
22. Adverse effects, topical neomycin sulfate (Neosporin)	________
23. Adverse effects, laxatives, therapeutic	________
24. Lithium, taken as directed	________
25. Adverse effects, bee sting	________
26. Elevated blood pressure reading	________
27. Hypertensive renal disease	________
28. Secondary hypertension from Cushing's disease	________
29. Hypertension from polycystic kidney disease	________
30. Intraocular hypertension	________
31. Squamous cell carcinoma in situ, floor of mouth	________
32. Metastatic malignant melanoma from left lateral chest wall to axillary lymph node	________
33. Carcinoma, rectosigmoid junction and prostate	________
34. Adenocarcinoma, right upper lobe, lung, with metastases to mediastinal lymph nodes	________
35. Breast mass	________

Practical Application

Review the documents on the following pages and assign ICD-9-CM codes as appropriate.

1. Progress note

PROGRESS NOTE

Date:	**Vital signs:** T	R
Chief complaint:	P	BP

63-year-old female who has taken Norvasc for approximately the past five years for hypertension presents for evaluation and urinary tract symptoms and nausea. She is on no other medications, and has had hypertension for approximately the past two decades.
Social History/Past Medical History:
Non-smoker, non-drinker. Past surgeries include three cesarean sections, a hysterectomy in 1999, cholecystectomy in 2001.

Physical examination:

She is afebrile. Vital signs are stable. Color normal, she is not diaphoretic. Neck is supple, carotids are normal. Chest is clear, with good air movement. Abdomen, soft and nontender. Pulses are normal.

LABS:
CBC and Comprehensive Metabolic Panel revealed patient in renal failure.

Assessment:

IMPRESSION:
Hypertension, acute renal failure

Plan:

Arrangements will be made for the patient to begin dialysis ASAP. Continue hypertension medications and we will consider additional medications after dialysis has improved her renal function somewhat.

Maurice Doater, MD

Patient name:
DOB:
MR/Chart #:

GODFREY REGIONAL OUTPATIENT CLINIC
3122 Shannon Avenue • Aldon, FL 77712 • (407) 555-7654

Codes: ____________________

2. Progress note

PROGRESS NOTE

Date:	**Vital signs:** T R
Chief complaint:	P BP

A 68-year-old male presents for evaluation of increasing shortness of breath over the past several weeks. He has experienced no other symptoms other than feeling a bit run down and lethargic over the past several days. Feels effort must be taken to complete daily tasks and feels exhausted when he returns from work.
Past Medical History: History of smoking 2 packs per day/20 years. Ceased smoking in 1998 following a scare with a lung mass that was thought to be malignant, however, repeat x-rays revealed poor x-ray technique and no mass could be appreciated after multiple repeated x-rays.
Patient works in the sales field, traveling from city to city, and a great deal of driving is involved.

Examination:

This gentleman appears short winded and a bit anxious. Color is good, P 84, R 12, BP 120/80. Chest: Lungs bilaterally clear to auscultation. Heart: Regular rate and rhythm. Abdomen: Postive bowel sounds, soft and nontender. Extremities: normal strength and sensation with no cyanosis and a minimal pitting edema around the ankles. He reports that he has some edema as the result of sitting and driving for many hours a day. This has been present for years.

Chest x-ray was performed, which revealed a mass in the left lower lobe of the lung. We will schedule for additional testing to include a CT Scan as well as an MRI to determine primary site and any other possible involvement.

Impression:

Lung mass, suspicious for malignant neoplasm

Plan:

Stacy Kraft, MD

Patient name:
DOB:
MR/Chart #:

GODFREY MEDICAL ASSOCIATES
1532 Third Avenue, Suite 120 • Aldon, FL 77713 • (407) 555-4000

Codes: ______________________________

3. Progress note

PROGRESS NOTE

Chief complaint: ______________________________

Date: ______________

Vital signs: BP_____ P_____ R_____

History:

SUBJECTIVE:
68-year-old male returns following initial evaluation for shortness of breath which revealed a suspicious lesion in the left lower lobe of the lung. CT Scan and MRI were ordered to determine primary site and any other possible involvement. MRI of the bone was performed that was positive for metastases to the bone. CT of the lung confirmed a malignant oat cell carcinoma of the left lower lobe. MRI of the brain also revealed metastatic involvement in the brain as well.

Exam:

OBJECTIVE:
68-year-old male who appears anxious for his test results.
He is informed that the diagnosis is guarded, with primary oat cell carcinoma of the left lower lobe with metastatic changes in the brain and bone.

Diagnosis/assessment:

ASSESSMENT:
Primary oat cell carcinoma
Metastatic to brain and bone

PLAN:
Will refer to Oncologist for intervention probably to include both chemotherapy and radiation therapy. Offer reassurance, however, explained that the prognosis was guarded until oncologist has ability to evaluate.

Jay Corman MD

Godfrey Medical Associates

Patient name: ______________________________

Date of service: ______________

GODFREY MEDICAL ASSOCIATES
1532 Third Avenue, Suite 120 • Aldon, FL 77713 • (407) 555-4000

Codes: ______________________________

4. Progress note

PROGRESS NOTE

Date:	**Vital signs:** T	R
Chief complaint:	P	BP

Patient is a 12-month-old active female who presents with a rash over the trunk and lower extremities. She was in approximately 1 week ago with complaints of sore throat, fever and cough and was diagnosed with an upper respiratory infection. She was prescribed penicillin for her URI at that time.

Allergies: None reported

Examination:

She appears to be an active, normal healthy 12-month-old female in no acute distress. She does continue to cough and her upper respiratory infection is not resolved. Lungs, congested. HEENT: Normal. Heart, normal rate and rhythm. Abdomen: soft and non-tender. Coarse rash over the lower trunk and lower extremities that seems to have spread diffusely. Mom indicates no new foods, detergents or lotions have been introduced in the past couple weeks.

Impression:

Non-resolved URI
Allergic reaction to Penicillin

Plan:

Will switch to Keflex for 10 day course

Felix Washington MD

Patient name:
DOB:
MR/Chart #:

GODFREY REGIONAL OUTPATIENT CLINIC
3122 Shannon Avenue • Aldon, FL 77712 • (407) 555-7654

Codes: ______________________

5. Progress note

PROGRESS NOTE

Date:	**Vital signs:** T	R
Chief complaint:	P	BP

34-year-old female presents for extremely anxious feelings. Reports that she takes Solumedrol for her asthma and accidentally took twice the normal dosage recommended and prescribed. She has had asthma since the age of 8 and uses Solumedrol and inhaler therapy to keep her asthma under control.

Examination:

Anxious appearing 34-year-old female who appears in no acute distress. Her breathing is rapid, however, her lungs are clear and her asthma appears to be well-controlled at this time. HEENT normal. Vital signs are stable. PERRLA, neck, soft. Abdomen, soft and nontender. Heart, regular rate and rhythm.

Impression:

Accidental overdose of Solumedrol
Asthma, under control

Plan:

Patient is cautioned about adhering to the correct dosages for her medications and not to overdose even when her asthma is not well-controlled. She should seek medical attention when her medications are not controlling her asthma rather than taking additional dosages.

Stacy Kraft, MD

Patient name:
DOB:
MR/Chart #:

GODFREY REGIONAL OUTPATIENT CLINIC
3122 Shannon Avenue • Aldon, FL 77712 • (407) 555-7654

Codes: ______________________

6. Emergency room record

EMERGENCY ROOM RECORD

Name:	**Age:** **DOB:**	**ER physician:**

Allergies/type of reaction:	**Usual medications/dosages:**

Triage/presenting complaint: 24-year-old male presents to the ER via ambulance in a non-responsive state. He is accompanied by friends who indicate he had been drinking this evening, several beers and a few mixed drinks. He returned home, and was unable to sleep, so he took some prescribed Valium to sleep.

Initial assessment:

Time	T	P	R	BP	Other:					

Medication orders:

Lab work:

X-Ray:

Physician's report:

24-year-old male who presents in a non-arousable state after ingesting alcohol and prescription sleeping medications. Pulse is rapid and irregular, BP 80/60. Patient is intubated and his stomach contents lavaged. Following treatment, the patient became arousable, began to improve and his pulse became regular, his BP stabilized to 120/80 over a period of approximately 4 hours in the ER.

Diagnosis:	**Physician sign/date**
ASSESSMENT: Adverse reaction to alcohol and prescription sleeping aids PLAN: Patient will be discharged with follow-up to an outpatient alcohol treatment facility as he indicates he is binge drinking on a fairly regular basis, at least 2–3 times weekly.	Nancy Connolly MD
Discharge **Transfer** **Admit** **Good** **Satisfactory** **Other:**	

GODFREY REGIONAL HOSPITAL
123 Main Street • Aldon, FL 77714 • (407) 555-1234

Codes: ______________________

7

Coding Special Complexities

LEARNING OBJECTIVES

After completing this chapter, the student will be able to:

- Understand the rules and guidelines for assigning codes for pregnancy and pregnancy complications.
- Comprehend the correct usage of V codes for pregnancy conditions and their outcomes and deliveries.
- Use the decision tree for pregnancy and postpartum conditions (Tool 7-1).
- Discern the different types of fractures and dislocations.
- Understand the importance of identifying the most significant injury as the chief reason for encounter and listing it first in the coding sequence.
- Comprehend the correct terminology of burns and the ICD-9-CM codes that specify severity.
- Discern the different types of mental disorders defined for ICD-9-CM.
- Understand the coding concepts for coding special complexities from each body area and organ system.
- Apply ICD-9-CM coding concepts for diagnostic complexities to practical coding scenarios.

CODING REFERENCE TOOLS

Tool 7-1
Pregnancy/Postpartum Coding Guidelines

Tool 7-2
Guidelines for Coding Trauma and Injuries

Tool 7-3
Injury, Trauma, and Burn Index

Tool 7-4
Injury and Trauma Coding Matrix

KEY TERMS

Alcohol Abuse
Alcohol Dependence
Closed Fracture
Compression Fracture
Full-Thickness Burn
Myocardial Infarction (MI)
Normal Delivery
Open Fracture
Partial-Thickness Burn
Rule of Nines
Superficial Burn
Type 1 Diabetes
Type 2 Diabetes

Several areas of diagnostic coding require special attention because of their complexity. Because special circumstances surround each of these areas, they are addressed individually. Some of these areas, such as drugs and chemicals, hypertension, and neoplasms, are presented in table format in the ICD-9-CM book and are discussed in Chapter 6 of this text. This chapter deals with other ICD-9-CM diagnostic coding complexities, which are presented by system in the order they appear in the ICD-9-CM code book. You will note numerous references to *Coding Clinic* as well as *ICD-9-CM Official Guidelines for Coding and Reporting* in this section, which direct the coder to the most accurate coding assignment for the specific scenarios. As previously mentioned, care should be taken to use only definitive, credible resources for coding assignments.

Documentation Guidelines for Coding Complexities

Guidelines for coding medical complexities vary from one section to another within the ICD-9-CM code book. Documentation drives the coding process, and specific diagnoses can only be used when supporting documentation is present in the medical record. In instances when specific documentation does not exist, it is necessary to use an unspecified code.

The coder should keep in mind that part of her or his responsibility is to educate. The coder should not simply assign the unspecified code, but should also educate the provider on the appropriate information needed to code the diagnosis to the highest level of specificity.

INFECTIOUS AND PARASITIC DISEASES (CODES 001-139)

When codes are assigned for infectious and parasitic diseases, the medical record must be reviewed for body site, severity of disease (acute vs. chronic), the specific organism involved (unspecified if not known), cause of the infection (if known), and any associated signs and symptoms.

In Chapter 1 of the ICD-9-CM book (Infectious and Parasitic Diseases), many conditions are covered by one combination code that identifies both the condition and the specific organism. Consider the following examples:

034.0 Streptococcal sore throat
038.2 Pneumococcal septicemia

Many conditions in this section, however, require two codes: one to describe the condition and the other to describe the organism.

599.0 Urinary tract infection
041.4 *E. coli*

In Chapter 1 (Infectious and Parasitic Diseases), the following conditions can be located:

Infectious gastroenteritis (003-008). Inflammation of the gastrointestinal (GI) tract caused by different organisms such as bacteria, viruses, or parasites.

Tuberculosis (010-018). Acute or chronic infection resulting from *Mycobacterium tuberculosis.* The fifth digit for tuberculosis (TB) is determined by the method used for confirming this disease, as in the following examples:

0 Unknown
1 Bacteriologic/histologic examination

Codes from the Nonspecific Abnormal Findings section of ICD-9-CM are used when the condition is only reported as an abnormal finding rather than confirmation of the TB bacteria.

795.5 Positive PPD test, without diagnosis of TB

Streptococcal sore throat (034). Infection from beta-hemolytic *Streptococci* organism. The following conditions are assigned codes from the 034 series of the infectious and parasitic disease category:

Streptococcal pharyngitis
Streptococcal laryngitis
Streptococcal tonsillitis
Septic sore throat

Septicemia (038). Defined as the entrance of bacteria into the bloodstream; extreme caution should be taken when assigning these codes. Infection alone does not constitute septicemia, and these codes should be used only when the record indicates clinical evidence of this condition.

Care should be taken to determine whether sepsis should be used as a primary or secondary diagnosis. Per the *ICD-9-CM Official Guidelines for Coding and Reporting,* if sepsis is present at the time of the encounter or admission, the underlying systemic infection should be assigned as the primary diagnosis, or reason for the visit or admission, followed by 995.91, systemic inflammatory response syndrome.

In most instances a code from the septicemia category 038 will be assigned in conjunction with a code from the 995.9 category. If the record states that the condition is diagnosed as streptococcal sepsis, code 038.0 should be assigned along with 995.91 as a secondary diagnosis. Sepsis or systemic inflammatory response syndrome must be documented to assign a code from the category 995.9x. These terms indicate that the patient's infection has advanced into a systemic infection, and therefore the systemic infection should be sequenced before any localized infection.

In instances in which severe sepsis is documented, the code for the systemic infection—from the 038.xx or other area of systemic infection or trauma—should be sequenced first, followed by either 995.92 for systemic inflammatory response syndrome due to organ dysfunction or 995.94 for systemic inflammatory response with organ dysfunction.

According to the ICD-9-CM Official Guidelines, septic shock cannot occur without severe sepsis. Codes from the 995.9 series would therefore be sequenced first before the septic shock code, followed by the additional codes necessary to complete the diagnostic statement.

Meningitis (036). This code is for meningitis caused by bacterial infections. Codes from the 321 series, meningitis due to other organisms, should be assigned if the causal agent is other than bacteria.

HIV (042). Care should be taken in the assignment of the human immunodeficiency virus (HIV) code. Category 042 includes the following:

Human immunodeficiency virus
AIDS-related complex
Symptomatic HIV infection

Other diagnostic codes used for HIV, exposure to acquired immunodeficiency syndrome (AIDS), and other associated diagnoses are as follows:

V73.89	Testing to determine HIV status
V08	Asymptomatic HIV status when patient tests positive with no symptoms
V01.7	Exposure to AIDS
795.71	Inconclusive serologic test for HIV
V69.8	Other problems related to lifestyle for asymptomatic patient in known high-risk group for HIV
V65.44	Counseling for HIV status

According to the ICD-9-CM Official Guidelines, any patient diagnosed with an HIV illness should always be assigned 042 on any subsequent visits or encounters. These patients should never be assigned a diagnosis from the V08 or 795.71 series once they have been diagnosed with code 042.

Childhood communicable disease (052-056). Examples include the following:

052	Varicella (chickenpox)
055	Measles
056	Rubella (German measles)

Herpes (053-054). Herpes zoster (053), known as *shingles,* is caused by the varicella zoster virus. Herpes simplex (054) is a recurrent viral infection resulting from the herpes virus hominis.

Viral hepatitis (070). There are five forms of hepatitis in this category:

Type A (HAC)
Type B (HBV)
Type C (HCV)
Type D (HDV-δ)
Type E (HEV)

Sexually transmitted diseases (090-099). Diseases from this section are also known as *venereal diseases* and are usually spread through sexual intercourse or genital contact. Some examples are the following:

Syphilis
Gonorrhea
Chlamydia

SPECIFIC DOCUMENTATION ISSUES

Caution should be taken in the assignment of infectious and parasitic disease codes to observe the appropriate order for code assignment. The coder must keep in mind the primary guideline discussed in general ICD-9-CM coding guidelines; that is, assign the chief reason for the encounter. If the infectious or parasitic disease is not the chief reason for the encounter, it would not be coded first. Consider the following examples:

EXAMPLE 1

Patient presents 24 weeks pregnant with complaints of sore throat, fever, and chills. Laboratory tests reveal streptococcal sore throat.

Coding would be as follows:

647.61	Other viral/parasitic disease in pregnancy complicating pregnancy
034.0	Streptococcal sore throat

EXAMPLE 2

Patient with AIDS seen by physician for acute lower abdominal pain. Studies reveal acute cholecystitis.

Coding would be as follows:

575.0	Acute cholecystitis
042	AIDS

STOP AND PRACTICE

Assign ICD-9-CM code(s) as appropriate for the following diagnoses:

1. Poliomyelitis ______________
2. Acute streptococcal pharyngitis ______________
3. Viral hepatitis, type C ______________
4. Gastroenteritis due to *Salmonella* infection ______________
5. Gastroenteritis, probably viral ______________
6. Varicella ______________
7. Pneumonia due to *E. coli* ______________
8. Encephalitis due to malaria ______________
9. Bacterial meningitis ______________
10. Asymptomatic HIV infection ______________

Neoplasms (Codes 140-239)

Neoplasms are discussed in Chapter 6 because these codes are presented in ICD-9-CM in a table format.

Endocrine, Nutritional, and Metabolic Diseases and Immunity Disorders (Codes 240-279)

The most common and perhaps complicated diagnostic coding from this section involves the correct assignment of codes for diabetes mellitus. Diabetes is classified by a fifth digit that indicates the type of diabetes and whether the current status of diabetes is controlled or uncontrolled. The fifth digits for diabetes are as follows:

0	Type 2 unspecified type, not stated as uncontrolled
1	Type 1 juvenile type, not stated as uncontrolled
2	Type 2 or unspecified type, uncontrolled
3	Type 1 juvenile type, uncontrolled

Type 1 diabetes includes the following:
- Juvenile type
- Insulin dependent
- Ketosis prone

Type 2 diabetes includes the following:
- Non–insulin dependent
- Adult onset, maturity onset
- Not otherwise specified (NOS)

When patients with diabetes receive insulin during hospitalization, it should NOT be assumed that the patient is insulin dependent. It is not unusual for patients with type 2 diabetes to require short-term administration of insulin for regulation of diabetes.

Many complications occur as sequelae of diabetes mellitus. Acute metabolic changes arise but do not require assignment of an additional code. When conditions occur in other body areas or organ systems as the result of diabetes, two codes are required: one for the diabetic complication and one for the manifestation. Because the diabetes occurs and is responsible for the manifestations, the diabetes code should be assigned first, followed by the manifestation code(s). Instructions in ICD-9-CM indicate coding the underlying condition (diabetes) first. Manifestations for these conditions are as follows:

249.xx	Secondary diabetes
250.1x	Diabetes with ketoacidosis
250.2x	Diabetes with hyperosmolarity
250.3x	Diabetes with other coma
250.4x	Diabetes with renal manifestations
250.5x	Diabetes with ophthalmic manifestations
250.6x	Diabetes with neurologic manifestations
250.7x	Diabetes with peripheral circulatory disorders
250.8x	Diabetes with other specified manifestations
250.9x	Diabetes with unspecified complications

Further explanation of some of the most common complications follows. Fifth digits are required.

DIABETES WITH KETOACIDOSIS (250.1X)

Diabetic ketoacidosis occurs because of a lack of insulin. Most often this condition occurs in patients with type 1 diabetes. For that reason, code 250.11 should be assigned unless the medical documentation specifically states non-insulin-dependent diabetes.

DIABETES WITH RENAL MANIFESTATIONS (250.4X)

Conditions related to the kidneys are coded with 250.4x as well as a manifestation code of 583.81 (nephritis and nephropathy, not specified as acute or chronic, in diseases classified elsewhere). When the renal condition has progressed to reported chronic renal failure (CRF), codes 585.9 (chronic renal failure) and 250.4x would be assigned with the diabetes assigned as the primary code. It is not necessary to assign the additional code of 583.81.

DIABETES WITH OPHTHALMIC MANIFESTATIONS (250.5X)

Another manifestation of diabetes is the development of diabetic cataract, also referred to as a *snowflake cataract*. Senile cataracts occur frequently in patients with diabetes but are not a result of the diabetic condition. Therefore a regular diabetes code, 250.0x, and a regular ICD-9-CM code for the cataract, such as 366.10, would be assigned.

DIABETIC FOOT ULCERS (250.6X-250.8X)

Foot complications, most commonly foot ulcers, are a common condition among people with diabetes. In many instances these foot ulcers result from peripheral vascular disease and peripheral neuropathy. When documentation supports that the ulcer results from existing peripheral vascular disease, codes from the 250.6 and 250.7 series are used. If documentation does not specify whether the ulcer is caused by peripheral vascular disease, a code from the 250.8 series, other specified manifestations, is appropriate.

DIABETES AND PREGNANCY (648.0X)

Codes from the 600 series are assigned for conditions that arise or require treatment during pregnancy. Therefore the 250.0x codes would not apply during the antepartum and postpartum periods.

OTHER CONDITIONS

Hyperthyroidism and hypothyroidism are conditions listed in this section. Hypothyroidism is coded to category 244, whereas hyperthyroidism is categorized to 242. The most common form of hyperthyroidism is known as Graves disease and is characterized by goiter, weight loss, sweating, diarrhea, tremor, palpitations, and heat intolerance.

STOP AND PRACTICE

Assign ICD-9-CM code(s) as appropriate to the following diagnoses:

1. Diabetes, type 1 ________
2. Diabetes, type 2 ________
3. Hypothyroidism ________
4. Hyperthyroidism ________
5. Diabetes mellitus with hypoglycemic coma ________
6. Iatrogenic hypothyroidism ________
7. Hyperlipidemia ________
8. Diabetic ophthalmic neuropathy ________
9. Diabetic nephritic syndrome ________
10. Cystic fibrosis with pulmonary exacerbation ________

Blood, Blood-Forming Organs (Codes 280-289)

Chapter 4 of ICD-9-CM contains codes related to blood and the blood-forming organs, such as anemias, coagulation defects, and other disorders associated with hemorrhage. The most common condition in this chapter is anemia, which has multiple causes. Anemia is defined as a decrease in red blood cells, the quantity of hemoglobin, or the volume of red blood cells contained in the blood.

Types of anemias contained in Chapter 4 include the following:

280-281	Deficiency anemia
282-283	Hemolytic anemia
284	Aplastic anemia
285	Unspecified anemia

Two issues of *Coding Clinic* specific to the assignment of anemia codes state the following:

Anemia after surgery without documentation due to blood loss should be assigned as 285.1 (*Coding Clinic*, 2nd Quarter, 1992).

Postoperative anemia as a complication of a surgical procedure should be assigned to 998.11 (*Coding Clinic*, 2nd Quarter, 1992).

STOP AND PRACTICE

Assign ICD-9-CM code(s) to the following diagnoses:

1. Iron-deficiency anemia ________
2. Iron-deficiency anemia due to blood loss ________
3. Sickle cell anemia ________
4. Sickle cell anemia in crisis ________
5. Screening for iron-deficiency anemia ________
6. Acquired aplastic anemia ________
7. Atypical anemia ________
8. Nutritional anemia ________
9. Eosinophilia ________
10. Chronic lymphadenitis ________

Mental Disorders (Codes 290-319)

The types of mental disorders classified in this section are categorized in the following sections.

ORGANIC BRAIN SYNDROME

Organic brain syndrome (OBS) may be psychotic or nonpsychotic depending on the level of distortion of reality. The symptoms associated with OBS are related to impaired cerebral function. Levels of OBS range from acute and reversible to chronic and irreversible and are considered when this disorder is coded. Keep in mind the same rules already learned for diagnostic coding. Only the documentation listed may be used for diagnostic coding purposes. If the provider does not document the specific type of OBS, a nonspecific code may be required.

Remember that caution should be used in assigning nonspecific codes because of their effect on reimbursement. As previously mentioned, unspecified or nonspecific codes may be reimbursed in some instances; however, insurance carriers are less likely to reimburse nonspecific diagnostic statements made by the specialist. For instance, if the family practitioner makes the initial diagnosis of OBS, he or she quite possibly could be reimbursed for this diagnostic statement. In contrast, the psychiatrist, psychologist, and other professional specializing in the field of psychiatry would be expected to specify the level of this disorder.

When a provider in the psychiatry field does not specify this information, the coder should compile a list of diagnoses or diagnostic statements that will be acceptable for coding, billing, and reimbursement.

ALZHEIMER'S DISEASE

Alzheimer's disease is coded as 331.0. This disease is a progressive atrophic process that involves the degeneration of nerve cells. As the disease progresses, mental changes occur that range from mild or moderate intellectual deterioration to full-blown dementia.

Keep in mind that the patient with Alzheimer's disease is usually elderly and may be receiving treatment for several diseases. Alzheimer's disease must be documented as the confirmed disease when this condition is coded. If the diagnosis has not been made, only signs, symptoms, or conditions such as dementia can be coded. If the patient with Alzheimer's disease seeks medical care for a laceration or illness, the chief reason for the encounter—not Alzheimer's disease—would be coded. In this case, Alzheimer's disease would be coded as a secondary diagnosis only if the condition is involved in the encounter.

METABOLIC ENCEPHALOPATHY

Metabolic encephalopathy is an altered state of consciousness. This disease process is often associated with delirium and may involve treatment by professionals other than psychiatrists, such as critical care specialists.

TRANSIENT GLOBAL AMNESIA

The diagnosis of transient global amnesia is not considered psychiatric and is therefore not coded as such. Code 437.7 is used for this condition, which may be the result of trauma, accident, or injury and usually lasts only for a few hours. Because this code is not considered psychiatric, the reimbursement guidelines followed by third-party carriers are the usual reimbursement guidelines rather than those subject to the limitations that a psychiatric diagnosis might have.

SCHIZOPHRENIC DISORDERS

Schizophrenic disorders are coded to category 295. The fourth and fifth digits for schizophrenic disorders delineate the type of schizophrenia and the level of the condition. Fifth digits for schizophrenic disorders are defined as follows:

0 Unspecified
1 Subchronic
2 Chronic
3 Subchronic with acute exacerbation
4 Chronic with acute exacerbation
5 In remission

Most psychiatrists are aware of the specific level of coding necessary for psychiatric diagnoses. If the psychiatric providers do not use fifth digits other than unspecified, consider developing a tool for guidance. The coder may not be able to determine the level of the condition on the basis of review of the documentation. The provider should include this information in the diagnostic statement.

AFFECTIVE DISORDERS

Coded to category 296, affective disorders are characterized by mood changes that recur on a cyclical basis. The patient experiences highs and lows that vary from periods of deep depression to periods of elation.

Affective disorders are diagnosed when mood disorders are beyond the usual range of mood swings. If in addition to this cyclical mood disorder the patient has manic and depressive periods, the disorder would be further diagnosed as circular or bipolar. The fifth digit for this category determines the level of the condition:

0 Unspecified
1 Mild
2 Moderate
3 Severe, without mention of psychotic behavior
4 Severe, specified as with psychotic behavior
5 In partial or unspecified remission
6 In full remission

PSYCHOPHYSIOLOGIC DISORDERS

This type of disorder arises from mental factors such as hyperventilation or paralysis and manifests itself with physiologic malfunctions. Psychophysiologic disorders are assigned code 306.

REACTIONS TO STRESS

Only acute and adjustment reactions to stress are categorized for this disorder. The psychiatric specialist must categorize the levels of reaction to stress. Code 308 is used for acute reactions to stress, and code 309 is used for adjustment reactions.

SUBSTANCE ABUSE DISORDERS

Probably the most common coding error made in this category is the coding of alcoholism, or **alcohol dependence**, compared with alcohol abuse. In most cases, the confusion is the result of inadequate or incomplete documentation.

Alcoholism, or alcohol dependence, is seen in the patient who is dependent on alcohol and is unable to control his or her drinking. As with all diagnostic codes, the physician or provider must place the patient within this category. The most common codes for this category are the following:

303.0 Alcohol dependence syndrome
303.0 Alcohol dependence syndrome, acute alcoholic intoxication

303.0	Patient presents for care in an intoxicated state; specified by the provider or physician
303.9	Other and unspecified alcoholism

The other disorder, **alcohol abuse,** is defined as problem drinking that has not been documented as physical dependence. In many cases, the patient may, in fact, be alcohol dependent; however, the treating provider does not have sufficient history or documentation to state this diagnostically. Code 305.0 is used for alcohol abuse with the following fifth digit:

0	Unspecified
1	Continuous
2	Episodic
3	In remission

As with the alcohol diagnostic codes, drug dependence and drug abuse are different. Drug dependence is seen in patients who are dependent on drugs and are unable to stop using drugs, as diagnostically stated by the physician. Drug abuse is coded for patients who have a drug problem but in whom drug dependence has not been and cannot be diagnosed at the time of the specific encounter.

SUBSTANCE-RELATED PSYCHOSIS

Many patients in whom substance and alcohol abuse or dependence are diagnosed will have additional physical conditions or problems that include psychotic symptoms. Alcohol-related psychosis is coded to category 291; drug-related psychosis is coded to 292.

SPECIFIC DOCUMENTATION ISSUES

Care should be used in assigning diagnostic codes for psychiatric conditions. Keep in mind that the chief reason for the encounter or service should always be the primary diagnosis for each procedure or service provided.

When using diagnostic codes from the mental illness section (290-319) the coder must realize that the attachment of a mental disorder diagnosis will trigger third-party attention. Third-party reimbursement for mental disorders may be limited under many health insurance contracts. All services reported with a mental disorder diagnosis will be attached to the maximum amount per calendar year or contract period.

For example, when a patient presents with a problem of upper respiratory infection (URI) and mentions that he or she is depressed, unless the physician incorporates the depressive disorder diagnosis in the diagnostic statement, the depression should not be coded. When the physician actually treats the depression (e.g., by prescription or hospital orders) and includes this information in the diagnostic statement, the coder should include the appropriate mental disorder codes. The codes must be placed in the correct order. Remember that if the patient presents with URI and indicates depression, the chief reason for the encounter is the URI, with a secondary diagnosis of depression.

Keep the basic ICD-9-CM coding rules in mind; always code the chief reason for the encounter as primary. Mental disorder codes are treated no differently than other diagnostic codes.

The mere mention by the patient of a "depressed" feeling or state does not require coding for "depressive disorder" unless documented by the physician or provider. When the chief reason for the encounter is an injury that was inflicted because of a mental disorder, the chief reason for the encounter is the injury, followed by the mental disorder.

Psychiatric coding is a specialty all its own. In addition to the ICD-9-CM coding book, psychiatric practices typically use the *Diagnostic and Statistical Manual of Mental Disorders, 4th Edition, Text Revision* (DSM-IV-TR) for diagnostic purposes.

The primary rules of coding apply to the patient with a psychiatric disorder. All encounters must be coded with the chief reason for that encounter, admission, or visit. In some instances the visit will be for the evaluation and treatment of the mental disorder. In other instances the patient will present for another problem, unassociated or perhaps associated with the mental disorder, and the problem would be coded as the principal diagnosis. The mental disorder or associated problem would be coded as a secondary or contributory diagnosis only if that disorder is also treated or is part of the clinical consideration for the presenting problem.

ICD-10-CM Implementation Impact

The ICD-9-CM chapter titled "Mental Disorders" was expanded in the ICD-10-CM to "Mental Disorders and Behavioral Disorders." With this expansion, specific disorders are arranged differently in ICD-10-CM and more clinical details have been added.

A number of additional codes for conditions that are drug induced have been added in ICD-10-CM, such as the following:

292.2	Pathologic drug intoxication
292.81	Drug-induced delirium
292.82	Drug-induced dementia
292.83	Drug-induced amnestic syndrome
292.84	Drug-induced organic affective syndrome

STOP AND PRACTICE

Code the following ICD-9-CM exercises for mental disorders:

1. Severe manic disorder, recurrent ____________
2. Bipolar disorder, manic phase, mild ____________
3. Bipolar disorder, atypical ____________
4. Psychogenic paralysis ____________
5. Schizophrenia, subchronic ____________
6. Depression with anxiety, dependent personality ____________
7. Anxiety reaction ____________
8. Anxiety reaction manifested by tachycardia ____________
9. Psychotic depression reaction ____________
10. Aggressive personality, adjustment reaction ____________

Nervous System and Sense Organs (Codes 320-389)

Codes from these chapters deal with diseases of the nervous system and sense organs. Subcategories for Chapter 6 of the ICD-9-CM code book include the following:

320-326	Inflammatory diseases of the central nervous system
330-337	Hereditary and degenerative diseases of the central nervous system
340-349	Other disorders of the central nervous system
350-359	Disorders of the peripheral nervous system
360-379	Diseases of the eye and adnexa
380-389	Diseases of the ear and mastoid process

NERVOUS SYSTEM

The nervous system, which is composed of the central (brain and spinal cord) and peripheral nervous systems, is covered in Chapter 6 of ICD-9-CM. One of the most common conditions in this section is epilepsy, defined as any disorder or condition characterized by recurrent seizures. The assignment of code(s) for epilepsy would include one of the following fifth-digit categories:

0	Without mention of intractable epilepsy
1	With intractable epilepsy

The statement of intractable epilepsy would need to be documented in the medical order for "1" to be assigned.

SPECIFIC DOCUMENTATION ISSUES

Several types of epilepsy, such as *grand mal* and *petit mal*, may be assigned codes. None of the specific types of epilepsy may be assigned codes without the appropriate medical documentation.

Physicians may document terms such as *recurrent seizure* or *seizure disorder*. It should not be assumed that either of these statements is intended to be coded as epilepsy unless documented by the physician.

SENSE ORGANS

The eyes and ears are categorized as sense organs and are included in Chapter 6 of ICD-9-CM. One of the most common disorders is cataract, which is opacity of the lens of the eye or its capsule. Congenital cataracts are not included with other cataracts but are assigned codes from the 743 series because they are congenital anomalies. When specific documentation of the nature of the cataract is not present, the condition is coded as 366.9, cataract, unspecified.

The ear is also considered a sensory organ and is also included in Chapter 6. Otitis media and otitis externa are both common conditions of the ear. Otitis media, or inflammation of the middle ear, is often categorized further as follows:

381.00	Acute nonsuppurative otitis media, unspecified
381.01	Chronic serous otitis media
381.10	Chronic serous otitis media, simple/unspecified
381.3	Other/unspecified chronic nonsuppurative otitis media
381.4	Nonsuppurative otitis media, not specified as acute/chronic
382.00	Acute suppurative otitis media without spontaneous rupture eardrum
382.01	Acute suppurative otitis media with spontaneous rupture eardrum
382.3	Unspecified chronic suppurative otitis media
382.4	Unspecified suppurative otitis media
382.9	Unspecified otitis media

ICD-10-CM Implementation Impact

In addition to the creation of separate chapters for eye and ear, additional categories for intraoperative, complications, and postprocedural disorders were created in ICD-10-CM.

STOP AND PRACTICE

Assign the appropriate ICD-9-CM code(s) to the following diagnoses:

1. Otitis media, NOS ________
2. Chronic suppurative otitis media ________
3. Senile cataract ________
4. Cataract, NOS ________
5. Migraine headache ________
6. Trigeminal neuralgia ________
7. Parkinson's disease ________
8. Bell's palsy ________
9. Congenital hereditary muscular dystrophy ________
10. Reflex sympathetic dystrophy ________

Circulatory System (Codes 390-459)

Chapter 7 of ICD-9-CM includes codes for the cardiovascular or circulatory system. Subcategories for this section include the following:

390-392	Acute rheumatic fever
393-398	Chronic rheumatic heart disease
401-405	Hypertensive disease
410-414	Ischemic heart disease
415-417	Diseases of pulmonary circulation
420-429	Other forms of heart disease
430-438	Cerebrovascular diseases
440-448	Diseases of arteries, arterioles, capillaries
451-459	Diseases of veins, lymphatics, other diseases of the circulatory system

Hypertension is included in diseases of the circulatory system, so codes are provided in table format in the ICD-9-CM book and are therefore discussed in Chapter 6 of this book.

Rheumatic fever typically occurs after a streptococcal infection such as a sore throat. It is included in the circulatory system section because of the possibility for collateral heart damage. Rheumatic fever can recur, so categories are included for acute rheumatic fever and chronic rheumatic heart disease.

Ischemic heart disease, also known as *arteriosclerotic heart disease* or *coronary artery disease,* is included in the circulatory system. Three forms of heart disease are classified under ischemic heart disease: angina, chronic ischemic heart disease, and **myocardial infarction (MI)**.

MI is the sudden inadequate flow of blood to the heart. Code 410 is assigned for the diagnosis of MI, with a fourth digit describing the specific location as follows:

0	Anterolateral wall
1	Other anterior wall
2	Inferolateral wall
3	Inferoposterior wall
4	Other inferior wall
5	Other lateral wall
6	True posterior wall
7	Subendocardial infarction
8	Other specific site(s)
9	Unspecified site(s)

Fifth digits are assigned based on the episode of care as follows:

0	Episode of care unspecified
1	Initial episode of care—newly diagnosed MI without regard to the number of times the patient is seen or transferred
2	Subsequent episode of care—after the initial episode of care and during which the patient is seen or admitted for additional care or observation for the previously diagnosed MI within an 8-week period

When a patient has a history of MI, it is NOT coded as 410.xx but is assigned 412. Code 412 would not be used as a primary diagnosis because this code indicates there are no signs or symptoms of MI present.

Angina, or cardiac chest pain, is assigned codes from this section as well. Unlike chest pain (786.50), angina indicates that the chest pain has been determined to be cardiac in nature. A number of codes are assigned for angina, including the following:

411.1	Preinfarction angina
411.1	Crescendo angina
411.1	Unstable angina
413.9	Stable angina

Heart failure, or the inability of the heart to pump blood effectively, is assigned a code from the following areas:

428.2x	Systolic heart failure
428.3x	Diastolic heart failure
428.4x	Combined systolic and diastolic heart failure
428.9	Unspecified heart failure
428.0	Congestive heart failure

CHRONIC ISCHEMIC HEART DISEASE

Both arteriosclerosis and atherosclerosis are the narrowing of the arterial wall by the deposit of plaque. This condition is the major cause of ischemia and is reported as 414.0 with the following fifth digit(s):

0	Unspecified type of vessel
1	Native coronary artery
2	Autologous vein bypass graft
3	Nonautologous biologic bypass graft
4	Artery bypass graft
5	Unspecified type of graft

If medical documentation does not reflect that the disease is present in a native vessel or graft, the fifth digit "0" should be assigned.

CARDIAC DYSRHYTHMIAS

Cardiac dysrhythmias are defined as disturbances in the electrical activity of the heart muscle. When additional information regarding the nature of the disturbance is not available, code 427.9 would be assigned. Specific cardiac dysrhythmias include the following:

427.31	Atrial fibrillation
427.32	Atrial flutter
427.41	Ventricular fibrillation
427.0	Paroxysmal supraventricular tachycardia
427.81	Sick sinus syndrome
426.11	First-degree heart block
426.12	Second-degree heart block, type I
426.13	Second-degree heart block, type II
426.0	Third-degree heart block

CEREBROVASCULAR DISEASE

Any condition that pertains to the blood vessels or blood flow to the brain is classified as a cerebrovascular disease. The 430 series of ICD-9-CM covers codes for cerebrovascular diseases and identifies specific conditions. Subcategories are as follows:

430	Subarachnoid hemorrhage
431	Intracerebral hemorrhage
432	Other/unspecific intracranial hemorrhage
433	Occlusion/stenosis of precerebral arteries
434	Occlusion, cerebral arteries
435	Transient cerebral ischemia
436	Acute, ill-defined, cerebrovascular disease
437	Other, ill-defined, cerebrovascular disease
438	Late effects of cerebrovascular disease

Make certain that when fourth and fifth digits are necessary, such as with codes 433 and 434, that the additional digits are assigned appropriately.

PHLEBITIS AND THROMBOPHLEBITIS

Phlebitis, or inflammation of the vessels, leads to thrombophlebitis or thrombus formation in the deep or superficial veins. Category 451 is assigned for these conditions, with additional digits to classify the specific vessel(s) or site(s) involved. specify what vein

SPECIFIC DOCUMENTATION ISSUES

Documentation issues associated with hypertension are discussed in Chapter 6 of this text. Those codes are presented in table format.

MI should always be coded with a five-digit ICD-9-CM diagnostic code that identifies both the site and the episode of care. In the outpatient setting, the fifth digit assigned will typically be a 2.

ICD-10-CM Implementation Impact

Codes for transient cerebral ischemia included in ICD-9-CM in the Circulatory System have been moved to the Nervous System in ICD-10-CM as a more appropriate location.

STOP AND PRACTICE

Assign the appropriate ICD-9-CM diagnostic code(s) to the following diagnoses:

1. Mitral valve stenosis 394.0
2. Old MI 412
3. Myocardial infarction, NOS 410.90
4. Congestive heart failure 428.0
5. Thrombophlebitis, deep femoral vein 451.11
6. Cerebrovascular accident 434.91
7. Arteriosclerosis 440.9
8. Unstable angina 411.1
9. Cardiomegaly 429.3
10. Atrioventricular block, first degree 426.11

Diseases of the Respiratory System (Codes 460-519)

Chapter 8 of ICD-9-CM covers infections and other diseases associated with the respiratory system. A brief review of the codes is provided here.

BRONCHITIS

Bronchitis, or inflammation of the bronchi, can be classified as either acute or chronic. Acute bronchitis, coded to 466.0, includes the following:

- Acute tracheobronchitis
- Viral bronchitis
- Pneumococcal bronchitis
- Membranous bronchitis
- Septic bronchitis

UPPER RESPIRATORY INFECTION

When diagnosis of upper respiratory infection is made, code 465.9 is appropriate. However, if viral respiratory infections are specified, codes are as follows:

480.1	Bronchopneumonia
466.1	Bronchiolitis
466.0	Tracheobronchitis
460	Acute nasopharyngitis
460	Cold-like syndrome

CHRONIC OBSTRUCTIVE PULMONARY DISEASE

Coded to 496 when no further specification is available, chronic obstructive pulmonary disease (COPD) associated with other respiratory conditions is assigned codes as follows:

491.20	Obstructive chronic bronchitis without acute exacerbation Chronic asthmatic bronchitis Emphysema with chronic bronchitis
491.21	Chronic obstructive bronchitis with acute exacerbation Acute exacerbation of COPD Acute bronchitis with COPD Acute and chronic obstructive bronchitis Chronic asthmatic bronchitis with acute exacerbation Emphysema with acute and chronic bronchitis
492.8	COPD with emphysema
493.2x	COPD with asthma

PNEUMONIA

Specific codes for pneumonia, or inflammation of the lung, are assigned according to the underlying cause (e.g., bacterial, viral). Viral pneumonia (category 480) is further divided according to the identity of the virus.

Pneumococcal pneumonia (category 481) is used when pneumonia results from pneumococcal bacteria. Category 482 is used for other bacterial infections that cause pneumonia. When pneumonia is a secondary diagnosis to an infectious disease, the underlying disease code and a code from category 484 are assigned. When the record lacks identification of a specific organism, 485, pneumonia, organism unspecified would be assigned.

Specific *Coding Clinic* guidelines for pneumonia-related conditions are as follows:

Pneumonia and COPD should be assigned two codes (*Coding Clinic*, 3rd Quarter, 1997).

Lobar pneumonia should be assigned codes from the 481 series (*Coding Clinic*, 4th Quarter, 1985).

When available, the etiology or organism should also be coded, such as:

428.30	Pneumonia due to *Streptococcus*
482.0	Pneumonia due to *Klebsiella*

ASTHMA

When the condition *reactive airway disease* is documented, the diagnosis of asthma would be appropriate. Specific types of asthma are assigned a fourth digit as follows:

0	Extrinsic asthma
1	Intrinsic asthma
2	Chronic obstructive asthma
3	Unspecified

A required fifth-digit classification, indicating whether the patient was in status asthmaticus, is assigned as follows:

0	Without mention of status asthmaticus
1	With mention of status asthmaticus
2	With acute exacerbation

For status asthmaticus to be assigned, one or more of the following conditions must be documented:

Prolonged, severe intractable wheezing despite treatment

Prolonged severe respiratory distress

Respiratory failure

Absence of breath sounds

Lethargic, confused state due to prolonged asthmatic attack

ICD-10-CM Implementation Impact

Asthma codes in ICD-10-CM have been completely restructured. For example:

ICD-9-CM

493.0x	Extrinsic asthma
493.1x	Intrinsic asthma
493.2x	Chronic obstructive asthma
493.9x	Asthma, unspecified

ICD-10-CM

J45.0	Predominantly allergic asthma
J45.1	Nonallergic asthma
J45.8	Mixed asthma
J45.9	Asthma, unspecified

STOP AND PRACTICE

Assign ICD-9-CM diagnostic code(s) as appropriate to the following diagnoses:

1. Tonsil hypertrophy ______
2. Pneumonia, NOS ______
3. Viral pneumonia ______
4. Chronic respiratory failure ______
5. Asthma ______
6. Acute respiratory distress syndrome ______
7. COPD with bronchitis ______
8. URI ______
9. Lower respiratory infection ______
10. Sinusitis ______

Diseases of the Digestive System (Codes 520-579)

The category of digestive diseases is subdivided as follows:

520-529	Diseases of the oral cavity, salivary glands, jaws
530-537	Diseases of the esophagus, stomach, and duodenum
540-543	Appendicitis
550-553	Hernia of the abdominal cavity
555-558	Noninfectious enteritis and colitis
450-569	Other diseases of the intestine and peritoneum
570-579	Other digestive diseases

The following diseases are classified within the digestive disease section.

GASTROINTESTINAL ULCERS

Ulcers are further classified as inflammatory or necrotic. The specific location of the ulcers (e.g., gastric, duodenal, peptic, gastrojejunal) should also be given.

HERNIAS

Numerous types of hernias are assigned codes from the digestive disease section of ICD-9-CM. The appropriate codes are assigned based on the following:

- Location of hernia (e.g., inguinal, umbilical, hiatal)
- Severity (unspecified, strangulated, incarcerated)

GASTROENTERITIS

Gastroenteritis, or inflammation of the stomach, small intestine, and colon, may be caused by a number of factors. Codes are based on the nature of the inflammation as follows:

003.0	Due to *Salmonella* infections
005.9	Food poisoning
008.8	Viral gastroenteritis NEC
009.0	Infectious gastroenteritis
556.9	Ulcerative colitis
558.3	Allergic gastroenteritis and colitis
558.9	Other/unspecified noninfectious gastroenteritis

CHOLECYSTITIS AND CHOLELITHIASIS

Cholecystitis, or inflammation of the gallbladder, is assigned codes from the 575 series of ICD-9-CM. When gallstones are also involved, codes from the 574 series are assigned as a combination code for this disorder.

APPENDICITIS

Inflammation of the appendix, or appendicitis, is classified to the 540 series of ICD-9-CM. Additional digits are assigned for complications such as perforation, abscess, and peritonitis. When an appendectomy has been performed and the pathology report reflects a normal appendix, symptom code(s) that prompted the surgery, such as abdominal pain, should be used (*Coding Clinic*, 2nd Quarter, 1990).

DIVERTICULOSIS VERSUS DIVERTICULITIS

Care should be taken to distinguish diverticulosis from the condition of diverticulitis. Typically, the patient's condition starts with the condition known as *diverticulosis*, or the abnormal development of lesions or pockets in the wall of the colon. Left untreated, undiagnosed, or unsuccessfully treated, the condition may develop into diverticulitis, in which the lesions or pockets develop inflammation, possibly causing bleeding.

STOP AND PRACTICE

Assign ICD-9-CM diagnostic code(s) as appropriate for the following diagnoses:

1. Inguinal hernia ______
2. Gastroenteritis, probably viral ______
3. Nausea and vomiting with gastroenteritis ______
4. Recurrent inguinal hernia, with strangulation ______
5. Reflux esophagitis ______
6. Acute pancreatitis ______
7. Acute cholecystitis with cholelithiasis ______
8. Hematemesis ______
9. GI hemorrhage ______
10. Anal fistula ______

Diseases of the Genitourinary System (Codes 580-629)

Diseases of the genitourinary system include the following:

580-589	Nephritis, nephrotic syndrome, and other kidney diseases
590-599	Diseases of the urinary system
600-608	Diseases of the male genital organs
610-611	Breast disorders
614-616	Female pelvic organ inflammatory diseases
617-629	Other disorders of the female genital tract

Listings in this section of ICD-9-CM include diseases and disorders of the urinary, female, and male systems. Some of the diseases included in this section are listed in the following paragraphs.

CHRONIC RENAL FAILURE

Usually the result of progressive loss of renal function, CRF is assigned code 585.9. This is one of the few codes in ICD-9-CM that does not require five digits. Additional ICD-9-CM codes may be required for additional complications or manifestations that often occur with CRF.

Care should be taken to assign CRF only when appropriate. Acute (series 584) should be assigned when documentation does not support the use of CRF.

CHRONIC KIDNEY DISEASE

Chronic kidney disease is categorized by the level of disease and damage as follows:

Stage I	Kidney damage with glomerular filtration rate 90 or greater
Stage II	Kidney damage with mild decrease in GFR 60-89
Stage III	Kidney damage with moderate decrease in GFR 30-59
Stage IV	Kidney damage with severe decrease in GFR 15-29
Stage V	Kidney damage with kidney failure, GFR less than 15 or dialysis

GFR stands for *glomerular filtration rate*, which is an indication of the level of kidney failure obtained from a blood or urine test.

URINARY TRACT DISORDERS

Disorders of the urinary tract can include pyelonephritis (590.xx series), cystitis (595.xx series), calculus of the urinary system (592.x to 594.x series), and urinary tract infection (599.x). Pyelonephritis usually involves an infection that moves from the lower urinary tract into the kidneys. Cystitis involves infection or inflammation of the urinary bladder and ureters. The fourth digit assigned for cystitis identifies the type, severity, and location of the infection:

0	Acute
1	Chronic interstitial
2	Other chronic
3	Trigonitis
4	Cystitis in diseases classified elsewhere
8	Other specified types
9	Unspecified

When a specific organism is identified, code(s) from the infectious and parasitic disease section should also be assigned. Consider the following example:

UTI due to *E. coli*

599.0	Urinary tract infection
041.4	E. coli

Calculi are stones that form in the kidney, ureter, or bladder. Fourth digits are assigned based on the location as follows:

592.0	Kidney
592.1	Ureter
592.9	Urinary calculus, unspecified
594.0	Diverticulum of bladder
594.1	Other calculus of bladder
594.2	Urethra
594.8	Other lower urinary tract
594.9	Lower urinary tract, unspecified

SYMPTOMS OF THE URINARY TRACT

In many instances, signs and symptoms of the urinary tract are reported when a specified diagnosis has not been determined at the conclusion of the encounter. Consider the following examples:

599.7	Hematuria
788.20-788.29	Urinary retention
788.1	Urinary dysuria
788.3	Urinary incontinence
788.41	Urinary frequency
788.42	Polyuria
788.43	Nocturia
788.5	Oliguria

HYPERPLASIA OF THE PROSTATE

Code 600, hyperplasia of the prostate, includes a number of forms of prostatic enlargement, such as the following:

600.0	Benign hypertrophy
600.1	Nodular prostate
600.2	Benign localized hyperplasia
600.3	Cyst
600.9	Unspecified hyperplasia

BREAST DISORDERS

Breast disorders that are not defined as neoplasms are listed in categories 610 and 611 of the genitourinary system. Examples include the following:

- Inflammatory diseases of the breast
- Hypertrophy of the breast
- Lump or mass in breast
- Fibroadenosis
- Fibrosclerosis
- Mastodynia

INFLAMMATORY DISEASE OF THE FEMALE PELVIC ORGANS

Codes from 614 through 616 are assigned for inflammatory diseases of the female pelvic organs. An additional code is assigned when the organism causing the inflammation is identified. Consider the following example:

Acute inflammatory uterine infection due to streptococcal infection

615.0	Acute inflammatory uterine infection
041.00	Unspecified streptococcal infection

GYNECOLOGIC DISORDERS NOT RELATED TO REPRODUCTION

Codes from 616 through 626 are assigned for gynecologic disorders not related to reproduction. Examples from this section include the following:

617.x	Endometriosis
616.0	Cervicitis
618.x	Genital prolapse
622.1	Cervical dysplasia
620.x	Ovarian cyst
626.x	Disorders of menstruation/abnormal bleeding

STOP AND PRACTICE

Assign ICD-9-CM diagnostic code(s) to the following diagnoses:

1. Hematuria ____________
2. Acute renal failure ____________
3. Amenorrhea ____________
4. Polycystic kidney disease ____________
5. Interstitial cystitis ____________
6. Endometriosis, ovaries ____________
7. Breast mass ____________
8. Acute prostatitis ____________
9. Benign hypertrophy of the prostate ____________
10. Ureter calculus ____________

Complications of Pregnancy, Childbirth, and the Puerperium (Codes 630-679)

Conditions usually classified elsewhere that complicate the obstetric condition are listed in Chapter 11 of ICD-9-CM. Conditions that occur during pregnancy are assumed to arise as the result or a complication of pregnancy unless otherwise specified by the provider. This guideline differs from instances other than pregnancy because in those cases, the coder will assign the least significant service or diagnosis codes when documentation does not clarify otherwise.

When the provider indicates that the obstetric condition is coincidental, the diagnosis code of V22.2, pregnancy state, incidental, will be used after the primary diagnoses are coded.

Codes from Chapter 11 of the ICD-9-CM take priority over codes from other sections. Codes from other chapters may be listed as additional codes only when necessary or when they add to the diagnostic statement for the encounter.

Codes from Chapter 11 of the coding book are subdivided into the following categories:

640-648	Complications related mainly to pregnancy
650-659	Normal delivery; other indications for care in pregnancy, labor, and delivery
660-669	Complications occurring mainly during the course of pregnancy
670-677	Complications of puerperium

These codes are used for the period that begins with conception and ends 6 weeks after delivery.

Fourth digits for this section typically provide additional information regarding complications that have occurred during the specified pregnancy period. The fifth digit contains information specific to the episode of care, as indicated in the following list:

1	Delivered, with or without mention of antepartum condition
2	Delivered, with mention of postpartum complication
3	Antepartum condition or complication, not delivered
4	Postpartum condition or complication, delivery occurred during previous episode of care

Make certain that the fifth digit chosen for the pregnancy condition is allowed for the diagnosis selected. Some diagnostic codes in this section typically take place during a specific period only, such as postpartum hemorrhage.

Tool 7-1 provides a decision tree for determining the appropriate diagnosis to be used in pregnancy and postpartum coding. This tool, which will assist the coder in assignment of numeric as well as V codes, will prove invaluable for the specialty coder in obstetrics and gynecology.

TOOL 7-1

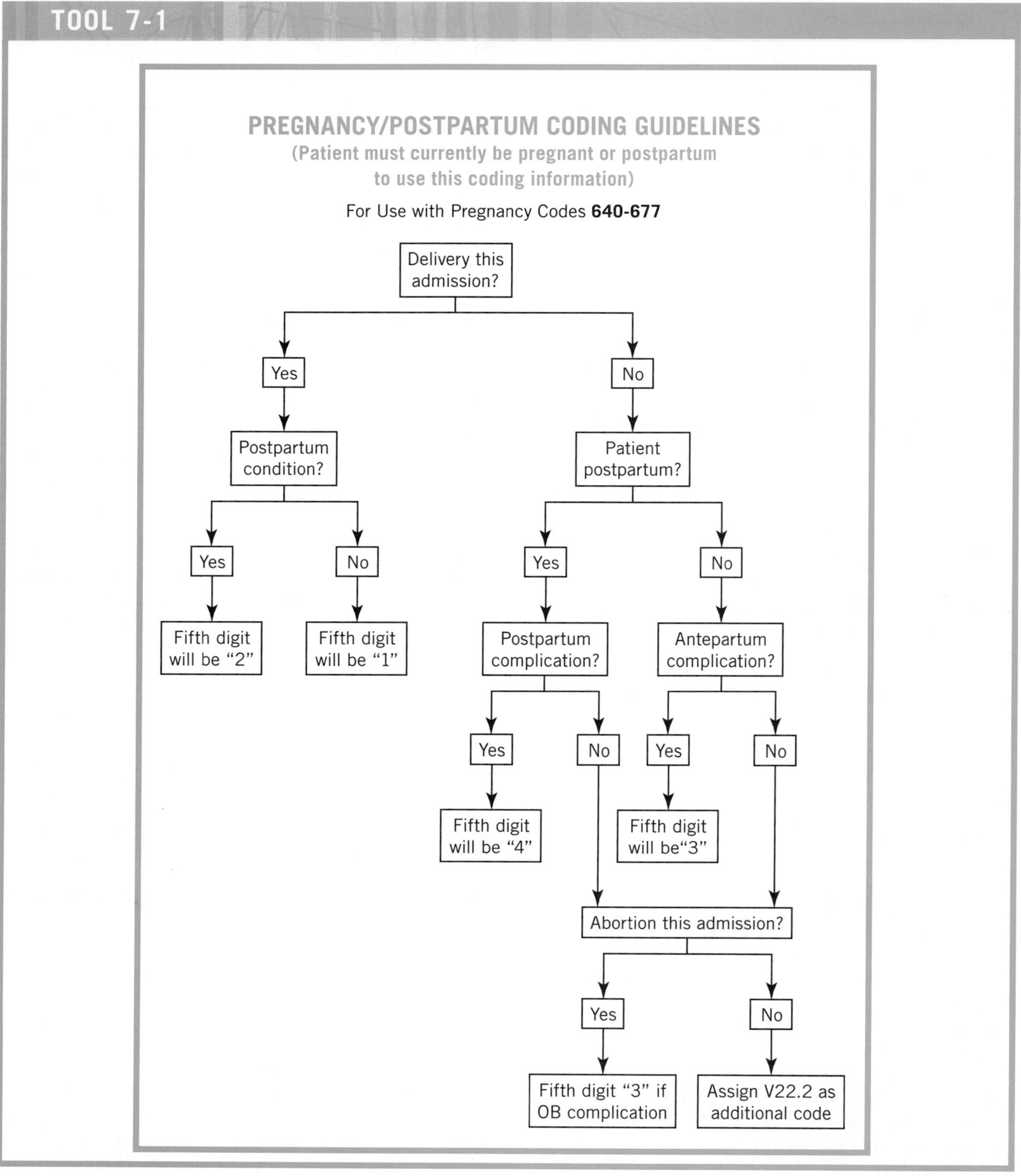
PREGNANCY/POSTPARTUM CODING GUIDELINES
(Patient must currently be pregnant or postpartum to use this coding information)
For Use with Pregnancy Codes 640-677
Delivery this admission?
Yes
No
Postpartum condition?
Patient postpartum?
Yes
No
Fifth digit will be "2"
Fifth digit will be "1"
Yes
No
Postpartum complication?
Antepartum complication?
Yes
No
Yes
No
Fifth digit will be "4"
Fifth digit will be"3"
Abortion this admission?
Yes
No
Fifth digit "3" if OB complication
Assign V22.2 as additional code

OTHER MATERNITY CODING ISSUES

Normal Delivery

Code 650 is used for coding an admission and the subsequent delivery of a baby. This code is used only when the entire delivery is normal and yields a single liveborn outcome. Code 650 cannot be used with any other code from the categories 630 through 677; these codes indicate other than completely normal deliveries.

Conditions that existed during the pregnancy but are not present during the delivery admission would not be coded. Code 650, **normal delivery**, could still be used as long as there were no other complications.

For code 650 to be used, all the following conditions must be met:

- Presentation must be head/occipital.
- Abnormalities during labor and/or delivery cannot exist.
- Complications of the antepartum period cannot be present at the time of the delivery admission.
- Single live birth can be the only delivery. Multiple births or stillbirth cannot be coded as 650.
- No obstetric procedures can be performed other than episiotomy, amniotomy, manually assisted delivery, fetal monitoring, or sterilization.

Fetal Abnormality Affecting Management of the Mother

Codes from the 655 section may be used only when the condition of the fetus is responsible for affecting the usual obstetric care of the mother. If no change is made in the mother's care, the codes from this section should not be used.

When conditions in other sections of ICD-9-CM complicate pregnancy, childbirth, or puerperium, they are coded from Chapter 11.

Preexisting hypertension is considered a complication of pregnancy, childbirth, and puerperium. Coding is changed from the 400 series hypertension codes to category 642 as follows:

642.00-642.04	Benign essential hypertension
642.10-642.14	Hypertension secondary to renal disease
642.20-642.24	Other preexisting hypertension

Other complications of hypertension may develop during pregnancy, such as eclampsia or preeclampsia. When these conditions arise, they are coded based on the preexistence of hypertension before the pregnancy.

642.4-642.6	Without preexisting hypertension
642.7x	With preexisting hypertension

As with the coding of hypertension in the nonpregnant patient, hypertension in the pregnant patient may be coded only when the diagnosis has been made. Elevated blood pressure or abnormal findings alone do not constitute justification for coding hypertension in the pregnant or nonpregnant patient.

Postpartum Conditions and Complications

Postpartum conditions and complications are defined as problems arising during the 6-week postpartum period. If the condition occurs during the delivery admission, the fifth digit "2" is assigned. Fifth digit "4" identifies those complications occurring after discharge and during the postpartum period.

Outcome of Delivery

V27 codes should be assigned to designate the delivery consequences (e.g., single liveborn) and therefore would be coded only to the mother's diagnostic statement.

Sterilization

Typically, the coder tries to avoid the use of a V code as a primary diagnostic code; however, when sterilization is coded, category V25 is appropriate. Although the service for the delivery may indicate the code 650, normal delivery, and V27.0, single liveborn, the service for sterilization has a different primary diagnosis. This series of V25 codes may be used as a primary or a secondary diagnosis when appropriate. The hospital will code the previous case as follows:

650	Primary diagnosis for admission
V27.0	Single liveborn
V25.2	Sterilization

STOP AND PRACTICE

Code the following maternity cases:

1. Hypertension in pregnancy ____________
2. Preeclampsia, delivered ____________
3. Cephalopelvic disproportion ____________
4. Fetal distress, delivered ____________
5. Uterine fibroids, pregnant ____________
6. Poor fetal growth ____________
7. Post dates, delivered ____________
8. Premature rupture of membranes, not delivered ____________
9. Retention of placenta, postpartum ____________
10. False labor, not delivered ____________

Diseases of the Skin and Subcutaneous Tissue (Codes 680-709)

Chapter 12 of the ICD-9-CM book describes conditions of the skin, hair, and nails, all of which are components of the integumentary system. Inflammation is perhaps the most common problem with the skin and subcutaneous tissue. This may take the form of cellulitis, an acute localized inflammation of superficial tissue, or dermatitis, an inflammation of the skin. Codes for cellulitis are assigned on the basis of the location of the infection (e.g., arm [682.3], breast [611.0], cervix [616.0], eyelid [373.13], neck [682.1]). When a specific organism is involved, an additional code(s) should be assigned to identify the causal pathogen.

Chronic ulcers of the skin are assigned codes from the 707 category. Decubitus ulcers, or ulcerations from prolonged pressure such as a bedsore, are assigned the code 707.0 without regard to the site involved.

STOP AND PRACTICE

Assign ICD-9-CM diagnostic code(s) to the following diagnoses:

1. Cellulitis, arm ________
2. Allergic urticaria ________
3. Ingrown toenail ________
4. Decubitus ulcer ________
5. Contact dermatitis due to perfume ________
6. Abscess of the arm ________
7. Impetigo ________
8. Pilonidal cyst ________
9. Psoriasis ________
10. Keloid scar ________

Diseases of the Musculoskeletal System (Codes 710-739)

Chapter 13 of ICD-9-CM covers diseases of the musculoskeletal system. Injuries to the musculoskeletal system, including fractures, open wounds (lacerations), contusions, abrasions, sprains, and dislocations, are covered in Chapter 17 (Injuries, Poisonings, and Adverse Effects). Musculoskeletal injuries are covered later.

Subsections for Chapter 13 include the following:

710-719	Arthropathies and related disorders
720-724	Dorsopathies
725-729	Rheumatism, excluding the back
730-739	Osteopathies, chondropathies, acquired musculoskeletal deformities

Diseases and conditions of the musculoskeletal system are discussed in the following sections.

SYSTEMIC LUPUS ERYTHEMATOSUS

Systemic lupus erythematosus is assigned to code 717.0. Because this disease is systemic, additional code(s) may be necessary for additional manifestations.

ARTHRITIS

The various types of arthritis are classified to the following codes:

711	Arthropathy associated with infections
712	Crystal arthropathies
713	Arthropathies associated with disorders classified elsewhere
714	Rheumatoid arthritis
715	Osteoarthrosis and associated disorders
716	Other/unspecified arthropathies

OTHER JOINT DISORDERS

Category 719 covers other or unspecified joint disorders such as the following:

719.0	Effusion of the joint
719.1	Hemarthrosis
719.2	Villonodular synovitis
719.3	Palindromic rheumatism
719.4	Pain in joint
719.5	Stiffness in joint
719.6	Symptoms referable to joint
719.7	Difficulty walking

ACQUIRED MUSCULOSKELETAL DEFORMITIES

Bone deformities acquired from fractures caused by disease or from nonunion or malunion of a fracture are coded from this section.

Pathologic fractures (733.1x) result from an existing disease process or occur spontaneously. Malunions, classified to 733.81, arise when fragments or ends of a fractured bone are not aligned and thereby heal improperly. Nonunion, the failure of fractured bone fragments or ends to unite, is classified to 733.82.

STOP AND PRACTICE

Assign appropriate ICD-9-CM diagnostic code(s) to the following:

1. Dupuytren's contracture ________
2. Acute osteomyelitis ________
3. Systemic lupus erythematosus ________
4. Rheumatoid arthritis, hand ________
5. Osteoarthritis, knee ________
6. Pain, knee ________
7. Fracture, vertebra, pathologic ________
8. History of arthritis ________
9. Nonunion of femur fracture ________
10. Chondromalacia, knee ________

Congenital Anomalies and Certain Conditions Originating in the Perinatal Period (Codes 740-779)

The perinatal period begins at birth and lasts through the 28th day after birth. Congenital abnormalities are present at, and exist from, the time of birth. An appropriate code from the 740-759 series of ICD-9-CM should be assigned for each of these conditions. When the condition presents itself during the admission when the child is born, the congenital anomaly code(s) would be assigned in addition to the primary diagnosis of V30-V39, liveborn infant categorization.

Liveborn female infant born with spina bifida at the hospital

V30.00	Liveborn infant born at hospital
741.0	Unspecified spina bifida

Specific conditions contained in this section include the following.

SPINA BIFIDA

Spina bifida is defined as a defective or incomplete closure of the vertebral column. With the exception of spina bifida occulta, spina bifida is assigned as 741. Further digits describe the presence or absence of hydrocephalus and the site of the spina bifida. Other conditions, such as hydrocephalus, are commonly associated with spina bifida and are assigned additional codes accordingly.

CARDIAC DEFECTS AND ABNORMALITIES

Congenital heart defects are categorized according to anomalies of the cardiac septal closure and of the heart. Category 745, cardiac septal closure anomalies, includes such common congenital disorders as the following:

745.1x	Transposition of great vessels
745.2	Tetralogy of Fallot
745.3	Ventricular septal defect

CLEFT LIP AND CLEFT PALATE

Cleft lip and cleft palate are the two most common congenital anomalies of the upper body. Cleft palate is categorized to 749.0x; cleft lip is categorized to 749.1x. A combination code, 749.2x, is used for cleft lip and palate occurring together.

MATERNAL CAUSES OF PERINATAL MORBIDITY AND MORTALITY

When a medical condition or complication of pregnancy, labor, or delivery results in conditions that affect the newborn, codes from section 760-763 should be assigned. If the condition does not cause adverse affects in the newborn, it is not necessary to assign codes. Consider the following example:

Mother consumes alcohol during pregnancy but child does not have any adverse effects.
Code only the liveborn infant code V30.00

For codes from these categories to be assigned, the condition(s) must develop at birth or within 28 days of birth. If a condition develops after this time, codes from the usual ICD-9-CM chapters would be used. Consider the following example:

3-month-old female has strep throat

034.0	Streptococcal sore throat

Note that no codes from this section (760-763) would be assigned because the condition did not develop within 28 days after birth.

Signs, Symptoms, and Ill-Defined Conditions (Codes 780-799)

When a specific diagnosis is not available at the conclusion of the encounter, code(s) from the signs, symptoms, and ill-defined conditions section would be appropriate. Codes from this section are assigned in the following instances:

- No further diagnosis can be made at the conclusion of the encounter.
- Signs and symptoms are transient and cannot be determined at the time of the encounter.
- Patient is referred for further treatment or evaluation.
- Signs and symptoms did not have the workup necessary to establish a definitive diagnosis at the conclusion of the encounter.

The use of signs and symptoms is discussed in Chapter 3 of this text, "Determining Physician Diagnoses."

Codes from categories 790-796 (Nonspecific Abnormal Findings) are required for findings on laboratory, radiography, and other diagnostic tests when the results are inconclusive and a definitive diagnosis cannot be made at the conclusion of the encounter. These codes should only be used when a diagnosis is not possible. In many cases codes from this section are necessary to justify additional testing necessary to either rule out or diagnose a condition.

Codes from 797-799 (Ill-Defined and Unknown Causes of Morbidity and Mortality) are assigned when additional information is not available in the medical record. Consider the following examples:

799.0	Asphyxia
799.1	Respiratory arrest
799.4	Cachexia

Codes from the Common Signs and Symptoms category are assigned to signs and symptoms that do not have a definitive diagnosis, and they do not represent a significant finding over and above the underlying cause or disease.

Examples of common signs and symptoms would be the following:

780.2	Syncope
780.31-780.39	Convulsions/seizures
780.4	Dizziness and giddiness
782.0	Disturbance of skin sensation
784.7	Epistaxis
785.1	Palpitations
786.01	Hyperventilation
786.05	Shortness of breath
786.07	Wheezing
786.2	Cough
786.50	Chest pain, unspecified
787.0x	Nausea and vomiting
787.1	Heartburn
787.2	Dysphagia
787.91	Diarrhea
789.0x	Abdominal pain

Codes were added in ICD-9-CM for 2007 to classify pain as acute, chronic, or due to neoplasms. These codes are due to be expanded even further with the implementation of ICD-10-CM.

ICD-10-CM Implementation Impact

Additional codes for the description of pain will be added to the ICD-10-CM, including the following:

R52.00	Acute pain, unspecified
R52.01	Acute postoperative pain
R52.02	Acute pain in neoplastic disease
R52.09	Other acute pain
R52.10	Chronic intractable pain, unspecified
R52.11	Chronic intractable postoperative pain
R52.12	Chronic intractable pain in neoplastic disease
R52.19	Other chronic intractable pain

STOP AND PRACTICE

Assign ICD-9-CM diagnostic code(s) to the following:

1. RUQ pain ~~789~~ 789.01
2. Abdominal pain, NOS 789.00
3. Abnormal chest x-ray 793.1
4. Cough 786.2
5. Abnormal Pap smear 795.00
6. Dyspnea 786.09
7. Hemoptysis 786.3
8. Respiratory arrest 799.1
9. Seizures 780.39
10. Urinary incontinence 788.30

Injuries, Poisonings, and Adverse Effects (Codes 800-999)

Perhaps the most difficult part of coding injuries and trauma is the identification of the type of injury. As mentioned in the musculoskeletal chapter discussion, diagnoses that occur as the result of an injury, such as fractures, intracranial injuries, open wounds, and dislocations, are located in Chapter 17 of ICD-9-CM. Of course, most of the codes assigned from this section will necessitate the addition of an E code to describe the external or environmental cause of the injuries. Some examples of conditions included in this section are listed in the following paragraphs.

FRACTURES

Different types of fractures are specified by the following definitions:

Open: A wound resulting in direct contact of the bone and tissues with the environment. Typical descriptors for open fractures include the following terminology:
- Compound
- Infected
- Puncture

Closed: The integrity of the overlying muscle and skin has not been breached. Any fracture not specified as open is classified as closed. Typical descriptors for closed fractures include the following terminology:
- Comminuted
- Depressed
- Greenstick
- Simple
- Spiral

Pathologic: Bones weakened by disease
Compression: Attributable to disease or trauma
Vertebral: Involves spinal cord injury
Skull: Fifth digit specifies level of consciousness

Fractures attributable to birth injuries are classifiable elsewhere. Fractures that are not classified as open or closed are always coded as closed. The coder always assumes the lowest, least complex service or encounter and the least complicated diagnosis when specific information is not available.

Coding Clinic guidelines specific to fractures include:

Multiple fracture code should be utilized when insufficient detail in the record as to specific locations, multiple trauma transferred to another facility, or insufficient space on claim to list each fracture (*Coding Clinic*, 1st Quarter, 2005).

Admissions for therapy in conjunction with fracture coded to orthopedic aftercare (*Coding Clinic*, 4th Quarter, 1999).

Encounters for cast removal assigned as V54.8 (*Coding Clinic*, 1st Quarter, 1990).

INTRACRANIAL INJURIES

Intracranial injuries include the following conditions and diagnoses:

- Concussion
- Cerebral laceration or contusion
- Intracranial hemorrhage

Code 850 is used for concussions, with the fifth digit used for coding the level of consciousness associated with the injury.

INTERNAL INJURIES

Codes from this category include injury to internal organs such as:

- Heart
- Lung
- Liver
- Kidney
- Pelvic organs

Internal injuries constitute a variety of wounds such as lacerations, tears, traumatic rupture, penetrating wounds, blunt trauma, and other open wounds. The fourth digit for internal injuries specifies whether there is an associated open wound.

OPEN WOUNDS

This classification includes all open wounds other than those caused by internal injury. Included are injuries or wounds to the skin, tendon, or muscle. They may be caused by laceration, puncture, trauma, or avulsion. Open wounds may be classified as complicated or uncomplicated. For open wound injuries to be classified as complicated, medical documentation and the diagnostic statement must specify delayed healing or treatment, the presence of a foreign body, or infection. The fourth digit indicates whether the wound is simple or complicated or whether there is tendon involvement.

BLOOD VESSEL AND NERVE INJURIES

These codes are used when a primary injury results in minor damage to peripheral nerves or blood vessels. Injuries to nerves or the spinal cord are coded with codes 950-957. Blood vessel injuries are coded with codes 900-904.

SUPERFICIAL INJURIES

These codes include injuries that involve blisters, abrasions, and friction burns.

CONTUSIONS

Contusions include bruises and hematoma without a fracture or open wound. If a fracture or open wound occurs at the same time, the coder should code whichever is the most significant injury to that site—the fracture or the open wound.

CRUSH INJURY

Crush injuries include injuries not complicated by concussion, fracture, injury to internal organs, or intracranial injury.

DISLOCATION

This injury includes subluxation or displacement. As with fractures, dislocations may be open or closed. If not specified, the dislocation should be coded to the least specific level of closed.

SPRAIN OR STRAIN

Sprain or strain injuries can occur to joint capsules, ligaments, muscles, and tendons. The rules listed in Tool 7-2 for coding injuries and trauma may help correctly assign ICD-9-CM codes for these cases. In addition, Tool 7-3 is an index for locating the proper injury, trauma, and burn codes. The type of injury has been defined so that the coder may select the proper category for coding the injury. Additional information regarding the injury involves the location and complications.

The coder may wish to develop an injury or trauma "coding matrix" such as Tool 7-4. Keep in mind that this matrix should be developed according to the diagnoses most commonly used in the coder's practice. Also remember that this matrix, as well as others that have been developed, serves as a reference tool and should be updated with each new edition of ICD-9-CM and Current Procedural Terminology books. As with any coding matrix that has been developed, the codes should be cross-referenced in the alphabetical and numeric indexes of ICD-9-CM until every code has been verified. The coder may wish to mark codes in the ICD-9-CM code book after they have been cross-referenced. After completion of cross-reference verification, the coder should document the verification of this information and keep a copy of this information on file.

STOP AND PRACTICE

Assign the appropriate ICD-9-CM codes to these injury and trauma cases:

1. Paralysis of right wrist ______
2. Nonunion of fracture, neck of femur ______
3. Fracture, pelvis, right femur, right foot ______
4. Contusions, right cheek/right forearm/right hand ______
5. Open wound, right thigh and knee ______
6. Fracture, left hip ______
7. Compound fracture, left tibia/fibula ______
8. Fracture, left pelvic ______
9. Pneumothorax trauma w/o mention of open wound ______
10. Stab wound of abdominal wall, infected ______

TOOL 7-2

GUIDELINES FOR CODING TRAUMA AND INJURIES

1. Primary axis indicates the type of injury (e.g., fracture).
2. Injuries classifiable to more than one subcategory should be coded separately unless a combination code is available.
3. Always code the most severe injury as primary diagnosis.
4. Late effect injury codes are always coded after the residual condition.
5. Assign V codes for aftercare required for wires, pins, plates, and external fixation devices.
6. Assign E codes for accidents.

TOOL 7-3

INJURY, TRAUMA, AND BURN INDEX

Fractures	820-829
Dislocations	830-839
Sprains/Strains	840-848
Intracranial Injuries	850-854
Internal Injuries	860-869
Open Wounds	870-897
Blood Vessel Injuries	900-904
Late Effects of Injuries	905-909
Superficial Injuries	910-919
Contusions	920-924
Crushing Injuries	925-929
Foreign Body Entering Through Orifice	930-939
Burns	940-949
Nerve/Spinal Cord Injuries	950-957
Complications of Trauma and Unspecified Injuries	958-959

BURNS

All burns (except friction burns and sunburn, which are not considered burns) are classified to categories 940-949. Friction burns are classified as superficial injuries. Sunburn is coded to 692.71, inflammatory conditions of skin and subcutaneous tissues.

Categorization of Burns

When coding burns, remember the following information regarding the degree of burn:

Superficial burn	Erythema
Partial-thickness burn	Blistering
Full-thickness burn	Full-thickness (muscle) involvement

In burn codes, the numbers identify and code the following:

First axis	Identifies the anatomic site
Fourth digit	Identifies the depth of the burn
Fifth digit	Provides more specified site information

With burns of more than one site, code the most severe burn first. When the body service area codes are used, the **rule of nines** applies.

Each arm	9%
Each leg	18%
Anterior trunk	18%
Posterior trunk	18%
Genitalia	9%

When full-thickness burns are coded, it is necessary to code the body surface area involved. Code 958.3 should be used for posttraumatic wound infection not elsewhere classified.

TOOL 7-4

INJURY AND TRAUMA CODING MATRIX

Site	Contusion	Superficial Injury*	Wound, Open: Uncomplicated	Wound, Open: Complicated	Sprain/ Strain	Fracture: Closed	Fracture: Open	Dislocation: Closed	Dislocation: Open	Burns: Superficial	Burns: Partial-Thickness	Burns: Full-Thickness
Abdomen	922.2	911	879.2	879.3	848.8	N/A	N/A	N/A	N/A	942.13	942.23	942.33
Ankle	924.21	916	891.0	891.1	845.00	824.8	824.9	837.0	837.1	945.23	945.23	945.33
Arm	923.9	913	884.0	884.1	840.9	818.0	818.1	839.8	839.9	943.10	943.20	943.30
Shoulder												
Humerus												
Elbow												
Forearm												
Wrist												
Finger(s)												
Back	922.31	911	876.0	876.1	847.9	805.8	805.9	839.8	839.9	942.14	942.24	942.34
Cervical	922.31	911	876.0	876.1	847.0	805.0	805.1	839.00	839.10	942.14	942.24	942.34
Coccyx	922.32	911	876.0	876.1	847.4	805.6	805.7	839.41	839.51	942.14	942.24	942.34
Dorsal	922.31	911	876.0	876.1	847.1	805.2	805.3	839.21	839.31	942.14	942.24	942.34
Lumbar	922.31	911	876.0	876.1	847.2	805.4	805.5	839.20	839.30	942.14	942.24	942.34
Leg												
Femur												
Knee												
Tibia												
Fibula												

*Superficial injuries require fourth digit for 910-917, 919:
0: Abrasion/friction burn, no infection
1: Abrasion/friction burn, with infection
2: Blister, no infection
3: Blister, with infection
4: Insect bite, nonvenomous, no infection
5: Insect bite, nonvenomous, infection
6: Superficial foreign body, no infection
7: Superficial foreign body, infection

NOTE: Always develop any coding matrix tools directly from your current ICD-9-CM manual. Keep in mind these codes should be used ONLY when no additional coding documentation to code to a higher level of specificity is available.

STOP AND PRACTICE

Complete these ICD-9-CM burn exercises. Remember to use E codes when appropriate.

1. Superficial and partial-thickness burns, thumbs and two fingers, from kitchen fire ________________
2. Partial-thickness burns in factory fire, determined to be arson ________________
3. Burns 30% of body (10% full-thickness, 20% partial-thickness), firefighter in forest fire ________________
4. Severe sunburn of face, neck, shoulders ________________
5. Full-thickness burns, shoulder, upper arm, elbow, garage fire ________________
6. Superficial burn of left foot, partial-thickness burn of toes, bonfire ________________
7. Burn of trachea from accidental ingestion of caustic substance ________________
8. Allergic dermatitis, face ________________
9. Superficial and partial-thickness burns of arm ________________
10. Partial- and full-thickness burns of lower leg, house fire ________________

Chapter in Review

Certification Review

- Normal delivery diagnostic codes are used when the entire delivery process is normal, there are no additional diagnostic problems, and the delivery results in a single liveborn only.
- All deliveries should include the outcome of delivery code.
- Fractures are classified as either open and closed. The coder should code the least significant (closed) injury when diagnostic information does not state the category.
- Lacerations are defined in ICD-9-CM as open wounds; therefore they are located under the category "wound, open (site)."
- Burns are classified into three categories: superficial (erythema), partial-thickness (blisters), and full-thickness (muscle involvement) burns.
- Alcohol or drug dependence is defined as the inability to cease the intake of alcohol or drugs; this must be designated by physician documentation for coding purposes.
- Alcohol or drug abuse is defined as problem drinking and drug use that has not been given the diagnosis of dependence in the physician diagnostic statement.
- Fifth digits for substance abuse codes define the period of the abuse, such as continuous, episodic, or in remission. These must be stated as such by the physician diagnosis statement.
- Codes for specific diagnoses by body area and organ system are defined by the guidelines for the specific chapter in which they are found.

Student Assignments

- Study Chapter 7.
- Review the Learning Objectives for Chapter 7.
- Complete the Stop and Practice exercises.
- Complete the Certification Review for Chapter 7.
- Complete the Chapter Review exercise to reinforce concepts learned in this chapter.
- Complete the practice exercises on the companion Evolve site to reinforce the concepts contained in Chapter 7.
- Complete the Practical Application exercise in Chapter 7.
- Complete the Workbook exercises in Chapter 7 as assigned by your instructor, or independently for additional practice.

Chapter Review Exercise

Provide codes for the following:

	ICD-9-CM Code(s)
1. Maternal venereal disease, not delivered	________
2. Twin pregnancy	________
3. Threatened abortion	________
4. Breech presentation, delivered	________
5. Mild concussion following accidental fall down steps, no loss of consciousness	________

ICD-9-CM Code(s)

6. Head injury ______
7. Laceration to hand ______
8. Contusions to left elbow ______
9. Sprained ankle ______
10. Burns to left cheek from stove ______
11. Superficial burns, 10% body surface, arm ______
12. Obsessive-compulsive disorder ______
13. Depressive disorder ______
14. Hyperventilation syndrome ______
15. Failed attempted abortion ______
16. Fetal disproportion ______
17. Rh incompatibility ______
18. Four rib fractures ______
19. Burns to left lower extremity, hand ______
20. Sternoclavicular joint sprain ______
21. Shoulder laceration ______
22. Corneal foreign body ______
23. Depression ______
24. Antisocial personality ______
25. Paranoid reaction ______
26. Separation anxiety ______
27. Abdominal mass ______
28. Cervical cancer ______
29. Uterine cancer, squamocolumnar junction ______
30. Maternal venereal disease ______
31. Varicose veins/legs in pregnancy ______
32. Umbilical cord around neck with compression ______
33. Concussion with less than 1 hour loss of consciousness ______
34. Knee laceration ______
35. Dislocation, metacarpophalangeal joint ______
36. Chemical burns of eyelids ______
37. Sander's disease ______
38. Schizophrenia ______
39. Juvenile delinquency ______
40. Multiple personality disorder ______
41. Spontaneous abortion ______
42. Insect bite, leg ______
43. Traumatic pneumothorax ______
44. Elbow dislocation, lateral ______
45. Bimalleolar fracture ______
46. Coin in nostril ______
47. Mental retardation ______

ICD-9-CM Code(s)

48. Drug addiction ______
49. Psychogenic asthenia ______
50. Arthritis, ankle ______
51. Type 1 diabetes ______
52. Hyperthyroidism ______
53. Nonvenomous insect bite, elbow, infected ______
54. Gestational diabetes ______
55. Acute pyelonephritis due to *E. coli* ______
56. Fibroadenosis of breast ______
57. Anorexia nervosa ______
58. Simple greenstick fracture, radius ______
59. Laceration of wrist with tendon involvement ______
60. Compound fracture, proximal end of ulna ______
61. Traumatic laceration of kidney ______
62. Aortic stenosis ______
63. Ventricular septal defect ______
64. Diverticulosis of colon ______
65. Maternal drug dependency ______
66. Fetal distress ______
67. Postpartum cardiomyopathy ______
68. Abrasion, finger ______
69. Skull base fracture ______
70. Open C1 fracture ______
71. Infected insect bite, finger ______
72. Acid burns to cornea ______
73. Brief depressive reaction ______
74. Developmental dyslexia ______
75. Cocaine dependency ______
76. Hysterical paralysis ______
77. Hiatal hernia ______
78. Alcohol liver cirrhosis ______
79. Aortic valve insufficiency ______
80. Hypoglycemia ______
81. Triplet pregnancy ______
82. Third-degree perineal laceration ______
83. Traumatic amputation of leg, below knee ______
84. Lung contusion ______
85. Attention deficit disorder ______
86. Aggressive personality ______
87. Viral hepatitis ______
88. Bacterial meningitis ______
89. Hepatitis B ______

ICD-9-CM Code(s)

90. Placenta previa ______

91. Antepartum hemorrhage 641.93

92. Gestational hypertension ______

93. Anxiety reaction ______

94. Septicemia due to streptococcus 038.0

95. Right lower extremity paralysis 344.30

96. Gouty arthritis ______

97. Acute alcoholic intoxication ______

ICD-9-CM Code(s)

98. Chronic alcohol abuse ______

99. Barbiturate abuse, episodic ______

100. Separation anxiety disorder ______

Practical Application

Review the following medical charts. Determine the appropriate ICD-9-CM diagnostic code(s) and arrange them in the appropriate order.

1. Progress note

PROGRESS NOTE

Chief complaint: ____________________

Date: ____________

Vital signs: BP_____P_____R_____

History:

SUBJECTIVE:
35-year-old with known history of asthma presents with shortness of breath, feeling of tightness and inability to move air. She has experienced these symptoms in the past when her asthma has not been under good control.

Exam:

OBJECTIVE:
35-year-old female in slight distress, obviously anxious. BP 120/80, pulse 70, R20 and shallow. Heart, normal rate and rhythm, HEENT, normal, PERRLA, normal, neck, soft and supple. Lungs have coarse rhonchi which cleared with bronchodilator treatments X 2.

Diagnosis/assessment:

ASSESSMENT:
Acute exacerbation of asthma

PLAN:
Treated with two bronchodilator treatments, prescribed antibiotics and IV steroids.

Jay Corman MD
Godfrey Medical Associates

Patient name: ____________________

Date of service: ____________

GODFREY MEDICAL ASSOCIATES
1532 Third Avenue, Suite 120 • Aldon, FL 77713 • (407) 555-4000

Codes: ____________________

2. Progress note

PROGRESS NOTE

Date:	**Vital signs:** T	R
Chief complaint:	P	BP

58-year-old male presents with complaints of abdominal pain for the past 24–48 hours. States somewhat nauseated, however, no vomiting. No fever, chills or other symptoms. No unusual foods during the past 24–48 hour period.

Past history: History of Cholelithiasis

Examination:

58-year-old in no acute distress. BP 128/82, Pulse 71, Temperature 98.2. Color is good, HEENT normal. Abdomen, guarded but soft and tender. Heart, normal rate and rhythm. Lungs are clear to auscultation.
Labs indicated elevated liver function is a patient with known cholelithiasis.

Impression:

Abnormal Liver Function, possibly due to cholelithiasis

Plan:

Patient name:
DOB:
MR/Chart #:

GODFREY REGIONAL OUTPATIENT CLINIC
3122 Shannon Avenue • Aldon, FL 77712 • (407) 555-7654

Codes: ____________________

3. Progress note

PROGRESS NOTE

Date:	**Vital signs:** **T**	**R**
Chief complaint:	**P**	**BP**

SUBJECTIVE:
Patient presents with history of 3–4 weeks of headaches, fever and chills. Was prescribed antibiotics for an apparent viral infection, however, little or no improvement over the past few weeks. He has finished the antibiotic regimen, and still experiences fever and headaches, nonchanged from his original complaint(s) 3–4 weeks ago. No history of hypertension, diabetes, infections, cardiac problems. Has been apparently in good health until this incident 3–4 weeks ago.

Physical examination:

OBJECTIVE:
Patient exam reveals a 37-year-old male in slight distress, probably from anxiety but appearing worn from his recent illness period. Vital signs are stable, HEENT normal, abdomen soft and nontender, heart regular rate and rhythm.

Labs show WBC 12.3, hemoglobin 13.2, Hepatitis B panel is positive. Chest x-ray was returned as normal.

Assessment:

Hepatitis B

Plan:

Will admit for inpatient treatment to stabilize his condition with IV antibiotics and IV fluids.

Willem Obst MD

Patient name:
DOB:
MR/Chart #:

GODFREY REGIONAL OUTPATIENT CLINIC
3122 Shannon Avenue • Aldon, FL 77712 • (407) 555-7654

Codes: ______________________________

4. Progress note

PROGRESS NOTE

Chief complaint: ______________________________

Date: ______________

Vital signs: BP_____ P_____ R_____

History:

SUBJECTIVE:
Patient is known-diabetic who presents with nausea and vomiting over the past week. No shortness of breath, no palpitations, however reports nausea and vomiting as well as increased urination over the past 24–48 hours.

Exam:

OBJECTIVE:
Pleasant appearing 39-year-old female who appears in no acute distress. Vital signs are normal. Appears pale, with multiple episodes of vomiting while in the office. Lungs are clear to ausculation, neck soft and supple. HEENT normal. PERRLA. Neurologically intact. Abdomen is tender from multiple episodes of vomiting, positive for bowel sounds, soft and tender apparently only from the vomiting.

Labs indicated blood sugar over 600 is a patient with known Type I diabetes mellitus.

Diagnosis/assessment:

Diabetes Type I
Diabetic Ketoacidosis

Maurice Doater, MD
Godfrey Regional Outpatient Clinic

Patient name: ______________________________

Date of service: ______________

GODFREY MEDICAL ASSOCIATES
1532 Third Avenue, Suite 120 • Aldon, FL 77713 • (407) 555-4000

Codes: ______________________________

5. Progress note

PROGRESS NOTE

Chief complaint: ______________________

Date: __________

Vital signs: BP_____ P_____ R_____

History:

SUBJECTIVE:
Patient presents with fever and chills 3 days prior to presenting to office. She has experienced nausea, vomiting, fever and chills for several days with shortness of breath over the past 24 hours.

PAST MEDICAL HISTORY:
She is a known hypertensive, with unstable blood pressure readings in the past. She also had a myocardial infarction approximately 4 weeks ago and is continuing to be followed.

Exam:

OBJECTIVE:
Upon examination, she appears ill, with shortness of breath noted. Her vital signs are stable, except for her blood pressure reading which was 190/117; however, as mentioned, her BP readings have been unstable in the past. She is not experiencing chest pain, however, has had anxiety problems in the past, and appears anxious. Heart, normal rate and rhythm. HEENT normal, neck soft and supple. Abdomen, soft and non-tender. Her lungs had bilateral crackles upon ausculation.

Chest x-ray revealed bilateral lower lobe pneumonia.

Diagnosis/assessment:

Bilateral lower lobe pneumonia, old myocardial infarction, hypertension, anxiety state

Stacy Kratt, MD

Godfrey Medical Associates

Patient name: ______________________

Date of service: __________

GODFREY MEDICAL ASSOCIATES
1532 Third Avenue, Suite 120 • Aldon, FL 77713 • (407) 555-4000

Codes: ______________________

6. Progress note

PROGRESS NOTE

Date:	**Vital signs:** T	R
Chief complaint:	P	BP

79-year-old female presents with 3 days history of severe epigastric pain associated with considerable nausea, minimal vomiting. Patient has no history of food reactions, or consumption of any unusual foods over the past few days. Denied melena, shortness of breath, diarrhea, constipation, or fever.

Medications: The patient takes hypertensive medication however does not remember the name of the medication.

Examination:

Normal appearing 79-year-old female who appears pale in color and anxious. Vital signs are stable, HEENT normal, PERRLA. Abdomen is non-tender with normal bowel sounds. The pain appears to be high in the abdominal area rather than in the actual abdominal area. Extremities are normal with no clubbing or cyanosis. Heart and lungs are normal.

Impression:

Will order gall bladder ultrasound to rule out possible cholecystitis and upper GI for possible stomach ulcer.

Plan:

Patient will have tests performed at the hospital on an outpatient basis and return as soon as tests are completed for further evaluation and treatment.

Stacy Kraatt, MD

Patient name:
DOB:
MR/Chart #:

GODFREY REGIONAL OUTPATIENT CLINIC
3122 Shannon Avenue • Aldon, FL 77712 • (407) 555-7654

Codes: ______________________________

7. Progress note

PROGRESS NOTE

Chief complaint: ______________________

Date: ______________

Vital signs: BP_____ P_____ R_____

History:

SUBJECTIVE:
25-year-old patient presents for routine prenatal visit with complaints of hyperemesis. This is her first pregnancy and 24 weeks and she continues to have intermittent nausea and vomiting throughout her pregnancy. On her last visit, she was informed that she was anemic and should carefully watch her intake of food and vitamins.

Exam:

OBJECTIVE:
25-year-old female who appears in no distress. 24-week gestation with normal development. Fetal heart tones appear normal. CBC indicates that the patient continues to be anemic, and we will supplement her vitamins with additional medications as she appears unable to hold down food on a regular basis. She will also report to the OB Unit at the hospital for IV hydration at which time a Fetal Non-Stress test will also be performed.

Diagnosis/assessment:

Anemia
Hyperemesis Gravidarum

Felix Washington MD
Godfrey Medical Associates

Patient name: ______________________

Date of service: ______________

GODFREY MEDICAL ASSOCIATES
1532 Third Avenue, Suite 120 • Aldon, FL 77713 • (407) 555-4000

Codes: ______________________

8. Progress note

PROGRESS NOTE

Date:	Vital signs: T	R
Chief complaint:	P	BP

23-year-old patient presents 4 days postoperative for cesarean section at 39 weeks for fetal distress. She delivered a healthy 6 pound 14 ounce female, with apgars of 6 and 8 and both the mother and child are doing fine.

Examination:

Her temperature is normal, vital signs are stable. The wound shows no signs of infection and is healing nicely. She is encouraged to apply lotion to the area and warned of lifting anything heavy for the next several weeks. Staples are removed and she is to return at 6 weeks for her postpartum re-check and discharge.

Impression:

Normal postpartum check and suture removal

Plan:

Return at six weeks postpartum for re-check and discharge.

Adam Westy MD

Patient name:
DOB:
MR/Chart #:

GODFREY MEDICAL ASSOCIATES
1532 Third Avenue, Suite 120 • Aldon, FL 77713 • (407) 555-4000

Codes: ______________________________

9. Emergency room record

EMERGENCY ROOM RECORD

Name:	**Age:**	**ER physician:**
	DOB:	
Allergies/type of reaction:	**Usual medications/dosages:**	

Triage/presenting complaint: Patient presents to the Emergency Room having been involved in a minor automobile accident. He went to his family physician complaining of left leg pain and the physician noted the left lateral leg to be swollen, pain to touch and sent the patient to the Emergency Room for further evaluation and x-ray.

Initial assessment:

Time	**T**	**P**	**R**	**BP**	**Other:**					

Medication orders:

Lab work:

X-Ray:

Physician's report:

The patient appears in no acute distress. Vital signs are normal. Leg appears swollen, painful to touch and an x-ray is ordered that reveals a small fracture of the proximal tibia. Splint is placed and the patient is instructed to non-weight bear for approximately 7 days and then partial weight-bearing for approximately 3–4 weeks. Patient should return to his physician for further follow-up.

Diagnosis:	**Physician sign/date**
ASSESSMENT: Proximal Tibia Fracture PLAN: Follow up with physician in approximately 6 weeks for further evaluation and treatment.	Robert Rai MD
Discharge **Transfer** **Admit** **Good** **Satisfactory** **Other:**	

GODFREY REGIONAL HOSPITAL
123 Main Street • Aldon, FL 77714 • (407) 555-1234

Codes: ____________________________

10. Progress note

PROGRESS NOTE

Date:	**Vital signs:** T R
Chief complaint:	P BP

SUBJECTIVE:
14-year-old presents to the physician's office for evaluation and treatment following an altercation with his brother at home. He complains of multiple injuries consisting of bruises, cuts and scrapes and his mother requests evaluation and appropriate treatment. He denies any loss of consciousness, double vision or any other symptoms. Apparently the altercation was more of a wrestling match and neither party appeared to have been injured significantly.

Physical examination:

OBJECTIVE:
14-year-old in no acute distress who presents with multiple cuts and scrapes on his upper extremities. Head is atraumatic, neck soft and supple, PERRLA. His left upper extremity has multiple contusions on the anterior surface, with a minimal laceration to the lower part of his upper extremity which does not require suturing or treatment. His right upper extremity has an area of swelling with discoloration but not open wounds or concerns.

Assessment:

Abrasions to upper extremities
Contusion to R upper extremity
Open wound to arm
Resulting from altercation

Plan:

Willem Obst MD

Patient name:
DOB:
MR/Chart #:

GODFREY REGIONAL OUTPATIENT CLINIC
3122 Shannon Avenue • Aldon, FL 77712 • (407) 555-7654

Codes: ____________________

Additional Practical Exercises

Take the practical exercises completed at the end of Chapter 3, where you identified the diagnostic statements necessary to identify WHY the services were provided, and assign the appropriate ICD-9-CM code(s). Please note that the "header" identifying each case scenario is NOT the diagnosis(es) appropriate for each scenario. Assign all appropriate ICD-9-CM code(s) including V codes and E codes.

1. Borderline hypercholesterolemia
   ICD-9-CM code(s): ____________________
2. Shortness of breath versus angina
   ICD-9-CM code(s): ____________________
3. Pain in chest
   ICD-9-CM code(s): ____________________
4. Slow heartbeat
   ICD-9-CM code(s): ____________________
5. Motor vehicle accident
   ICD-9-CM code(s): ____________________
6. Chest pain in elderly patient
   ICD-9-CM code(s): ____________________
7. Upper abdominal pain
   ICD-9-CM code(s): ____________________
8. Severe headache
   ICD-9-CM code(s): ____________________
9. Finger laceration
   ICD-9-CM code(s): ____________________
10. Shortness of breath
    ICD-9-CM code(s): ____________________
11. Chest discomfort
    ICD-9-CM code(s): ____________________
12. Injury trauma
    ICD-9-CM code(s): ____________________
13. History of bipolar disorder
    ICD-9-CM code(s): ____________________
14. Admitted patient with chills
    ICD-9-CM code(s): ____________________
15. Shortness of breath this evening, emergency department visit
    ICD-9-CM code(s): ____________________
16. Episode of dyspnea
    ICD-9-CM code(s): ____________________
17. Radiology report, venous Doppler ultrasound
    ICD-9-CM code(s): ____________________
18. Note
    ICD-9-CM code(s): ____________________
19. Fever of unknown origin
    ICD-9-CM code(s): ____________________
20. Bilateral pedal edema
    ICD-9-CM code(s): ____________________

8

ICD-10-CM

LEARNING OBJECTIVES

After completing this chapter, the student will be able to:

- Understand the changes that will be effective with the introduction of ICD-10-CM.
- Comprehend the basic layout of ICD-10-CM.
- Understand the concepts of code families and service categories with the implementation of ICD-10-CM.

Introduction to ICD-10-CM

EXPECTED DATE

An update to ICD-9-CM is expected in approximately 2013. The information contained in this chapter regarding ICD-10-CM may change in some respects. Make certain to check the final information in ICD-10-CM when it is published.

The rules and guidelines currently used for coding purposes will likely not change significantly. Significant content and format changes will be noted in ICD-10-CM. These changes are presented in some detail later in the chapter.

LAYOUT AND CONVENTIONS

The ICD-10-CM is scheduled to be divided into chapters:

Chapter 1: Tabular List
Chapter 2: Instruction Manual (may not be included in ICD-10-CM)
Chapter 3: Alphabetical Index (by diagnosis)

ICD-10-CM coding will begin with A00 and will end with Z99. Codes are scheduled to include a maximum of seven digits (those currently used in ICD-9-CM include no more than five digits). Therefore many facilities will need to reformat their computerized billing and coding systems to accommodate the increased number of digits.

The content of ICD-10-CM will be expanded to 21 chapters from the 17 chapters that make up ICD-9-CM.

The new chapters and the code families or blocks of three-digit categories included in each chapter proposed for ICD-10-CM are listed in Table 8-1.

NEW FEATURES OF ICD-10-CM

The added features of ICD-10-CM are important because of their impact on medical practices and hospitals. These changes are as follows:

- More complete descriptions of disorders and treatments will be included.
- Postprocedural disorders for each specific body system will be listed at the end of each chapter.
- The book will be organized into ICD-10-CM blocks; that is, each chapter will begin with a list of subchapters or "blocks" of three-character origin.
- Mental Disorders will become Mental and Behavioral Disorders; this section will expand from three to 11 subchapters.
- Injury, poisoning, and other externally caused illnesses will be grouped under body region, then type of injury. These were previously classified only by type of injury.
- Victim mode of transportation will be revised in the section titled External Causes of Morbidity/Mortality.

TABLE 8-1 ICD-10-CM CHAPTER LIST

CHAPTER	BLOCKS	TITLE
I	A00-B99	Certain infectious and parasitic diseases
II	C00-D48	Neoplasms
III	D50-D89	Diseases of the blood and blood-forming organs and certain disorders involving the immune mechanism
IV	E00-E90	Endocrine, nutritional, and metabolic diseases
V	F00-F99	Mental and behavioral disorders
VI	G00-G99	Diseases of the nervous system
VII	H00-H59	Diseases of the eye and adnexa
VIII	H60-H95	Diseases of the ear and mastoid process
IX	I00-I99	Diseases of the circulatory system
X	J00-J99	Diseases of the respiratory system
XI	K00-K93	Diseases of the digestive system
XII	L00-L99	Diseases of the skin and subcutaneous tissue
XIII	M00-M99	Diseases of the musculoskeletal system and connective tissue
XIV	N00-N99	Diseases of the genitourinary system
XV	O00-O99	Pregnancy, childbirth, and the puerperium
XVI	P00-P96	Certain conditions originating in the perinatal period
XVII	Q00-Q99	Congenital malformations, deformations, and chromosomal abnormalities
XVIII	R00-R99	Symptoms, signs, and abnormal clinical and laboratory findings, not elsewhere classified
XIX	S00-T98	Injury, poisoning, and certain other consequences of external causes
XX	V01-Y98	External causes of morbidity and mortality
XXI	Z00-Z99	Factors influencing health status and contact with health services
XXII	U00-U99	Codes for special purposes

- Laterality codes will be indicated in the final character of the code as follows:
  1: right side
  2: left side
  3: bilateral
  0 or 9: unspecified
- Trimester specificity will be included for obstetric coding.
- Expansion changes of the Alcohol/Drug codes will include:
  Fourth digit—Effects (dependence, abuse)
  Fifth digit—Aspects of use (withdrawal)
  Sixth digit—Manifestations (delirium)

- Expansion of injury codes will include type and site of injury:

S51.034	Puncture wound, without foreign body (FB), elbow
S51.031	Puncture wound, without FB, elbow, right
S51.032	Puncture wound, without FB, elbow, left
S51.039	Puncture wound, without FB, elbow, unspecified

- New combination codes will be included; common signs, symptoms, and complications will be added as a fifth digit.
- Manifestation codes have been eliminated through the use of combination codes that encompass the condition and the source.
- Postoperative complication codes will be expanded.
- Deactivation of some codes will take place. Consider the following:
  Immunizations will be coded differently (e.g., there will be only one code for "encounter for immunization").
  Nonspecific codes (unspecified diabetes, multiple superficial injuries) will be deleted from ICD-10-CM.
- **Code families** will be introduced. Each chapter will contain a three-character category:

C	Neoplasm/(**C**)ancer
E	(**E**)ndocrine Disorders
N	(**N**)ephrology Disorders
O	(**O**)bstetrical Conditions/Disorders
P	(**P**)erinatal Conditions/Disorders

The proposed code families for ICD-10-CM are listed in Table 8-2.

Implementation Planning for ICD-10-CM

Because many changes will come with the introduction of ICD-10-CM, both the coder and medical facilities must prepare for quick implementation.

Comparison of ICD-9-CM and ICD-10-CM

A comparison of ICD-9-CM with ICD-10-CM appears in Table 8-3, which also presents issues that may need to be resolved before the implementation of ICD-10-CM.

TABLE 8-2 ICD-10-CM CODE FAMILIES

Chapter I: Certain Infectious and Parasitic Diseases (A00-B99)			
A00-A09	Intestinal infectious diseases		
A15-A19	Tuberculosis		
A20-A28	Certain zoonotic bacterial diseases		
A30-A49	Other bacterial diseases		
A50-A64	Infections with a predominantly sexual mode of transmission		
A65-A69	Other spirochaetal diseases		
A70-A74	Other diseases caused by chlamydiae		
A75-A79	Rickettsioses		
A80-A89	Viral infections of the central nervous system		
A90-A99	Arthropod-borne viral fevers and viral hemorrhagic fevers		
B00-B09	Viral infections characterized by skin and mucous membrane lesions		
B15-B19	Viral hepatitis		
B20-B24	Human immunodeficiency virus (HIV) disease		
B25-B34	Other viral diseases		
B35-B49	Mycoses		
B50-B64	Protozoal diseases		
B65-B83	Helminthiases		
B85-B89	Pediculosis, acariasis, and other infestations		
B90-B94	Sequelae of infectious and parasitic diseases		
B95-B97	Bacterial, viral, and other infectious agents		
B99	Other infectious diseases		
Chapter II: Neoplasms (C00-D48)			
C00-C97	Malignant neoplasms		
	C00-C75	Malignant neoplasms, stated or presumed to be primary, of specified sites, except of lymphoid, hematopoietic, and related tissue	
		C00-C14	Lip, oral cavity, and pharynx
		C15-C26	Digestive organs
		C30-C39	Respiratory and intrathoracic organs
		C40-C41	Bone and articular cartilage
		C43-C44	Skin

Continued

TABLE 8-2 ICD-10-CM CODE FAMILIES—cont'd

		C45-C49	Mesothelial and soft tissue
		C50	Breast
		C51-C58	Female genital organs
		C60-C63	Male genital organs
		C64-C68	Urinary tract
		C69-C72	Eye, brain, and other parts of central nervous system
		C73-C75	Thyroid and other endocrine glands
	C76-C80	Malignant neoplasms of ill-defined, secondary, and unspecified sites	
	C81-C96	Malignant neoplasms, stated or presumed to be primary, of lymphoid, hematopoietic, and related tissue	
	C97	Malignant neoplasms of independent (primary) multiple sites	
D00-D09	In situ neoplasms		
D10-D36	Benign neoplasms		
D37-D48	Neoplasms of uncertain or unknown behavior		
Chapter III: Diseases of the Blood and Blood-Forming Organs and Certain Disorders Involving the Immune Mechanism (D50-D89)			
D50-D53	Nutritional anemias		
D55-D59	Hemolytic anemias		
D60-D64	Aplastic and other anemias		
D65-D69	Coagulation defects, purpura, and other hemorrhagic conditions		
D70-D77	Other diseases of blood and blood-forming organs		
D80-D89	Certain disorders involving the immune mechanism		
Chapter IV: Endocrine, nutritional, and metabolic diseases (E00-E90)			
E00-E07	Disorders of thyroid gland		
E10-E14	Diabetes mellitus		
E15-E16	Other disorders of glucose regulation and pancreatic internal secretion		
E20-E35	Disorders of other endocrine glands		
E40-E46	Malnutrition		
E50-E64	Other nutritional deficiencies		
E65-E68	Obesity and other hyperalimentation		
E70-E90	Metabolic disorders		
Chapter V: Mental and Behavioral Disorders (F00-F99)			
F00-F09	Organic, including symptomatic, mental disorders		
F10-F19	Mental and behavioral disorders due to psychoactive substance use		
F20-F29	Schizophrenia, schizotypal and delusional disorders		
F30-F39	Mood (affective) disorders		
F40-F48	Neurotic, stress-related, and somatoform disorders		
F50-F59	Behavioral syndromes associated with physiological disturbances and physical factors		
F60-F69	Disorders of adult personality and behavior		
F70-F79	Mental retardation		
F80-F89	Disorders of psychological development		
F90-F98	Behavioral and emotional disorders with onset usually occurring in childhood and adolescence		
F99	Unspecified mental disorder		
Chapter VI: Diseases of the Nervous System (G00-G99)			
G00-G09	Inflammatory diseases of the central nervous system		
G10-G13	Systemic atrophies primarily affecting the central nervous system		
G20-G26	Extrapyramidal and movement disorders		
G30-G32	Other degenerative diseases of the nervous system		
G35-G37	Demyelinating diseases of the central nervous system		
G40-G47	Episodic and paroxysmal disorders		
G50-G59	Nerve, nerve root, and plexus disorders		
G60-G64	Polyneuropathies and other disorders of the peripheral nervous system		
G70-G73	Diseases of myoneural junction and muscle		
G80-G83	Cerebral palsy and other paralytic syndromes		
G90-G99	Other disorders of the nervous system		

Continued

TABLE 8-2 ICD-10-CM CODE FAMILIES—cont'd

Code	Description
Chapter VII: Diseases of the Eye and Adnexa (H00-H59)	
H00-H06	Disorders of eyelid, lacrimal system, and orbit
H10-H13	Disorders of conjunctiva
H15-H22	Disorders of sclera, cornea, iris, and ciliary body
H25-H28	Disorders of lens
H30-H36	Disorders of choroid and retina
H40-H42	Glaucoma
H43-H45	Disorders of vitreous body and globe
H46-H48	Disorders of optic nerve and visual pathways
H49-H52	Disorders of ocular muscles, binocular movement, accommodation, and refraction
H53-H54	Visual disturbances and blindness
H55-H59	Other disorders of eye and adnexa
Chapter VIII: Diseases of the Ear and Mastoid Process (H60-H95)	
H60-H62	Diseases of external ear
H65-H75	Diseases of middle ear and mastoid
H80-H83	Diseases of inner ear
H90-H95	Other disorders of ear
Chapter IX: Diseases of the Circulatory System (I00-I99)	
I00-I02	Acute rheumatic fever
I05-I09	Chronic rheumatic heart diseases
I10-I15	Hypertensive diseases
I20-I25	Ischemic heart diseases
I26-I28	Pulmonary heart disease and diseases of pulmonary circulation
I30-I52	Other forms of heart disease
I60-I69	Cerebrovascular diseases
I70-I79	Diseases of arteries, arterioles and capillaries
I80-I89	Diseases of veins, lymphatic vessels, and lymph nodes, not elsewhere classified
I95-I99	Other and unspecified disorders of the circulatory system
Chapter X: Diseases of the Respiratory System (J00-J99)	
J00-J06	Acute upper respiratory infections
J09-J18	Influenza and pneumonia
J20-J22	Other acute lower respiratory infections
J30-J39	Other diseases of upper respiratory tract
J40-J47	Chronic lower respiratory diseases
J60-J70	Lung diseases due to external agents
J80-J84	Other respiratory diseases principally affecting the interstitium
J85-J86	Suppurative and necrotic conditions of lower respiratory tract
J90-J94	Other diseases of pleura
J95-J99	Other diseases of the respiratory system
Chapter XI: Diseases of the Digestive System (K00-K93)	
K00-K14	Diseases of oral cavity, salivary glands, and jaws
K20-K31	Diseases of esophagus, stomach, and duodenum
K35-K38	Diseases of appendix
K40-K46	Hernia
K50-K52	Noninfective enteritis and colitis
K55-K63	Other diseases of intestines
K65-K67	Diseases of peritoneum
K70-K77	Diseases of liver
K80-K87	Disorders of gallbladder, biliary tract, and pancreas
K90-K93	Other diseases of the digestive system
Chapter XII: Diseases of the Skin and Subcutaneous Tissue (L00-L99)	
L00-L08	Infections of the skin and subcutaneous tissue
L10-L14	Bullous disorders

Continued

TABLE 8-2 ICD-10-CM CODE FAMILIES—cont'd

L20-L30	Dermatitis and eczema	
L40-L45	Papulosquamous disorders	
L50-L54	Urticaria and erythema	
L55-L59	Radiation-related disorders of the skin and subcutaneous tissue	
L60-L75	Disorders of skin appendages	
L80-L99	Other disorders of the skin and subcutaneous tissue	
Chapter XIII: Diseases of the Musculoskeletal System and Connective Tissue (M00-M99)		
M00-M25	Arthropathies	
	M00-M03	Infectious arthropathies
	M05-M14	Inflammatory polyarthropathies
	M15-M19	Arthrosis
	M20-M25	Other joint disorders
M30-M36	Systemic connective tissue disorders	
M40-M54	Dorsopathies	
	M40-M43	Deforming dorsopathies
	M45-M49	Spondylopathies
	M50-M54	Other dorsopathies
M60-M79	Soft tissue disorders	
	M60-M63	Disorders of muscles
	M65-M68	Disorders of synovium and tendon
	M70-M79	Other soft tissue disorders
M80-M94	Osteopathies and chondropathies	
	M80-M85	Disorders of bone density and structure
	M86-M90	Other osteopathies
	M91-M94	Chondropathies
M95-M99	Other disorders of the musculoskeletal system and connective tissue	
Chapter XIV: Diseases of the Genitourinary System (N00-N99)		
N00-N08	Glomerular diseases	
N10-N16	Renal tubulo-interstitial diseases	
N17-N19	Renal failure	
N20-N23	Urolithiasis	
N25-N29	Other disorders of kidney and ureter	
N30-N39	Other diseases of urinary system	
N40-N51	Diseases of male genital organs	
N60-N64	Disorders of breast	
N70-N77	Inflammatory diseases of female pelvic organs	
N80-N98	Noninflammatory disorders of female genital tract	
N99	Other disorders of genitourinary tract	
Chapter XV: Pregnancy, Childbirth, and the Puerperium (O00-O99)		
O00-O08	Pregnancy with abortive outcome	
O10-O16	Edema, proteinuria, and hypertensive disorders in pregnancy, childbirth, and the puerperium	
O20-O29	Other maternal disorders predominantly related to pregnancy	
O30-O48	Maternal care related to the fetus and amniotic cavity and possible delivery problems	
O60-O75	Complications of labor and delivery	
O80-O84	Delivery	
O85-O92	Complications predominantly related to the puerperium	
O94-O99	Other obstetric conditions, not elsewhere classified	
Chapter XVI: Certain Conditions Originating in the Perinatal Period (P00-P96)		
P00-P04	Fetus and newborn affected by maternal factors and by complications of pregnancy, labor, and delivery	
P05-P08	Disorders related to length of gestation and fetal growth	
P10-P15	Birth trauma	
P20-P29	Respiratory and cardiovascular disorders specific to the perinatal period	
P35-P39	Infections specific to the perinatal period	
P50-P61	Hemorrhagic and hematological disorders of fetus and newborn	

Continued

TABLE 8-2 ICD-10-CM CODE FAMILIES—cont'd

P70-P74	Transitory endocrine and metabolic disorders specific to fetus and newborn
P75-P78	Digestive system disorders of fetus and newborn
P80-P83	Conditions involving the integument and temperature regulation of fetus and newborn
P90-P96	Other disorders originating in the perinatal period
Chapter XVII: Congenital Malformations, Deformations, and Chromosomal Abnormalities (Q00-Q99)	
Q00-Q07	Congenital malformations of the nervous system
Q10-Q18	Congenital malformations of eye, ear, face, and neck
Q20-Q28	Congenital malformations of the circulatory system
Q30-Q34	Congenital malformations of the respiratory system
Q35-Q37	Cleft lip and cleft palate
Q38-Q45	Other congenital malformations of the digestive system
Q50-Q56	Congenital malformations of genital organs
Q60-Q64	Congenital malformations of the urinary system
Q65-Q79	Congenital malformations and deformations of the musculoskeletal system
Q80-Q89	Other congenital malformations
Q90-Q99	Chromosomal abnormalities, not elsewhere classified
Chapter XVIII: Symptoms, Signs, and Abnormal Clinical and Laboratory Findings, Not Elsewhere Classified (R00-R99)	
R00-R09	Symptoms and signs involving the circulatory and respiratory systems
R10-R19	Symptoms and signs involving the digestive system and abdomen
R20-R23	Symptoms and signs involving the skin and subcutaneous tissue
R25-R29	Symptoms and signs involving the nervous and musculoskeletal systems
R30-R39	Symptoms and signs involving the urinary system
R40-R46	Symptoms and signs involving cognition, perception, emotional state, and behavior
R47-R49	Symptoms and signs involving speech and voice
R50-R69	General symptoms and signs
R70-R79	Abnormal findings on examination of blood, without diagnosis
R80-R82	Abnormal findings on examination of urine, without diagnosis
R83-R89	Abnormal findings on examination of other body fluids, substances, and tissues, without diagnosis
R90-R94	Abnormal findings on diagnostic imaging and in function studies, without diagnosis
R95-R99	Ill-defined and unknown causes of mortality
Chapter XIX: Injury, Poisoning, and Certain Other Consequences of External Causes (S00-T98)	
S00-S09	Injuries to the head
S10-S19	Injuries to the neck
S20-S29	Injuries to the thorax
S30-S39	Injuries to the abdomen, lower back, lumbar spine, and pelvis
S40-S49	Injuries to the shoulder and upper arm
S50-S59	Injuries to the elbow and forearm
S60-S69	Injuries to the wrist and hand
S70-S79	Injuries to the hip and thigh
S80-S89	Injuries to the knee and lower leg
S90-S99	Injuries to the ankle and foot
T00-T07	Injuries involving multiple body regions
T08-T14	Injuries to unspecified part of trunk, limb, or body region
T15-T19	Effects of foreign body entering through natural orifice
T20-T32	Burns and corrosions
	T20-T25 Burns and corrosions of external body surface, specified by site
	T26-T28 Burns and corrosions confined to eye and internal organs
	T29-T32 Burns and corrosions of multiple and unspecified body regions
T33-T35	Frostbite
T36-T50	Poisoning by drugs, medicaments, and biological substances
T51-T65	Toxic effects of substances chiefly nonmedicinal as to source
T66-T78	Other and unspecified effects of external causes
T79	Certain early complications of trauma
T80-T88	Complications of surgical and medical care, not elsewhere classified
T90-T98	Sequelae of injuries, poisoning, and other consequences of external causes

Continued

TABLE 8-2 ICD-10-CM CODE FAMILIES—cont'd

Chapter XX: External Causes of Morbidity and Mortality (V01-Y98)

Code	Code	Code	Description
V01-X59			Accidents
	V01-V99		Transport accidents
		V01-V09	Pedestrian injured in transport accident
		V10-V19	Pedal cyclist injured in transport accident
		V20-V29	Motorcycle rider injured in transport accident
		V30-V39	Occupant of three-wheeled motor vehicle injured in transport accident
		V40-V49	Car occupant injured in transport accident
		V50-V59	Occupant of pickup truck or van injured in transport accident
		V60-V69	Occupant of heavy transport vehicle injured in transport accident
		V70-V79	Bus occupant injured in transport accident
		V80-V89	Other land transport accidents
		V90-V94	Water transport accidents
		V95-V97	Air and space transport accidents
		V98-V99	Other and unspecified transport accidents
	W00-X59		Other external causes of accidental injury
		W00-W19	Falls
		W20-W49	Exposure to inanimate mechanical forces
		W50-W64	Exposure to animate mechanical forces
		W65-W74	Accidental drowning and submersion
		W75-W84	Other accidental threats to breathing
		W85-W99	Exposure to electric current, radiation, and extreme ambient air temperature and pressure
		X00-X09	Exposure to smoke, fire, and flames
		X10-X19	Contact with heat and hot substances
		X20-X29	Contact with venomous animals and plants
		X30-X39	Exposure to forces of nature
		X40-X49	Accidental poisoning by and exposure to noxious substances
		X50-X57	Overexertion, travel, and privation
		X58-X59	Accidental exposure to other and unspecified factors
X60-X84			Intentional self-harm
X85-Y09			Assault
Y10-Y34			Event of undetermined intent
Y35-Y36			Legal intervention and operations of war
Y40-Y84			Complications of medical and surgical care
	Y40-Y59		Drugs, medicaments, and biological substances causing adverse effects in therapeutic use
	Y60-Y69		Misadventures to patients during surgical and medical care
	Y70-Y82		Medical devices associated with adverse incidents in diagnostic and therapeutic use
	Y83-Y84		Surgical and other medical procedures as the cause of abnormal reaction of the patient, or of later complication, without mention of misadventure at the time of the procedure
Y85-Y89			Sequelae of external causes of morbidity and mortality
Y90-Y98			Supplementary factors related to causes of morbidity and mortality classified elsewhere

Chapter XXI: Factors Influencing Health Status and Contact with Health Services (Z00-Z99)

Code	Description
Z00-Z13	Persons encountering health services for examination and investigation
Z20-Z29	Persons with potential health hazards related to communicable diseases
Z30-Z39	Persons encountering health services in circumstances related to reproduction
Z40-Z54	Persons encountering health services for specific procedures and health care
Z55-Z65	Persons with potential health hazards related to socioeconomic and psychosocial circumstances
Z70-Z76	Persons encountering health services in other circumstances
Z80-Z99	Persons with potential health hazards related to family and personal history and certain conditions influencing health status

Chapter XXII: Codes for Special Purposes (U00-U99)

Code	Description
U00-U49	Provisional assignment of new diseases of uncertain etiology
U80-U89	Bacterial agents resistant to antibiotics

TABLE 8-3 ICD-9-CM AND ICD-10-CM COMPARISON

ISSUE	ICD-9-CM	ICD-10-CM	CONVERSION ISSUE
Number of characters	3-5	3-7	Additional field
Type of characters	Numeric only (except V and E codes)	Alphanumeric	Allow for alphanumeric system; will need to distinguish between 0/1 and O/I (numbers vs. letters)
Decimals	Allow third character	Allow third character	ICD-10-CM: decimals
Descriptions	Tabular list show partial descriptions, fourth and fifth digits	Stand-alone descriptions	Length of field must accommodate longer descriptions
Hierarchy	Fourth- and fifth-digit codes have hierarchical relations within 3-character category	Fourth-, fifth-, and sixth-digit codes have hierarchical relations within 3-character category	
Quantity	>15,000 codes in volumes 1 and 3	>24,000 codes; ICD-10-PCS >20,000 codes	More codes, more space
Format availability	Print and various computerized electronic formats	Print only; no electronic format at this time	May need to reformat to accept electronic file(s) in a different format

Chapter in Review

Certification Review

- The format of ICD-10-CM will change significantly; however, many rules for assigning codes will remain much the same.
- ICD-10-CM codes will be assigned with six alphanumeric digits.
- V codes and E codes will be incorporated into the regular alphabetical, and tabular sections of ICD-10-CM, thereby eliminating the indexes that are used in ICD-9-CM.
- Because the codes will become more specific, the coder will be able to designate right, left, bilateral, and unspecified.
- Manifestation codes will be eliminated through the use of combination codes when necessary.
- Unspecified codes (i.e., those currently listed in ICD-9-CM as unspecified) will be eliminated.
- One code will be assigned for all immunizations, regardless of which specific immunization is administered.
- Facilities must begin preparation for ICD-10-CM implementation by identifying potential problems, eliminating staff shortages, and resolving other matters of concern before the official introduction.

Student Assignments

- Study Chapter 8.
- Review the Learning Objectives for Chapter 8.
- Complete the Certification Review for Chapter 8.
- Complete the Chapter Review exercise to reinforce concepts learned in this chapter.

Chapter Review Exercise

Answer the following questions.

1. ICD-10-CM codes will be:
   a. alphabetical
   b. numeric
   c. alphanumeric
2. There will be no additional chapters in ICD-10-CM than were in ICD-9-CM.
   a. True
   b. False
3. Define *code families.*
   ____
   ____
4. Define *service categories.*
   ____
   ____
5. List three significant changes that will be made with the introduction of ICD-10-CM to the coding world.
   ____
   ____
   ____
6. List three significant issues facilities face in implementing ICD-10-CM.
   ____
   ____
   ____

Identify what chapter and code family the following diagnoses will be found in ICD-10-CM.

7. Acute bacterial meningitis
   Chapter __________ Code family ______________
8. Urolithiasis
   Chapter __________ Code family ______________
9. Burns of the eye
   Chapter __________ Code family ______________
10. Contraceptive management
    Chapter __________ Code family ______________

SECTION 3

CPT and HCPCS Procedural Coding

Section III of this text discusses coding for procedures or services for physicians and other providers. Each of these services is billed according to specific coding guidelines outlined in the Current Procedural Terminology (CPT) book. Whereas physician and outpatient facility services are reimbursed based on the code assignments from the CPT coding system, inpatient facility services are reimbursed based on *International Classification of Diseases*, 9th Revision, Clinical Modification (ICD-9-CM) diagnostic coding. During the discussion of the reimbursement process later in this text, why this distinction is necessary will become apparent.

Documentation plays a vital role in the assignment of CPT and Healthcare Common Procedure Coding System (HCPCS) codes for services. A review of this documentation involves reading and interpreting progress notes, medical histories, physical examination results, and operative reports. From these documents, the key elements needed to assign the proper CPT codes must be extracted. Such elements will differ greatly on the basis of coding guidelines for each chapter of the CPT coding book. An important consideration is that the CPT and HCPCS books differ somewhat from ICD-9-CM, for which the rules remain essentially the same from one chapter to the next. In contrast, CPT guidelines differ to some degree from section to section. For this reason, information in this section of the text is presented by CPT chapter. The documents necessary for obtaining the information for coding, the specific rules for assigning codes for those services, and coding assignment exercises are introduced accordingly.

CPT, currently in the fourth edition, is used in much the same way as the ICD-9-CM coding book. CPT, however, provides standardization for coding billable services and procedures (i.e., WHAT was performed) rather than explanations of the medical necessity or diagnosis for the encounter. The information coded from CPT is also used for standardization in billing and compilation of statistical information in much the same way as ICD-9-CM information is used.

It is important to emphasize that only by using ICD-9-CM and CPT and HCPCS coding for provider services does the coder get the opportunity to describe WHAT (procedure: CPT) service took place, as well as justify WHY (diagnosis: ICD-9-CM) the service took place. Claim forms do not give the coder or biller the opportunity to explain the circumstances surrounding a particular service. This explanation must be clearly and concisely provided with the use of CPT and ICD-9-CM codes.

The information contained in the summary of CPT and ICD-9-CM and HCPCS codes should "tell the story" of what services were performed and why those services were medically necessary. If this is successfully accomplished, appropriate reimbursement will be the result. ■

9

Determining Codeable Services and Applying Modifiers

LEARNING OBJECTIVES

After completing this chapter, the student will be able to:

- Understand the key elements of physician documentation that drive the assignment of Current Procedural Terminology (CPT) codes.
- Follow the basic steps in the CPT coding process.
- Comprehend the difference between diagnostic codes and procedural codes.
- Understand how the proper use of both diagnostic and procedural codes "tells the story" of what services were performed and gives the medical necessity (diagnosis) for those services.
- Understand the importance of properly matching the descriptions (codes) for WHAT services were performed (CPT) with those explaining WHY (*International Classification of Diseases*, 9th Revision, Clinical Modification [ICD-9-CM]) services were performed.
- Understand the global surgical concept and what the terms *bundled* and *unbundled* refer to in relation to this process.
- Understand the concept of "separate procedure" in CPT use.
- Comprehend the rules and application of modifiers to the coding process.
- Know the proper application of each modifier.
- Understand the appropriate reason for applying modifiers to services.
- Grasp the reimbursement significance of proper modifier code(s) submission.
- Apply modifier coding concepts to practical coding scenarios.

CODING REFERENCE TOOLS

Tool 9-1
CPT Coding Steps

Tool 9-2
CPT Coding Guidelines

Tool 9-3
Proper Use of Modifiers

Tool 9-4
CPT Modifier Coding Reference Tool

KEY TERMS

Bilateral

Bundled

Current Procedural Terminology (CPT)

Evaluation and Management Codes

Global Procedure

Healthcare Common Procedure Coding System (HCPCS)

Incidental Procedure

Modifier Code

Modifiers

KEY TERMS—*cont'd*

- National Correct Coding Initiative (NCCI)
- Pathology
- Professional Component
- Radiology
- Separate Procedure
- Surgery
- Technical Component
- Unbundled
- Unlisted Procedure

The Concept of Codeable Services

In the world of Current Procedural Terminology (CPT) coding, information on WHAT services may be coded and billed is located in specific sections or chapters of CPT, where individualized guidelines for specific types of service to be followed may also be found.

GENERAL DOCUMENTATION GUIDELINES

Only services that have been documented may be coded and billed (as is the case with ICD-9-CM diagnostic coding). In addition, signature requirements for documentation, as discussed in Section 1 of this text, apply to services as well. Services from any section of CPT may be billed by any licensed professionals with the credentials to perform those services in their respective state or area. There are no restrictions on specific physicians or specialties coding and billing only from a specific section of the CPT book. The student will, however, see in an in-depth discussion of each CPT section that certain specialties and professionals will use certain sections of the CPT book more than others. For instance, an orthopedic surgeon will most commonly use the musculoskeletal surgical section of CPT; however, if the surgeon performs a nerve block (located in the nervous system section of CPT), use of that code by the orthopedic surgeon would be appropriate. In addition, the orthopedic surgeon may use evaluation and management codes for visits or encounters with the patient, radiology codes for performing or interpreting radiologic studies, pathology codes when interpreting laboratory testing, as well as medicine codes when performing diagnostic studies.

At a minimum, the service must be documented according to guidelines pertaining to that procedure, and it must be authenticated, or signed, by a physician. In addition, for the physician service or procedure to be billed, the provider must document his or her interpretation of these services and meet signature requirements.

Perhaps the most difficult part of CPT procedural coding is identifying the key words in the document so that documentation requirements for the CPT descriptor may be satisfied. Because a number of CPT procedural codes describe service(s) provided, each code needs to be considered carefully; the CPT descriptor needs to be compared with the information contained in the medical documentation.

The process of extracting chart information needed for coding procedures with CPT is discussed later in this chapter.

MATCHING SERVICES AND DIAGNOSTIC CODES

The order of services provided is important for CPT coding (as it is with ICD-9-CM). The order of CPT and ICD-9-CM codes together can make the difference between reimbursement and denial of payment. As mentioned throughout this text, the correct order for each procedure is critical.

> Patient presents to the *physician's office* because of an ongoing problem with cough, fever, and cold symptoms. *Chest x-ray* and *complete blood count (CBC)* are ordered, which indicate the presence of an *upper respiratory infection*. In addition, the patient complains of urinary frequency; therefore a *urinalysis* is performed and a diagnosis of *urinary tract infection* is made.

Review the "story" of what services were provided and why those services were performed.

Services (WHAT)	Diagnosis (WHY)
Physician office visit	Upper respiratory infection
	Urinary tract infection
Urinalysis	Urinary tract infection
CBC	Upper respiratory infection
Chest x-ray	Upper respiratory infection

Diagnoses and procedural codes must coincide for proper reimbursement. Medical necessity is also justified when the appropriate diagnostic codes are assigned for each service (CPT code) provided.

NOTE: There will always be a WHAT (procedure or service) necessitated by at least one WHY (diagnosis or medical necessity).

Take another look at the above example and demonstrate what happens when services are matched with an inappropriate diagnosis:

> Patient presents to the *physician's office* because of an ongoing problem with cough, fever, and cold symptoms. *Chest x-ray* and *CBC* are ordered, which indicate the

presence of an *upper respiratory infection.* In addition, the patient complains of urinary frequency; therefore a *urinalysis* is performed and a diagnosis of ***urinary tract infection*** is made.

Services (WHAT)	Diagnosis (WHY)
Physician office visit	Upper respiratory infection
	Urinary tract infection
Urinalysis	Upper respiratory infection
CBC	Urinary tract infection
Chest x-ray	Urinary tract infection

As the result of the above inappropriate assignment or "matching" of diagnoses to services performed, the information given to the insurance company and the outcome would be as follows:

The patient came to the physician's office to be evaluated for an upper respiratory infection and urinary tract infection.

PAID services are supported as medically necessary.
A urinalysis was performed and was diagnostic of an upper respiratory infection.
A urinalysis is an analysis of urine and would not provide information regarding the presence or absence of an upper respiratory infection.
DENIED as the charge is "not medically necessary" or "diagnosis does not match services performed."
A CBC revealed a urinary tract infection.
The CBC would be obtained from a blood specimen, which would not indicate the presence of a urinary tract infection.
DENIED as "not medically necessary" or "diagnosis does not match services performed."
Chest x-ray findings indicated the presence of a urinary tract infection.
The chest x-ray, which is a radiologic image, would reveal findings only of the respiratory system and, more specifically, the lungs. Therefore the diagnosis of a urinary tract infection could not be made based on a chest x-ray.
DENIED for the same reason as above, "not medically necessary" or "diagnosis does not match services performed."

In summary, four services were provided during the above encounter. When the diagnoses are not appropriately matched to the services, only one of the four services, or 25% of the services coded and billed, will be paid by the insurance carrier. Obviously, this type of error could represent a significant loss of revenue for the practice. You will learn later that resubmissions and corrections of these types of errors are costly and often overlooked until time limitations established by the carriers have expired. As a result, many providers never receive reimbursement for the additional 75% of services.

STOP AND PRACTICE

Part I: Matching Services and Medically Necessary Diagnoses

Match the following services with the appropriate diagnoses. More than one diagnosis may be appropriate, and each diagnosis can be used more than once if necessary.

1. Computed tomography (CT), abdomen
2. Pulmonary function test
3. Colonoscopy
4. Incision and drainage, finger abscess
5. Thyroid-stimulating hormone test
6. Bronchoscopy
7. Removal of foreign body (FB), finger
8. Tetanus immunization
9. Open reduction internal fixation (ORIF), distal radius
10. Esophagoscopy with FB removal
11. Removal impacted ear cerumen
12. Circumcision
13. Vaginal delivery
14. Well-baby exam
15. Urinalysis
16. Pap smear
17. Annual exam
18. Amniocentesis
19. Biopsy skin
20. Visual acuity exam

a. Diarrhea
b. Chronic obstructive pulmonary disease
c. Hyperthyroidism
d. Abdominal pain
e. Pulmonary fibrosis
f. General medical exam
g. Fetal abnormality
h. Finger abscess
i. Prophylactic immunization for tetanus
j. FB, finger
k. Normal pregnancy
l. Hematuria
m. Well-woman exam
n. Skin lesion
o. Excessive foreskin
p. Myopia
q. Fracture, distal radius
r. FB esophagus
s. Six-month baby checkup
t. Impacted cerumen

STOP AND PRACTICE—cont'd

Part II: Identify WHAT Services and WHY

For the following progress notes, identify services (WHAT) and WHY the services are medically necessary based on the documentation provided.

Chart 1

S: This 14-year-old female presents after hurting her left thumb. She states she was in a basketball game last night and she fell. She has not taken any medications for pain. Patient is right-handed and wants to make sure her thumb is not broken because she has another game tomorrow evening.

O: Vital signs normal. Left hand has slight swelling over the distal phalanx of the thumb. No erythema present. In addition, she has a 2-cm laceration to the second digit that will require repair.

Radiology of thumb shows no acute bony abnormality.

A: Sprain of left thumb, open wound second finger

P: Patient given thumb splint and advised to take ibuprofen. Repair of 2-cm simple laceration was completed before discharge. Wound was sutured and bandaged with Kerlix.

Services (WHAT)	Medical Necessity or Diagnosis (WHY)
__________	__________
__________	__________
__________	__________
__________	__________
__________	__________
__________	__________
__________	__________

Chart 2

This 5-year-old female comes in with her mother over concerns regarding an ear infection. She has also been having abdominal pain. Her last ear infection was approximately 2 months ago. She has no fever or chills. She has slight abdominal pain, more abdominal cramping, off and on, for the past several weeks. Currently she is on no medications.

On exam, the left ear has slight erythema. The right ear is more erythematous than the left. PERRLA (pupils equal, round, reactive to light and accommodation), no discharge. Abdomen: bowel sounds present, soft, not tender, no rigidity, although no complaints of abdominal pain at the current time.

We will get abdominal x-rays to rule out any GI abnormality and treat ear infection.

Assessment:

Abdominal x-rays are negative. Treat otitis media with erythromycin.

Services (WHAT)	Medical Necessity or Diagnosis (WHY)
__________	__________
__________	__________
__________	__________
__________	__________
__________	__________
__________	__________
__________	__________

Chart 3

Four-year-old brought in by mother with concerns of fever. Mother states child was seen in the emergency room approximately 7 days ago, diagnosed with bronchitis and given a Z-pack. She states he has not gotten any better and, in fact, is probably worse. He does have an Albuterol nebulizer. States he has a cough; however, uncertain whether productive or not. States temperature has been running 101 to 102 at home.

We will go ahead and get a chest x-ray and CBC.

HEENT (head, ears, eyes, nose, throat) normal, GI normal, all other systems normal. Temperature at time of exam was 101.2; however, Tylenol given approximately 30 minutes before exam. Chest x-ray normal, CBC normal.

Impression:

Bronchitis

Fever

Services (WHAT)	Medical Necessity or Diagnosis (WHY)
__________	__________
__________	__________
__________	__________
__________	__________
__________	__________
__________	__________
__________	__________

Chart 4

Patient here today accompanied by mother. Says he has pain in the right shoulder after falling off his bike and striking the right shoulder and head. Patient indicates he blacked out for a brief period of time; however, it was an unwitnessed event, so unsure of duration of loss of consciousness (LOC).

Alert, responsive, cooperative. Musculoskeletal: shoulders are symmetrical, without contusion or abrasions. No superficial scratches, deformity, or redness of shoulder area. However, there is significant joint effusion of the right elbow that requires drainage.

STOP AND PRACTICE—cont'd

Labs and x-ray: right clavicle x-ray is negative for fracture, CT head negative.
Assessment:
Right shoulder pain, status post-fall
Joint effusion, right elbow
Closed head injury with brief LOC
Plan:
Will give ibuprofen 400 mg to use 1 every 4 to 6 hours as needed for pain. We also tapped the elbow joint and aspirated a significant amount of fluid. Will send for cytology and contact patient for any abnormalities.

Services (WHAT)	Medical Necessity or Diagnosis (WHY)
______________	______________
______________	______________
______________	______________
______________	______________
______________	______________
______________	______________
______________	______________

Chart 5

83-year-old female with complaints of urinary symptoms. Quite a list of medications and quite a long list of complaints, most of them chronic. Her main complaint when she comes in today is burning and frequency, a little nausea, just in general not feeling well. Has chronic backache, hypertension, hypothyroidism, anxiety, and depression.
Physical exam:
She is afebrile. HEENT unremarkable. Chest: lungs clear. Heart regular rate and rhythm. Abdomen: soft, active bowel sounds, a little suprapubic tenderness. Extremities appear normal.
Labs and x-rays:
Urinalysis was positive for urinary tract infection.
Plan:
We will give her a dose of Rocephin IM 500 mg and Cipro 500 mg bid for 7 days. Push fluids and follow up in 7 to 10 days for repeat urinalysis.

Services (WHAT)	Medical Necessity or Diagnosis (WHY)
______________	______________
______________	______________
______________	______________
______________	______________
______________	______________
______________	______________
______________	______________

Basic Steps in Coding Services

Now that you have learned to distinguish diagnoses from services, we can begin looking at the information needed to assign codes for the services performed.

The basic steps for procedural coding are similar to those for diagnostic coding. The basic difference in CPT coding is to determine from which chapter of the book services will be coded.

Tool 9-1 summarizes the individual steps necessary for assigning codes from each section or chapter of the CPT book. When we begin looking at the assignment of actual CPT codes in Chapter 10, it will become apparent why a systematic approach is necessary in narrowing down the correct code selections.

Step 1: Determine the Appropriate Chapter from Which Services Will Be Assigned

Although each chapter of CPT will be discussed in detail in the text chapters that follow, a general understanding of the type of services found in each section is necessary.

Chapter 1: Evaluation and Management

Services in this chapter represent encounters or visits typically between the provider and patient. Because the majority of physicians and providers will use evaluation and management codes on a regular basis, this section appears first in the CPT book despite numeric sequence.

Examples of services

- Office visits
- Nursing home visits
- Consultations
- Hospital visits
- Preventive medicine visits

Chapter 2: Anesthesia

Anesthesia services typically represent services provided by the anesthesiologist or certified nurse anesthetist for pain relief, either during surgical procedures or as part of a pain management program.

Examples of services

- Epidural during delivery
- General anesthesia

TOOL 9-1

CPT CODING STEPS

Service Type	E & M	Anesthesia	Surgery	Radiology	Pathology	Medicine
Step 1: Identify chapter	Visits/encounters	General, regional, spinal	Definitive, restorative, invasive	X-rays, MRI/CT, ultrasounds, nuclear medicine	Study of body substances	Diagnostic therapy
Range of codes	99201-99499	00100-01999; 99100-99140	10021-69990	70010-79999	80048-89399	90281-99199; 99500-99600
Step 2: Determine type/location	Location: office, hospital	Anatomic location: head, upper extremities	Anatomic system: integumentary, respiratory	Type of service: diagnostic, ultrasound	Type of service: chemistry, hematology	Specialty type: allergy, pulmonary
Step 3: Specific type	Patient, new patient, established	Body area: eye, thyroid	Anatomic part: skin, finger	Anatomic part: chest, lower extremity	Specific test: hemoglobin, hematocrit	Specific test: pulmonary function test
Step 4: Specific procedure information	Level of service	Procedure: open, closed	Procedure: excision, incision	Views/contrast, 2 views with contrast	Auto/manual, automated manual	Tests with contrast
Step 5: Extent/ additional specifics	Time/other guidelines, 45 min	Specifics extent: XXXXX	Extent: procedure, size/cm	Additional guidelines	Additional guidelines	Additional guidelines

E & M, Evaluation and management.

- Endotracheal anesthesia
- Monitored anesthesia care
- Epidural injections for pain

Chapter 3: Surgery

Services in this chapter of CPT are typically defined as invasive, restorative, or definitive in nature. Many services the layperson would typically not consider as "surgical" are contained in this section because they meet one or more of the above three definitions.

Examples of services

- Tonsillectomy
- Excision of benign lesion
- Laceration, repairs or closures
- Cataract extractions
- Removal of foreign body
- Colonoscopy

Chapter 4: Radiology

The radiology chapter contains codes that typically involve imaging, such as x-ray examination or other imaging services. Different methods of imaging are represented in this section.

Examples of services

- Chest x-ray
- Bone x-rays (e.g., radius, clavicle, fibula, femur, pelvis)
- Ultrasounds
- Nuclear medicine
- Radiation oncology

Chapter 5: Pathology

Examination and study of bodily fluids and other body substances are included in the pathology chapter of CPT.

Examples of services

- CBC
- Urinalysis
- Pap smear
- Surgical pathology
- Drug screens
- Chemistry
- Hematology
- Immunology

Chapter 6: Medicine

Services contained in the medicine chapter of CPT are most commonly diagnostic or therapeutic in nature. Not to be confused with the surgery chapter, most of the procedures in the medicine chapter aid in the diagnosis of the patient or provide therapy for the condition rather than provide a definitive solution to the presenting problem.

Examples of services

- Immunizations
- Injections
- Infusions
- Allergy testing
- Audiology testing
- Cardiology testing
- Physical therapy

A step-by-step process is imperative to correct coding, so following is a review of key concepts and some medical and anatomic terminology.

STOP AND PRACTICE

Step 1: Identify Chapter

For the following services, state the chapter they would be found in CPT.

Service	Chapter
1. CT, abdomen	______
2. Pulmonary function test	______
3. Colonoscopy	______
4. Incision and drainage, finger abscess	______
5. Thyroid-stimulating hormone test	______
6. Bronchoscopy	______
7. Removal of FB, finger	______
8. Tetanus immunization	______
9. ORIF, distal radius	______
10. Esophagoscopy with FB removal	______
11. Removal impacted ear cerumen	______
12. Circumcision	______
13. Vaginal delivery	______
14. Well-baby exam	______
15. Urinalysis	______
16. Pap smear	______
17. Annual exam	______
18. Amniocentesis	______
19. Biopsy skin	______
20. Visual acuity exam	______

By using the first step of this systematic process, the student considerably narrows down the possibility of code selections, eliminating approximately five sixths of the codes in the CPT book. The student will see how, as the result of each step of the process, additional section or code selections are eliminated. When the final steps of the process are completed, only a few code selections are possible.

Step 2: Identify the Key Words and Phrases Necessary to Assign Codes for Services

Important components of the documentation include information regarding location of services (e.g., hospital, office, inpatient or outpatient facility) and anatomic site for which the patient received service (e.g., humerus, radius, femur, tibia, fibula). To find the correct codes in the CPT book, a basic knowledge of human anatomy is essential.

A glossary of body systems, major components, and major functions has been provided as a basic review and reference guide in Chapter 1 of this text.

As you can see by the matrix provided in Tool 9-1, the details of each step vary somewhat, but the level of detail becomes greater with each step of the process.

Within the surgery chapter of CPT, for example, Tool 9-1 indicates we will identify the anatomic system where the service was performed. This, again, will continue to narrow down the possible CPT code selections. By selecting one specific anatomic system, the process eliminates the other 15 systems identified in the CPT surgery chapter.

This step, as well as step 3, requires knowledge of medical terminology and human anatomy to make the correct selection(s). Some practice in this area will be provided before we attempt to apply step 2 and step 3 of this process to an actual medical report.

Table 9-1 summarizes outlining anatomic systems and anatomic parts.

Step 3: Identify Specifics about the Procedure or Service Being Performed

Specifics required in step 3 include information such as new or established patient or the specific body area or test. For a surgical procedure, this step identifies the specific body area or anatomic part for the procedure or service performed.

For example, for the procedure ORIF of the distal radius, the anatomic system would be musculoskeletal (step 2) and the specific body area or part within the musculoskeletal system would be the radius (step 3). Additional specifics, such as the fact that the fracture is to the *distal* radius, will be identified in future steps.

STOP AND PRACTICE

Part 1 Anatomic System and Body Parts

Identify the anatomic system and specific body part within that system for each of the following from the surgery chapter of CPT. Refer to Table 9-1 for reference purposes.

	Anatomic System	Specific Body Part
1. Laryngectomy	______	______
2. Excision of lesion, arm	______	______
3. Arthroscopy, knee	______	______
4. Tenotomy, extensor tendon	______	______
5. Thoracentesis	______	______
6. Nasal endoscopy, ethmoidectomy	______	______
7. Pacemaker insertion	______	______
8. Cystourethroscopy	______	______
9. Prostatectomy	______	______
10. ORIF, radius or ulna	______	______
11. Laceration repair or closure, arm	______	______
12. Carpal tunnel repair	______	______
13. Nerve block, peripheral	______	______
14. Circumcision	______	______
15. Vasectomy	______	______
16. Colposcopy	______	______
17. Total abdominal hysterectomy/ bilateral salpingo-oophorectomy	______	______
18. Transurethral resection of the prostate	______	______
19. CABG, venous, 1 vessel	______	______
20. Extracapsular cataract extraction with intraocular lens	______	______

A review of medical terms, prefixes, and suffixes might be appropriate at this time. You may want to refer to the tables in Chapter 1 and spend additional time reviewing these terms. Also, you will note that a number of surgical services are represented by abbreviations or acronyms and often are not spelled out in the operative reports. You may wish to spend additional time reviewing these from Chapter 1 as well. This additional time will prove worthwhile as we start looking at progress notes and operative reports.

STOP AND PRACTICE—cont'd

Part 2: Practical Application

After becoming more familiar with systems and specific areas within each anatomic system, take a look at the following surgical reports and identify the anatomic system and specific body part to which services were provided. Step 1 (identifying the chapter from CPT) has already been determined because all the following are surgical in nature and therefore would be taken from the surgery chapter of CPT.

Chart 1

Procedure: Flexible sigmoidoscopy

With the patient in the left lateral recumbent position, the rectum was lubricated with Xylocaine viscous and the colonoscope was inserted and passed with minimal difficulty to the cecum. The scope was withdrawn and the mucosa inspected. No significant abnormalities were seen. No polyps, lesions, obstructions, or other abnormalities appeared to be present. No diverticula were present. There were some mild to moderate internal hemorrhoids as well as some external hemorrhoids present, but none appeared to be inflamed or bleeding. Procedure was then terminated and the patient tolerated the procedure well.

Step 1: CPT chapter: Surgery
Step 2: Anatomic system: ____________________
Step 3: Specific organ or body part: ____________________

Chart 2

Procedure: Thoracentesis

Patient was brought to the operating room and positioned on the table. The back was prepped and draped over a marker that had been placed on the left posterior chest to mark the level of the pleural effusion. The area of skin was anesthetized with 1% lidocaine.

With a 22-gauge needle, the pleural space was infiltrated and approximately 100 to 120 mg of straw-colored pleural fluid was aspirated. The needle was removed and a small dressing was placed over the puncture site. Pleural fluid sample was sent for studies. A postthoracentesis chest x-ray revealed no pneumothorax. Patient tolerated the procedure well.

Step 1: CPT chapter: Surgery
Step 2: Anatomic system: ____________________
Step 3: Specific organ or body part: ____________________

Chart 3

Procedure: Right inguinal hernia repair

Right groin incision was made and carried through the subcutaneous tissue. The external oblique fascia was opened from the internal inguinal ring to the external inguinal ring. The cord was mobilized and the defect identified medially. This was a direct inguinal hernia recurrence. The floor was entirely opened up, and a hernia repair was carried out by reapproximating the conjoined tendon down to Cooper's ligament with a running 0 Prolene stitch. The external oblique was closed over the cord with a running 3-0 Vicryl suture, the subcutaneous tissue with 3-0 plain, and the skin with running 4-0 subcuticular Dexon stitch. The patient's wound was dressed, and he was sent to the recovery room in satisfactory condition.

Step 1: CPT chapter: Surgery
Step 2: Anatomic system: ____________________
Step 3: Specific organ or body part: ____________________

Chart 4

Procedure: Dual-chamber transvenous pacemaker placement

Patient was prepped and draped in the usual manner. With the use of sedation and 1% Xylocaine anesthesia, an infraclavicular incision was made. The pocket was carried down to the fascia and placed subfascially. Then the subclavian vein was located with a needle and a guide wire placed into the vein. Two introducers were placed over this wire, and the atrial and ventricular leads were placed into the superior vena cava. Then the atrial lead was put into place and leads were screwed in. Then the ventricular lead was placed in the ventricular apex.

Leads were checked for length on fluoroscopy and then attached into the pocket around a collar with a 2-9 silk suture. The leads and generator were connected together and the pacemaker placed in the pocket. Thresholds were measured and found to be adequate.

Step 1: CPT chapter: Surgery
Step 2: Anatomic system: ____________________
Step 3: Specific organ or body part: ____________________

Chart 5

Mass in left thigh

The left thigh and leg were prepped and draped. Using a no. 15 blade scalpel, a 5-cm incision was made over the mass and the mass removed. The mass was approximately 2 × 2 cm and a lipoma-type mass. It was excised completed through the fascial layer. The 2-cm fascial defect was closed using 3-0 silk. The subcutaneous layer was closed using 3-0 silk as well as the skin. The patient tolerated the procedure well without complications.

Step 1: CPT chapter: Surgery
Step 2: Anatomic system: ____________________
Step 3: Specific organ or body part: ____________________

TABLE 9-1 MAIN BODY SYSTEMS

SYSTEM	COMPONENTS	MAJOR COMBINING FORM	MAJOR FUNCTIONS
Integumentary	Skin	cutaneo/dermo	Protection of body, temperature, and water regulation
	Sweat glands	hidro	
	Nails	onycho	
Musculoskeletal	Bones	osteo	Support, shape, protect, store minerals, locomotion, hold body erect, movement of body fluids, generate body heat
	Joints	arthro	
	Cartilage	chondro	
	Muscles	myo	
	Fascia	fascio	
	Tendon	tendo/tendino	
Cardiovascular	Heart	cardio	Pump blood through circulatory system
	Arteries	arterio	
	Veins	veno/phlebo	
	Blood	hemo/hemato	
Respiratory	Nose	naso/rhino	Bring oxygen into body for transportation to the cells; move carbon dioxide and water waste from body
	Pharynx	pharyngo	
	Trachea	tracheo	
	Larynx	laryngo	
	Lungs	pneumo	
Digestive	Mouth	oro/stomato	Digestion of food, absorption of digested food, elimination of solid wastes
	Esophagus	esophago	
	Stomach	gastro	
	Small intestine	entero	
	Large intestine	colo/colono	
	Liver	hepato	
	Pancreas	pancreato	
	Appendix	appendico	
	Gallbladder	cholecysto	
Endocrine	Adrenals	adreno	Glandular and hormonal regulation and growth of the body
	Pituitary	pituito	
	Thyroid	thyroido	
	Thymus	thymo	
Urinary	Kidneys	nephro/reno	Filtration of blood to remove waste, maintain electrolyte balance, regulate fluid balance within body
	Ureters	uretero	
	Urine	urino	
	Urethra	urethro	
	Bladder	cysto	
Reproductive (male and female)	Testes	orchio/orchido	Production of new life
	Prostate	prostato	
	Ovary	oophoro	
	Uterus	hystero	
	Fallopian tubes	salpingo	
Nervous and sense organs	Nerves	neuro	Coordination mechanism, reception of stimuli, transmission of messages
	Brain	encephalo	
	Spinal cord	myelo	
	Eye	oculo/ophthalmo	
	Ear	acousto/oto	

Step 4: Determine Additional Specific Information Regarding the Services

Additional information includes documentation that addresses the level of complexity and specific technique or approach for a surgical procedure.

In the case of the surgery section of CPT, step 4 identifies the specific approach for the procedure. Remember that in steps 1 through 3 we identified the procedure as surgery, the anatomic system, and the specific body part or organ within that anatomic system.

Step 4 for the surgery section identifies the technique for or nature of the surgical procedures, such as the following:

- Incision
- Excision
- Introduction or removal
- Fracture or dislocation (when applicable)
- Repair or reconstructions
- Endoscopy

Keep in mind that it is the definitive, restorative procedure being identified. For instance, when it is necessary to make an incision to remove the tonsils, as is the case with a tonsillectomy, the approach would be by incision; but the definitive, restorative procedure is performed by excision, and therefore the procedure will be located under the excision heading.

Step 5: Provide Information that Supports or Clarifies

Any additional specifics should be included, such as extent of the procedure, open versus closed or, regarding fracture, with or without fixation.

In the surgery section, this step usually identifies specifics about the surgery, such as the size of the lesion, the approach of the fracture repair (open or closed), specific information regarding the location (distal or proximal), and other information specific to the surgical procedure. This step will be explored further in Chapter 13 in an in-depth discussion of the surgery chapter of CPT.

For purposes of the general exercises in this text, we are attempting to pull out key information that may be necessary for appropriate coding. As the material gets more specific, some unnecessary terms will be eliminated.

The goal of the coder is to read the report one time, identify and list the key words, then work from that key word list when looking up the appropriate code(s) in the CPT book. This eliminates unnecessary time reviewing or re-reviewing extensive reports for necessary information.

On completion of this chapter, you should be capable of reading a medical report and making that list of key words necessary for coding before advancing to Chapter 10, where the key words will be used for obtaining the correct code from the CPT book.

STOP AND PRACTICE

Let's take the same reports you completed for steps 1, 2, and 3 and identify the technique or approach used for each procedure as well as specifics regarding the procedure itself. You have provided some answers in the previous Stop and Practice exercise. Keep in mind that when reading operative reports, "findings" or "observations" of the anatomic site are not services provided, but diagnostic information. This information is needed for diagnostic purposes but does not need to be captured in CPT coding.

Once you have mastered both ICD-9-CM coding and CPT coding, all the coding systems will be put together so you can envision the complete coding of a medical chart.

Chart 1

Procedure: Flexible sigmoidoscopy

With the patient in the left lateral recumbent position, the rectum was lubricated with Xylocaine viscous and the colonoscope was inserted and passed with minimal difficulty to the cecum. The scope was withdrawn and the mucosa inspected. No significant abnormalities were seen. No polyps, lesions, obstructions, or other abnormalities appeared to be present. No diverticula were present. There were some mild to moderate internal hemorrhoids as well as some external hemorrhoids present, but none appeared to be inflamed or bleeding. Procedure was then terminated and the patient tolerated the procedure well.

Step 1: CPT chapter: Surgery
Step 2: Anatomic system: ________
Step 3: Specific organ or body part: ________
Step 4: Technique or approach: ________
Step 5: Additional specifics: ________ ________
________ ________

STOP AND PRACTICE—cont'd

Chart 2

Procedure: Thoracentesis

Patient was brought to the operating room and positioned on the table. The back was prepped and draped over a marker that had been placed on the left posterior chest to mark the level of the pleural effusion. The area of skin was anesthetized with 1% lidocaine.

With a 22-gauge needle, the pleural space was infiltrated and approximately 100 to 120 mg of straw-colored pleural fluid was aspirated. The needle was removed with a small dressing placed over the puncture site. Pleural fluid sample was sent for studies, and a postthoracentesis chest x-ray revealed no pneumothorax. Patient tolerated the procedure well.

Step 1: CPT chapter: Surgery
Step 2: Anatomic system: ____________
Step 3: Specific organ or body part: ____________
Step 4: Technique or approach: ____________
Step 5: Additional specifics: ____________ ____________
____________ ____________

Chart 3

Procedure: Right inguinal hernia repair

Right groin incision was made and carried through the subcutaneous tissue. The external oblique fascia was opened from the internal inguinal ring to the external inguinal ring. The cord was mobilized and the defect identified medially. This was a direct inguinal hernia recurrence. The floor was entirely opened up, and a hernia repair was carried out by reapproximating the conjoined tendon down to Cooper's ligament with a running 0 Prolene stitch. The external oblique was closed over the cord with a running 3-0 Vicryl suture, the subcutaneous tissue with 3-0 plain, and the skin with running 4-0 subcuticular Dexon stitch. The patient's wound was dressed, and he was sent to the recovery room in satisfactory condition.

Step 1: CPT chapter: Surgery
Step 2: Anatomic system: ____________
Step 3: Specific organ or body part: ____________
Step 4: Technique or approach: ____________
Step 5: Additional specifics: ____________ ____________
____________ ____________

Chart 4

Procedure: Dual chamber transvenous pacemaker placement

Patient was prepped and draped in the usual manner. With the use of sedation and 1% Xylocaine anesthesia, an infraclavicular incision was made. The pocket was carried down to the fascia and placed subfascially. Then the subclavian vein was located with a needle and a guide wire placed into the vein. Two introducers were placed over this wire, and the atrial and ventricular leads were placed into the superior vena cava. Then the atrial lead was put into place and leads were screwed in. Then the ventricular lead was placed in the ventricular apex.

Leads were checked for length on fluoroscopy and then attached into the pocket around a collar with a 2-9 silk suture. The leads and generator were connected together and the pacemaker placed in the pocket. Thresholds were measured and found to be adequate.

Step 1: CPT chapter: Surgery
Step 2: Anatomic system: ____________
Step 3: Specific organ or body part: ____________
Step 4: Technique or approach: ____________
Step 5: Additional specifics: ____________ ____________
____________ ____________

STOP AND PRACTICE—cont'd

Chart 5

Mass in left thigh

The left thigh and leg were prepped and draped. With a no. 15 blade scalpel, a 5-cm incision was made over the mass and the mass removed. The mass was approximately 2 × 2 cm and a lipoma-type mass. It was excised completed through the fascial layer. The 2-cm fascial defect was closed using 3-0 silk. The subcutaneous layer was closed using 3-0 silk as well as the skin. The patient tolerated the procedure well and without complications.

Step 1: CPT chapter: Surgery
Step 2: Anatomic system: ____________
Step 3: Specific organ or body part: ____________
Step 4: Technique or approach: ____________
Step 5: Additional specifics: ____________ ____________ ____________ ____________

Let's take all the steps learned in this chapter and apply them to the medical report in Figure 9-1. Take the operative report, step by step, and capture the information as covered in the discussion of steps 1 through 5. Keep in mind that there will often be information that is not necessary for capturing data for assigning codes. Also remember that any observations or findings not captured for purposes of CPT coding will be needed for assigning ICD-9-CM codes. For purposes of these beginning exercises, do not capture diagnostic information or assign ICD-9-CM codes.

Step 1: CPT Section or Chapter

The choices are as follows:

Chapter 1: Evaluation and Management	Visit or encounter with physician
Chapter 2: Anesthesia	Typically provided by anesthesiologist or certified nurse anesthetist to provide pain relief or as part of pain management
Chapter 3: Surgery	Invasive, restorative, definitive procedure
Chapter 4: Radiology	X-rays and other imaging
Chapter 5: Pathology	Examination of bodily fluids and body substances
Chapter 6: Medicine	Diagnostic, therapeutic services

Because the procedure is definitive and restorative, the code assignment will be taken from the Surgery chapter of CPT (step 1).

Step 2: Anatomic System

Once you have determined that the surgery chapter is appropriate for the procedure, the next step is to determine the anatomic system in which the procedure was performed. The choices are as follows:

Integumentary	Skin, hair, nails, sweat glands
Musculoskeletal	Bones, joints, cartilage, muscles, fascia, tendons
Cardiovascular	Heart, arteries, veins, blood
Respiratory	Nose, pharynx, trachea, larynx, lungs
Digestive	Mouth, esophagus, stomach, intestines, liver, pancreas, appendix, gallbladder
Endocrine	Adrenals, pituitary, thyroid, thymus
Urinary	Kidneys, ureters, urethra, bladder
Reproductive (male or female)	Testes, prostate, ovary, uterus, fallopian tubes
Nervous or sense organs	Nerves, brain, spinal cord, eyes, ears

Because the procedure performed is the extraction, or removal, of a cataract the procedure is being performed on the eye. Therefore the anatomic system within the surgery chapter (step 2) will be the *nervous* or *sense organ* system.

As a result of the above process, we have narrowed down the areas within CPT to look for the correct codes to the surgery chapter, nervous or sense organ subsection.

Step 3: Specific Organ or Body Part

Within the nervous or sense organ section, which would be the appropriate organ or body part on which the procedure is being performed?

- Nerves
- Brain
- Spinal cord
- Eyes
- Ears

OPERATIVE REPORT

Patient information:

Patient name:
DOB:
MR#:

Preoperative diagnosis:

Cataract, OS

Postoperative diagnosis:

Cataract, OS

Procedure(s) performed:

Phacoemulsification Cataract with IOL Implantation

Complications: None

Anesthesia:

Assistant surgeon:

Description of procedure:

After written informed consent was obtained, the patient was brought to the operating room where he was given Topical Lidocaine jelly to the eye. The right eye was then prepped and draped in the usual sterile fashion. A wire lid speculum was placed in the eye. Lidocaine followed by Vitrax viscoelastic was injected in the anterior chamber. A corneal groove was created, where a capsulorrhexis was then performed. The lens was hydrodissected and removed utilizing phacoemulsification technique. The wound was enlarged, Gel viscoelastic was injected into the capsular sac. An AR 40 acrylic diopter 22.5 lens was injected into the capsular bag where it was unfolded and centered without any complications. The wounds were hydrated and no leaks were noted. Topical Oxuflox was placed on the eye and the patient was taken to the recovery room in excellent condition.

Linda Patrick MD

GODFREY REGIONAL HOSPITAL
123 Main Street • Aldon, FL 77714 • (407) 555-1234

FIGURE 9-1. Sample medical report.

Looking at the operative report, the procedure was performed on the "OD," which is the medical acronym for *right eye*. Therefore the anatomic part in step 3 is the eye.

Step 4: Technique or Approach

Step 4 of the process identifies what was performed to the organ or body part identified in step 3. Therefore we are looking for WHAT was performed on the right eye during the operative session. Review of the operative report reveals the following information:

> The lens was hydrodissected and removed.

The lens of the eye was removed, thereby removing or "extracting" a cataract. Notice that the procedural heading indicates "Phacoemulsification cataract with IOL implantation," which is, in fact, the extraction or removal of a cataract by phacoemulsification technique with intraocular lens (IOL) implantation. The operative report further describes or confirms that the "phacoemulsification" technique was indeed used to remove the cataract.

Care should be taken to NOT use diagnostic or procedural headings in the operative report solely for determining the information necessary for coding. Although they can be used as a starting point, all the information gathered for coding purposes must be confirmed in the operative report itself.

Therefore the technique or approach (step 4) would be *extraction* or *removal* of *cataract by phacoemulsification technique.*

Step 5: Additional Specifics

The last step of gathering data from the operative report involves collecting other information that may be necessary to assign an appropriate code(s) for the procedure. Although this step may involve gathering information that may eventually be eliminated during the coding process, gathering more information than necessary is better than having to return repeatedly to the operative report for needed information. Therefore gather data you believe may be necessary; you can filter out unnecessary information as the process advances.

Take another look at the operative report and identify information regarding the procedure that may or may not be necessary; capture only those key words.

> After written informed consent was obtained, the patient was brought to the operating room where he was given topical lidocaine jelly to the eye. The **right** eye was then prepped and draped in the usual sterile fashion. A wire lid speculum was placed in the eye. Lidocaine followed by Vitrax viscoelastic was injected in the anterior chamber. A corneal groove was created, where a **capsulorrhexis** was then **performed**. The **lens** was hydrodissected and **removed utilizing the phacoemulsification technique**. The wound was enlarged, and gel viscoelastic was injected into the capsular sac. An AR 40 acrylic diopter 22.5 **lens was injected** into the capsular bag where it was unfolded and centered without any complications. The wounds were hydrated and no leaks were noted. Topical Oxuflox was placed on the eye and the patient was taken to the recovery room in excellent condition.

Summarize the key words identified:

- Right eye
- Capsulorrhexis was performed
- Lens removed utilizing phacoemulsification technique
- Lens was injected

Note that "lens removed utilizing the phacoemulsification technique" has already been captured, so the only additional information gathered is as follows:

- Right eye
- Capsulorrhexis was performed
- Lens was injected

In summary, the following information was gathered from the documentation:

Step 1: CPT chapter or section:	Surgery
Step 2: Anatomic system:	Nervous or sense organs
Step 3: Specific organ or body part:	Eye
Step 4: Technique or approach:	Extraction or removal cataract by phacoemulsification
Step 5: Additional specifics:	Right eye Capsulorrhexis Lens injected

This is all the information necessary to locate the code(s) necessary for coding or billing the services performed. At this point the operative report has been reviewed and all pertinent data captured. Therefore no additional time with the operative report is necessary. The report itself can be set aside, and only the captured information used when assigning code(s) from the CPT book in the last steps of the process (discussed in Chapter 10).

STOP AND PRACTICE

As in the sample exercise, extract the information necessary from the following charts to assign appropriate CPT codes. Note that different reports have been used, so you may need to refer to Tool 9-1 to determine the appropriate steps based on the chapter or section chosen. For this reason, the descriptors for steps 2 through 5 have been left blank for you to fill in.

Chart 1. Finger laceration

EMERGENCY ROOM RECORD

Name:	**Age:**	**ER physician:**
	DOB:	

Allergies/type of reaction:	**Usual medications/dosages:**
No known drug allergies	He is on no medications

Triage/presenting complaint: Laceration between 4th/5th fingers of right hand

Initial assessment:

Alert and cooperative, appearing queasy with sitting on exam gurney. Resolved when lying down supine. There is a 1.5 cm laceration between the interspace of the 4th/5th finger which is deep into the subcutaneous layer.

Tetanus greater than 5 years ago. Quit smoking 2-3 years ago.

Time	**T:** 98.2	**P:** 76	**R:** 20	**BP:** 114/84	**Other:**				

Medication orders:

Lab work:

X-Ray:

Physician's report:

Patient is an 18-year-old male, who was on the job as a welder, standing in front of a palette to move it onto the fork palates. His co-worker was driving a fork truck when his foot slipped off the brake and the truck moved forward catching the patient's right hand between the corner of the palette and the fork. The form went into his hand, and the co-worker was able to reverse the forklift. Denies any injuries to his arm. Did not fall or loss any consciousness. Rates his pain on a 7-8 out of 0-10 pain scale.

Review of Systems: Denies any forearm or elbow pain. Denies any fever or chills. No mental depression, easy or frequent bleeding or bruising. Denies wounds that will not heal.

Wound was repaired in layers, subcutaneous layers with subcutaneous sutures and additional closure of the skin. Dressing applied and patient Instructed to return In 2 days for wound check.

Diagnosis:	**Physician sign/date**
	Nancy Connelly MD
Discharge Transfer Admit Good Satisfactory Other:	

GODFREY REGIONAL HOSPITAL
123 Main Street • Aldon, FL 77714 • (407) 555-1234

Step 1: __________
Step 2: __________
Step 3: __________
Step 4: __________
Step 5: __________ __________
__________ __________

Chart 2. Epigastric pain

OPERATIVE REPORT

Patient information:

Patient name:
DOB:
MR#:

Preoperative diagnosis:

Epigastric pain with anemia

Postoperative diagnosis:

Epigastric pain with anemia and gastritis

Procedure(s) performed:

Esophagastroduodenoscopy

Anesthesia:

Assistant surgeon:

Description of procedure:

Patient was brought to the main endoscopic are and given Tetracaine gargle. He was placed in the left lateral decubitus position. Endoscope was inserted into the oral cavity. No abnormality was noted in the oropharynx or esophagus. The GE junction was at 40 cm from the incisor and there was no evidence of esophagitis, regurgitation, or hiatal hernia. Scope was advanced into the stomach where mild gastritis was noted. The scope was then further advanced into the duodenum where multiple pictures were obtained. The scope was withdrawn and the patient was taken to the recovery room in satisfactory condition.

Rachel Perez MD

GODFREY REGIONAL HOSPITAL
123 Main Street • Aldon, FL 77714 • (407) 555-1234

Step 1: ______________

Step 2: ______________

Step 3: ______________

Step 4: ______________

Step 5: ______________ ______________

______________ ______________

Chart 3. Annual examination

OFFICE NOTE

Chief complaint: ____________

Date: ____________

Vital signs: BP______ P______ R______

History:

This is a 45-year-old female here for her annual well woman exam. Menses are regular without intermenstrual bleeding. When seen a year ago, she felt fatigued. Blood work at that time showed her to be hypokalemic. She took a potassium supplement at that time and felt much better. She has no headaches. She had some vaginal itching and discharge off and on during the summer but currently does not have this complaint. She has never had a mammogram.

Exam:

Breasts without masses. No axillary adenopathy. Abdomen soft and nontender. Pelvic: External genitalia normal. Vaginal rugous, with a small amount of yellow discharge. Cervix clean. Uterus anterior, mobile, nontender, normal in size, shape, and consistency. Adenxa clear, nontender. Pap smear was obtained.

Diagnosis/assessment:

Well woman

Willen Obst MD

Patient name: ____________

Date of service: ____________

GODFREY MEDICAL ASSOCIATES
1532 Third Avenue, Suite 120 • Aldon, FL 77713 • (407) 555-4000

Step 1: ____________
Step 2: ____________
Step 3: ____________
Step 4: ____________
Step 5: ____________ ____________
____________ ____________

Chart 4. Rectal bleeding

OPERATIVE REPORT

Patient information:

Patient name:
DOB:
MR#:

Preoperative diagnosis:

Rectal Bleeding

Postoperative diagnosis:

Lesion at 55 cm of left colon

Procedure(s) performed:

Colonoscopy and multiple biopsies

Anesthesia:

Assistant surgeon:

Description of procedure:

Patient was placed in the left lateral Sims position. The anus was digitally dilated and the colonoscope was passed up through the rectum, sigmoid colon into the descending colon. At 55 cm, a colonic lesion was encountered. It was snared and removed in toto. No tumor nodules or masses were found. The mucosa appeared to be somewhat constricted, however, we were able to advance the scope to the cecum. Postoperative condition was satisfactory.

Adam Westgate MD

GODFREY REGIONAL HOSPITAL
123 Main Street • Aldon, FL 77714 • (407) 555-1234

Step 1: ____________
Step 2: ____________
Step 3: ____________
Step 4: ____________
Step 5: ____________ ____________
____________ ____________

Chart 5. Discharge summary

DISCHARGE SUMMARY

Admitted:
Discharged:

Discharge diagnoses:

Discharge Medications:
Potassium 10 mEq 2 tablets bid
Prednisone 15 mg daily
Lasix 40 mg 1 In the morning 1/2 In the afternoon
Vitamin D and Calcium daily

History:

Laboratory and radiology studies:

Hospital course:

The patient was admitted with dehydration, weakness and hypokalemia. She was treated with IV fluids, IV potassium as she was hypokalemic. She improved slowly but steadily on the second hospital day and on the third hospital day actually ended fluid overloaded for which she received IV Lasix. On the day of discharge, she was able to eat breakfast without difficulty. While still weak she was able to be up safely with assistance and will be discharged for follow-up as an outpaitent.

GODFREY REGIONAL HOSPITAL
123 Main Street • Aldon, FL 77714 • (407) 555-1234

Step 1: __________
Step 2: __________
Step 3: __________
Step 4: __________
Step 5: __________ __________
__________ __________

CPT Concepts

In addition to gathering key elements needed to assign the appropriate CPT codes for services performed, you must master a number of key concepts to determine which codes should be included and excluded in your final selection.

CPT GUIDELINES

To select the appropriate CPT codes, the coder should know some definitions of terms and concepts provided in CPT. The coder also must understand CPT guidelines (see Tool 9-2) because they are essential for correctly coding documentation so that reimbursement is timely and correct.

CPT guidelines are section specific. The coder must identify the procedure, ascertain which section contains the appropriate code, and follow the individual guidelines for that section.

DEFINITIONS OR CONCEPTS

Global Procedures "Package Concept"

The **global procedure** concept is probably the most difficult concept to grasp in coding. Global procedures are defined by both insurance carriers and CPT as those that follow a predetermined outline that specifically addresses services necessary to complete a surgical procedure, including preoperative and postoperative care. More specifically, they include the following:

Preoperative Care

Preoperative care includes visits or care provided up to 1 day before and the day of the surgical procedure—as long as the care is performed by the actual surgeon. In instances in which the service provided during this time frame are for the purposes of "decision for surgery," these services are codeable with the use of a modifier code, which is explained later in this chapter.

Intraoperative Services or Surgery

Intraoperative services include the surgery itself as well as the following:

- Cleaning, shaving, prepping of skin
- Draping and positioning of the patient
- Insertion of intravenous access for medication administration
- Sedative administration by physician performing surgery
- Local, topical, or regional anesthesia administered by physician performing surgery
- Surgical approach
- Surgical cultures
- Wound irrigation
- Insertion or removal of drain
- Surgical closures and dressing
- Surgical supplies
- Preoperative, intraoperative, and postoperative documentation, including photographs

TOOL 9-2

CPT CODING GUIDELINES

1. Identify the key words and phrases for coding purposes. Use medical term(s) for coding procedures and services.
2. Identify procedural statements and services to be used for coding purposes.
3. Determine the correct order for billing services and procedures.
   Make certain the correct primary diagnosis (WHY) has been matched to the correct procedure (WHAT). Determine the most significant service provided for a given date as the primary procedure.
4. Select the correct code(s) from CPT/HCPCS using the following steps:
   - Locate the main term for the procedure or service in the index.
   - Locate each code listed in the CPT book.
   - Follow all notes and cross-references to ensure correct selection.
   - Follow the rules for inclusion/exclusion as well as surgical packages (global).
   - Determine whether a modifier code is necessary.
   - Make certain the correct guidelines and modifiers are used by checking the code selected and verifying which section of CPT this code originated from. Follow those guidelines and rules ONLY.

Normal Uncomplicated Postoperative Care

These postoperative services are defined as follow-up visits or services during the postoperative period of surgery related to the recovery from surgery. If services or visits are performed during this postoperative period are considered "complicated" or "unrelated," they may be codeable or billable with the use of a modifier code.

For example, only one repair method can be reported for a single organ or body part. Therefore if one method is attempted but proves unsuccessful, only the method that successfully accomplishes the intent of the surgical procedure is reported. An example would be a surgical procedure attempted laparoscopically, but the repair proves unsuccessful and thus is converted to an open surgical procedure. In this instance only the open surgical procedure would be reportable.

The difficulty in understanding the global procedures concept arises when it is implemented by third-party insurance carriers. Consider the concept of global services applied to purchasing an automobile. When an automobile is purchased, it comes equipped with a number of specified items that are a part of the package price, such as a steering wheel, tires, wheels, seats, and so forth. Extras, or upgrades, such as a CD player or leather seats, are not included in the package price. Therefore they are charged individually when chosen (Fig. 9-2). Envisioning the concept of the car purchase may help the coder when attempting to determine whether services are included, or **bundled**.

Global packages for procedures are much the same as the package price for an automobile. Certain items are included in the package, but extras must be noted as such by proper modifier codes. The difficulty comes from the many interpretations by third-party insurance carriers of this package concept. In the scenario of the car purchase, one dealer may include a CD player as part of the sticker package; another may not. Leather seats may be included in the package in some instances but not in others. This inherent variability applies to third-party insurance carriers and the services and procedures they may or may not reimburse.

Postoperative, or follow-up, periods may be defined differently by different carriers. For instance, Medicare defines procedures as either major, which have a 90-day postoperative period, or minor, which have a 10-day postoperative period. To identify the global period for any surgical procedure, refer to the Medicare Physician Fee Schedule database at www.cms.hhs.gov/physicians/mpfsapp/step0.asp.

Other insurance carriers either follow the Medicare guidelines or use the resource-based relative value scale (RBRVS), which lists each CPT code and the follow-up days allowed for

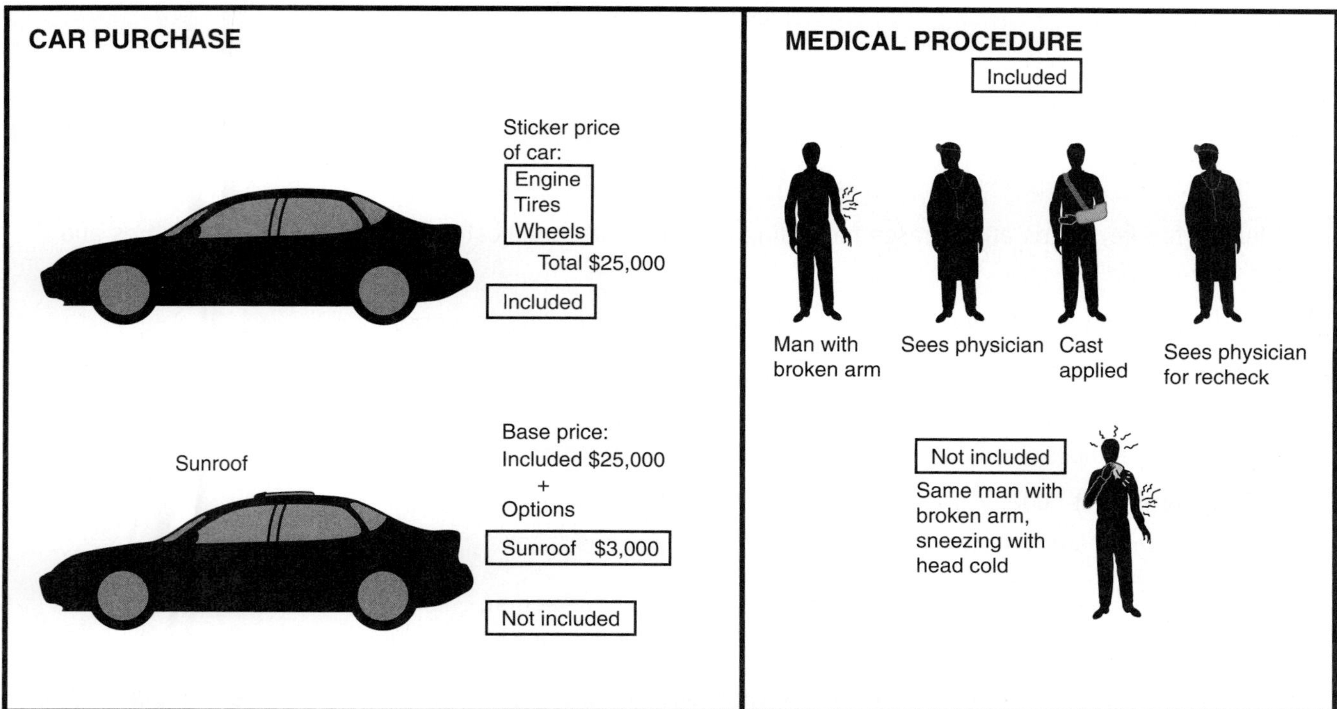

FIGURE 9-2. Compare the package concept of an automobile purchase to the package concept of global medical procedures.

each procedure. Other valuable information is included in the RBRVS, such as whether an assistant surgeon is an appropriate caregiver in a procedure as well as the relative value for the procedure, which helps the providers and insurance carriers determine appropriate payment. RBRVS is discussed further in Chapter 19.

The following services are typically not considered part of the global package concept and, in most instances, are separately reportable or billable:

- Visits unrelated to the diagnosis for which the surgical procedure is performed unless the visit occurs as a result of complications of the surgery.
- Treatment for an underlying condition or an added treatment that is not part of the normal recovery for the surgical procedure.
- Diagnostic tests and procedures, including radiologic services.
- Distinct surgical procedures.
- Treatment for postoperative complications requiring a return to the operating room.

Concept of Bundling or Unbundling of Global Procedures

The Centers for Medicare and Medicaid Services (CMS) instituted the **National Correct Coding Initiative** (**NCCI**) to clarify coding guidelines. The *NCCI edits*, as they are referred to, are based on the coding conventions outlined in the CPT book, providing additional information regarding specifics on those procedures considered included, or bundled, in the global service package concept. When procedures typically considered integral to the global procedures are coded and billed, this practice is referred to as **unbundling**. Detailed information regarding the NCCI policies can be found online at the CMS website (www.cms.hhs.gov) or simply by using a search engine and entering "NCCI coding edits."

Some basic concepts apply to global package services as defined by the NCCI edits, including the following:

- A provider should not report multiple CPT codes when a single comprehensive code would describe the services (an excellent example of unnecessary unbundling).
- A provider should not fragment a procedure into component parts.
- A provider should not unbundle a bilateral procedure into two unilateral procedures.
- A provider should not unbundle services integral to a more comprehensive procedure. For example, surgical approach is always integral to a surgical procedure. Therefore if a physician performs an exploratory laparotomy (CPT code 49000) as well as a total abdominal hysterectomy (CPT code 58150), the laparotomy would be the approach by which the hysterectomy was performed and therefore considered bundled. It would be inappropriate to code or bill for both services.

Most Extensive Procedure

Codes grouped together in CPT are similar in content, differing only in complexity or extent. Unless procedures are performed on separate anatomic sites or during a separate encounter, the following guidelines apply:

"Simple" procedures are included in those described as "complex."

"Simple" procedures are included in those described as "complicated."

"Limited" procedures are included in those described as "complete."

"Intermediate" procedures are included in those described as "comprehensive."

"Superficial" procedures are included in those described as "deep."

"Incomplete" procedures are included in those described as "complete."

"External" procedures are included in those described as "internal."

Keep in mind that the basic coding or documentation concept of "If it isn't documented, it didn't happen" applies in the selection of CPT codes as well. Therefore if a procedure is not documented as "complex," for example, it would be considered "simple."

More specific NCCI policies are discussed in detail in subsequent chapters.

Incidental Procedures

Incidental procedures are performed at the same time as a more complex primary procedure. They typically require few, if any, additional physician resources and are generally not considered integral to the performance of the primary procedure. When incidental procedures are performed during a primary surgical procedure, they are not reimbursable and are considered bundled.

One example is an asymptomatic appendectomy performed during a hysterectomy. In this instance, the appendectomy would be considered bundled and not separately reimbursable or codeable.

Integral procedures are performed as part of a more complex primary procedure. One example is when a transurethral incision of the prostate is performed at the same time as a cytourethroscopy. The cystourethroscopic procedure is considered integral to the primary procedure—transurethral incision of the prostate—and is therefore bundled and not codeable.

Unlisted Procedures

When no specific procedural code has been assigned, the procedure is listed as "unspecified" or "unlisted." Because several procedures without a specific code could be noted as "unlisted respiratory conditions," the coder should include a report for such a procedure, an explanation of the procedure, and its name. With these data, the insurance carrier accumulates information about each specific procedure. At a later date the carrier will be able to assign specific codes for high-volume procedures.

The significance of this designation for a third-party insurance carrier is that the unlisted procedure code(s) provided in each anatomic section of CPT should be used ONLY when no other valid CPT code is available. If the insurance carrier decides there is an appropriate code for the service, it may be recoded accordingly. Again, because this type of service may encompass several procedures ranging from minor to major, a detailed report of the procedure must be attached.

Separate Procedure

A number of procedures, especially in the surgical section of CPT, have the designation **separate procedure** after the description. This notes a procedure that may be assigned a code ONLY if it is the only procedure from within that section of codes; thus it is a "separate" procedure. If other codes from within that subcategory are assigned, the procedure with this designation is considered included or incidental.

Codes designated as separate procedures may not be additionally reported when the procedure is an integral component of another. For example, code 29870 describes a knee arthroscopy, diagnostic, with or without synovial biopsy. When performed alone—that is, separate—this procedure is codeable or billable. However, when the diagnostic knee arthroscopy serves as the approach for a surgical arthroscopic procedure of the knee, it is NOT codeable or billable. An example is when a meniscectomy, lateral (code 29881) is performed, code 29870 (described above) would not be reported because it is no longer a separate procedure performed alone without any other procedures in the knee arthroscopy section. The student will see this concept frequently when reading and assigning codes for surgical services in future chapters of this text.

However, codes designated as separate procedures may be reported additionally when they are performed to unrelated or distinct sites or during separate and distinct encounters.

CPT Modifiers

Modifiers are the means by which the physician indicates that a service or procedure has been altered in some manner. Although the code itself does not change, the procedure has been modified in some respect, and an explanation of this change is required. CPT modifiers are 2-digit numeric indicators—with the exception of anesthesia *physical status modifiers,* which begin with the letter P and are followed by a single digit between 1 and 6.

The CPT code and modifier are reported as one line on the claim form. For example: CPT code 45378, colonoscopy, diagnostic and modifier 52 would be listed on the claim as:

45378 52

The coder may describe provided services using only CPT codes. Therefore any changes must also be described by codes, numbers, or assignment of modifiers.

Modifier codes may be used by adding a 2-digit numeric code after the CPT code to represent the modifier. Additional modifier codes found in the **Healthcare Common Procedure Coding System (HCPCS)**, level II, which is discussed in Chapter 18, are represented by alpha or alphanumeric 2-digit codes for clarification of services. The most common HCPCS modifier codes are included later in this chapter in the discussion regarding modifiers.

Note that individual modifiers may be used only for specific sections of the CPT. Unfortunately, the newest edition of CPT does not indicate for which section(s) each modifier is appropriately used. Coders may use the "Appendix on Modifiers" located in the back of the CPT book or the materials provided in this chapter to develop their own coding reference tools.

THIRD-PARTY OR INSURANCE CARRIER SIGNIFICANCE

The use of a modifier code indicates to the insurer that the CPT codes reported are not reflected in the third-party fee calculations used for averaging and statistical record keeping of charges. Modifiers also indicate that changes were made to a usual procedure, so there may be differences between the usual reimbursement rate for that specific service and the reimbursement amount requested by a provider for services.

By placing the modifier code after a procedure code, the coder specifies that there has been a recognized exception or change in the procedure, so the request for payment differs from the usual reimbursement. Such modifiers explain the changes and indicate to the insurance carrier that this altered service should, in fact, be considered for payment.

Think of this coding principle as follows:

CPT Code + Modifier Code = CPT Code (WHAT was provided) + (But) Modifier Code (special consideration should be made for the services or reasons identified)

As with other services, those with appended modifier codes must be substantiated by documentation that supports the request for payment in extenuating circumstances. For instance, the use of modifier 22, unusual procedural services, suggests that the services performed were beyond the normal scope of the CPT descriptor and justify additional reimbursement consideration. Without proper documentation, the services will receive only the usual reimbursement for the CPT code listed. Unusual circumstances that create additional complexity during the procedure, such as complications or hemorrhage, must be documented with an explanation of why services outside the norm were rendered and should be considered for additional payment.

Once the coder has decided that a modifier code is necessary for billed services to be considered for reimbursement, he or she must gather some additional information regarding the service, such as the following:

- What type of service was provided (which chapter guidelines are appropriate)?
- Are the services listed as physician or outpatient surgery (separate modifiers for physician versus outpatient)?
- When needed, does documentation reflect the unusual circumstances (e.g., greater than usual service)?
- Does the service require a report and manual billing?

Tool 9-3 provides guidelines for when to consider the use of a modifier code as well as rules for using modifier codes appropriately.

TOOL 9-3

PROPER USE OF MODIFIERS

1. Use a modifier when further explanation of performed services is necessary.
2. Use a modifier when a service typically would not be reimbursable by the carrier but extenuating circumstances should override.
3. Remember that services usually bundled or included in the global surgical procedure are NOT typically considered without the use of a modifier.
4. Remember that insurance carrier software "blocks out" payment for ANY services performed by that provider during the global period unless a modifier is added.
5. Modifiers are assigned by section within CPT, and only modifiers for that specific section should be used.
6. Modifier 59 should be used when appropriate, but only when no other modifier is appropriate.
7. Multiple modifiers require the use of modifier 99 followed by a listing of the appropriate modifiers.
8. Medicare allows up to two modifiers to be used in the modifier section of the claim form before modifier 99 is required. A revision to the claim form is currently underway that will allow for the reporting of up to four modifiers without the use of modifier 99.

GUIDELINES FOR USING MODIFIER CODE(S)

1. Make certain that "extenuating circumstances" billed with the modifier code selected are documented or clearly evident.
   - For example, "significantly separately identifiable" is easier to justify if a separate surgical or procedure report is included, rather than leaving information intermingled with the visit description.
   - Services greater than usual should be explained in the medical documentation.
   - Discontinued procedures should clearly indicate what portion of the procedure was completed so that partial reimbursement for services performed can be received.
2. Reimbursement may be affected by the use of the modifier code. Depending on the modifier used, reimbursement may be increased or decreased proportionately.
3. Some third-party carriers do not recognize SOME or ANY modifiers on claims. A review process will be necessary to justify why these services are "outside the norm."
4. Carefully review the carrier's Explanation of Benefits to make certain that allowances have been made for services with modifiers, when appropriate.
5. Check the modifier list to ensure that codes used are applicable to the services billed. (Outpatient surgery modifiers are different than physician service modifiers.)
6. Check carrier specifications regarding HCPCS modifiers taken from CPT.

As with other ICD-9-CM and CPT codes, the use of a modifier is supported by the documentation whether coding or billing for more or reduced services. Typically, services coded with the use of a modifier code may be subject to manual review by the carrier, and a copy of the documentation that substantiates the request for payment may be requested. The assignment of an appropriate modifier code is essential to proper reimbursement. Documentation is even more vital to receiving reimbursement for services coded with a modifier.

TYPES OF MODIFIERS

One of the last steps in correct procedure coding is determining whether a modifier code is appropriate and which modifier(s) are appropriate. Conditions that typically require a modifier code include the following:

- Professional versus technical component(s)
- Services provided by more than one physician or more than one location
- Services greater or less than level usually provided
- Partial service or one portion of service performed
- Additional services performed in conjunction with major service
- Bilateral services provided
- Services or procedure performed more than once
- Services outside those ordinarily provided within global period

Professional versus Technical Component(s)

Certain procedures are a combination of a physician component and technical component. When only the professional portion of those services are performed, modifier 26 would be appended to those services to indicate that the global service for that CPT code descriptor is not complete.

More Than One Physician or Location

When the same service is supplied by more than one physician or is repeated by the same physician, a modifier indicates that the service listed is not a duplicate or an error in billing. Without the use of the modifier code, the insurance carrier assumes an error in billing or a duplicate of the same service. Without such a modifier, claims with the same procedure code on the same day of service by the same provider will be disallowed or denied.

Service Performed at a Different Level Than Usual

When a service is provided at a level greater or less than usual, the change can be indicated by the appropriate modifier code. The use of this modifier is not intended to denote an increase or decrease in the amount charged but rather a change in the level or type of service provided. These modifiers are typically used when the greatest or least level of service has been selected but additional description or clarification is needed. Special documentation may be required to justify the medical necessity of increased service and the requested increase in reimbursement.

Partial Service or One Portion of a Service Performed

When the service described is inclusive of several components but not all components were performed, a modifier indicates which portion was completed. Because the total service was not performed, total reimbursement would not be appropriate. Instead, only a portion of the total reimbursement may be expected. For many years, insurance carriers did not reimburse for procedures that were started but not completed. With the introduction of a modifier code to describe this situation, however, insurance carriers now recognize that even when the procedure was not completed, the preparation and medical decision making involved should be given consideration for at least partial payment. The provider must document what portion of the service was performed.

Additional Services Performed in Conjunction with Major Service

When coding for surgical procedures, the coder must frequently use multiple procedural codes to adequately describe the surgical case. The coder must specify the primary procedure, the secondary procedure, and contributing procedures. Proper use of modifiers is important because additional procedures following the first will usually be significantly discounted for reimbursement. Thus the most significant service must be listed as the primary service. Although this service will frequently also be the most substantial charge, the coder should make certain not to select primary procedures on the basis of the charge but on their medical significance.

Bilateral Services Provided

When services are provided to both right and left extremities or to other body areas considered **bilateral**, the coder must use a modifier code to indicate that charges are not a duplication of billing but are two separate and legitimate charges.

Service or Procedure Performed More Than Once

Repeat procedures must be indicated as such so that insurance carriers will not deny reimbursement for duplication of services. For instance, when a patient with myocardial infarction undergoes multiple electrocardiograms throughout the course of treatment during a given day, the coder must indicate, by the use of a modifier, that the multiple charges are NOT a duplication error, but rather that repeat services were medically necessary.

Services Outside Those Ordinarily Provided

In some situations the normal postoperative period is interrupted by another procedure that may or may not have relevance to the original procedure. In other instances additional procedures intended to be performed as part of the overall surgery plan may be performed during what would otherwise be considered the postoperative period. Modifiers can explain these unusual circumstances or exceptions, which should be considered for reimbursement.

CPT MODIFIER CODE LISTING

A complete listing of modifier codes and a discussion of their proper use is included in Table 9-2 and Tool 9-4.

HCPCS Modifier Codes

Level II (HCPCS) modifiers are also available for use in coding. Before using any of these modifiers, the coder must ascertain whether specific carriers accept these codes. When the carrier accepts both CPT and HCPCS codes and modifiers, the guidelines dictate that the highest level of specificity should be indicated. HCPCS codes (level II codes) permit greater specificity than CPT codes (level I).

COMMON HCPCS MODIFIER CODES

The most common level II HCPCS modifier codes are listed below. A complete listing is presented in Table 9-3.

LT	Left side of body
RT	Right side of body
E1	Upper left, eyelid
E2	Lower left, eyelid
E3	Upper right, eyelid
E4	Lower right, eyelid
FA	Left hand, thumb
F1	Left hand, second digit
F2	Left hand, third digit
F3	Left hand, fourth digit
F4	Left hand, fifth digit
F5	Right hand, thumb
F6	Right hand, second digit
F7	Right hand, third digit
F8	Right hand, fourth digit
F9	Right hand, fifth digit
TA	Left foot, great toe
T1	Left foot, second digit
T2	Left foot, third digit
T3	Left foot, fourth digit
T4	Left foot, fifth digit
T5	Right foot, great toe
T6	Right foot, second digit
T7	Right foot, third digit
T8	Right foot, fourth digit
T9	Right foot, fifth digit
LC	Left circumflex coronary artery
LD	Left anterior descending coronary artery
RC	Right coronary artery
QM	Ambulance service provided under arrangement with provider of services
QN	Ambulatory service provided directly by provider of services
QR	Repeat laboratory test on same day

SPECIFIC MODIFIER ISSUES

Right or Left Modifier(s)

Right (RT) and left (LT) anatomic modifiers should be appended when the *CPT descriptor* describes an anatomic site that ONLY has a right and left side. Consider the following examples:

Code 25600 Closed treatment of distal radial fracture

There are two radii, right and left. The anatomic RT or LT modifier should be appended for this procedure.

Code 12001 Simple repair, superficial wounds of scalp, neck, axillae, external genitalia, trunk, and/or extremities (including hands/feet) 2.5 cm or less

Multiple anatomic sites are listed in the CPT code 12001, so appending anatomic RT or LT to this procedure code would not clarify the exact location. It would NOT be appropriate to append an RT or LT for this procedure.

Anatomic Modifiers (FA-F9, TA-T9, E1-E4)

Certain modifiers are used to identify specific fingers (FA-F9), specific toes (TA-T9), or specific eyelids (E1-E4) that have been treated. As previously outlined, anatomic modifiers should only be used when the CPT descriptor is specific to that body area or part.

When the CPT descriptor describes only two locations, RT or LT would still be appropriate. Consider the following example:

Code 28505 Open treatment of a great toe fracture

There is only a right (RT) great toe and a left (LT) great toe, so an RT or an LT modifier would be appropriate.

TOOL 9-4

PHYSICIAN CPT-4 MODIFIER CODING REFERENCE TOOL

Modifier Code	Description	E & M	Anesthesia	Surgery	Radiology	Pathology	Medicine	ASC/Outpatient Surgery
21	Prolonged evaluation and management service	X						
22	Unusual procedural services		X	X	X	X	X	
23	Unusual anesthesia services		X					
24	Unrelated evaluation and management service same physician, global/postoperative period	X						
25	Significantly separately identifiable E & M service, same physician, same day	X						
26	Professional component service only			X	X	X	X	
32	Mandated service	X	X	X	X	X	X	
47	Anesthesia service performed by surgeon			X				
50	Bilateral procedure			X				X
51	Multiple procedures performed during one operative session		X	X	X		X	
52	Reduced service	X	X	X	X	X	X	X
53	Discontinued procedure		X	X	X	X	X	
54	Surgical care of global package only performed			X				
55	Postoperative care of global package only performed			X			X	
56	Preoperative care of global package only performed			X			X	
57	Decision made during E & M for surgical service	X						
58	Related/staged procedure, same physician during global surgical period			X	X		X	
59	Distinct procedure service		X	X	X	X	X	X
62	Two surgeons			X	X			
63	Procedures performed on infants <4 kg			X			X	
66	Surgical team			X			X	
73	Discontinued ASC procedure/before anesthesia							X
74	Discontinued ASC procedure/after anesthesia							X
76	Same physician repeats procedure			X	X		X	X
77	Different physician repeats procedure			X	X		X	X
78	Need for return to the OR for related procedure during global/postoperative period			X	X		X	
79	Need for unrelated procedure/service, same physician during global/postoperative period			X	X		X	
80	Assistant surgeon services			X	X			
81	Minimum assistant surgeon services			X				
82	Assistant surgeon services provided because qualified resident not available			X				
90	Services referred to outside to reference laboratory			X	X	X	X	
91	Repeat pathology service same day					X		X
99	Use of multiple modifiers for service billed			X	X		X	

E & M, Evaluation and management; *ASC*, ambulatory surgery center; *OR*, operating room.

TABLE 9-2 CPT MODIFIER CODES

MODIFIER	DESCRIPTION AND USE	EXAMPLE	SERVICE TYPE
22	Unusual procedural services beyond the usual scope of description	Increased difficulty in performing procedural services is encountered, such as extensive lysis of adhesions during the performance of an abdominal hysterectomy	Anesthesia, surgery, radiology, pathology, medicine
23	Unusual anesthesia services beyond the usual scope of description; may indicate greater service or general anesthesia for a procedure that typically does not require it.		Anesthesia services only
24	Unrelated E & M services by same physician during a predetermined follow-up postoperative period, which requires a modifier to justify the circumstances. Further justification is typically displayed in a diagnosis code for the E & M service unrelated to the global service.	When a postoperative patient encounters a problem during the postoperative period such as infection, fever, or bleeding, these visits do not classify as "normal postoperative care" and may be coded and billed with this modifier.	E & M services only
25	Significantly separately identifiable E & M services by same physician on same day. Diagnosis for the two separate services is typically different; however, coding guidelines specify this will not always be the case. Make certain the primary diagnosis for each service is, in fact, the primary reason for that encounter.	A patient arrives at the physician's office for E & M of pharyngitis and repair of an open wound of the finger. The physician documentation should reflect the E & M service with a primary diagnosis of pharyngitis and, preferably, a procedure note for the finger wound repair.	E & M services only
26	Applicable only when the physician provides a professional interpretation and report and the technical component is provided by the facility or another entity.		Surgery, radiology, pathology, medicine
32	Mandated service required by a third party such as an insurance carrier or a physician review organization.		All CPT services
47	Anesthesia service (regional or general) performed by surgeon rather than an anesthesiologist. Only codes from the surgery section should be used for these services. No anesthesia codes should be used with this modifier.		Surgery codes only
50	For identical services performed bilaterally that are not specified as such in the CPT descriptions. Controversy exists regarding the correct use of this modifier code; the coder must ascertain the preferred method for each third-party carrier to ensure proper coding. Some carriers require that the procedure be listed twice—once without the modifier and then as an additional code with the modifier. Other carriers want the procedure code listed only once, with modifier 50 added to indicate that the procedure was performed bilaterally. Make certain the charge amount corresponds with the billing method accepted by the third-party carrier. If the carrier wants the code to be listed only once, then the charge will typically be double the usual, single-procedure price.		Surgery, radiology, outpatient surgery

Continued

TABLE 9-2 CPT MODIFIER CODES—cont'd

MODIFIER	DESCRIPTION AND USE	EXAMPLE	SERVICE TYPE
51	Multiple procedures during same operative session by the same physician(s), with each **subsequent** procedure having this modifier Each subsequent procedure reimbursement is dramatically reduced because the preoperative approach has already been considered in the primary procedure reimbursement. Correctly listing the most significant primary procedure first is imperative for proper reimbursement.		Anesthesia, surgery, radiology, medicine
52	Services provided are atypical for the procedure. Remember that the coder should not assign a lower level of service with a requested decrease in charge but should charge the correct level of service with this modifier and bill the appropriate charge. This modifier should also be used when the service was not completed for reasons unrelated to the physician's decision or the patient's medical condition.	A colonoscopy could not be completed because of the inability of the scope to pass through the splenic flexure. The reduced service in this procedure was not from physician decision or medical condition.	All physician services; outpatient surgery
53	Physician decision to terminate the procedure before completion. This may occur because of changes in the patient's status or an inability to complete the procedure for other reasons. Not to be used for ambulatory/hospital outpatient coding (see modifiers 73 and 74).	A colonoscope cannot advance past a certain point, and the surgical procedure is halted because of patient hypotension.	Anesthesia, surgery, radiology, pathology, medicine
54	When only the surgical component of a global surgery procedure is performed by one physician. This results in a significant decrease in reimbursement because the global (preoperative, postoperative, and surgical) components were not performed.		Surgery codes only
55	When only the postoperative care of a global procedure is performed, designating only the usual uncomplicated follow-up postoperative care. If the surgeon providing the postoperative management encounters complications outside the normal global concept, those services may be billed additionally.		Surgery codes only
56	When only the preoperative component of a global surgery procedure is provided.	Preoperative clearance visits	Surgery codes only
57	The E & M service provided to determine that surgery is necessary. If not used, the service will be considered as preoperative care within the global package.		E & M services only
58	Staged or related procedure by same physician during the global operative period; when the physician plans to provide additional procedure(s) related to the initial procedure during the global postoperative period or is required to perform additional, more extensive surgery than was originally performed.		Surgery, radiology, medicine

59	When procedural services are distinct from other procedures performed on the same day by the same physician. In some instances this may be the result of two distinct surgical services (e.g., repair of hernia, repair of fractured humerus), different sessions or encounters (e.g., laceration repair in the morning, removal of foreign body from the eye in the evening), or different excisions or incisions (e.g., lesion removals). Use only if another modifier has not already been used to describe the circumstances.		Surgery, radiology, pathology, medicine, outpatient surgery
62	Two surgeons; when two surgeons worked together to perform one primary procedure, each physician should report the same procedural code with this modifier. As a general rule, the third-party carrier pays approximately 125% of the total allowance, with each physician receiving approximately 62.5% of the allowance. If one of the physicians bills this service incorrectly, only one physician will be paid.	Two surgeons are involved in a cochlear implant surgery, and each bills the same CPT code with modifier 62 for services described.	Surgery and radiology codes
63	Procedure performed on infants <4 kg; when procedures are performed on infants, some carriers will require the addition of this modifier. Many carriers, however, will not require the addition of this modifier. Other modifiers that may be applicable should still be assigned in addition to this modifier code.		
66	Surgical team; use this modifier when the skills of more than two physicians, as well as a team of highly skilled technical employees, are required to perform a procedure.	Transplant teams for kidney, heart, and lung operations.	Surgery, radiology
73	Discontinued outpatient hospital or ambulatory surgery center procedure before administration of anesthesia; when the procedure performed in the outpatient hospital or ambulatory surgery center setting is terminated after the preparation for surgery, but before the administration of anesthesia, this modifier should be appended to the surgical procedure code. These procedures may be cancelled for a number of reasons, including concern for the welfare of the patient and extenuating circumstances, but not because the patient has elected to terminate the procedure. The facility will be reimbursed a proportionate amount for that portion of the procedure performed. It is necessary to document at what point the procedure was terminated and why. The third-party carrier may request documentation before considering services with this modifier attached for reimbursement.		Outpatient surgery codes only

Continued

TABLE 9-2 CPT MODIFIER CODES—cont'd

MODIFIER	DESCRIPTION AND USE	EXAMPLE	SERVICE TYPE
74	Discontinued outpatient hospital or ambulatory surgery center procedure after administration of anesthesia; when a procedure scheduled in the outpatient hospital or ambulatory surgery center is terminated after the administration of anesthesia, that proportionate amount of service performed will be considered for reimbursement with the use of this modifier. Again, documentation regarding the progression of the surgery, as well as why the procedure was terminated, is necessary for reimbursement consideration. Elective termination by the patient will not be considered.		Outpatient surgery codes only
76	Repeat procedure by same physician; this modifier is used to indicate that the same procedure was performed more than once by the same physician in a given day. Each additional repeat procedure must be listed with the addition of this modifier.		Surgery, radiology, medicine codes Outpatient surgery codes
77	Repeat procedure by another physician; when the same procedure must be performed on the same day on which it was already performed by another physician, modifier 77 should be used. Both modifiers 76 and 77 are most commonly used for repeat procedures such as ECGs and chest x-rays, when periodic reevaluations during the course of a given day are necessary for the appropriate treatment or care of the patient.		Surgery, radiology, medicine codes Outpatient surgery codes
78	Return to the operating room for related procedure during the postoperative period; when related procedures are necessary during the postoperative period of the initial procedure, the related procedure must have this modifier added. This is necessary only for subsequent surgical procedures performed in the operating suite.		Surgery, radiology, medicine codes
79	Unrelated procedure/service by same physician during postoperative period. When an additional surgical procedure is performed by the same physician during the postoperative period of the first procedure, the subsequent procedure must be explained with the use of this modifier.	If a patient initially has a hernia repair performed by the surgeon on January 1 with a planned postoperative period of 30 days and returns to the general surgeon for outpatient clinic removal of a ganglion cyst during that 30-day period, the second procedure must have modifier 79 added to be considered for payment. This, of course, must be further justified by a diagnosis code unrelated to the primary diagnosis code.	Surgery, radiology, medicine codes
80	Assistant surgeon; when surgical assistant services are required to perform a given surgical procedure, the assistant surgeon should code the identical surgery code(s) as the primary surgeon, with this modifier added. If the second surgeon performed services in conjunction with the primary surgeon, this modifier would be appropriate.		Surgery, radiology codes

	Assistant surgeons not needed to perform a particular service typically are not reimbursed by third-party carriers. Third-party guidelines, as well as guidelines from the RBRVS, assist the coder in applying for reimbursement for these services.	
81	Minimum assistant surgeon; when only minimal services are required from the assistant surgeon, modifier 81 is appropriate. Because the reimbursement for assistant surgeon is typically 10% to 20% of the allowance for the primary surgeon, the allowance for the minimum assistant surgeon will be even less.	Surgery codes only
82	Assistant surgeon (when qualified resident surgeon not available); when hospital guidelines require the presence of an assistant surgeon and a qualified resident is not available to provide that service because of scheduling problems, emergency services, or lack of residents within that facility, this information must be communicated to the third-party carrier with the addition of this modifier.	Surgery codes only
90	Reference (outside) laboratory; when laboratory services are billed by the provider yet performed by an outside laboratory or other entity, these services should be listed, and modifier 90 should be added to each service. Remember that Medicare law does not allow any entity to bill for a service that it has not provided; therefore modifier 90 should NEVER appear on a Medicare claim.	Surgery, radiology, pathology, medicine codes
91	Repeat pathology services same day; when repeat laboratory services are designated as medically necessary on the same date as the original service, modifier 91 should be appended to subsequent listings of the same laboratory CPT code. This modifier was added in the 2000 version of CPT; it is not intended for repeat services necessary because of inadequate specimen(s).	
99	Multiple modifiers; when the use of multiple modifier codes is necessary to adequately explain more than one extenuating circumstance, modifier 99 must be appended to the procedure code, and a description of the multiple modifiers must be attached. Medicare allows up to two modifiers following a procedure code before multiple modifier 99 must be attached.	

E & M, Evaluation and management; *ECG,* electrocardiogram; *PRO,* physician review organization; *RBRVS,* resource-based relative value scale.

TABLE 9-3 LEVEL II HCPCS MODIFIERS

MODIFIER	DESCRIPTION
A1	Dressing, one wound
A2	Dressing, two wounds
A3	Dressing, three wounds
A4	Dressing, four wounds
A5	Dressing, five wounds
A6	Dressing, six wounds
A7	Dressing, seven wounds
A8	Dressing, eight wounds
A9	Dressing, nine or more wounds
AA	Anesthesia services performed personally by anesthesiologist
AB	Medical direction of own employee(s) (no more than four) by anesthesiologist
AC	Medical direction of other than own employee(s) (no more than four) by anesthesiologist
AD	Medical supervision by a physician: more than four employees concurrently
AE	Direction of residents in furnishing not more than two concurrent anesthesia services (attending physician relationship met)
AF	Anesthesia complicated by total body hypothermia
AG	Anesthesia for emergency surgery on patient who is moribund or who has an incapacitating systemic disease that is a constant threat to life
AH	Clinical psychologist
AJ	Clinical social worker
AK	Nurse practitioner, rural team member
AL	Nurse practitioner, nonrural team member
AM	Physician team member service
AN	Physician assistant services for other than assistant-at-surgery; nonteam member
AS	Physician assistant services for assistant-at-surgery
AT	Acute treatment (used with A2000 for acute treatment)
AU	Items furnished in conjunction with urologic, ostomy, or tracheostomy supply
AV	Items furnished in conjunction with prosthetic device, prosthetic, or orthotic
AW	Items furnished in conjunction with surgical dressing
AX	Items furnished in conjunction with dialysis services
BA	Items in conjunction with parenteral and enteral services
BO	Orally administered nutrition
BP	Beneficiary informed of purchase and rental options and has elected to purchase item (DME)
BR	Beneficiary informed of purchase and rental options and has elected to rent item (DME)
BU	Beneficiary informed of purchase and rental options and after 30 days has not informed supplier of decision
CC	Procedure code change Used when procedure code submitted was changed for administrative reasons or because of filing of incorrect code
DD	Powdered enteral formula
E1	Upper left eyelid
E2	Lower left eyelid
E3	Upper right eyelid
E4	Lower right eyelid
EJ	Subsequent claim (Epoetin ALFA [EPO] injection only)
EM	Emergency reserve supply (ESRD benefit only)
EP	Service provided as part of EPSDT program
ET	Emergency treatment (dental emergencies)
EY	No physician or licensed health care provider order
FA	Left hand, thumb
F1	Left hand, second digit
F2	Left hand, third digit
F3	Left hand, fourth digit
F4	Left hand, fifth digit
F5	Right hand, thumb
F6	Right hand, second digit

TABLE 9-3 LEVEL II HCPCS MODIFIERS—cont'd

MODIFIER	DESCRIPTION
F7	Right hand, third digit
F8	Right hand, fourth digit
F9	Right hand, fifth digit
FP	Services provided by Medicaid Family Planning Program
GA	Waiver of liability on file/ABN
GN	Service delivered under outpatient speech language pathology plan of care
GO	Service delivered under outpatient occupational therapy plan of care
GP	Service delivered under outpatient physical therapy plan of care
JW	Drug amount discarded/not administered to any patient
K Modifiers for Use with DME Claims Only	
KA	Add-on option/accessory wheelchair
KB	16 square inches or less
KC	More than 16 but ≤48 in^2
KD	More than 48 in^2
KE	1 Ounce
KF	1 Linear yard
KG	1 Cubic centimeter
KH	DMEPOS item, initial claim, purchase or first month rental
KI	DMEPOS item, second or third month rental
KJ	DMEPOS item, parenteral enteral nutrition pump or capped rental
KK	Inhalation solution compounded for FDA-approved formulation
KL	Product characteristics defined in medical policy have been met
KO	Lower extremity prosthesis functional level 0; no ability to ambulate or transfer with or without assistance; prosthesis does not enhance quality of life or mobility
K1	Lower extremity prosthesis functional level 1 Ability or potential to use prosthesis for transfers and/or ambulation on level surface Limited and unlimited household ambulator
K2	Lower extremity prosthesis functional level 2 Ability or potential to use prosthesis for ambulation and low-level environmental barriers (curbs, stairs) Typical limited community ambulator
K3	Lower extremity prosthesis functional level 3 Ability or potential to use prosthesis for ambulation and to cross most environmental barriers; may allow vocational, therapeutic, or exercise activity beyond simple locomotion
K4	Lower extremity prosthesis level 4 Ability or potential to use prosthesis exceeding basic ambulation skills; exhibiting high impact, stress, or energy levels Child, active adult, athlete
LL	Lease/rental; when DME rental is applied against purchase price
LR	Laboratory round trip
LS	FDA-monitored intraocular lens implant
LT	Left side of body
MS	Six-month maintenance and service fee for parts and labor not covered under any warranty
NR	New when rented; when DME, which was new at the time of rental, is subsequently purchased
NU	New equipment
PL	Progressive addition lenses
PS	Professional component charge for separate specimen
Q3	Live kidney donor surgery and related services
QB	Physician providing service in rural health professional shortage area
QC	Single-channel monitoring
QD	Recording/storage solid-state memory by a digital recorder
QE	Prescribed amount of oxygen less than 1 LPM
QF	Prescribed amount of oxygen exceeds 4 LPM and portable oxygen is prescribed
QG	Prescribed amount of oxygen exceeds 4 LPM
QH	Oxygen-conserving device being used with oxygen delivery system
QI	Deleted and replaced with modifier 57

Continued

TABLE 9-3 LEVEL II HCPCS MODIFIERS—cont'd

MODIFIER	DESCRIPTION
QJ	Medically directed by physician: two concurrent procedures
QK	Medical direction of two, three, or four concurrent anesthesia procedures involving qualified individuals
QM	Ambulance service provided under arrangement by hospital
QN	Ambulance service furnished directly by hospital
QO	Medically directed by physician: three concurrent procedures
QQ	Medically directed by physician: four concurrent procedures
QS	Monitored anesthesia care service (can be billed by certified registered nurse anesthetist or physician)
QT	Recording and storage of tape by analog tape recorder
QU	Physician providing services in urban HPSA
QX	CRNA service: with medical direction by physician
QZ	CRNA service: without medical direction by physician
Q1	Evidence of mycosis of toenail causing marked limitation of ambulation (for podiatry codes)
Q2	CMS demonstration project procedure/service
Q3	Live kidney donor; services associated with postoperative complications directly related to donor
Q4	Referring/ordering physician has no financial relationship with performing/billing entity
Q5	Service furnished by substitute physician under a reciprocal agreement
Q6	Service furnished by locum tenens physician
Q7	One class A finding (podiatry)
Q8	Two class A findings (podiatry)
Q9	One class B and two class A findings (podiatry)
RP	Replacement and repair; may be used to indicate replacement of DME, orthotic, or prosthetic device
RR	Rental (DME)
RT	Right side of body
SF	Second opinion ordered by PRO
SG	Ambulatory surgical center facility service
SK	Member high-risk population
SL	State supplied vaccine
ST	Related to trauma/injury
SU	Procedure performed in physician's office (to denote use of facility/equipment)
TA	Left foot, great toe
T1	Left foot, second digit
T2	Left foot, third digit
T3	Left foot, fourth digit
T4	Left foot, fifth digit
T5	Right foot, great toe
T6	Right foot, second digit
T7	Right foot, third digit
T8	Right foot, fourth digit
T9	Right foot, fifth digit
TC	Technical component
TS	Follow-up service
TT	Individual services provided to more than one patient/same setting
TU	Special payment rate, overtime
UE	Used DME rental
VP	Aphakic patient
YY	Second surgical opinion
ZZ	Third surgical opinion

ABN, Advanced beneficiary notice; *CME,* continuing medical education; *CRNA,* certified registered nurse anesthetist; *DME,* durable medical equipment; *DMEPOS,* durable medical equipment, prosthetics, orthotics, and supplies; *ESRD,* end-stage renal disease; *EPSDT,* early periodic screening, diagnosis, and treatment; *FDA,* Food and Drug Administration; *HCPCS,* Healthcare Common Procedure Coding System; *HPSA,* Healthcare Population Shortage Area; *LPM,* liters per minute; *PRO,* physician review organization.

STOP AND PRACTICE

Identify the correct modifier code(s) and give an example of each.

	Modifier	Example Code
1. Services greater than usually performed	______	______
2. Services less than usually performed	______	______
3. Office visit **for** laceration repair, 2.5 cm, eyebrow	______	______
4. Office visit **with** laceration repair, 2.5 cm, eyebrow	______	______
5. Office visit for postoperative follow-up	______	______
6. Office visit for postoperative complication	______	______
7. Repeat chest x-ray, same day, same physician	______	______
8. Repeat ECG, same day, different physician	______	______
9. Office visit during which decision for surgery is made	______	______
10. Consult during which decision for surgery is made	______	______
11. Hospital admission during which decision for surgery is made	______	______
12. Multiple procedures performed to same site	______	______
13. Multiple procedures performed, different operative site	______	______
14. Two surgeons performing same procedures	______	______

Identify the service billed, where in CPT the service is located, and whether a modifier is appropriate. You do not have to select the code itself. If no modifier code is appropriate, answer "none" or "NA."

15. A patient with fracture repair of the clavicle performed 10 days before presents for evaluation to the same physician for a sore throat.
    Service(s): _____
    CPT chapter: _____
    Modifier? Y N
    Modifier code: _____
16. A patient with a 1.2-cm laceration repair performed 3 days before presents for a recheck of suture repair.
    Service(s): _____
    CPT chapter: _____
    Modifier? Y N
    Modifier code: _____
17. A patient with fracture repair of the humerus performed 15 days earlier presents to the orthopedist for evaluation and repair of a clavicular fracture.
    Service(s): _____
    CPT chapter: _____
    Modifier? Y N
    Modifier code: _____
18. A laboratory service is not performed by the physician's office; however, the laboratory bills the physician's office and the physician's office bills the third-party carrier.
    Service(s): _____
    CPT chapter: _____
    Modifier? Y N
    Modifier code: _____
19. Two procedures are provided during one surgical session: abdominal hysterectomy and omentectomy.
    Service(s): _____
    CPT chapter: _____
    Modifier? Y N
    Modifier code: _____
20. Two surgical procedures are performed during the same surgical session: repair of inguinal hernia and repair of metacarpal fracture.
    Service(s): _____
    CPT chapter: _____
    Modifier? Y N
    Modifier code: _____
21. A patient presents after ORIF of a humerus fracture for evaluation and treatment of an ankle sprain.
    Service(s): _____
    CPT chapter: _____
    Modifier? Y N
    Modifier code: _____
22. A colonoscopy scheduled to be performed is canceled at the patient's request.
    Service(s): _____
    CPT chapter: _____
    Modifier? Y N
    Modifier code: _____
23. A colonoscopy that could not be completed because of the inability to advance the scope further.
    Service(s): _____
    CPT chapter: _____
    Modifier? Y N
    Modifier code: _____

Chapter in Review

Certification Review

- Matching of diagnostic and procedural codes is imperative for correct coding.
- Coding for physician services must always include a statement of services that specifies a diagnosis (WHY) and a procedure (WHAT).
- Procedural coding differs from diagnostic coding in that guidelines and rules are different for each section of the CPT manual.
- Listing CPT codes on the claim form in the most significant order is critical to for reimbursement.
- Modifier codes should be used to explain unusual circumstances for services.
- Modifier codes justify services that may not otherwise be considered for payment.
- Diagnosis codes that indicate medical necessity do not alone garner reimbursement for services typically included in the global surgical component unless the use of a modifier code designates the need for additional consideration.
- Modifier codes that should be used with CPT codes are included in the CPT coding book.
- Additional modifier codes, known as *HCPCS modifier codes,* are used by some carriers to designate more specific information. For instance, CPT modifier 50 indicates bilateral, and HCPCS modifiers RT/LT specify right and left.
- The global surgical concept includes all services performed as part of a surgical package.
- Separate procedures may only be coded when performed independently.

Student Assignments

- Review the Learning Objectives for Chapter 9.
- Complete the Certification Review for Chapter 9.
- Complete the Chapter Review exercise to reinforce concepts learned in this chapter.
- Complete the practice exercises on the companion Evolve site that accompanies this text for reinforcement of modifier coding concepts.
- Complete the Workbook exercises as assigned by your instructor.

Coding Review

Many of the case exercises include the assignment of modifier code(s). Although no exercises are specifically identified for modifier use, many contain multiple services, or services performed during the global postoperative period, that require the assignment of modifier code(s). No specific section of the coding certification examination covers modifier code use. These are included in the surgical, evaluation and management, and other services in the coding certification examination and exercises.

Chapter Review Exercises

Match the following services (procedures) to their appropriate diagnoses.

Services	Diagnosis
1. Chest x-ray	Anemia
2. CBC	Pneumonia
3. Wound repair	Bacterial infection
4. Injection antibiotic	COPD
5. Electrocardiogram	Schizophrenia
6. Bronchospasm	Open wound, arm evaluation
7. Psychotherapy, 45 min	Chest pain
8. Wrist x-ray	Coronary artery disease
9. Mammogram	Wrist sprain
10. Cardiac catheterization	Fibrocystic breast disease

Practical Application

For the following exercises, provide the following:

- All services performed and the reason (diagnosis) for each service. Do not assign ICD-9-CM codes.
- Steps 1 through 5 of the coding process. Use the grid in Tool 9-1 to determine the steps specific to the section or chapter of CPT. Also determine whether modifiers, if any, would be applied.

1. Discharge summary

DISCHARGE SUMMARY

Admitted: 05/07/xx
Discharged: 05/11/xx

Discharge diagnoses:

History:

Patient is a 34-year-old male who stated he was assaulted the evening of admission by several men. The patient stated he was struck by an object on the right side of the back and the groin. He came to the ER complaining of right testicular pain to the groin. Patient denied burning, frequency or urgency. Denied loss of consciousness or head trauma. No past medical, social or family history.

PHYSICAL EXAM:
Fair amount of swelling in the right scrotal sac. Right testicle is tender to palpation and tender in the right inguinal area. Prostate smooth but extremely tender and mildly enlarged. Remainder of physical exam is unremarkable.

Laboratory and radiology studies:

Significant for WBC of 11.8. All other labs returned normal

Hospital course:

Patient was admitted to the Urology Service and placed on intravenous antibiotics. A testicular nuclear medicine scan was obtained which revealed normal blood flow to both testicles. There was increased uptake in the epididymis of the affected testicle, interpreted as traumatic epididymitis. This was followed by a small scrotal hematoma. NO evidence of ruptured testicle was found.

Patient was maintained on IV antibiotics. Improved significantly over the course of his admission.

He will be discharged with a prescription for Vibramycin and will be on regular diet with activities as tolerated. He will follow up in the urological clinic in one week.

Felix Washburn MD

GODFREY REGIONAL HOSPITAL
123 Main Street • Aldon, FL 77714 • (407) 555-1234

Services Provided ______________

Diagnosis or Medical Necessity ______________

Step 1: CPT chapter: ______________

Step 2: ______________

Step 3: ______________

Step 4: ______________

Step 5: ______________

Modifier code: Y/N

Code: ______________

2. Office consultation

OFFICE CONSULTATION

Indication for consultation:

This is a 47-year-old male, lifelong smoker, referred to me. He complains of 2 week history of dry cough associated with dull discomfort and dyspnea. Otherwise, he has been free of any other associated symptoms. He denied any preceding cold, flu or allergic exposure symptoms. He denies any fever, chills, night sweats or weight loss.

History:

Has traveled extensively throughout the US, admits to having childhood asthma. He has not had pneumonia vaccine. Had a TB skin test 10 years ago and flu vaccine 3 years ago.

Exam:

Blood pressure, 150/85, pulse 80, respiratory rate, 20, temperature 98.3. Chest exam is completely normal, with no rales, wheezes, rhonchi, or rubs. Even on forced exhalation there was no cough or prolongation. Cardiac exam showed a regular rate and rhythm with no murmur or gallop.

Laboratory Data:
PA Chest is remarkable for a new interstitial infiltrate seen in both mid-lung zones with some shagging of the cardiac borders, indicating involvement of the lingual and right middle lobe.

Spirometry before and after bronchodilator shows a vital capacity of 3.79 or 69% after an 11% improvement with bronchodilator.

Diagnosis/assessment:

Differential Diagnosis includes the following:
Hypersensitivity pneumonia
Mycoplasmal pneumonia

John Palermo

Patient name: ______

Date of service: ______

GODFREY MEDICAL ASSOCIATES
1532 Third Avenue, Suite 120 • Aldon, FL 77713 • (407) 555-4000

Services Provided ______

Diagnosis or Medical Necessity ______ ______ ______

Step 1: CPT chapter:
Step 2:
Step 3: ______
Step 4: ______
Step 5: ______
Modifier code: Y/N Code: ______

3. Bronchoscopy

OPERATIVE REPORT

Patient information:

Patient name:
DOB:
MR#:

Preoperative diagnosis:

The patient had a right lower lobe lung nodule.

Postoperative diagnosis:

Procedure(s) performed:

Bronchoscopy

The video Olympus bronchoscope with small diameter was used.

Anesthesia:

IV conscious sedation at .5 mg and 1 mg titrations.

Assistant surgeon:

Description of procedure:

The bronchoscope was passed via the left nares without difficulty. The epiglottis and aryepiglottic folds were normal in appearance and color. The vocal cords moved equally and approximated with phonation. The bronchoscope was then passed into the tracheobronchial tree. The mucosa at the level of the carina was normal in appearance and color. The right upper lobe, right middle lobe and right lower lobe were all patent, no endobronchial lesions seen. The bronchoscope was taken to the left tracheobronchial tree. The left lower lobe and left upper lobe were patent with no endobronchial lesion seen.

The bronchoscope was then taken to the right lower lobe anterior basal segment and multiple transbronchial brushings and biopsies obtained with fluoroscopic guidance. Scant bleeding stopped spontaneously.

CONCLUSIONS:
Peripheral nodule in the right lower lobe, anterior basal segment. Transbronchial biopsies obtained without difficulty. The patient tolerated the procedure well.

Adam Westy MD

GODFREY REGIONAL HOSPITAL
123 Main Street • Aldon, FL 77714 • (407) 555-1234

Services Provided	Diagnosis or Medical Necessity		
______________	______________	Step 3:	______________
Step 1: CPT chapter:	______________	Step 4:	______________
Step 2:	______________	Step 5:	______________
		Modifier code: Y/N	Code: ______________

4. Cholecystectomy

OPERATIVE REPORT

Patient information:

Patient name:
DOB:
MR#:

Preoperative diagnosis:

Cholelithiasis, chronic cholecystitis

Postoperative diagnosis:

Same

Procedure(s) performed:

Laparoscopic Cholecystectomy

Anesthesia:

Assistant surgeon:

Description of procedure:

After satisfactory general anesthesia was accomplished, a nasogastric tube was placed. The anterior abdominal wall was sterilely prepped and draped. An infraumbilical incision was made and pneumoperitoneum was established. The camera was placed through the trocars. An epigastric port was placed and two 5 mm ports were placed in the subcostal plane. Graspers were placed through the lateral ports and used to retract the fundus of the gallbladder.

The cystic artery and duct were isolated and doubly slipped. Dissection commenced with the gallbladder removed from the hilar structures of the fundus. The gallbladder was removed through the umbilical port. The gallbladder was inspected. There was an approximately 2 cm stone in the gallbladder.

The lateral ports were removed and revealed no bleeding. The epigastric port was removed and also revealed no bleeding. The pneumoperitoneum was evacuated and sutures placed at the umbilical fascia to close the fascial defect and skin incisions closed with a running subcuticular 4-0 Vicryl suture. Steri-strips were applied.

The patient tolerated the procedure well and was returned to the recovery room in stable condition. Rachel Perez MD

GODFREY REGIONAL HOSPITAL
123 Main Street • Aldon, FL 77714 • (407) 555-1234

Services Provided	Diagnosis or Medical Necessity
Step 1: CPT chapter:	
Step 2:	
Step 3:	
Step 4:	
Step 5:	
Modifier code: Y/N	Code:

5. Colonoscopy and polypectomy

OPERATIVE REPORT

Patient information:

Patient name:
DOB:
MR#:

Preoperative diagnosis:

History of Colonic Polyps

Postoperative diagnosis:

Colonic Polyp

Procedure(s) performed:

Colonoscopy and polypectomy

Anesthesia:

Assistant surgeon:

Description of procedure:

The patient was brought to the endoscopy suite and placed in the supine position. The colonoscope was introduced and passed through all flexures into the cecum. Position in the cecum was identified by the ileocecal valve. The scope was then withdrawn visualizing all the sites of the colon. The patient had a small ulcerated polyp in the proximal ascending colon. Using snare polypectomy, it was removed in piecemeal fashion.

The patient tolerated the procedure well and was transferred to the Same Day Surgery in stable condition.

Adam Westy MD

GODFREY REGIONAL HOSPITAL
123 Main Street • Aldon, FL 77714 • (407) 555-1234

Services Provided	Diagnosis or Medical Necessity		
______	______	Step 3:	______
Step 1: CPT chapter:	______	Step 4:	______
Step 2:	______	Step 5:	______
		Modifier code: Y/N	Code: ______

10

Using CPT

LEARNING OBJECTIVES

After completing this chapter, the student will be able to:

- Understand the levels of Healthcare Common Procedure Coding System (HCPCS) codes used.
- Comprehend the basic concept and format of the Current Procedural Terminology (CPT) coding book.
- Understand that all services in CPT are broken down into six chapters, with specific guidelines for each group.
- Identify and understand the significance of signs and symbols used in the CPT coding book.
- Grasp the concept of modifiers and explain their proper application to the CPT coding system.

KEY TERMS

Add-on Procedure

American Medical Association (AMA)

Anesthesiology

Bullet

Current Procedural Terminology (CPT)

Evaluation and Management (E & M)

Healthcare Common Procedure Coding System (HCPCS)

Medicine

Pathology

Radiology

Surgery

During the early 1980s, the **American Medical Association (AMA)**, with the assistance of a physician editorial panel, developed a coding method to standardize reporting of procedures and services, much like the standardized diagnostic coding of the ICD-9-CM. Since that time, third-party carriers have required that this procedural coding be used in billing for physician services. Effective August 2000, this methodology became required on outpatient facility (hospital) claims as well. This coding system, **Current Procedural Terminology** (**CPT**), is only one part of a third-party coding system, the **Healthcare Common Procedure Coding System** (**HCPCS**). These two levels are as follows:

Level 1	CPT
Level 2	National codes (referred to as HCPCS level II)

With the implementation of the Health Insurance Portability and Accountability Act (HIPAA) of 1996 and its subsequent updates, codes specific to individual regions became obsolete. Under HIPAA, the law dictates that all third-party carriers in the United States must use the same code sets for billing and coding services; thus local codes are no longer applicable.

General Documentation Requirements for CPT Coding

The assignment of CPT codes is perhaps the simplest part of the coding process. The process of extracting the key words needed to assign the appropriate CPT code(s) is discussed in Chapter 9. This chapter deals with taking that information gathered and assigning the appropriate CPT code(s) and modifiers for those services.

After a brief overview of the layout and format of the CPT book, steps 6 through 8 of the CPT coding selection process will be discussed. These steps describe how to select the code(s) and modifier(s) for the services provided.

LAYOUT

General

The CPT coding book is divided into six chapters (listed below); each uses a distinctly separate set of guidelines. This was discussed briefly in Chapter 9; however, a more in-depth discussion is necessary to narrow the selection process.

Evaluation and management (visits)	99201-99499
Anesthesiology	00100-01999 99100-99140
Surgery	10000-69999
Radiology	70000-79999
Pathology/laboratory	80000-89999
Medicine	90700-99199

The layout is based on the "step" method of identifying the correct section within CPT and the correct components and eventually narrowing the possible selections down to only the correct code. Each section within the CPT book is divided into subsections by anatomic, pr
descriptor subheadings. Procedures
sented in numeric order EXCEPT f
and management section, which is p
the CPT book. It is the most comm
used by every provider.

Each section is prefaced with codi
that section. Modifier codes are li
section as well as any instructions u
assigning appropriate codes.

Each section of CPT is unique reg
for assigning codes from that secti
process remains the same. The intri
CPT are discussed in individual cha
a snapshot of the components need
Tool 9-1, which shows the basic steps
each section of CPT. In this chapt
through 8 to that process, finishing
CPT code assignment.

EVALUATION AND MANAGE
99201-99499)

This section was specifically design
provided directly by the physician or
visits or evaluation services. The spe
medical information for coding evalu
services (steps 1 through 5 of the pr
as follows:

Identify CPT chapter:	Services
Identify type/location:	Inpatient consult
New/established:	New pati initial
Level of service:	Level 1 Level 2 Level 3 Level 4 (Level 5 (

This information is necessary to c
agement services as well as all other
CPT codes. As with ICD-9-CM codi
on the documentation by the provid
not documented, the coder or bil
knowledge of the services and may n
than was actually provided.

Because all codes in the evalua
section begin with the number 99, t
simply as level 1, level 2, level 3, le
notation is commonly used throug
likely be encountered in physician a

The CPT section titled Evaluatio
vices is subsectioned as follows:

- Outpatient/Office Visits
- Hospital Observation Services

spital Inpatient Services
nsultations
ergency Department Services
tical Care Services
onatal/Pediatric Intensive Care Services
rsing Facility Services
miciliary, Rest Home, Custodial Services
longed Services
ysician Standby Services
se Management Services
re Plan Oversight Services
ventive Medicine Services
unseling/Risk Factor Services
wborn Care
cial Evaluation and Management Services

code services from the evaluation and management n of CPT, the coder must capture specific information he documentation. The steps listed in Tool 9-1 neces- o capture information for assigning evaluation and gement codes are as follows.

1: Determine Chapter or Section of CPT

tion and Management

2: Type/Location

/outpatient
tal observation
tal inpatient
ltations
gency department services
ric critical care patient transport
l care
ent neonatal and pediatric critical care services
g facility services
iliary, rest home, or custodial care services
services
ged services
management services
lan oversight services
ntive medicine services
l evaluation and management services

Step 3: Patient Status

New/established
Initial/subsequent

Step 4: Level of Service

Level 1
Level 2
Level 3
Level 4 (when applicable)
Level 5 (when applicable)

These levels will be determined by documentation pulled from the report that supports the following:

- History: Information gathered regarding the patient's description of the current illness, a review of systems as well as past medical, family, and social history.
- Exam: Clinical examination of the patient to include all pertinent and negative findings of the affected body systems or body areas.
- Medical decision making: The extent of diagnosis and management options considered by the physician in making a final diagnosis, data considered, and the risk of morbidity/mortality for the condition(s) of the patient.

Step 4 is discussed in Chapter 11 regarding details of specific information for evaluation and management services.

Step 5: Determine Whether Time or Other Guidelines Are Applicable

This step will be discussed in Chapter 11 in the in-depth discussion of evaluation and management services.

Example of the abstracting of an evaluation and management service would be as follows:

Type/location:	Outpatient
New/established:	Established patient
Level:	Level 3; based on documentation of history, exam, medical decision making (see Chapter 11)
Code assignment:	99213

This method of assigning the correct evaluation and management level of service is discussed in depth in Chapter 11. This chapter only discusses determining which range of codes will be used for assignment.

P AND PRACTICE

ew the following evaluation and management ces and determine the appropriate range of codes for assignment. Further code selection will be ned based on history, exam, and medical decision- ng information taken from the report (discussed in ter 11).

1. Outpatient office visit for an established patient
   Step 1: Chapter of CPT: Evaluation and Management
   Step 2: Type/location: ____________
   Range of codes: ____________
   Step 3: Patient status: ____________
   Range of codes: ____________
   Code range selection: ____________

STOP AND PRACTICE—cont'd

2. Initial hospital visit
   Step 1: Chapter of CPT: Evaluation and Management
   Step 2: Type/location: ____
   Range of codes: 99221-99223
   Step 3: Patient status: ____
   Range of codes: ____
   Code range selection: ____
3. Initial inpatient consultation
   Step 1: Chapter of CPT: Evaluation and Management
   Step 2: Type/location: ____
   Range of codes: ____
   Step 3: Patient status: ____
   Range of codes: ____
   Code range selection: ____
4. Preventive medicine visit for new patient, age 50 years
   Step 1: Chapter of CPT: Evaluation and Management
   Step 2: Type/location: ____
   Range of codes: ____
   Step 3: Patient status: ____
   Range of codes: ____
   Code range selection: ____
5. Subsequent nursing facility visit
   Step 1: Chapter of CPT: Evaluation and Management
   Step 2: Type/location: ____
   Range of codes: ____
   Step 3: Patient status: ____
   Range of codes: ____
   Code range selection: ____
6. Home visit, new patient
   Step 1: Chapter of CPT: Evaluation and Management
   Step 2: Type/location: ____
   Range of codes: ____
   Step 3: Patient status: ____
   Range of codes: ____
   Code range selection: ____
7. Hospital discharge visit/services
   Step 1: Chapter of CPT: Evaluation and Management
   Step 2: Type/location: ____
   Range of codes: ____
   Step 3: Patient status: ____
   Range of codes: ____
   Code range selection: ____
8. New patient office visit
   Step 1: Chapter of CPT: Evaluation and Management
   Step 2: Type/location: ____
   Range of codes: ____
   Step 3: Patient status: ____
   Range of codes: ____
   Code range selection: ____
9. Observation care discharge visit
   Step 1: Chapter of CPT: Evaluation and Management
   Step 2: Type/location: ____
   Range of codes: ____
   Step 3: Patient status: ____
   Range of codes: ____
   Code range selection: ____
10. New office consultation
    Step 1: Chapter of CPT: Evaluation and Management
    Step 2: Type/location: ____
    Range of codes: ____
    Step 3: Patient status: ____
    Range of codes: ____
    Code range selection: ____

STOP AND PRACTICE

Review the following evaluation and management services and determine the appropriate range of codes used for assignment. As in the previous Stop and Practice exercise, further code selection will be assigned based on history, exam, and medical decision-making information taken from the report (discussed in Chapter 11).

1. Chest pain

HISTORY AND PHYSICAL EXAMINATION

Godfrey Regional Hospital History & Physical
Admission: 11/17/xx

CHIEF COMPLAINT: Chest Pain

HISTORY OF PRESENT ILLNESS: 65-year-old female admitted with chest pain on night of admission. This lasted off and on for some time, probably several hours. It was not relieved by nitroglycerin. She also has Type 1 Diabetes and her sugars are sporadically in the 300-400 range. She has been unable to lose weight and is grossly obese.

Past medical history:

Please see old records

Family and social history

Please see old records

Review of systems:

Essentially unchanged from last admission. She has occasional headaches. She has cough and congestion but no pneumonia or TB. Appetite and digestion have been good, and she has had no GI bleeding. No urgency, frequency, dysuria. Positive for arthritis.

Physical exam

Vital Signs: BP 140/80, Pulse 88 and regular, respirations 16
General: Well developed female complaining of chest pain and shortness of breath
HEENT: Head normocephalic.
Lungs: Reveal scattered wheezes and basiliar rales
Heart: Regular sinus rhythm.
Abdomen: No masses felt. Nontender
Extremities: Unremarkable except 1+ dema.
Neuro: Reflexes equal and active

Laboratory/radiology:

Labs: Abnormal Labs, WBC
ECG: Normal

X-ray:

Assessment:

Chest Pain

Plan:

Will admit, try trial of Nitroglycerin and Morphine and recheck cardiac enzymes and ECG. Will schedule cardiac stress test for the morning and proceed based on findings.

GODFREY REGIONAL HOSPITAL
123 Main Street • Aldon, FL 77714 • (407) 555-1234

Step 1: Chapter of CPT: Evaluation and Management

Step 2: Type/location: ____________
Range of codes: ____________

Step 3: Patient status: ____________
Range of codes: ____________

Code range selection: ____________

2. Reaction to erythromycin

OFFICE NOTE

Chief complaint: Rash

Date: ________________

Vital signs: BP______P______R______

History:

Exam:

The patient has had what appears to be a significant reaction to Erythromycin. He has a total body rash which has not responded to antihistamines. He has marked swelling of the right arm within the last 24 hours. The right forearm is warm, red and has a severe dermatitis.

Diagnosis/assessment:

Severe allergic reaction to Erythromycin

PLAN: I have advised the patient to contact the dermatologist for further treatment and referral.

William Obert MD

Patient name: ________________

Date of service: ________________

GODFREY MEDICAL ASSOCIATES
1532 Third Avenue, Suite 120 • Aldon, FL 77713 • (407) 555-4000

Step 1: Chapter of CPT: Evaluation and Management

Step 2: Type/location: ________________
Range of codes: ________________

Step 3: Patient status: ________________
Range of codes: ________________

Code range selection: ________________

3. Consultation for bladder output obstruction

CONSULTATION

Indication for consultation:

Follow up for bladder outlet obstruction

History:

Patient is a 64-year-old treated last week for urinary retention. He has an indwelling Foley but it is unclear when it was first inserted.

Exam:

Well developed, well nourished male in no apparent distress. He has an indwelling Foley with some erosion of the urethra. The prostate exam failed to reveal any obvious nodularity.

IMPRESSION:
Indwelling Foley catheter
Urethral erosion
Urinary tract infection

Diagnosis/assessment:

While the patient is still in the hospital, we might as well give him a voiding trial.

Maurice Doder, MD

Patient name: ______________________

Date of service: ______________

GODFREY MEDICAL ASSOCIATES
1532 Third Avenue, Suite 120 • Aldon, FL 77713 • (407) 555-4000

Step 1: Chapter of CPT: Evaluation and Management

Step 2: Type/location: ______________
Range of codes: ______________

Step 3: Patient status: ______________
Range of codes: ______________

Code range selection: ______________

4. Discharge summary

DISCHARGE SUMMARY

Patient name, MR#
DOB:

Admitted:
Discharged:

Discharge diagnoses:

Discharged in satisfactory condition.

History:

29-year-old severely mentally retarded female admitted for left breast biopsy for breast mass found on routine physical exam. No past surgical history, medications or allergies.

PHYSICAL EXAM: A severely contracted female in no apparent distress. She was afebrile with stable vital signs. Patient had a 2 X 3 cm irregular mobile mass in the left breast. The rest of her exam was unremarkable.

Laboratory and radiology studies:

Hospital course:

Breast biopsy was performed under local anesthesia. She was brought to the floor postoperatively with stable vital signs. She was able to tolerate a diet and void without difficulty. The patient is being discharged and transferred back to the development center for following up in the general surgery clinic.

D:
T:

GODFREY REGIONAL HOSPITAL
123 Main Street • Aldon, FL 77714 • (407) 555-1234

Step 1: Chapter of CPT: Evaluation and Management

Step 2: Type/location: __________
Range of codes: __________

Step 3: Patient status: __________
Range of codes: __________

Code range selection: __________

5. Possible seizure

OFFICE NOTE

Chief complaint: ____________________

Date: ____________

Vital signs: BP______ P______ R______

History:

Seven year old brought in by mother with complaint of possible seizure. According to mother, first episode was witness by sister a couple months ago while sleeping. Patient has a history of nightmares, night terrors and sleepwalks. Last night he had a similar episode with moving and frothing at the mouth. It was difficult to wake him, and he had no postictal state. Denies any incontinence. Denies biting his tongue. Denies any history of falls, medication changes or any similar episodes.

No medications or allergies.

Exam:

Alert and oriented X 3. No acute distress. Vital signs, stable. Very interactive. Understands and answers questions appropriately. Does not appear to be in postictal state by any means. No tongue trauma or bruise marks. HEENT, PERRLA, EOMI, Throat clear. Chest: clear. Abdomen: Soft, nontender. Extremities: No edema, no cyanosis. CNS: Grossly intact with no focal deficit.

Diagnosis/assessment:

Questionable seizure activity versus night terrors. Reassured parents. Need to follow up with neurologist for further diagnosis.

Stacy Kraatt, MD

Patient name: ____________________

Date of service: ____________

GODFREY MEDICAL ASSOCIATES
1532 Third Avenue, Suite 120 • Aldon, FL 77713 • (407) 555-4000

Step 1: Chapter of CPT: Evaluation and Management

Step 2: Type/location: ____________
Range of codes: ____________

Step 3: Patient status: ____________
Range of codes: ____________

Code range selection: ____________

ANESTHESIOLOGY (CODES 00100-01999/99100-99140)

Services performed by the anesthesiologist or the certified nurse anesthetist (under the supervision of the anesthesiologist) are listed in the **anesthesiology** section. Keep in mind that the anesthesiology provider may also perform services outside the anesthesia section, such as an injection made into the spinal column and nerves for pain management. The code for this service would be found in another section of CPT.

Codes in the anesthesia section of CPT are assigned according to anatomic location of the surgery and are arranged in "anatomic order," starting at the head and progressing down the body, except for a few sections that cannot be organized in this fashion. Procedures performed on the head and neck, for example, are found in the front portion of the anesthesia section. Keep in mind that these codes are for analgesic medications used during surgical procedures; the surgeon performing the actual surgery will use other codes, usually found in the surgery section.

The anesthesia codes found in this section are easily distinguishable from surgical codes for the same procedures because all codes found in the anesthesia section begin with a zero. It is clear when reviewing a claim form that a procedure code beginning with a zero is for anesthesia services only and not the surgery itself. The following example demonstrates how to code for anesthesia by taking one step at a time:

Identify chapter:	Anesthesia
Anatomic location:	Where surgical procedure is being performed Listed as general areas such as head/neck, lower/upper abdomen
Specific location:	Codes sometimes are specific to one body area or region (e.g., radius, ulna, femur, fibula, tibia)
Specific procedure:	Descriptions of specifically what is performed, such as fracture treatment/resection/reduction/incision
Specifics:	Open/closed reduction

The information necessary to code or bill for anesthesia services is typically contained in the anesthesia billing card completed by the provider at the time of service. It is then returned to the provider's office for coding and billing. In addition to the above information, many carriers require the physical status of the patient, any "qualifying" circumstances, and the anesthesia time, typically reported in "start/stop" times. This information is discussed in depth in Chapter 12. Keep in mind that the coder and biller are responsible for making certain that appropriately signed documentation exists for all services being billed.

STOP AND PRACTICE

Review the following examples of anesthesia services and determine what code(s) would be appropriate. After mastering the selection of CPT codes by the breakdown process, you will look at that same process with a sample medical report. Most of the additional information needed for assigning all the codes for anesthesia services will be captured from the anesthesia billing card, which is reviewed in Chapter 12.

1. Knee arthroscopy
   Step 1: Identify chapter: ____________
   Step 2: Anatomic location: ____________
   Step 3: Body area/organ: ____________
   Step 4: Specific procedure: ____________
   Step 5: Additional specifics: ____________
   Anesthesia procedure code assignment: ____________
2. Closed reduction femur fracture
   Step 1: Identify chapter: ____________
   Step 2: Anatomic location: ____________
   Step 3: Body area/organ: ____________
   Step 4: Specific procedure: ____________
   Step 5: Additional specifics: ____________
   Anesthesia procedure code assignment: ____________
3. Radical mastectomy
   Step 1: Identify chapter: ____________
   Step 2: Anatomic location: ____________
   Step 3: Body area/organ: ____________
   Step 4: Specific procedure: ____________
   Step 5: Additional specifics: ____________
   Anesthesia procedure code assignment: ____________
4. Blepharoplasty
   Step 1: Identify chapter: ____________
   Step 2: Anatomic location: ____________
   Step 3: Body area/organ: ____________
   Step 4: Specific procedure: ____________
   Step 5: Additional specifics: ____________
   Anesthesia procedure code assignment: ____________
5. Repair of cleft palate
   Step 1: Identify chapter: ____________
   Step 2: Anatomic location: ____________
   Step 3: Body area/organ: ____________
   Step 4: Specific procedure: ____________
   Step 5: Additional specifics: ____________
   Anesthesia procedure code assignment: ____________

STOP AND PRACTICE—cont'd

6. Permanent intravenous pacemaker placement
   Step 1: Identify chapter: ____________
   Step 2: Anatomic location: ____________
   Step 3: Body area/organ: ____________
   Step 4: Specific procedure: ____________
   Step 5: Additional specifics: ____________
   Anesthesia procedure code assignment: ____________
7. Amniocentesis
   Step 1: Identify chapter: ____________
   Step 2: Anatomic location: ____________
   Step 3: Body area/organ: ____________
   Step 4: Specific procedure: ____________
   Step 5: Additional specifics: ____________
   Anesthesia procedure code assignment: ____________
8. Radical prostatectomy
   Step 1: Identify chapter: ____________
   Step 2: Anatomic location: ____________
   Step 3: Body area/organ: ____________
   Step 4: Specific procedure: ____________
   Step 5: Additional specifics: ____________
   Anesthesia procedure code assignment: ____________
9. Extracorporeal shock wave lithotripsy
   Step 1: Identify chapter: ____________
   Step 2: Anatomic location: ____________
   Step 3: Body area/organ: ____________
   Step 4: Specific procedure: ____________
   Step 5: Additional specifics: ____________
   Anesthesia procedure code assignment: ____________
10. Total wrist arthroplasty
   Step 1: Identify chapter: ____________
   Step 2: Anatomic location: ____________
   Step 3: Body area/organ: ____________
   Step 4: Specific procedure: ____________
   Step 5: Additional specifics: ____________
   Anesthesia procedure code assignment: ____________

SURGERY (CODES 10000-69999)

Procedures that the layperson may not consider surgical may have surgical codes in CPT (e.g., laceration repairs). The **surgery** section is composed of services that typically are invasive, restorative, or definitive. In other words, for the services to be performed, "invading" or entering the body by some method is typically required. The procedure performed may also be definitive or corrective for the problem being treated. When codes from the surgery section are assigned, all guidelines and modifiers for that section should be used when applicable. Because of the size of the section, it is imperative that the coder use the breakdown method built into the CPT layout.

Identify chapter: Surgery considered invasive, definitive, or corrective in nature
Anatomic system
- Integumentary
- Musculoskeletal
- Respiratory
- Cardiovascular
- Hematologic and lymphatic
- Mediastinum and diaphragm
- Digestive system
- Urinary system
- Male genital system
- Intersex surgery
- Female genital system
- Maternity care and delivery
- Endocrine system
- Nervous system
- Eye and ocular adnexa
- Auditory system

Anatomic part
- Examples: Radius, breast, eye, ear

Type of procedure
- Incision
- Excision
- Fracture/dislocation
- Repair, reconstruction
- -Scopy
- Introduction/removal
- Arthrodesis
- Amputation

Extent of procedure
- Examples: Fracture, closed/open
- With/without manipulation
- With/without fixation

Many of the exercises in Chapter 9 involved surgical procedures, one of the most difficult sections in CPT. Following is a surgical procedure and the breakdown process:
Procedure: Mastectomy
Chapter: Surgery
Anatomic system: Integumentary
Anatomic part: Breast
Procedure: Excision
Extent: Breast lesion

The code(s) for mastectomy are in the 19140-19240 range. After reviewing the operative report for information such as the extent of the excision, the specific mastectomy code is selected. This process is explored in Chapter 13.

STOP AND PRACTICE

Following are a few practice exercises in breaking down the information for CPT code assignment for the surgery section by using sample operative reports.

1. Chronic adenotonsillitis

OPERATIVE REPORT

Patient information:

Patient name:
DOB:
MR#:

Preoperative diagnosis:

Chronic Adenotonsillitis

Postoperative diagnosis:

Chronic Adenotonsillitis

Procedure(s) performed:

Tonsillectomy and Adenoidectomy

Anesthesia:

Assistant surgeon:

Description of procedure:

The patient was taken to the operating room where in a supine position under general anesthesia, the patient was prepped and draped in a sterile manner. The ring mouth gag was placed in position. The oropharynx was exposed. The left tonsil was grasped with a tonsil tenaculum. Using a modified Harris dissector, the tonsillar capsule was exposed from the anterior pillar. Using blunt dissection, the tonsil was then dissected and excised with Metzenbaum scissors. This procedure was then repeated on the right side. The naasopharynx was inspected and there was not significant adenoid tissue present. All bleeding vessels were cauterized to maintain hemostasis.

This was then repeated on the right fossa. Final inspection of both fossa did not reveal any bleeding. Nasopharynx was inspected and there was a large amount of adenoid tissue present. This was removed with adenotome and adenoid curet. Cotton sponges with 1% Neo-Synephrine were inserted in the nasopharynx to promote hemostasis.

Rachel Perez MD

GODFREY REGIONAL HOSPITAL
123 Main Street • Aldon, FL 77714 • (407) 555-1234

Step 1: CPT chapter: ________
Step 2: Anatomic system: ________
Step 3: Organ/body part: ________
Step 4: Technique/approach: ________
Step 5: Additional specifics: ________ ________ ________ ________

2. Lymphadenopathy

OPERATIVE REPORT

Patient information:

Patient name:
DOB:
MR#:

Preoperative diagnosis:

Right inguinal lymphadenopathy, history of lymphoma

Postoperative diagnosis:

Right inguinal lymphadenopathy, history of lymphoma, rule out persistent lymphoma

Procedure(s) performed:

Excision of inguinal lymph node

Anesthesia:

Assistant surgeon:

Description of procedure:

With the patient in supine position, the right inguinal area was widely prepared with Betadine and draped. After administration of local anesthesia, a transverse incision was made. Incision was carried through Scarpa's fascia with cautery until the lymph node was encountered. The lymph node was then carefully dissected from surrounding vascular and areolar attachments. Hemostasis was obtained using cautery. Hemostasis was good after the lymph node was excised. The wound was closed in layers using interrupted 3-0 plain catgut to approximately Scarpa's fascia and interrupted 5-0 Vicryl subcuticular sutures to approximate the skin. Wound was dressed with Xeroform gauze, dry sterile dressing and tegaderm.

Adam Westgate MD

GODFREY REGIONAL HOSPITAL
123 Main Street • Aldon, FL 77714 • (407) 555-1234

Step 1: CPT chapter: ____________
Step 2: Anatomic system: ____________
Step 3: Organ/body part: ____________
Step 4: Technique/approach: ____________
Step 5: Additional specifics: ____________ ____________ ____________ ____________

3. Gastrostomy tube placement

OPERATIVE REPORT

Patient information:

Patient name:
DOB:
MR#:

Preoperative diagnosis:

The patient is an 83-year-old female with a gastrostomy tube removed for an unknown amount of time. Attempts at placement in the ER failed, and, the patient is admitted with reinsertion of the tube.

Postoperative diagnosis:

Procedure(s) performed:

Gastrostomy tube placement

Anesthesia:

Assistant surgeon:

Description of procedure:

Patient placed on the operating table in supine position, general anesthesia induced, and abdomen prepped and draped in usual sterile manner. A paramedian incision was made and the skin, subcutaneous tissue and fascia were incised. The rectus muscle was incised and peritoneum entered. Feeding gastrostomy was placed with two rows of pursestring 2-0 silk sutures in the anterior wall of the stomach. The stomach was incised and a small catheter introduced. The catheter was brought out through a separate stab wound incision in the upper quadrant of the abdomen. The gastrostomy tube was placed with drainage to a Foley bag. Abdomen was closed in layers using interrupted sutures of 2-0 silk. The skin was closed with interrupted mattress sutures of 4-0 silk. Sterile dressings were applied. The patient tolerated the procedure well.

Patrick Olson MD

GODFREY REGIONAL HOSPITAL
123 Main Street • Aldon, FL 77714 • (407) 555-1234

Step 1: CPT chapter: ____________
Step 2: Anatomic system: ____________
Step 3: Organ/body part: ____________
Step 4: Technique/approach: ____________
Step 5: Additional specifics: ____________ ____________
____________ ____________

4. Chondromalacia patella

OPERATIVE REPORT

Patient information:

Patient name:
DOB:
MR#:

Preoperative diagnosis:

Chondromalacia patella, lateral patellar tilt and lateral retinacular tightness

Postoperative diagnosis:

Same

Procedure(s) performed:

Right knee arthroscopy and chondroplasty patella. Right knee arthroscopic lateral release

Anesthesia:

Assistant surgeon:

Description of procedure:

After suitable general anesthesia had been achieved, patient's right knee was prepped and draped in the usual manner. Prior to prepping, a thigh tourniquet was applied and after draping, inflated to 300 mm of Mercury. Inflow cannula was inserted in to the suprapatellar pouch on the medial side. The arthroscope was inserted through an anterior lateral portal. The medial compartment was intact with stable medial meniscus and intact articular surfaces. Examination of the lateral compartment revealed intact articular surfaces and stable lateral meniscus. Examination of the patellofemoral joint revealed localized chondromalacia at the lateral aspect of the inferior pole of the patella. This was smoothed with a shaver and further smoothing was done using Oratec Probe. Using an arthroscopic cautery arthroscopic lateral release was done from the superior pole of the patella to the joint line. The knee joint was thoroughly irrigated and arthroscope removed. Patient tolerated the procedure well and was returned to the Recovery Room in satisfactory condition.

GODFREY REGIONAL HOSPITAL
123 Main Street • Aldon, FL 77714 • (407) 555-1234

Step 1: CPT chapter: ____________
Step 2: Anatomic system: ____________
Step 3: Organ/body part: ____________
Step 4: Technique/approach: ____________
Step 5: Additional specifics: ____________ ____________ ____________ ____________

5. Colonoscopy

OPERATIVE REPORT

Patient information:

Patient name:
DOB:
MR#:

Preoperative diagnosis:

Surveillance colonoscopy for colon cancer
S/P colon cancer with hemicolectomy

Postoperative diagnosis:

Same

Procedure(s) performed:

Colonoscopy

Anesthesia:

Assistant surgeon:

Description of procedure:

After obtaining informed consent, patient was put in the left lateral position. IV sedation was given, and vital signs monitored throughout the procedure. Digital rectal examination was normal and the colonoscope was introduced and advanced all the way to the ileocecal anastomosis without difficulty. The anastomosis looked clean. No masses, no tumors and no polyps were seen. The scope was withdrawn carefully, watching all of the colonic mucosa. There were a few pockets of liquid stools which were washed away and examined carefully. Small internal hemorrhoids were observed in the rectum. The scope was withdrawn.

Patrick Olson MD

GODFREY REGIONAL HOSPITAL
123 Main Street • Aldon, FL 77714 • (407) 555-1234

Step 1: CPT chapter: ____________
Step 2: Anatomic system: ____________
Step 3: Organ/body part: ____________
Step 4: Technique/approach: ____________
Step 5: Additional specifics: ____________ ____________
____________ ____________

RADIOLOGY (CODES 70000-79999)

The radiology section includes codes for services when imaging is performed to determine the scope or extent of a medical problem. Imaging may be performed by a number of methods, so the proper coding for **radiology** requires the following determinations in order:

Determine chapter: Radiology
Type of service: Diagnostic (x-ray, computed tomography [CT], magnetic resonance imaging [MRI])
Ultrasound
Radiation therapy
Nuclear medicine
Anatomic part: Body area imaged
Number of views/contrast: 2 views, 3 views
With/without contrast

The services found in the radiology section could include a simple chest x-ray (diagnostic section), a fetal ultrasound (ultrasound section), radiation therapy (radiation oncology), or bone scan (nuclear medicine). Information regarding the anatomic location and view/contrast information will depend on the radiologic report because the actual films are not part of the medical record. Chapter 15 contains information about radiologic reports and their necessity on reports for coding and billing purposes.

STOP AND PRACTICE

Radiologic reports tend to not be as extensive as evaluation and management and surgical reports. Review the following simple radiologic reports, extract the key information, and assign CPT codes for these services.

1. Ultrasonography of the kidneys

RADIOLOGY REPORT

MR#:
DOB:
Dr. Smith

Clinical summary:

Abdomen:

Conclusion:

Patient: John Doe

Dear Dr. Smith:

The following radiologic procedure was performed on your patient:
Ultrasonography of the Kidneys

A real-time ultransonic examination of the kidneys was performed. The kidneys are normal in size measuring approximately 11-11.5 cm in length. There was no evidence of hydronephrosis, calculi or renal mass seen. There were no perinephric fluid collections.

Ddt/mm

D:
T:

Date

GODFREY REGIONAL HOSPITAL
123 Main Street • Aldon, FL 77714 • (407) 555-1234

Step 1: CPT chapter: ____________
Step 2: Type of service: ____________
Step 3: Anatomic part: ____________
Step 4: # Views/limited/complete: ____________
Step 5: Additional guidelines: ____________

2. Chest posteroanterior and lateral

RADIOLOGY REPORT

MR#:
DOB:
Dr.

Clinical summary:

EXAM: Chest PA and Lateral

Abdomen:

Conclusion:

There are degenerative changes of the dorsal spine. Postoperative changes are noted. There is increased density in the infrahilar region seen on the lateral film. This may be in the right infrahilar region. The prior film is somewhat overexposed however the increased density in the right infrahilar regional appears to be new. Follow up is suggested. No hemo or pneumothorax is identified.

IMPRESSION: Prominence in the right infrahilar region is of uncertain significance. This may be related to some mild atelectasis. Clinical correlation and follow-up is recommended.

Ddt/mm

D:
T:

Date

GODFREY REGIONAL HOSPITAL
123 Main Street • Aldon, FL 77714 • (407) 555-1234

Step 1: CPT chapter: ____________
Step 2: Type of service: ____________
Step 3: Anatomic part: ____________
Step 4: # Views/limited/complete: ____________
Step 5: Additional guidelines: ____________

3. Bilateral mammography

RADIOLOGY REPORT

MR#:
DOB:
Dr.

Clinical summary:

CLINICAL INFORMATION: Area seen on CT Scan

BILATERAL MAMMOGRAPHY: Exam was performed to evaluate a questioned nodular density described on CT of chest performed earlier.

Abdomen:

Conclusion:

Two thirds of each breast is occupied by parenchyma which is fairly symmetric in the two breasts. In the upper outer quadrant of the right breast, there is a relatively dense parenchymal collection measuring 2 cm. This would correspond to the density found on the CT scan. There are no abnormal calcifications. There has been no change from previous exams. There are no radiographic signs of breast carcinoma.

Ddt/mm

D:
T:

Date

GODFREY REGIONAL HOSPITAL
123 Main Street • Aldon, FL 77714 • (407) 555-1234

Step 1: CPT chapter: __________
Step 2: Type of service: __________
Step 3: Anatomic part: __________
Step 4: # Views/limited/complete: __________
Step 5: Additional guidelines: __________

4. Brain CT scan

RADIOLOGY REPORT

MR#:
DOB:
Dr.

Clinical summary:

Brain CT Scan

CLINICAL INFORMATION: Motor vehicle accident with head pain and brief LOC

Abdomen:

Conclusion:

Multiple spirally acquired 5.0 mm section axial images through the brain were obtained without the use of intravenous contrast.

The ventricles appeared unremarkable. There are no abnormal hypodensities. There is no bleed. There is no mass effect, midline shift or extra-axial fluid collection. The visualized paranasal sinuses, mastoid air cells and osseous structures appear within normal limits

Ddt/mm

D:
T:

Date

GODFREY REGIONAL HOSPITAL
123 Main Street • Aldon, FL 77714 • (407) 555-1234

Step 1: CPT chapter: __________
Step 2: Type of service: __________
Step 3: Anatomic part: __________
Step 4: # Views/limited/complete: __________
Step 5: Additional guidelines: __________

5. Renal ultrasound/intravenous pyelogram

RADIOLOGY REPORT

MR#:
DOB:
Dr.

Clinical summary:

DIAGNOSIS: Hematuria
PART TO BE EXAMINED: Renal ultrasound/IVP

Abdomen:

Conclusion:

EXCRETORY UROGRAM WITH TOMOGRAPHY: Following injection of contrast, both kidneys are well visualized on the tomograms and are of normal size and shape. Prompt function of normal appearing collecting systems bilaterally. Urinary bladder is not optimally opacified or distended but there is evidence of a large filling defect, base of urinary bladder, consistent with a considerable enlarged prostate gland.

ULTRASOUND OF KIDNEYS AND URINARY BLADDER: Both kidneys are of normal size and shape with no evidence of mass, obstruction or calcification. Quite a bit of nonspecific enlargement of prostate gland. The prostate gland is lobulated and measures at least 5 cm in diameter.

Ddt/mm

D:
T:

Date

GODFREY REGIONAL HOSPITAL
123 Main Street • Aldon, FL 77714 • (407) 555-1234

Step 1: CPT chapter: ______________
Step 2: Type of service: ______________
Step 3: Anatomic part: ______________
Step 4: # Views/limited/complete: ______________
Step 5: Additional guidelines: ______________

PATHOLOGY AND LABORATORY (CODES 80000-89399)

Services in the **pathology** or laboratory section typically include procedures to obtain specimens and their subsequent analysis. Such specimens may include blood, urine, cervical and vaginal fluids, semen, mucus, and other bodily fluids as well as biopsy specimens sent to the laboratory for analysis and diagnosis. Because many of these tests may be performed by a number of different methods, care must be taken to select a code on the basis of the specimen and the method (e.g., automated, manual, dipstick).

Subsections for the pathology section are as follows:

- Organ or Disease Oriented Panels
- Drug Testing
- Therapeutic Drug Assays
- Evocative/Suppression Testing
- Consultations (Clinical Pathology)
- Urinalysis
- Chemistry
- Hematology and Coagulation
- Immunology
- Transfusion Medicine
- Microbiology
- Anatomic Pathology
- Cytopathology
- Cytogenetic Studies
- Surgical Pathology
- Reproductive Medicine Procedures

To code services from the pathology section of CPT, the coder must capture the following information:

Identify chapter:	Pathology
Procedure performed:	Transfusion, microbiology, surgical pathology
Specific procedure:	Complete blood count, blood typing
Extent/specifics:	Automated, manual

The majority of laboratory and pathology services will be captured by a laboratory order form or laboratory slip. Chapter 16 takes an in-depth look at coding for a laboratory and discusses these specialized services.

MEDICINE (CODES 90701-99199)

The **medicine** section encompasses a variety of specialty services and procedures that do not meet the criteria of surgery in nature or visits/encounters. It is sometimes difficult to differentiate between medical procedures and surgical procedures. If the coder keeps in mind that codes in the surgical section specify procedures that are invasive, definitive, or restorative in nature, and that those in the medicine section are diagnostic or therapeutic in nature, differentiation becomes straightforward. The medicine section encompasses the following services:

- Immune globulins
- Vaccines/toxoids
- Injections
- Psychiatry
- Dialysis
- Gastroenterology
- Ophthalmology
- Ears, nose, and throat (ENT)
- Cardiovascular
- Pulmonary
- Allergy
- Neurology
- Osteopathic procedures
- Chiropractic services

A number of specialties are represented in the previous list. The procedures listed under each specialty are diagnostic or therapeutic in nature; that is, they do not meet the criteria for surgery or for evaluation and management. For example, such a procedure provided by a psychiatry specialist might include psychotherapy. Note this is a procedure and does not constitute an office visit. In the cardiovascular section are procedures, most of which are noninvasive, such as electrocardiograms (ECGs), cardiac stress testing, and cardiac catheterizations. In brief, the reason that cardiac catheterizations are located in the medicine section rather than the surgery section is because they are considered noninvasive and their primary purpose is for diagnosis. When cardiac catheterization involves the repair of a vessel (angioplasty), this procedure is also considered noninvasive because the advancement of a catheter is through a small incision. Compared with a coronary artery bypass graft or a pacemaker or defibrillator insertion, such procedures seem minor and nonsurgical.

For codes from the medicine section to be properly assigned, services should be broken down as follows:

Identify chapter:	Medicine
Identify specific specialty:	Gastroenterology, pulmonary, allergy, ophthalmology
Identify specific procedure:	Allergy testing
Allergy immunotherapy	
Preparation of allergen extract	
Identify specifics:	Age/minutes/level

Care should be taken to make certain that all services are documented as ordered and performed before CPT codes are assigned and services billed. Some of the services will be dictated as a separate report, such as audiology tests, electroencephalograms, and ECGs, whereas others, such as immunizations and injections, will be incorporated in the evaluation and management visit.

STOP AND PRACTICE

Complete the five steps of assigning CPT codes for the following exercises.

1. Psychotherapy, office, 45 minutes, insight oriented
   Step 1: CPT chapter: medicine
   Step 2: Identify specific specialty/subsection: psychiatry
   Step 3: Identify specific procedures: ______
   Step 4: Identify specifics of test: ______
   Step 5: Additional guidelines: ______
2. ECG, 12-lead, professional component only
   Step 1: CPT chapter: Medicine
   Step 2: Identify specific specialty/subsection: Cardiography
   Step 3: Identify specific procedures: ECG
   Step 4: Identify specifics of test: ______
   Step 5: Additional guidelines: 93010
3. Tetanus toxoid absorbed
   Step 1: CPT chapter: medicine
   Step 2: Identify specific specialty/subsection: ______
   Step 3: Identify specific procedures: ______
   Step 4: Identify specifics of test: ______
   Step 5: Additional guidelines: 90703
4. Intramuscular injection
   Step 1: CPT chapter: ______
   Step 2: Identify specific specialty/subsection: ______
   Step 3: Identify specific procedures: ______
   Step 4: Identify specifics of test: ______
   Step 5: Additional guidelines: ______
5. Transesophageal echocardiogram
   Step 1: CPT chapter: ______
   Step 2: Identify specific specialty/subsection: ______
   Step 3: Identify specific procedures: ______
   Step 4: Identify specifics of test: ______
   Step 5: Additional guidelines: ______

STOP AND PRACTICE

Using the breakdown process, review the following medicine service reports and identify the appropriate elements.

1. ECG

ELECTROCARDIOGRAM REPORT

MR#:
DOB:
Dr.

Clinical summary:

Atrial Rate: 100
PR Interval: Variable
Ventricular Rate: 80

The ST segments are sagging in leads I, II, V5 and V6 and are slightly depressed in V2-V4.The rhythm is Wenckebach. There is a second degree heart block. The T waves are low in leads I, V5 and V6.

Abdomen:

Impression:

1. 2nd degree heart block (Wenckebach)
2. Nonspecific ST segment and T wave changes
3. There is significant change since the last electrocardiogram.

Ddt/mm

D:
T:

_______________, M.D. Date

GODFREY REGIONAL HOSPITAL
123 Main Street • Aldon, FL 77714 • (407) 555-1234

Step 1: CPT chapter: ______________

Step 2: Identify specific specialty/ subsection: ______________

Step 3: Identify specific procedures: ______________

Step 4: Identify specifics of test: ______________

Step 5: Additional guidelines: ______________

2. Electroencephalogram report

ELECTROENCEPHALOGRAM REPORT

MR#:
DOB:
Dr.

Clinical summary:

Patient Age: 62 with seizure activity
Medications: Neurontin, Phenobarbital, Dilantin

There is a bioccipital rhythm, which is organized, of about 8 Hz. Frontal activity is a mixture of rapid and slow activity. Bifrontal spike and slow wave activities were noted, which have been noted on previous EEGs. High voltage delta slow waves are also noted intermittently in the frontal areas. Spike activity appears approximately every 2-3 minutes on the EEG. The high frequency delta waves are not as frequent. One episode, lasting up to 5 seconds is also noted. No clinical correlation was noted with this EEG by the EEG tech or patient. The patient is not photosensitive.

Abdomen:

Impression:

Compared to previous EEG, it is either unchanged or slightly better.

Ddt/mm

D:
T:

, M.D. Date

GODFREY REGIONAL HOSPITAL
123 Main Street • Aldon, FL 77714 • (407) 555-1234

Step 1: CPT chapter: ______________

Step 2: Identify specific specialty/subsection: ______________

Step 3: Identify specific procedures: ______________

Step 4: Identify specifics of test: ______________

Step 5: Additional guidelines: ______________

3. Electromyography

ELECTROMYOGRAPHY LABORATORY REPORT

Nerve conduction studies

Name: __________
Clinic number: __________ Age: ____
Birthdate: ________ Date: ________
Referring physician: __________

NR = No response
M = Motor
S = Sensory
Mx = Mixed
• = no increment after 10 sec. exercise
† = no decrement to 2/sec x3
X = Forearm median to ulnar crossover

Nerve stimulated	(Recording site)	Amplitude (Sensory = uV; Meter = mV) Distal Right	Left	Normal	Proximal Rt	Lt	Distal/peak latency (mSec) Rt	Lt	Normal	Conduction velocity (M/sec) Rt	Lt	Normal	F-wave latency (mSec) Rt	Lt	Normal
Lower right															
Sural (S) Pt.B	ankle														
Peroneal (M) knee	EDB														
Peroneal (M) ankle	EDB														
Posterior tibia (M) knee	AH														
Posterior tibia (M) ankle	AH														
H-reflex															
Med (s) wrist	1st														
Med (m) elbow	thenar														
Med (m) wrist	thenar														
Ulnar (s) wrist	5th														

Needle examination:

Summary:

Four limb motor and sensory NCV and EMG show widespread abnormalities consistent with neuropathy with the following results:

EMG: Left anterior leg compartment had fibrillations, positive sharp waves and insertional potentials
Both motor and sensory NCVs showed widespread but not universal abnormalities with marked variation from nerve to nerve
All F-waves were abnormal
The right median nerve had a reproducible conduction block at the elbow
Sural nerves had normal conduction velocity but small amplitude

Impression:

R/L Median Motor
R/L Ulnar Motor
R/L Orthodromic Median Sensory
R/L Orthodromic Ulnar Sensory
R/L Superficial Peroneal Sensory
R/L Sural Sensory

__________, M.D.

GODFREY CLINICAL LABORATORIES
465 Dogwood Court • Aldon, FL 77712 • (407) 555-9876

Step 1: CPT chapter: __________
Step 2: Identify specific specialty/subsection: __________
Step 3: Identify specific procedures: __________
Step 4: Identify specifics of test: __________
Step 5: Additional guidelines: __________

4. Cellulitis

EMERGENCY ROOM RECORD

Name:	Age:	ER physician: Nancy Connelly, MD
	DOB:	
Allergies/type of reaction:	**Usual medications/dosages:**	

Triage/presenting complaint: Patient presents to ED for additional IV Infusion of Rocephin for cellulitis of the arm.

Initial assessment:

Time	T	P 92	R 20	BP 150/72	Other:					

Medication orders: Infusion was begun at 10:00 AM In the L antecubital area without difficulty. IV Rocephin infusion was complete at 11:15 AM.

Lab work:

X-Ray:

Physician's report:

The patient was discharged in satisfactory condition and will return tomorrow for the next dosage of IV Rocephin.

Diagnosis:	Physician sign/date
	Nancy Connelly MD
Discharge Transfer Admit Good Satisfactory Other:	

GODFREY REGIONAL HOSPITAL
123 Main Street • Aldon, FL 77714 • (407) 555-1234

Step 1: CPT Chapter: ______________

Step 2: Identify specific specialty/ subsection: ______________

Step 3: Identify specific procedures: ______________

Step 4: Identify specifics of test: ______________

Step 5: Additional guidelines: ______________

5. Physical therapy visit

PROGRESS NOTE

Chief complaint: Physical therapy visit

Date: ________________

Vital signs: BP______ P______ R______

History:

This is the fourth PT visit for this patient with lower extremity ankle pain. She was involved in a motor vehicle accident approximately 2 months ago at which time she sustained a severe sprain of the right lateral malleous. She has continued to have difficulty ambulating. Swelling has continued, current 2 + edema.

Exam:

She presents for therapy to her ankle which consisted today of the following:

Supervised electrical stimulation for 16 minutes followed by attended ultrasound for 15 minutes.

Diagnosis/assessment:

The patient noted no pain or other complaints throughout the course of her therapy. She will return on Wednesday for additional treatment and therapy.

William Obert MD

Patient name: ________________

Date of service: ________________

GODFREY MEDICAL ASSOCIATES

1532 Third Avenue, Suite 120 • Aldon, FL 77713 • (407) 555-4000

Step 1: CPT chapter: ________________

Step 2: Identify specific specialty/subsection: ________________

Step 3: Identify specific procedures: ________________

Step 4: Identify specifics of test: ________________

Step 5: Additional guidelines: ________________

STOP AND PRACTICE

Take the following services and identify the information contained in each step of the coding process. Assign the appropriate CPT code when possible or assign a range of codes when adequate information is not available (e.g., evaluation and management codes).

Refer to the information listed earlier regarding specific information needed for each section of the CPT book or refer to Tool 9-1 for information needed.

1. Knee x-ray, right knee
   Step 1: CPT chapter: ________
   Step 2: ________
   Step 3: ________
   Step 4: ________
   Step 5: ________
2. New office visit
   Step 1: CPT chapter: ________
   Step 2: ________
   Step 3: ________
   Step 4: ________
   Step 5: ________
3. Drug assay, lithium
   Step 1: CPT chapter: Path / Lab
   Step 2: ________
   Step 3: ________
   Step 4: ________
   Step 5: 80178
4. Excision benign lesion, 4.0 cm, benign
   Step 1: CPT chapter: ________
   Step 2: ________
   Step 3: ________
   Step 4: ________
   Step 5: ________
5. ORIF (open reduction internal fixation), distal radius
   Step 1: CPT chapter: ________
   Step 2: ________
   Step 3: ________
   Step 4: ________
   Step 5: ________
6. Full body scan, Tc-99
   Step 1: CPT chapter: ________
   Step 2: ________
   Step 3: ________
   Step 4: ________
   Step 5: ________
7. Cardiac catheterization, left
   Step 1: CPT chapter: ________
   Step 2: ________
   Step 3: ________
   Step 4: ________
   Step 5: ________
8. Office consultation
   Step 1: CPT chapter: ________
   Step 2: ________
   Step 3: ________
   Step 4: ________
   Step 5: ________
9. Measles, mumps, rubella (MMR) immunization
   Step 1: CPT chapter: ________
   Step 2: ________
   Step 3: ________
   Step 4: ________
   Step 5: ________
10. Esophagogastroduodenoscopy
    Step 1: CPT chapter: ________
    Step 2: ________
    Step 3: ________
    Step 4: ________
    Step 5: ________

CPT Format

GENERAL

The CPT manual contains stand-alone descriptions of medical procedures. When an entry in the CPT book is followed by indented entries, the indented entries refer back to one or more common elements listed in the directly preceding entry. One of the tips for diagnostic coding from the ICD-9-CM code book is to refer back to the last entry that appears flush with the left margin. This allows the coder to ensure all components have been included; the same advice holds true for use of the CPT manual. Consider the following example:

58260	Vaginal hysterectomy;
58262	with removal of tube(s), and/or ovary(ies)
58263	with removal of tube(s), and/or ovary(ies) with repair of enterocele

All procedural codes listed here appear flush left; descriptors in subentries are indented past the margin of "vaginal hysterectomy." The semicolon, located immediately after the description of the primary service, indicates that everything before the semicolon is included in the descriptor for subsequent, indented service. The following would represent the complete descriptors if they were provided as such:

58260 Vaginal hysterectomy
58262 Vaginal hysterectomy with removal of tube(s), and/or ovary(ies)
58263 Vaginal hysterectomy with removal of tube(s), and/or ovary(ies) with repair of enterocele

SYMBOLS

Along with learning the format of CPT, the coder must become familiar with symbols used in the book. The following entries explain these symbols.

- • A **bullet** indicates that a code is a new addition to CPT with this edition.
- Δ A **triangle** indicates that the descriptive information for a CPT code has undergone revision.
- + **Add-on procedure** codes are only assigned when an initial code is assigned. Procedure codes should only be used in combination with another primary code(s). Add-on codes permit the reporting of significant supplemental services commonly performed in addition to the primary procedure.
- Ø Procedure code should NOT have a modifier 51 assigned despite the fact it would be appropriate according to CPT guidelines. Because these codes are usually assigned along with other CPT codes, CMS has stated modifier 51 would not be appropriate to assign in these instances.

Separate procedure: This designation is discussed in depth in Chapter 9. The use of this designation will become more apparent when we begin coding surgical procedures in Chapter 13.

Ea/Each: This designation is seen in CPT when the code descriptor is reported in units of service. For instance, the descriptor for code 26600 is:

Closed treatment of metacarpal fracture, single, without manipulation, each bone

In this case, when multiple metacarpal bones (e.g., "5") are treated, code 26600 will be coded/billed as 26600, unit "5" in the unit column of the Centers for Medicare and Medicaid Services claim form.

When services are designated as "each" or "each additional," care should be taken NOT to report on individual lines of the claim form, which will result in denial.

For purposes of coding, the coder typically writes the five closed metacarpal bone fracture treatments as follows:

26600 × 5

At data entry, the services will be entered as described here.

In addition to the main content of CPT, a number of appendixes are located at the back of the CPT book that provide additional information or clarification in assigning codes from the CPT book. They are as follows:

Appendix A: Modifiers (provides a listing of CPT modifiers and their definitions)
Appendix B: Summary of Additions, Deletions, and Revisions
Appendix C: Clinical Examples
Appendix D: Summary of CPT Add-on Codes
Appendix E: Summary of Modifier 51 Exempt CPT Codes
Appendix F: Summary of Modifier 63 Exempt CPT Codes
Appendix G: CPT Codes That Include Conscious Sedation
Appendix H: Performance Measures by Clinical Conditions
Appendix I: Genetic Testing Modifiers
Appendix J: Electrodiagnostic Medicine Listing of Sensory, Motor, and Mixed Nerves
Appendix K: Products Pending FDA [Food and Drug Administration] Approval
Appendix L: Vascular Family Listing

In addition to the actual CPT book, additional guidelines are offered by the AMA in the form of the monthly publication *CPT Assistant.* This newsletter, available in print and electronic formats, provides clarification to unique coding scenarios as well as updates to CPT coding policy and is available for purchase from the AMA. If you use a professional edition of CPT, you will see notations citing specific *CPT Assistant* articles relevant to CPT codes throughout the CPT book. Caution should be made to use only defensible sources for coding guidelines, such as *CPT Assistant*, Centers for Medicare and Medicaid Services, National Correct Coding Initiative, and *Coding Clinic for ICD-9-CM.*

Remaining Coding Steps

Steps 1 through 5 in coding for services performed were discussed in the previous chapter. Now that you have gathered all the information and key elements needed for assigning the appropriate codes and have learned the appropriate use of CPT code sections, let's discuss the last steps of the CPT code assignment process.

Step 6: Assign the Correct CPT Code(s) from the CPT Book

The basics of this step are similar throughout the CPT code book. Some variations occur depending on what chapter the appropriate codes are located. Although there are some exceptions or additional coding guidelines for specific services, the basic rules for assigning CPT codes have already been covered in steps 1 through 5.

The steps for identifying the elements necessary for assigning the CPT code were discussed in Chapter 9. With the information covered in Chapter 9 on coding guidelines, as well as the format, symbols, and how to look up CPT codes in the CPT book, you are ready to assign codes.

STOP AND PRACTICE

Take the exercises previously started and assign the appropriate CPT code(s) and modifier(s) when appropriate. If you are unable to identify a specific code because of inadequate information, simply list the code range encompassing the service.

1. Knee x-ray, right knee
   Step 1: CPT chapter: ______
   Step 2: ______
   Step 3: ______
   Step 4: ______
   Step 5: ______
   Step 6: CPT code(s): ______
2. New office visit
   Step 1: CPT chapter: ______
   Step 2: ______
   Step 3: ______
   Step 4: ______
   Step 5: ______
   Step 6: CPT code(s) ______
3. Drug assay, lithium
   Step 1: CPT chapter: ______
   Step 2: ______
   Step 3: ______
   Step 4: ______
   Step 5: ______
   Step 6: CPT code(s): ______
4. Excision benign lesion, 4.0 cm, benign
   Step 1: CPT chapter: ______
   Step 2: ______
   Step 3: ______
   Step 4: ______
   Step 5: ______
   Step 6: CPT code(s): ______
5. ORIF distal radius
   Step 1: CPT chapter: ______
   Step 2: ______
   Step 3: ______
   Step 4: ______
   Step 5: ______
   Step 6: CPT code(s): ______
6. Full body scan, Tc-99
   Step 1: CPT chapter: ______
   Step 2: ______
   Step 3: ______
   Step 4: ______
   Step 5: ______
   Step 6: CPT code(s): ______
7. Cardiac catheterization, left
   Step 1: CPT chapter: ______
   Step 2: ______
   Step 3: ______
   Step 4: ______
   Step 5: ______
   Step 6: CPT code(s): ______
8. Office consultation
   Step 1: CPT chapter: ______
   Step 2: ______
   Step 3: ______
   Step 4: ______
   Step 5: ______
   Step 6: CPT code(s): ______
9. MMR immunization
   Step 1: CPT chapter: ______
   Step 2: ______
   Step 3: ______
   Step 4: ______
   Step 5: ______
   Step 6: CPT code(s): ______
10. Esophagogastroduodenoscopy
    Step 1: CPT chapter: ______
    Step 2: ______
    Step 3: ______
    Step 4: ______
    Step 5: ______
    Step 6: CPT code(s): ______

Step 7: Determine the Correct Order for Billing Services and Procedures

Correct order of services is essential for proper reimbursement. Ensuring that services are listed in the proper order protects the interests of all involved—the patient, the provider, the place of service, and the insurer.

When multiple services are performed on the same date(s) of service, they should be listed in order of the most significant service. This concept was introduced with the discussion of modifier 59 in Chapter 9. In some instances, such as the case of an office visit with chest x-ray and laboratory values, the order may not be of importance; however, some carriers may only reimburse one service per day, so you will want the most significant service reimbursed in these instances.

Step 8: Determine Whether Modifier Code(s) Are Appropriate

The appropriate use of modifier code(s) assignment was discussed in Chapter 9.

APPLYING CODING STEPS 6 THROUGH 8

As previously discussed, the order of services may determine whether all services are paid or whether appropriate reductions are taken for procedures. Following are some examples of walking through the process in situations that involve more than one procedure. Read through the report in Figure 10-1. First determine what services were performed and which elements will need to be captured for each service. The services performed for this patient were as follows:

1. Laceration repair
2. ECG
3. Emergency room visit

Step 1: Determine Chapter of CPT

Laceration repair: Surgery
ECG: Medicine
Emergency room visit: Evaluation and management

Once this step has been determined, the appropriate steps for each procedure are established.

Service 1: Laceration Repair

Step 1: Chapter of CPT: Surgery
Step 2: Anatomic system: Integumentary
Step 3: Anatomic part: Skin
Step 4: Procedure: Laceration repair
Step 5: Additional specifics: Nose
Step 6: Assign CPT codes: 12011
Step 7: Appropriate order: 1
Step 8: Modifier(s) if appropriate: None

Service 2: ECG

Step 1: Chapter of CPT: Medicine
Step 2: Specialty type: Cardiology
Step 3: Specific test/procedure: ECG
Step 4: Additional specifics: Global procedures
Step 5: Additional guidelines: Office
Step 6: Assign CPT codes: 93000
Step 7: Appropriate order: 3
Step 8: Modifier(s) if appropriate: None

Service 3: Emergency Room Visit

Step 1: Chapter of CPT: Evaluation and Management
Step 2: Location/type: Emergency room
Step 3: Patient status: New/initial
Step 4: Level of service: (at this time only list range of codes)
Step 5: Additional guidelines: 99281-99285
Step 6: Assign CPT codes: (at this time only list range of codes)
(Additional review will follow in Chapter 11.)
Step 7: Appropriate order: 2
Step 8: Modifier(s) if appropriate: 25 (significantly separately identifiable evaluation and management)

Therefore the final answer for this scenario would be as follows:

12001
99281-99285-25
93000

Be sure enough diagnostic information is available to justify medical necessity for each of the services determined to be coded/billed:

12001	Laceration (open wound), nose
99281-99285-25	Syncope
	Open wound, nose
93000	Syncope

Using the sample exercise in Figure 10-2, make certain you understand the entire process before attempting to code a number of case scenarios.

Step 1: Determine Chapter of CPT

Diagnostic colonoscopy: Surgery
Colonoscopy with polypectomy by hot biopsy forceps: Surgery
Colonoscopy with biopsy: Surgery

Once this step has been determined, the appropriate steps for each procedure are established.

Service 1: Diagnostic Colonoscopy

Step 1: Chapter of CPT: Surgery
Step 2: Anatomic system: Digestive
Step 3: Anatomic part: Rectum
Step 4: Procedure: Endoscopy (colonoscopy)
Step 5: Additional specifics: Diagnostic
Step 6: Assign CPT codes: 45378
Step 7: Appropriate order: Indicated as "separate procedure" because no "separate procedure" will be included in other colonoscopy procedures
Step 8: Modifier(s) if appropriate: Not applicable

Service 2: Colonoscopy with Polypectomy by Hot Biopsy Forceps

Step 1: Chapter of CPT: Surgery
Step 2: Anatomic system: Digestive
Step 3: Anatomic part: Rectum
Step 4: Procedure: Endoscopy (colonoscopy)
Step 5: Additional specifics: With polypectomy by hot biopsy forceps
Step 6: Assign CPT codes: 45384
Step 7: Appropriate order: 1
Step 8: Modifier(s) if appropriate: Because this is the primary procedure, no modifier would be appropriate

EMERGENCY ROOM RECORD

Name:	Age:	ER physician:
	DOB:	Nancy Connelly, MD

Allergies/type of reaction:	**Usual medications/dosages:**
None	Neurontin, Meclizine, potassium, Fosamax, Lisinopril, Calcium, Vitamin B6, Lanoxin and Vitamin E

Triage/presenting complaint: Fall with laceration to the nose

Initial assessment: Patient was sitting in bathroom and fell, striking her head. There was no loss of consciousness, however, in addition to the laceration to the bridge of her nose she also sustained bruises and contusions to the face. No head injury, no neck injury. She indicated she experienced dizziness prior to and immediately after the fall.

Time	T	P 92	R 20	BP 150/72	Other:					

Medication orders: Laceration was infiltrated with 20 mg of 1% Lidocaine, primary closure was performed with five 5-0 Ethilon sutures. Polysporin and Band-Aid were applied to the wound.

Lab work:

X-Ray:

Physician's report:

PAST MEDICAL HISTORY: Chronic diarrhea, hypothyroidism, GERD, osteoporosis, peripheral neuropathy and depression

REVIEW OF SYSTEMS: Unremarkable other than as mentioned above

Examination of skin reveals 2 cm laceration on bridge of nose. There is some bleeding noted. When she arrived she was on a long board with C-collar. These were removed and with head support the neck was examined and is unremarkable. She states she has no pain. She has some generalized back pain which is apparently chronic. Heart: No murmurs. Lungs: Clear to auscultation. Abdomen: Soft and non-tender.

EKG reveals normal sinus rhythm with no irregularities.

Diagnosis:	**Physician sign/date**
ASSESSMENT: Syncope. Laceration to the bridge of nose. PLAN: Suture removal in one week. Return to nursing home.	Nancy Connelly MD
Discharge Transfer Admit Good Satisfactory Other:	

GODFREY REGIONAL HOSPITAL
123 Main Street • Aldon, FL 77714 • (407) 555-1234

FIGURE 10-1. Sample emergency department record.

OPERATIVE REPORT

Patient information:

Patient name:
DOB:
MR#:

Preoperative diagnosis:

INDICATIONS: Anemia

Prior to the procedure the risks, benefits, alternatives and discomfort were explained to the patient. Risks include but are not limited to perforation, bleeding, infection, need for IV antibiotics, blood transfusion or additional surgery. The patient understood, questions were answered and an informed consent was signed.

Postoperative diagnosis:

Procedure(s) performed:

Colonoscopy
The services performed for this patient were as follows:
1. Diagnostic colonoscopy
2. Colonoscopy with polypectomy by hot biopsy forceps
3. Colonoscopy with biopsy

Anesthesia:

Assistant surgeon:

Description of procedure:

Under MAC anesthesia the scope was passed all the way to the cecum. The cecum, and cecal vale were normal. Ascending colon, hepatic flexure, transverse colon, splenic flexure, and descending colon were normal. The sigmoid colon showed a polyp, approximately 3.0 mm size which was removed with hot biopsy forceps. An additional polyp was identified in the rectal area which was biopsied only. Otherwise, the rectum looked normal. Retroflex showed mild internal hemorrhoids.

Patient tolerated procedure well and left the endoscopy suite in satisfactory condition.

Patrick Olsen MD

GODFREY REGIONAL HOSPITAL
123 Main Street • Aldon, FL 77714 • (407) 555-1234

FIGURE 10-2. Sample operative report.

Service 3: Colonoscopy with Biopsy

Step 1: Chapter of CPT: Surgery
Step 2: Anatomic system: Digestive
Step 3: Anatomic part: Rectum
Step 4: Procedure: Endoscopy (colonoscopy)
Step 5: Additional specifics: With biopsy
Step 6: Assign CPT codes: 45380
Step 7: Appropriate order: 2
Step 8: Modifier(s) if appropriate: 51

Because this is a secondary procedure performed through the same incision, through the same approach, modifier 51 would be appropriate for all subsequent procedures. Therefore the final answer for this scenario would be as follows:

45384
45380-51
(Code 45378 would be "bundled" and not coded/billed.)

STOP AND PRACTICE

On the next page are exercises included in the Chapter Review for Chapter 9. Determine the appropriate assignment of CPT codes on the basis of information you have learned in this chapter. If you are unable to make a specific code assignment, indicate the range of codes that would be appropriate for the case scenario.

1. Discharge summary

DISCHARGE SUMMARY

Patient name, MR#
DOB:

Admitted: 05/07/xx
Discharged: 05/11/xx

Discharge diagnoses:

History:

Patient is a 34-year-old male who stated he was assaulted the evening of admission by several men. The patient stated he was struck by an object on the right side of the back and the groin. He came to the ER complaining of right testicular pain to the groin. Patient denied burning, frequency or urgency. Denied loss of consciousness or head trauma. No past medical, social or family history.

PHYSICAL EXAM: Fair amount of swelling in the right scrotal sac. Right testicle is tender to palpation and tender in the right inguinal area. Prostate smooth but extremely tender and mildly enlarged. Remainder of physical exam is unremarkable.

Laboratory and radiology studies:

Significant for WBC of 11.8. All other labs returned normal.

Hospital course:

Patient was admitted to the Urology Service and placed on intravenous antibiotics. A testicular nuclear medicine scan was obtained which revealed normal blood flow to both testicles. There was increased uptake in the epididymis of the affected testicle, interpreted as traumatic epididymitis. This was followed by a small scrotal hematoma. NO evidence of ruptured testicle was found.

Patient was maintained on IV antibiotics. Improved significantly over the course of his admission. He will be discharged with a prescription for Vibramycin and will be on regular diet with activities as tolerated. He will follow up in the urological clinic in one week.

D:
T:

Felix Wander MD

GODFREY REGIONAL HOSPITAL
123 Main Street • Aldon, FL 77714 • (407) 555-1234

Step 1: CPT chapter: ________________
Step 2: ____________________________________ (copy from Chapter 9 Chapter Review exercise)
Step 3: ____________________________________ (copy from Chapter 9 Chapter Review exercise)
Step 4: ____________________________________ (copy from Chapter 9 Chapter Review exercise)
Step 5: ____________________________________ (copy from Chapter 9 Chapter Review exercise)
Step 6: Assign CPT code(s): ________________________________
Step 7: Determine correct order for services: ___________________
Step 8: Assign modifier code(s) as appropriate: ________________

4. Operative report

OPERATIVE REPORT

Patient information:

Patient name:
DOB:
MR#:

Preoperative diagnosis:

Cholelithiasis, chronic cholecystitis

Postoperative diagnosis:

Same

Procedure(s) performed:

Laparoscopic Cholecystectomy

Anesthesia:

Assistant surgeon:

Description of procedure:

After satisfactory general anesthesia was accomplished, a nasogastric tube was placed. The anterior abdominal wall was sterilely prepped and draped. An infraumbilical incision was made and pneumoperitoneum was established. The camera was placed through the trocars. An epigastric port was placed and two 5 mm ports were placed in the subcostal plane. Graspers were placed through the lateral ports and used the retract the fundus of the gallbladder. The cystic artery and duct were isolated and doubly slipped. Dissection commenced with the gallbladder removed from the hilar structures of the fundus. The gallbladder was removed through the umbilical port. The gallbladder was inspected. There was an approximately 2 cm stone in the gallbladder. The lateral ports were removed and revealed no bleeding. The epigastric port was removed and also revealed no bleeding. The pneumoperitoneum was evacuated and sutures placed at the umbilical fascia to close the fascial defect and skin incisions closed with a running subcuticular 4-0 Vicryl suture. Steri-strips were applied. The patient tolerated the procedure well and was returned to the recovery room in stable condition.

Patrick Adams MD

GODFREY REGIONAL HOSPITAL
123 Main Street • Aldon, FL 77714 • (407) 555-1234

Step 1: CPT chapter: ___________________
Step 2: ______________________________________ (copy from Chapter 9 Chapter Review exercise)
Step 3: ______________________________________ (copy from Chapter 9 Chapter Review exercise)
Step 4: ______________________________________ (copy from Chapter 9 Chapter Review exercise)
Step 5: ______________________________________ (copy from Chapter 9 Chapter Review exercise)
Step 6: Assign CPT code(s): _________________________________
Step 7: Determine correct order for services: ___________________
Step 8: Assign modifier code(s) as appropriate: _________________

5. Operative report

OPERATIVE REPORT

Patient information:

Patient name:
DOB:
MR#:

Preoperative diagnosis:

History of colonic polyps

Postoperative diagnosis:

Colonic polyp

Procedure(s) performed:

Colonoscopy and polypectomy

Anesthesia:

Assistant surgeon:

Description of procedure:

The patient was brought to the endoscopy suite and placed in the supine position. The colonoscope was introduced and passed through all flexures into the cecum. Position in the cecum was identified by the ileocecal valve. The scope was then withdrawn visualizing all the sites of the colon. The patient had a small ulcerated polyp in the proximal ascending colon. Using snare polypectomy, it was removed in piecemeal fashion.

The patient tolerated the procedure well and was transferred to the Same Day Surgery in stable condition.

Patrick Adams MD

GODFREY REGIONAL HOSPITAL
123 Main Street • Aldon, FL 77714 • (407) 555-1234

Step 1: CPT chapter: ________________
Step 2: ________________________________ (copy from Chapter 9 Chapter Review exercise)
Step 3: ________________________________ (copy from Chapter 9 Chapter Review exercise)
Step 4: ________________________________ (copy from Chapter 9 Chapter Review exercise)
Step 5: ________________________________ (copy from Chapter 9 Chapter Review exercise)
Step 6: Assign CPT code(s): ____________________________
Step 7: Determine correct order for services: ________________
Step 8: Assign modifier code(s) as appropriate: ________________

STOP AND PRACTICE

Locate the appropriate CPT code(s) for the following procedure(s). Indicate the appropriate breakdown outlined in steps 1 through 8 for arriving at your answer. Assign a range of codes when more information is needed.

1. Chest x-ray, PA only
   Step 1: CPT chapter: ____________
   Step 2: ____________
   Step 3: ____________
   Step 4: ____________
   Step 5: ____________
   Step 6: ____________
   Step 7: ____________
   Step 8: ____________
2. CBC with differential
   Step 1: CPT chapter: ____________
   Step 2: ____________
   Step 3: ____________
   Step 4: ____________
   Step 5: ____________
   Step 6: ____________
   Step 7: ____________
   Step 8: ____________
3. Split-thickness skin graft, arm
   Step 1: CPT chapter: ____________
   Step 2: ____________
   Step 3: ____________
   Step 4: ____________
   Step 5: ____________
   Step 6: ____________
   Step 7: ____________
   Step 8: ____________
4. Pulmonary function testing
   Step 1: CPT chapter: ____________
   Step 2: ____________
   Step 3: ____________
   Step 4: ____________
   Step 5: ____________
   Step 6: ____________
   Step 7: ____________
   Step 8: ____________
5. Placement of gastrostomy tube
   Step 1: CPT chapter: ____________
   Step 2: ____________
   Step 3: ____________
   Step 4: ____________
   Step 5: ____________
   Step 6: ____________
   Step 7: ____________
   Step 8: ____________
6. Endoscopy, colon
   Step 1: CPT chapter: ____________
   Step 2: ____________
   Step 3: ____________
   Step 4: ____________
   Step 5: ____________
   Step 6: ____________
   Step 7: ____________
   Step 8: ____________
7. Tonsillectomy, age 7
   Step 1: CPT chapter: ____________
   Step 2: ____________
   Step 3: ____________
   Step 4: ____________
   Step 5: ____________
   Step 6: ____________
   Step 7: ____________
   Step 8: ____________
8. Cast application, lower leg
   Step 1: CPT chapter: ____________
   Step 2: ____________
   Step 3: ____________
   Step 4: ____________
   Step 5: ____________
   Step 6: ____________
   Step 7: ____________
   Step 8: ____________
9. Outpatient consultation
   Step 1: CPT chapter: ____________
   Step 2: ____________
   Step 3: ____________
   Step 4: ____________
   Step 5: ____________
   Step 6: ____________
   Step 7: ____________
   Step 8: ____________
10. Allergy immunotherapy only
    Step 1: CPT chapter: ____________
    Step 2: ____________
    Step 3: ____________
    Step 4: ____________
    Step 5: ____________
    Step 6: ____________
    Step 7: ____________
    Step 8: ____________
11. Psychotherapy, outpatient, 45 minutes
    Step 1: CPT chapter: ____________
    Step 2: ____________
    Step 3: ____________

STOP AND PRACTICE—cont'd

Step 4: ___
Step 5: ___
Step 6: ___
Step 7: ___
Step 8: ___

12. Immunization(s), MMR
Step 1: CPT chapter: ___
Step 2: ___
Step 3: ___
Step 4: ___
Step 5: ___
Step 6: ___
Step 7: ___
Step 8: ___

13. Abdominal hysterectomy
Step 1: CPT chapter: ___
Step 2: ___
Step 3: ___
Step 4: ___
Step 5: ___
Step 6: ___
Step 7: ___
Step 8: ___

14. Vaginal delivery only
Step 1: CPT chapter: ___
Step 2: ___
Step 3: ___
Step 4: ___
Step 5: ___
Step 6: ___
Step 7: ___
Step 8: ___

15. Hospital visit
Step 1: CPT chapter: ___
Step 2: ___
Step 3: ___
Step 4: ___
Step 5: ___
Step 6: ___
Step 7: ___
Step 8: ___

16. MRI, lower extremity
Step 1: CPT chapter: ___
Step 2: ___
Step 3: ___
Step 4: ___
Step 5: ___
Step 6: ___
Step 7: ___
Step 8: ___

17. Emergency department visit
Step 1: CPT chapter: ___
Step 2: ___
Step 3: ___
Step 4: ___
Step 5: ___
Step 6: ___
Step 7: ___
Step 8: ___

18. Allergy testing, scratch, 1 test
Step 1: CPT chapter: ___
Step 2: ___
Step 3: ___
Step 4: ___
Step 5: ___
Step 6: ___
Step 7: ___
Step 8: ___

19. Laceration repair, 2 cm, arm
Step 1: CPT chapter: ___
Step 2: ___
Step 3: ___
Step 4: ___
Step 5: ___
Step 6: ___
Step 7: ___
Step 8: ___

20. Nursing home visit
Step 1: CPT chapter: ___
Step 2: ___
Step 3: ___
Step 4: ___
Step 5: ___
Step 6: ___
Step 7: ___
Step 8: ___

21. Preventive medicine visit, age 50 years, new patient
Step 1: CPT chapter: ___
Step 2: ___
Step 3: ___
Step 4: ___
Step 5: ___
Step 6: ___
Step 7: ___
Step 8: ___

22. Antibiotic injection, intramuscular
Step 1: CPT chapter: ___
Step 2: ___
Step 3: ___

STOP AND PRACTICE—cont'd

Step 4: ______
Step 5: ______
Step 6: ______
Step 7: ______
Step 8: ______

23. Tetanus immunization
Step 1: CPT chapter: ______
Step 2: ______
Step 3: ______
Step 4: ______
Step 5: ______
Step 6: ______
Step 7: ______
Step 8: ______

24. Chemotherapy, infusion
Step 1: CPT chapter: ______
Step 2: ______
Step 3: ______
Step 4: ______
Step 5: ______
Step 6: ______
Step 7: ______
Step 8: ______

25. Repair of fracture, metacarpal
Step 1: CPT chapter: ______
Step 2: ______
Step 3: ______
Step 4: ______
Step 5: ______
Step 6: ______
Step 7: ______
Step 8: ______

Chapter in Review

Certification Review

- The coding system used to bill for procedures is known as the Healthcare Common Procedure Coding System (HCPCS).
- The HCPCS coding system consists of two levels:
  Level 1: CPT
  Level 2: National Codes
- CPT is divided into six sections with six distinctly separate sets of guidelines:
  Evaluation and Management
  Anesthesiology
  Surgery
  Radiology
  Pathology/Laboratory
  Medicine
- Evaluation and management services are listed first in CPT because of their universal use by most physicians. These codes are used for many different types and levels of physician encounters or visits.
- Anesthesiology codes are used only by the anesthesia physician or provider.
- Along with CPT modifiers, anesthesia codes require a physician status modifier and additional CPT codes to describe extenuating circumstances.
- The surgery section of CPT encompasses a vast number of procedures, including those that the layperson might not consider as surgery. As such, the rules and guidelines for surgical procedures apply to these services as well.
- Radiology services are categorized as diagnostic radiology, diagnostic ultrasound, radiation oncology, and nuclear medicine.
- Pathology services are performed with specimens obtained from the patient to perform diagnostic services.
- The medicine section of CPT includes services not considered surgical in nature and that do not fall under other sections of CPT.

Student Assignments

- Study Chapter 10.
- Review the Learning Objectives for Chapter 10.
- Complete the Stop and Practice exercises.
- Study the Certification Review for Chapter 10.
- Complete the Chapter Review exercise to reinforce concepts learned in this chapter.
- Complete the practice exercises on the companion Evolve site for reinforcement of coding concepts.
- Complete the Workbook exercises as assigned by your instructor, or individually for additional practice.

Chapter Review Exercise

Identify the sections and subsections where the following services are located as well as further breakdown as necessary.

	Chapter:			Subsection:	
Example: Vaginal hysterectomy	Surgery	Female	Corpus uteri	Excision	Vaginal genital
1. Chest x-ray, PA only					
2. CT scan, brain without contrast					
3. Electroencephalogram	Medicine			Neuro	
4. Emergency department visit	E+M			Emergency	
5. Epidural anesthesia	Anesthesia				
6. Repair, distal radius fracture	Surgery			Musculoskeletal	
7. Excision of lesion (skin)	Surgery			Integumentary	
8. Office visit	E+M			Office / Outpt.	
9. Mastectomy	Surg.			Integumentary	
10. ECG	Medicine			Cardiology	
11. Physical therapy	Medicine			Physical	
12. Manipulation, finger joint	Surgery			Musculoskeletal	
13. Bronchoscopy with biopsy	Surgery			Respiratory	
14. Tracheostomy, emergency	Surg			Resp	
15. Sinus endoscopy	Surg			Resp	
16. Insertion of pacemaker	Surg			Cardiology	
17. Colonoscopy w/removal of polyps	Surg			Digestive	
18. Cataract extraction	Surg			Eye	
19. Cytoscopy	Surg			Urinary	
20. Hospital visit	E+M			Hospital	

Practical Application

For the reports on the following pages, determine the appropriate steps necessary to assign the correct CPT code(s) as well as modifier(s).

1. Operative report

OPERATIVE REPORT

Patient information:

Patient name:
DOB:
MR#:

Preoperative diagnosis:

Weight loss
Abdominal pain
Vomiting

Postoperative diagnosis:

Colitis cecum
Gastritis
Duodenitis

Procedure(s) performed:

Colonoscopy with biopsy
EGD

Anesthesia:

Assistant surgeon:

Description of procedure:

Patient was brought to the Endoscopy Suite and placed in the left lateral position. IV sedation was given by anesthesia. After adequate sedation was obtained, Xylocaine cream was used in the perirectal area. Colonoscope was inserted and passed through all the flexures into the cecum. Position in the cecum was identified by ileocecal valve, and transillumination. No evidence of any malignant lesion in the cecum. Scope was retroflexed and found to be normal. Scope was then withdrawn.

Patient was turned around, Cetacaine spray was used in the throat. Gastroscope was introduced and passed through into the esophagus, stomach and duodenum. Patient had evidence of gastritis as well as inflammation of the duodenum.

Patient was transferred to the recovery area in stable condition.

Rachel Perez MD

GODFREY REGIONAL HOSPITAL
123 Main Street • Aldon, FL 77714 • (407) 555-1234

Step 1: CPT chapter: ______________________
Step 2: ______________________
Step 3: ______________________
Step 4: ______________________
Step 5: ______________________
Step 6: ______________________
Step 7: ______________________
Step 8: ______________________

2. Office note

OFFICE NOTE

Chief complaint: ____________________

Date: ____________

Vital signs: BP______ P______ R______

History:

This 45-year-old patient presents to the office for their weekly psychotherapy visit with me. Mary has been a patient for approximately 6 weeks, after experiencing a major depressive episode following marital discourse as well as significant financial difficulties.

Mary has begun to accept that her relationship is over and is working with the estranged husband in working out many of financial difficulties they have encountered.

Exam:

Diagnosis/assessment:

I have encouraged Mary to continue her ongoing discussions with her estranged to aid in coping with the end of her marital relationship.

Time spent in visit: 50 minutes
Return: 1 week

William Obert MD

Patient name: ____________________

Date of service: ____________

GODFREY MEDICAL ASSOCIATES
1532 Third Avenue, Suite 120 • Aldon, FL 77713 • (407) 555-4000

Step 1: CPT chapter: ____________________
Step 2: ____________________
Step 3: ____________________
Step 4: ____________________
Step 5: ____________________
Step 6: ____________________
Step 7: ____________________
Step 8: ____________________

3. Operative report

OPERATIVE REPORT

Patient information:

Patient name:
DOB:
MR#:

Preoperative diagnosis:

Intrauterine pregnancy at 40 weeks
Arrest of descent with 3 hours pushing in second stage

Postoperative diagnosis:

Same

Procedure(s) performed:

Primary low transverse cesarean section

Anesthesia:

Continuous lumbar epidural

Assistant surgeon:

Description of procedure:

Patient became exhausted after 3 hrs of pushing in the second stage. She had been on cefotetan since developing a fever in the second stage. After discussion of concerns and alternatives and an attempt at vacuum, she elected to proceed with cesarean section. Patient was prepped and draped in usual manner for abdominal procedure. Low transverse skin incision was made and the peritoneum was exposed and entered relatively high. Incision was extended superiorly and then inferiorly, the anterior leaf of the broad ligament was also incised. Incision was extended laterally in both directions and a bladder flap formed by a combination of sharp and blunt dissection. Uterine incision was made in the midline with the scalpel. This was extended both directions by gentle blunt traction. The vertex was found to be OT, +2 station and well wedged into the pelvis and was removed from the pelvis. Once it had been elevated, the delivery of the head was accomplished without difficulty. Shoulders and the remainder of the baby were delivered without difficulty, the cord clamped and cut, and the neonate handed off to the awaiting pediatrician. Female was delivered at 0211 with Apgars of 9 and 9 and a birth weight of 9 pounds 5 ounces. Placenta was delivered and the uterus was returned to the peritoneal cavity. Parietal peritoneum was closed with continuous 0 chromic sutures. Fascia was closed with 0 Vicryl and subcutaneous tissue irrigated and reapproximated with three 3-0 Vicryl subcutaneous sutures. Skin was closed with staples.

Felix Washington MD

GODFREY REGIONAL HOSPITAL
123 Main Street • Aldon, FL 77714 • (407) 555-1234

Step 1: CPT chapter: ____________________
Step 2: ____________________
Step 3: ____________________
Step 4: ____________________
Step 5: ____________________
Step 6: ____________________
Step 7: ____________________
Step 8: ____________________

4. Emergency room record

EMERGENCY ROOM RECORD

Name:	**Age:**	**ER physician:**
	DOB:	Nancy Connelly, MD

Allergies/type of reaction:	**Usual medications/dosages:**

Triage/presenting complaint:

Initial assessment:

Patient is seen today in the Emergency Room complaining of cough, headache and "bringing up some stuff" when she coughs. This has been going on for 3 days. She has had fever and been using over the counter medications with some relief. Her cough is hacky and productive, which is keeping her up at night.

Time	**T**	**P**	**R**	**BP**	**Other:**					

Medication orders:

Lab work:

X-Ray:

Physician's report:

She is overweight. No acute distress.
Vitals: Looks fine, afebrile
HEENT: Right TM is fairly normal looking as is the left. Throat is unremarkable
Lungs: Sound pretty clear with good air exchange
Heart: Regular rate and rhythm, except slight tachy with fever
Abdomen: Seems benign

Diagnosis:

ASSESSMENT: Bronchitis
PLAN: Z-Pack, Robitussin AC1. Return if not improving.

Discharge **Transfer** **Admit** **Good** **Satisfactory** **Other:**

Physician sign/date

Nancy Connelly MD

GODFREY REGIONAL HOSPITAL
123 Main Street • Aldon, FL 77714 • (407) 555-1234

Step 1: CPT chapter: ______________________
Step 2: ______________________
Step 3: ______________________
Step 4: ______________________
Step 5: ______________________
Step 6: ______________________
Step 7: ______________________
Step 8: ______________________

5. Radiology report

RADIOLOGY REPORT

MR#:
DOB:
Dr.

Clinical summary:

Cervical spine
MVA with neck pain

Abdomen:

Conclusion:

FINDINGS: Vertebral body heights are well maintained. There is no disk space narrowing, subluxation, or fracture. There is no foraminal narrowing. The soft tissues appear unremarkable.

IMPRESSION: Unremarkable cervical spine

D:
T:

Date

GODFREY REGIONAL HOSPITAL
123 Main Street • Aldon, FL 77714 • (407) 555-1234

Step 1: CPT chapter: ______________________
Step 2: ______________________
Step 3: ______________________
Step 4: ______________________
Step 5: ______________________
Step 6: ______________________
Step 7: ______________________
Step 8: ______________________

6. Hospital observation note

HOSPITAL OBSERVATION NOTE

Godfrey Regional Hospital Observation Note
Admission: 12/01/00

Admitting Diagnosis: Chest Pain

57-year-old with previous history of hypercholesterolemia, smoking, alcohol and drug abuse, history of hepatitis C.

Patient reports two prolonged episodes of chest pain that occurred with activity and exertion that lasted about 30 minutes each with relief by rest.

Past medical history:

Denies history of HTN, CVA, CAD or PVD.

Medications: Lorcet 7.5 mg, Soma one tab bid, Xanax 1 mg bid, sublingual Nitro, Toprol XL 25 mg, Lipitor 10 mg qhs

Family and social history

Heavy smoker, alcohol and drug abuse

Review of systems:

Physical exam

Vital signs: stable
HEENT: No JVD, no carotid bruits
Heart: Normal S-1, S-2, No gallops, no murmurs
Lungs: Clear
Abdomen: Soft, bowel sounds are positive, non tender to palpation, no rebound
Extremities: No pedal edema noted

Laboratory/radiology:

Creatinine 0.9, Potassium 3.7, Hemoglobin 15, Platelet Count 243,000, INR 1.1. All other labs normal.

ECG showed normal sinus rhythm, normal axis, QS morphology from V1 to V3 suspicious of anteroseptal MI.

X-ray:

Assessment:

Plan:

Discussed with him the need for cardiac catheterization. We will admit to observation, obtain a left heart cath in the morning. Continue current medical therapy.

Nath Brady MD

GODFREY REGIONAL HOSPITAL
123 Main Street • Aldon, FL 77714 • (407) 555-1234

Step 1: CPT chapter: ______________________
Step 2: ______________________
Step 3: ______________________
Step 4: ______________________
Step 5: ______________________
Step 6: ______________________
Step 7: ______________________
Step 8: ______________________

7. Radiology report

RADIOLOGY REPORT

MR#:
DOB:
Dr.

Clinical summary:

Examination of: Abdomen, 1 view
Clinical Symptoms: Abdominal pain, 1 day

Abdomen:

FINDINGS: One view of the abdomen was obtained. Non-obstructive bowel gas pattern. No calcification seen overlying the kidneys or course of ureters.

Conclusion:

IMPRESSION: No abnormality on one view of abdomen.

D:
T:

Date

GODFREY REGIONAL HOSPITAL
123 Main Street • Aldon, FL 77714 • (407) 555-1234

Step 1: CPT chapter: ______________________

Step 2: ______________________

Step 3: ______________________

Step 4: ______________________

Step 5: ______________________

Step 6: ______________________

Step 7: ______________________

Step 8: ______________________

8. Operative report

OPERATIVE REPORT

Patient information:

Patient name:
DOB:
MR#:

Preoperative diagnosis:

Symptomatic chronic cholecystitis and cholelithiasis

Postoperative diagnosis:

Same

Procedure(s) performed:

Cholecystectony with operative cholangiogram

Anesthesia:

Assistant surgeon:

Description of procedure:

Under satisfactory general anesthesia, the abdomen was prepped and draped and a right subcostal incision was made. On exploration, the liver margins were sharp and the gallbladder not thick-walled. It was somewhat tense and stones could not definitely be palpated within it. The cystic duct was fairly long and quite small in diameter and the common duct of normal size. The stomach, spleen, kidneys and pancreas were essentially normal to palpation, although the right kidney seemed quite small. The cystic artery was easily identified and the gallbladder dissected out from above and bleeders in the bed were electrocoagulated as they were encountered. A small opening was made in the cystic duct and with some difficulty a cystic duct cholangiocath was placed into the common duct and a special clamp used to hold it in place. Dye was injected and two films were taken. On the first film there was a suggestion of a round mass, not seen on subsequent films, so I was unable to confirm the presence of a definitive stone. Peritoneum and posterior rectum sheath were closed with running 0 Vicryl. Wound was irrigated and subcutaneous tissue approximated with interrupted 3-0 Vicryl and skin closed with clips. Patient's condition at conclusion of procedure was satisfactory. Estimated blood loss was 50 cc.

GODFREY REGIONAL HOSPITAL
123 Main Street • Aldon, FL 77714 • (407) 555-1234

Step 1: CPT chapter: ______________________
Step 2: ______________________
Step 3: ______________________
Step 4: ______________________
Step 5: ______________________
Step 6: ______________________
Step 7: ______________________
Step 8: ______________________

9. Operative report

OPERATIVE REPORT

Patient information:

Patient name:
DOB:
MR#:

Preoperative diagnosis:

Incomplete AB
INDICATIONS: The patient had an incomplete AB as confirmed on ultrasound. The patient was informed of the risks and benefits of waiting versus D & C and she chose the D & C.

Postoperative diagnosis:

Incomplete AB

Procedure(s) performed:

D & C

Anesthesia:

Assistant surgeon:

Description of procedure:

The patient was brought to the operating room and prepped and draped in the usual manner. The uterus was initially palpated with bimanual exam and found to be in the mid position. The size was consistent with approximately 7 week gestation. Weighted speculum was then placed in the vagina and uterus was sounded and appeared to be 3 ¾ inches deep. The cervix was grasped with a tenaculum forceps and progressively dilated without difficulty. The suction device was inserted into the uterus, and, suction was applied and rotated in a gentle manner. The retained products of conception were then removed. The uterus was then gently explored with a sharp curette, and no evidence of remaining tissue was found. Approximately 25 cc of blood loss noted. The products of conception were noted in the trap of the suction machine and sent to Pathology.

The patient tolerated the procedure well. Ten units of Pitocin were given after the procedure. The patient was taken to the Recovery Room in stable condition.

Rachel Perez MD

GODFREY REGIONAL HOSPITAL
123 Main Street • Aldon, FL 77714 • (407) 555-1234

Step 1: CPT chapter: ____________________
Step 2: ____________________
Step 3: ____________________
Step 4: ____________________
Step 5: ____________________
Step 6: ____________________
Step 7: ____________________
Step 8: ____________________

10. Operative report

Cardiac Catheterization Report

After informed consent, the patient was taken to the cardiac catheterization lab, right groin prepped and draped in the usual fashion under sterile conditions.

Under local anesthesia and conscious sedation with intravenous midazolam and fentanyl, right femoral arterial access was secured using Seldinger technique, a 6 French sheath was inserted into the femoral artery and flushed in the usual fashion. A left heart catheterization was successfully completed.

(**NOTE:** The remainder of this operative report has been omitted until the discussion of additional techniques necessary to code a complete cardiac catheterization. Code only for the actual heart catheterization performed.)

Step 1: CPT chapter: ______________________

Step 2: ______________________

Step 3: ______________________

Step 4: ______________________

Step 5: ______________________

Step 6: ______________________

Step 7: ______________________

Step 8: ______________________

11

Evaluation and Management Services

LEARNING OBJECTIVES

After completing this chapter, the student will be able to:

- Apply the concepts of evaluation and management (E & M) coding to practical cases.
- Understand the different types of E & M services.
- Grasp definitions of new and established patients for coding purposes.
- Know the differences between the 1995 and 1997 E & M guidelines.
- Identify and apply key concepts for determining E & M levels of service.
- Identify and apply correct modifiers to E & M service codes.
- Comprehend the relation of time to levels of service for E & M services.
- Understand the concept of "covering physician" as it relates to Current Procedural Terminology (CPT) E & M coding.
- Understand the concept of consultation as it relates to CPT E & M coding.
- Define critical care as it pertains to E & M services.

CODING REFERENCE TOOLS

Tool 11-1
New or Established Patient and Time-Driven Visit Codes

Tool 11-2
E & M Code Assignment Grid

Tool 11-3
History Guidelines

Tool 11-4
Examination Guidelines

Tool 11-5
Risk Grid (Medical Decision Making)

KEY TERMS

Coordination of Care
Counseling
Established Patient
History
History of Present Illness
Medical Decision Making
New Patient
Physical Examination
Review of Systems
Risk of Morbidity and Mortality

Documentation Guidelines

Documentation needs for physician services were discussed in Section 1 of this text. Evaluation and management (E & M) services are encounters or visits provided to the patient by the physician or physician extender. E & M services may be provided by any individual who is licensed to provide specified services in the state in which services are rendered. Documentation guidelines differ somewhat based on the provider (also discussed in Section 1). This chapter involves extensive work on identifying the key components in the physician encounter: **history**, **physical examination**, and **medical decision making**. These key elements are the individualized steps in the identification of the correct E & M procedure code for services performed.

E & M SERVICE CODES

Office and Outpatient Services	
New patient	99201-99205
Established patient	99211-99215
Hospital Observation Services	
Initial observation care	99218-99220
Observation discharge	99217
Observation/inpatient care/admit/ discharge same date	99234-99236
Hospital Inpatient Services	
Initial hospital care	99221-99223
Subsequent hospital care	99231-99233
Hospital discharge	99238-99239
Consultations	
Office consultations	99241-99245
Inpatient consultations	99251-99255
Emergency department services	99281-99285
Pediatric patient transport services	99289-99290
Critical Care Services	
Adult	99291-99292
Pediatric	99293-99294
Neonatal	99295-99296
Continuing intensive care services	99298-99300
Nursing Facility Services	
Initial nursing care	99304-99306
Subsequent nursing care	99307-99310
Nursing facility discharge	99315-99316
Other nursing facility	99318
Domiciliary, Rest Home, or Custodial Care Services	
New patient	99324-99328
Established patient	99334-99337
Oversight services, rest home, or home care	99339-99340
Home Services	
New patient	99341-99345
Established patient	99347-99350
Prolonged Services	
Direct patient contact	99354-99357
Without direct patient contact	99358-99539
Standby services	99360
Case Management Services	
Anticoagulation management	99363-99364
Medical team conferences	99366-99368
Care plan oversight services	99374-99380
Preventive Medicine Services	
New patient	99381-99387
Established patient	99391-99397
Individual counseling	99401-99404
Group counseling	99411-99412
Other	99420-99429
Newborn care services	99431-99440
Non–Face-to-Face Services	
Telephone services	99441-99443
Online medical evaluation	99444
Special E & M services	99450-99456
Other E & M services	99477-99499

Consistency is of the utmost importance in E & M coding. The coder must be able to substantiate the level of service coded on the basis of the documentation provided. The best way to achieve this consistency is to use some type of form to document how the coder arrives at a specific level of service. If a question arises at a later date, whether from a third-party audit or a patient inquiry, the practice or facility will be able to substantiate the level of service originally coded.

Other methods, such as developing specialty-specific coding guidelines, also help maintain consistency in E & M coding. Sample grids are included with the discussion of each type of E & M service.

Look again at the E & M portion of the table in Chapter 10 at the steps or components needed for CPT coding.

CPT CODING STEPS: E & M EXAMPLE

Step 1: Identify Chapter, Visit, and Encounter

Range of codes: 99201-99499

Step 2: Determine Location

Office
Hospital

Step 3: Determine Patient Type

New
Established

Step 4: Determine Level of Service

Level 1

Step 5: Identify Extent or Additional Specifics and Time or Other Guidelines

45 min

Step 6: Assign CPT Code(s)

Step 7: Put Codes in Appropriate Order

Step 8: Assign Modifier Code(s) if Appropriate

Take the sample E & M chart (Fig. 11-1) and evaluate it for the documentation components needed to appropriately assign the correct E & M level for the service.

CONSULTATION REPORT
GODFREY REGIONAL OUTPATIENT CLINIC

Patient:
Date of consultation: 05/14/XX
Consulting physician:
Referring physician:
Indication for consultation: Ventricular tachycardia

HPI (Quality)

History:

PMH

The patient is a 76-year-old female with known history of cardiac disease who underwent an outpatient knee arthroscopy yesterday. The procedure went well; however, during the postoperative period, the patient's cardiac rhythm was noted to have multiple runs of non-sustained ventricular tachycardia. The patient apparently remained asymptomatic and hemodynamically stable. Due to her significant cardiac history, it was felt she should follow up to rule out any cardiac abnormalities. Patient denies having any recent history of chest pain, PND, orthopnea, dyspnea on exertion, shortness of breath, palpitations, syncope/near syncope or lower extremity edema.

PMH PMH Chief Complaint

PMH — PAST MEDICAL HISTORY:
1. Coronary atherosclerotic heart disease
2. Status post myocardial infarction approximately 15 years ago
3. S/P PTCA

PMH — ALLERGIES: Iodine

PMH — MEDICATIONS:
1. Altace 10 mg qd
2. Aricept 5 mg qd
3. Amiodarone 100 mg qd
4. Clonazepam 5 mg qhs
5. Prevachol 40 mg qhs
6. Spironolactone 25 q tablet qhs

None — FAMILY HISTORY: Non-contributory
SOCIAL HISTORY: Non-contributory
REVIEW OF SYSTEMS: As stated in the HPI

1E Constitutional — **Exam:**

PHYSICAL EXAMINATION:
The patient is a well developed, elderly white female who is alert and oriented X3 in no acute distress with pleasant demeanor. She is afebrile with stable vital signs.

2E — HEAD: Normocephalic, atraumatic
3E — NECK: Supple without evidence of JCP, mass or bruit
4E — CHEST: Clear to auscultation
5E — CARDIAC: Normal carotid upstroke with normal contour – no evidence of peristernal Heave, lift, thrill. Auscultation reveals regular rate and rhythm without evidence of murmur, rub or gallop. Pulses are 1+ and symmetrical throughout.
6E — ABDOMEN: Soft, nontender, no evidence of pulsatile or palpable mass identified
GU: Deferred
7E — EXTREM: Showed no evidence of clubbing, cyanosis, or edema
8E — NEURO: Grossly intact, nonfocal
1M — EKG: Ectopic atrial rhythm with delayed precordial transmission and prolonged QT corrected interval. Telemetry shows no current findings suggestive of significant tachy or brady arrhythmia. No findings suggestive of any significant block or pause.
2M — LAB DATA: Hematology – WBC 4.5, hemoglobin 12.1, hematocrit 35.3, MCV 95.6, MCH 32.8, platelets 160,000. Glucose, 92, BUN 14, creatinine 1.0, calcium 8.6, alk phos 40, Potassium 3.5, Cardiac enzymes, CPK 88, CKMB 5, Troponin 0.5

Diagnosis/assessment:

IMPRESSION:
76-year-old female with known history of coronary atherosclerotic heart disease and atrial fibrillation, now presents with run of nonsustained V tach per report. Patient has remained hemodynamically stable, no evidence of persistent cardiac arrhythmia.

MDM Risk Low

We appreciate the opportunity to participate in the overall evaluation and management of this patient. We will continue the patient on her usual cardiac medications, and, should she experience any symptoms, she should follow-up immediately.

Maurice Doater, M.D

Patient name: ________
Date of service: ________

GODFREY REGIONAL OUTPATIENT CLINIC
3122 Shannon Avenue • Aldon, FL 77712 • (407) 555-7654

FIGURE 11-1. Sample consultation report.

CPT CODING STEPS

Step 1

Visit or encounter 99201-99499

Step 2

Hospital 99241-99275

Step 3

New patient 99241-99245

Step 4

Level of service Level 1

Step 5

Time/other guidelines 45 min

Steps 6 and 7

CPT code range 99241-99245

Step 8

Not necessary

At this point, an E & M code for this service would be assigned from the range between 99241 and 99245. The exact code would be assigned according to the level of service for the consultation. How to determine the level of service is discussed throughout this chapter. After the discussion, this chart is reconsidered and the key components extracted that are necessary to arrive at the exact CPT E & M code for this service.

General Coding Guidelines

DEFINITIONS

The specific definitions necessary for understanding E & M coding are as follows.

NEW PATIENT VISIT A patient who has not received any professional service from the physician or another physician of the same specialty in the same group over the past 3 years. New patient visits require all three key components be met.

ESTABLISHED PATIENT VISIT A patient who has received professional services from the physician or another physician of the same specialty in the same group during the past 3 years. Established or subsequent visits require only two of the three key components be met.

In the case of "on call" physicians, or "covering physicians," the E & M service is coded and billed with the same coding that would have been used by the physician who was not available. For example, if an established patient of a family practitioner is hospitalized and is seen by a covering physician, that E & M service would be billed as an established patient visit despite the fact the physician attending the patient may never have seen the patient in the past.

In most instances the physician may charge one level of service code per patient per day. Therefore when the patient is seen in the office and is referred to the hospital for admission, the provider may charge for only one service, that is, the office visit or the hospital admission.

INITIAL VISIT The initial, or first, visit during an episode of care. These visits typically occur during a stay in a hospital or nursing facility where the services typically last more than 1 day. An initial visit code is assigned for the first visit of the multiple days of care, despite the fact that the patient has seen the provider in the past. Remember, this visit is based on a new *stay,* not the new patient versus established patient guidelines. When initial visits are used, all three key components are required to meet the level of service.

SUBSEQUENT VISIT Visits after the initial, or first, visit during an episode of care. When a patient is confined for multiple days of services, such as a hospitalization or nursing home services, all dates of service after the initial or first date of service will be assigned subsequent visit codes. When subsequent visit codes are used, two of the three key components are necessary for assigning the level of service.

Tool 11-1 categorizes E & M codes that are used with new, established, initial, or subsequent visits, as well as time-driven codes, and how many key components are necessary for these services.

STOP AND PRACTICE

Read the following scenarios and determine whether they meet the criteria of new, established, initial, or subsequent patient status based on the definitions given above.

1. Patient has previously been seen at this practice for her chronic obstructive pulmonary disease. She is returning to the practice 2 years after having been seen by this physician.

   ___New ____ Established

2. Patient has been seen in the practice before by the internal medicine physician. Patient has been referred to the cardiologist in the practice for evaluation and treatment of the chronic condition of CHF.

   ___ New ____ Established

3. Patient has never been seen by Dr. Smith in the past. However, Dr. Smith is the covering physician for Dr. Jones, who saw the patient approximately 3½ years ago.

   ___ New ____ Established

STOP AND PRACTICE—cont'd

4. Patient is a regular patient with the family practice and usually saw Dr. Xavier. Dr. Xavier is no longer with the practice when the patient returns. She is scheduled to see another physician in the same practice.

   ___ New ____ Established

5. Patient has seen Dr. Jones on a regular basis over the past 2 to 3 years for her diabetes. She arrives in the emergency department reporting high blood sugar and is admitted to the service of Dr. Jones.

   ____ Initial ____ Subsequent

6 Patient is seen on his second day of hospitalization by his family medicine physician. The patient has not seen his family physician for approximately 2 or 3 months.

   ____ Initial ____ Subsequent

7. Patient is readmitted to a nursing facility after a hospitalization and stay at a rehabilitation center.

   ____ Initial ____ Subsequent

8. Patient is seen by Dr. Smith during a recent hospitalization. Patient is instructed to schedule a follow-up appointment with Dr. Smith in his office within 7 to 10 days. This will be the first time the patient has been seen in the physician's office.

   ___ New ____ Established

9. Patient was seen by her family physician at the office in the Westside clinic location. Patient indicates she can only come in for a visit on Thursdays, the day the Westside clinic location is closed. She schedules an appointment at the Northside clinic with the same physician on Monday.

   ___ New ____ Established

10. The family of the patient has been seen by Dr. Jones for several years. The family adopts a 2-year-old child and brings the child in for an annual check-up.

   ___ New ____ Established

TOOL 11-1

NEW OR ESTABLISHED PATIENT AND TIME-DRIVEN VISIT CODES

New/Initial Visits (3 of 3 Components Required)	Code Ranges
Office/outpatient	99201-99205
Hospital observation	99218-99220
Initial hospital care	99221-99223
Observation/inpatient admit/discharge same day	99234-99236
Office/outpatient consultations	99241-99245
Initial inpatient consultations	99251-99255
Emergency department services	99281-99285
Initial nursing facility care	99304-99306
Domiciliary, rest home, custodial care	99324-99328
Home services	99341-99345

Established/Subsequent Visits (2 of 3 Components Required)	Code Ranges
Office/outpatient	99211-99215
Subsequent hospital care	99231-99233
Subsequent nursing facility care	99307-99310
Domiciliary, rest home, custodial care	99334-99337
Home services	99347-99350

Time-Driven Codes	Code Ranges
Observation discharge services	99217
Hospital discharge services	99238-99239
Pediatric critical care transport	99289-99290
Critical care	99291-99292
Inpatient neonatal/pediatric critical care	99293-99296 (per-day codes)
Continuing intensive care	99298-99300 (per-day codes)
Nursing facility discharge services	99315-99316
Prolonged services	99354-99359
Physician standby services	99360
Case management services	99361-99362
Care plan oversight services	99374-99380
Counseling/risk factor intervention	99401-99412

BUNDLING AND UNBUNDLING ISSUES

Under general coding guidelines, E & M services may or may not be considered in other services such as surgical services. Although these guidelines differ from one insurance carrier to another, many carriers refer to the following National Correct Coding Initiative (NCCI) guidelines for general guidance.

- Physician may generally report one E & M service on a single date of service. There are a few exceptions, which are discussed later in this chapter. An example of an exception would be a patient who is seen in the office, referred to the emergency department, and admitted under the service of the physician seen earlier in the day at the office. This rule applies to each physician. Therefore multiple physicians may evaluate a patient in a given day as long as the service is medically necessary. However, the physician who saw the patient in the office and admitted the patient in the same day will typically be entitled to one E & M service for that date of service only.
- Digital rectal exams are considered a simple examination and are not codeable or billable when an E & M service is provided. In instances when it is the only service furnished or it is furnished as part of an otherwise noncovered service, it would be considered for payment.
- When major procedures (typically those with at least a 90-day global period) are provided on the same date of service as an E & M service, the E & M service is not payable unless it is performed solely for the purpose of deciding whether to perform the surgical procedure. In these instances, modifier 57 would be appropriate.
- When minor procedures (typically defined as having a 10-day global period) are provided on the same date as an E & M service, any decision to perform surgery for those minor procedures would be considered included, or bundled, in the procedure performed.
  However, in instances when a minor procedure or minor surgical service is performed as well as a "significantly separately identifiable E & M service" unrelated to the decision to perform the minor procedure, the minor procedure may be considered for coding and billing by appending modifier 25 to the E & M service.

NCCI further states that all procedural services involve some level of physician involvement or supervision that is considered integral to the service. In those instances a separate E & M service is not reportable.

It will become even more evident how some of these guidelines differ from carrier to carrier when reimbursement is discussed in relation to coding.

Modifier Usage

Although the general use of modifier codes has previously been discussed, a look at modifier use in relation to E & M services is also appropriate. Modifiers are summarized in Table 11-1.

MODIFIER 24—E & M SERVICES UNRELATED TO A GLOBAL OR POSTOPERATIVE PERIOD

With modifier 24 comes the concept of global procedures. Remember, when global procedures are performed, the normal preoperative, surgical, and postoperative services are included in the "package" price for that service. However, when E & M services are extras—that is, not included in the usual package price—the coder must indicate this by using a modifier that these services should be considered outside the normal global or postoperative package. An example would be follow-up visits during the postoperative period for completely unrelated services or complications.

Without the modifier code the carrier will NOT consider these services for payment. The modifier code tells the carrier that "This service is not usually covered; however, the service should be considered for payment because [modifier code]." A diagnosis code indicating that the chief reason for an encounter is unrelated to the initial service or that it is the

TABLE 11-1 MODIFIERS

MODIFIER	DESCRIPTOR	USE
24	E & M services unrelated to global or postoperative period	Services "outside" the global package
25	Significantly separately identifiable E & M at the time of another service	E & M services performed distinct to another service or procedure performed at the same encounter
32	Mandated services	Services requested by a third party
52	Reduced services	Services less than those typically performed with code assignment
57	Decision for surgery	E & M service performed for the sole purpose of determining whether surgery is medically indicated

result of a complication such as infection is usually necessary to justify payment for this modified service.

MODIFIER 25—E & M SERVICE THAT IS DISTINCT AND SEPARATE ("SIGNIFICANTLY SEPARATELY IDENTIFIABLE")

When the physician performs a procedure or service that is distinct and separate from the E & M service, it can be coded separately. Following is another instance in which medical necessity (diagnosis) is crucial to coding and reimbursement.

A patient visits the physician after an *automobile accident. Multiple contusions of the arms and legs, a painful shoulder,* and a head laceration are examined. Laceration repair is performed for the *open wound of the head.*

Services (What)	**Diagnosis (Why)**
Physician visit	Shoulder pain
	Multiple contusions, legs and arms
Laceration repair	Open wound of head

The chief reason for the encounter was the laceration repair of an open wound of the head. Because the open wound medically necessitated the laceration repair, the visit portion of the encounter focused on the evaluation and management specifically for shoulder pain and multiple contusions of the arms and legs.

NOTE: Modifier 25 is added to the E & M service code, NOT the surgical code.

MODIFIER 32—MANDATED SERVICES

When services are requested by a third party (e.g., a peer review organization) or a third-party carrier, the services should be designated as such with the modifier 32. Often this will be a request for an additional opinion regarding surgery. Insurance carriers may not pay for multiple physicians' opinions on the same problem; however, if insurance carriers dictate the necessity of an additional opinion, that E & M service should be coded with modifier 32.

MODIFIER 52—REDUCED SERVICES

Modifier 52 should NOT be used to reduce the charge for an E & M service. This modifier should be used to indicate that the level of a provided E & M service is partially reduced. Such an adjustment in the level of service should NOT be made for the purpose of adjusting the price for a particular service. Caution should be taken to ensure that services are billed at the level performed. If a particular service has been reduced or eliminated and a lower charge is appropriate, less may be charged with the same level of service coded and use of modifier 52. With the proper addition of modifier 52, the usual customary and reasonable reimbursement calculation for that level of service will not be affected. This was discussed in the use of the Table of Modifiers in our introduction to CPT coding.

For example, if a patient presents for an office visit and meets the criteria for a level 3, code 99213 visit but the visit is not as involved as the usual level 3, code 99213 visit, the coder should not assign a level 2, code 99212 or level 1, code 99211 level because the charge is significantly less. Rather, the coder should assign the appropriate level 3, code 99213 level of service based on the key components discussed below and assign modifier 52 to the E & M service.

MODIFIER 57—E & M SERVICE FOR PURPOSE OF DECISION FOR SURGERY

When an E & M service is performed and the determination is made during that E & M visit that surgery is necessary, the visit is NOT considered part of the preoperative global package; however, it may be considered for reimbursement by third-party carriers with the addition of modifier 57. Care should be taken to ensure that the service is not scheduled as a preoperative visit and that the decision to proceed with surgery has not already been made before the time of the visit. These E & M services are considered part of the global surgical package and would be considered as included, or *bundled.* If the surgical procedure is global and no modifier is appended to services, a visit on the same day or on the day(s) preceding surgery typically will be denied as part of the global surgical package.

Not all insurance carriers agree with the use of this modifier, and some may still include this visit as part of the global package. The discussion of bundled and unbundled services in Chapter 9 included the NCCI and Medicare guidelines for this modifier. Check the carrier's contract to determine how to categorize this service.

Remember that the coder should code and bill services according to CPT and not third-party guidelines. Despite the possibility that the carrier may include this service in the global package, the coder should code and bill the service if appropriate. Third-party carrier inclusion or exclusion of payment should not determine how services are coded.

E & M Service Determination

GENERAL GUIDELINES

CPT guidelines are given for each type and level of service. The E & M section offers perhaps the greatest coding diversity of any section in the CPT book. If the selection of codes from this section is made in a methodical step-by-step manner, then these services will be coded accurately.

The E & M section may also be the most controversial section of CPT. Many of the guidelines in this section are subject to interpretation, so the coder must be consistent and capable of documenting and defending his or her choice of codes. Despite accurate E & M coding, some insurance carriers will not pay for some services that have been coded and billed appropriately. Inclusion of codes in the CPT book does not necessarily mean that health insurance coverage will be provided for these services. These codes simply identify provided services; the medical necessity for those services is explained by the use of codes from the *International Classification of Diseases*, 9th Revision, Clinical Modification (ICD-9-CM).

Services within the E & M section are assigned levels. E & M services encompass those provided directly to the patient during a visit or encounter that does not involve diagnostic testing or services. This means that within the outpatient office visit section the patient may be given a numeric level, typically from 1 to 5, depending on what services are performed. Each E & M service is coded according to the following criteria:

- Location of service (e.g., outpatient, hospital, nursing home)
- New patient versus established patient status
- Level of service

Key E & M Components

The definitions of *new patient* and *established patient* have been discussed previously. Location of service, as it pertains to these definitions, is discussed later in the chapter. The key components that determine levels for all E & M services, despite new or established patient status and location of service, are as follows:

- History
- Physical examination
- Medical decision making

In certain instances other factors are taken into consideration as well. These include the following:

- Counseling
- Coordination of care
- Nature of presenting problem
- Time
- Centers for Medicare and Medicaid Services (CMS) "overarching" criteria

The first three components are considered *key components.* They are always considered in making the initial determination of level of service. The last four factors apply in certain circumstances discussed later.

Although CPT presents the determination of level of service from a basic approach, many carriers require more involved, specific guidelines for determining E & M levels of service.

Level of Service According to 1995 and 1997 Guidelines

Two separate sets of guidelines may be followed for determining the level of service. In 1995 guidelines were established that define history, physical examination, and medical decision-making components necessary for each level. New guidelines were introduced in 1997, but providers argued that these guidelines were exceedingly strict and difficult to meet; thus both the 1995 and the 1997 guidelines are considered acceptable for determining levels of services. According to the 1997 guidelines, history, physical examination, and medical decision-making criteria must still be met as outlined in the 1995 guidelines. In addition, specific elements or "bullets" must be present in the documentation for the minimum requirement for each level to be met. Under the 1997 guidelines, the provider has the choice of using the key elements or bullets from either the multisystem or body organ system review that are pertinent to the patient's complaint.

Figure 11-2 compares the 1995 and 1997 guidelines for outpatient office visits. The requirements of the 1995 and the 1997 guidelines are similar, except that the 1997 guidelines are more specific about the documentation that must be included. Because the 1995 guidelines are less specific, third-party carriers often disagree with the level the coder has assigned. Currently, the coder may use whichever guidelines he or she wishes to use for each case; however, it is advisable to stick with one set of guidelines to avoid confusion. Make certain that the physicians, the third-party carriers, and any entity performing chart audits are aware of which guidelines the facility has chosen to follow.

Facilities with many physicians may choose to use both sets of guidelines. A specific specialty or physician may choose to use the 1997 guidelines. Other providers in the same group may wish to follow the 1995 guidelines.

No matter which guidelines the facility or provider chooses to use for determining levels of service, the three primary factors of history, physical examination, and medical decision making still guide the assignment of those levels. Following is a discussion of the components needed in documentation so that E & M services can be coded appropriately.

Tool 11-2 will be used throughout this text as a mechanism for "counting" the components within each key component of E & M services. Although the tool may look a bit overwhelming at first glance, each key component of the form will be discussed separately and in depth. The grid will incorporate the 1995 E & M guidelines, which currently are the most commonly used.

A copy of the 1995 E & M guidelines from CMS is included on the companion Evolve site for further review and discussion.

HISTORY

History components provide information about the chief complaint and the history of the present illness, such as the following:

- Chief complaint
- History of present illness
- Review of systems
- Past medical, family, and social history

For specific examples of the documentation used to record these elements, refer to Tool 11-2.

1995/1997 E & M CODING GUIDELINES COMPARISON

OFFICE/OTHER OUTPATIENT SERVICES, NEW PATIENT

	1995 Guidelines	1997 Guidelines
99201 **History:**	CC/brief HPI	Same
Exam:	Limited exam of affected body area/organ system	1-5 bullet elements in >1 body area/organ system
MDM:	Dx/Mgt minimal; Quantity/complex data minimal/none Risk minimal	Same
99202 **History:**	CC/brief HPI/problem pertinent ROS	Same
Exam:	Limited exam of affected body area/organ system Other related/symptomatic system(s)	6 bullet elements in >1 body area/organ system
MDM:	Dx/Mgt minimal; Quantity/complex data minimal/none Risk minimal	Same
99203 **History:**	CC/extended HPI/problem pertinent ROS including review of limited number of additional systems	Same 2-9 systems ROS/PFSH 1 item any history area
Exam:	Pertinent PFSH directly related to problem(s) Extend exam of affected body area/organ system Other related/symptomatic system(s)	2 bullet elements in at least 6 body areas/organ systems OR 12 bullet elements in >2 body areas/organ systems Single system (eye/psych): 9 bullet items required
MDM:	Dx/Mgt limited; Quantity/complex data limited Risk low	Same
99204 **History:**	CC/extended HPI/problem pertinent ROS + review of all additional systems/complete PFSH	Same 4 elements of HPI or 3 chronic/inactive conditions ROS at least 10 body areas/organ systems
Exam:	General multisystem exam OR complete exam of one organ system	All bullet elements in at least 9 body areas/organ systems No fewer than 2 bullet elements in each area/system Single system: All bullet items in shaded boxes and at least one bullet in each unshaded box
MDM:	Dx/Mgt multiple; Quantity/complex data moderate Risk moderate	Same
99205 **History:**	CC/extended HPI/problem pertinent ROS + review of all additional systems/complete PFSH	Same 4 elements of HPI or 3 chronic/inactive conditions ROS at least 10 body areas/organ systems
Exam:	General multisystem exam OR complete exam of one organ system	All bullet elements in at least 9 body areas/organ systems No less than 2 bullet elements in each area/system Single system: All bullet items in shaded boxes and at least one bullet in each unshaded box
MDM:	Dx/Mgt extensive; Quantity/complex data extensive Risk high	Same

FIGURE 11-2. 1995 and 1997 E & M coding guidelines comparison.

1995/1997 E & M CODING GUIDELINES COMPARISON OFFICE/OTHER OUTPATIENT SERVICES, ESTABLISHED PATIENT	1995 Guidelines	1997 Guidelines
99211 **History:**	No key elements required	Same
Exam:	Problem severity does not require physician presence; however, service provided under physician's care	
MDM:	None specified	
99212 **History:**	CC/brief HPI	Same
Exam:	Limited exam of affected body area/organ system	1-5 bullet elements in >1 body area/organ system
MDM:	Dx/Mgt minimal; Quantity/complex data minimal/none Risk minimal	Same
99213 **History:**	CC/extended HPI/problem pertinent ROS	Same
Exam:	Limited exam of affected body area/organ system Other related/symptomatic system(s)	6 bullet elements in >1 body area/organ system
MDM:	Dx/Mgt limited; Quantity/complex data limited Risk low	Same
99214 **History:**	CC/extended HPI/problem pertinent ROS Review of limited additional systems Pertinent PFSH related to problem(s)	Same Document 2-9 systems for ROS PFSH document 1 item any history area
Exam:	Extend exam of affected body area/organ system Other related/symptomatic system(s)	2 bullet elements in at least 6 body areas/organ systems OR 12 bullet elements in >2 body areas/organ systems Single system (eye/psych): 9 bullet elements required and at least 1 bullet in each unshaded box
MDM:	Dx/Mgt multiple; Quantity/complex data moderate Risk moderate	Same
99215 **History:**	CC/extended HPI/problem pertinent ROS + review of all additional systems/complete PFSH	Same 4 elements of HPI or 3 chronic/inactive conditions ROS at least 10 body areas/organ systems
Exam:	General multisystem exam OR complete exam of one organ system	All bullet elements in at least 9 body areas/organ systems No fewer than 2 bullet elements in each area/system Single system: All bullet items in shaded boxes and at least one bullet in each unshaded box
MDM:	Dx/Mgt extensive; Quantity/complex data extensive Risk high	Same

FIGURE 11-2, cont'd.

TOOL 11-2

E & M CODE ASSIGNMENT GRID

Evaluation and Management Leveling Sheet: 1995 Guidelines **GODFREY MEDICAL GROUP**

Patient Name/ID:____________________ DOS:____________________ Chief Complaint:______________________________

	Final results for history (3 of 3 required)	Problem focused	Exp. problem focused	Detailed	Comprehensive
HISTORY	HPI: ☐ Location ☐ Timing ☐ Quality ☐ Associated signs and symptoms ☐ Severity ☐ Modifying factors ☐ Duration ☐ Context	Brief (1-3) ☐	Brief (1-3) ☐	Extended (4 or more) ☐	Extended (4 or more) ☐
	ROS: ☐ Constitutional (wt. loss, etc.) ☐ Integumentary (skin, breast) ☐ Endocrine ☐ All/Immunology ☐ ENM and T ☐ Eyes ☐ Cardio/Vasc ☐ Respiratory ☐ GI ☐ GU ☐ Musculoskeletal ☐ Psychiatric ☐ Hem/Lymph ☐ Neurological ☐ "All others negative"	None ☐	Pertinent to problem (1 system) ☐	Extended (2-9 systems including pertinent system) ☐	Complete (10 or more systems or pertinent systems with the statement "all others negative") ☐
	PFSH (past medical, family, social history): Past Hx. (the pts. past experience with illness, operations, and treatments) Family Hx. (a review of medical events in the pts. family) Social Hx. (an age appropriate review of past and current activities)	None ☐	None ☐	Pertinent *(1 or 2 history area) ☐	Complete *(2 or 3 history areas) ☐
EXAM	Body areas: ☐ Head, incl. face ☐ Chest, incl. breast and axillae ☐ Abdomen ☐ Neck ☐ Back, incl. spine ☐ Each extremity ☐ Genitalia, groin, buttocks Organ systems: ☐ Constitutional ☐ ENMT ☐ Respiratory ☐ Musculoskeletal ☐ Psych ☐ Eyes ☐ CV ☐ GI ☐ GU ☐ Skin ☐ Neurological ☐ Hem/lymph/imm	1 area or system ☐	2 to 4 areas or systems ☐	2 to 7 areas or systems MUST BE DETAILED ☐	8 or more systems or a complete exam of a single system ☐

*Complete PFSH - 2 Hx areas a) Estab pts Office (Output) care; domiciliary care; home care; b) Emergency Dept. c) Subsequent nursing facility care
3 Hx areas a) New pt. Office (Outpt) care; domiciliary care; home care; b) Consultations c) Initial hospital care d) hospital observation e) Comprehensive nursing facility assessments

Box A: Number of diagnosis or management options (NxP=R)

	Problems to Exam Physician	Number	Points	Results
MEDICAL	Self-limited or minor (stable, improved or worsening)	Max=2	1	
	Est. problem; stable, improved		1	
	Est. problem; worsening		2	
	New problem; no additional workup planned	Max=1	3	
	New problem; additional workup planned		4	
	Bring total to line A Box D		TOTAL	

	Box B: Amount and/or complexity of data to be reviewed	Points
DECISION	Review and/or order of clinical lab tests/procedures	1
	Review and/or order of tests/procedures in the radiology section of CPT	1
	Review and/or order of tests/procedures in the medicine section of CPT	1
	Discussion of diagnostic test results with performing physician	1
	Decision to obtain old records and/or obtain history from someone other than patient	1
	Review and summarization of old records and/or discussion of case with another health care provider	2
	Independent visualization of image, tracing, or specimen itself (not simply review of report)	2
	Bring total to line B Box D TOTAL	

Box D: Final result for complexity of medical decision making (2 of 3 required)

MAKING	A	Number of diagnosis or management options	≤1 minimal	2 limited	3 multiple	≥4 extensive
	B	Amount and complexity of data to be reviewed	≤1 minimal	2 limited	3 moderate	≥4 extensive
	C	Risk of complications and/or morbidity or mortality	Minimal	Low	Moderate	High
		Type of decision making	Straight-forward	Low Complex	Moderate Complex	High Complex

Lowest of the two chosen determines the medical decision making

Box C: Risk of complication and/or morbidity or mortality

Risk level	Presenting problem(s)	Diagnostic procedure(s) ordered	Management options selected
MINIMAL	• One self-limited or minor problem (ex. cold, insect bite, tinea corporis)	• Lab tests requiring venipuncture • Chest x-ray • EKG/EEG • Urinalysis • Ultrasound/Echo • KOH prep	• Rest • Gargles • Elastic bandages • Superficial dressings
LOW	• Two or more self-limited or minor problems • One stable chronic illness (ex. HTN, DM) • Acute uncomplicated illness or injury (ex. sprain, cystitis, rhinitis)	• Physiological test not under stress (ex. PFT) • Non-cardiovascular imaging studies with contrast (ex. barium enema) • Superficial needle biopsy • Clinical lab tests requiring arterial puncture • Skin biopsy	• Over the counter drugs • Minor surgery w/ no identified risk • PT/OT • IV fluids without additives
MODERATE	• One or more chronic illnesses with mild exacerbation, progression, or side effects of treatment • Two or more stable chronic illnesses • Undiagnosed new problem with uncertain prognosis (ex. lump in breast) • Acute illness with systemic symptoms (ex. pneumonitis, colitis) • Acute complicated injury (ex. head injury with brief LOC)	• Physiologic tests under stress (ex. cardiac stress test, fetal contraction stress test) • Diagnostic endoscopies with no identified risk factors • Deep needle or incisional biopsy • Cardiovascular imaging studies with contrast and no identified risk factors (ex. arteriogram, cardiac catheterization) • Obtain fluid from body cavity (ex. LP, thoracentesis)	• Minor surgery w/ identified risk factors • Elective major surgery (open, percutaneous, or endoscopic) with no identified risk factors • Prescription drug management • Therapeutic nuclear medicine • IV fluids with additives • Closed treatment of fracture or dislocation without manipulation
HIGH	• One or more chronic illnesses with severe exacerbation, progression, or side effects of treatment • Acute or chronic illnesses or injuries that pose a threat to life or bodily function (ex. multiple trauma, acute MI, pulm embolus, severe resp distress, progressive severe rheumatoid arthritis, ARF, psychiatric illness with potential threat to self or others, peritonitis) • An abrupt change in neurological status (ex. seizure, TIA, weakness, or sensory loss)	• Cardiovascular imaging studies with contrast with identified risk factors • Cardiac electrophysiological tests • Diagnostic endoscopies with identified risk factors • Discography	• Elective major surgery (open, percutaneous, or endoscopic) with identified risk factors • Emergency major surgery (open, endoscopic, percutaneous) • Parenteral controlled substances • Drug therapy requiring intensive monitoring for toxicity • Decision not to resuscitate or to de-escalate care because of poor prognosis

Bring results to line C in Box D (use the highest level chosen)

Hx Level:____________________ Exam Level:____________________ MDM Level:____________________

E & M CODE ASSIGNMENT GRID—cont'd

OFFICE/OUTPATIENT VISIT, NEW PATIENT: 3 OF 3 REQUIRED

E and M CODE	HISTORY	EXAM	MEDICAL DEC MAKING	AVERAGE TIME
99201	F	F	S	10
99202	E	E	S	20
99203	D	D	L	30
99204	C	C	M	45
99205	C	C	H	60

OFFICE/OUTPATIENT VISIT, ESTABLISHED PATIENT: 2 OF 3 REQUIRED

E and M CODE	HISTORY	EXAM	MEDICAL DEC MAKING	AVERAGE TIME
99211	N/A	N/A	N/A	5
99212	F	F	S	10
99213	E	E	L	15
99214	D	D	M	25
99215	C	C	H	40

OFFICE CONSULT, NEW OR ESTABLISHED PATIENT: 3 OF 3 REQUIRED

E and M CODE	HISTORY	EXAM	MEDICAL DEC MAKING	AVERAGE TIME
99241	F	F	S	15
99242	E	E	S	30
99243	D	D	L	40
99244	C	C	M	60
99245	C	C	H	80

ED VISIT, NEW OR ESTABLISHED PATIENT: 3 OF 3 REQUIRED

E and M CODE	HISTORY	EXAM	MEDICAL DEC MAKING	AVERAGE TIME
99281	F	F	S	N/A
99282	E	E	L	N/A
99283	E	E	M	N/A
99284	D	D	M	N/A
99285	C	C	H	N/A

INITIAL HOSPITAL CARE: 3 OF 3 REQUIRED

E and M CODE	HISTORY	EXAM	MEDICAL DEC MAKING	AVERAGE TIME
99221	D/C	D/C	S/L	30
99222	C	C	M	50
99223	C	C	H	70

SUBSEQUENT HOSPITAL CARE: 2 OF 3 REQUIRED

E and M CODE	HISTORY	EXAM	MEDICAL DEC MAKING	AVERAGE TIME
99231	F	F	S/L	15
99232	E	E	M	25
99233	D	D	H	35

INITIAL INPATIENT CONSULT: 3 OF 3 REQUIRED

E and M CODE	HISTORY	EXAM	MEDICAL DEC MAKING	AVERAGE TIME
99251	F	F	S	20
99252	E	E	S	40
99253	D	D	L	55
99254	C	C	M	80
99255	C	C	H	110

INITIAL OBSERVATION CARE: 3 OF 3 REQUIRED

E and M CODE	HISTORY	EXAM	MEDICAL DEC MAKING	AVERAGE TIME
99218	D/C	D/C	S/L	
99219	C	C	M	
99220	C	C	H	

INITIAL OBS/INPT SAME DAY IN/OUT CARE: 3 OF 3 REQUIRED

E and M CODE	HISTORY	EXAM	MEDICAL DEC MAKING	AVERAGE TIME
99234	D/C	D/C	S/L	
99235	C	C	M	
99236	C	C	H	

Code assignment:

Additional notes:

F - Prob Focused **D - Detailed** **S - Straightforward**
M - Moderate **E - Exp Prob Focused** **C - Comprehensive**
L - Low **H - High**

INITIAL NURSING FACILITY CARE: 3 OF 3 REQUIRED

E and M CODE	HISTORY	EXAM	MEDICAL DEC MAKING	AVERAGE TIME
99304	D/C	D/C	S/L	25
99305	C	C	M	35
99306	C	C	H	45

SUBSEQUENT NURSING FACILITY CARE: 2 OF 3 REQUIRED

E and M CODE	HISTORY	EXAM	MEDICAL DEC MAKING	AVERAGE TIME
99307	F	F	S	10
99308	E	E	L	15
99309	D	D	M	25
99310	C	C	H	35

DOMICILARY, REST HOME, BOARDING CARE, NEW PT: 3 OF 3 REQUIRED

E and M CODE	HISTORY	EXAM	MEDICAL DEC MAKING	AVERAGE TIME
99324	F	F	S	20
99325	E	E	L	30
99326	D	D	M	45
99327	C	C	M	60
99328	C	C	H	75

DOMICILARY, REST HOME, BOARDING CARE, EST PT: 2 OF 3 REQUIRED

E and M CODE	HISTORY	EXAM	MEDICAL DEC MAKING	AVERAGE TIME
99334	F	F	S	15
99335	E	E	L	25
99336	D	D	M	40
99337	C	C	H	60

HOME VISIT, NEW PATIENT: 3 OF 3 REQUIRED

E and M CODE	HISTORY	EXAM	MEDICAL DEC MAKING	AVERAGE TIME
99341	F	F	S	20
99342	E	E	L	30
99343	D	D	M	45
99344	C	C	M	60
99345	C	C	H	75

HOME VISIT, ESTABLISHED PATIENT: 2 OF 3 REQUIRED

E and M CODE	HISTORY	EXAM	MEDICAL DEC MAKING	AVERAGE TIME
99347	F	F	S	15
99348	E	E	L	25
99349	D/I	D	M	40
99350	C/I	C	H	60

By now it should be apparent why proper physician documentation is so crucial. If these elements of documentation are omitted or are not recorded adequately, the code assigned may reflect a reduced level of service and reimbursement may be adversely affected. Remember that the physician may bill only for what can be substantiated by the medical documentation. Tool 11-3 presents a list of elements that comprise all the history components of medical documentation.

History elements always give additional information regarding the present illness or injury as well as any contributing history factors such as past medical history, social history, and family history. They do NOT give information regarding the actual examination by the physician. These factors are included in the physical examination section.

Chief complaint has been previously defined as the chief reason for the encounter or service. This is usually information provided by the patient. The **history of present illness** gives additional details regarding the current illness or injury. Examples of history of present illness elements include location, quality, severity, associated signs and symptoms, timing, context, duration, and modifying factors. Descriptions of the type of information that would be contained in these elements are listed in Tool 11-2. The coder will find that individuals will identify elements of the record in different ways. For instance, one coder may assign the history of present illness element "location" for abdominal pain that radiates from one area to another, whereas another coder may assign this same information to the history of present illness element "quality," as the pain is described as burning from one area to another. The most important factor to keep in mind is consistency. Third-party carriers want to see the coder assigning the same elements for the same factors in similar instances. It is not the specific element that matters, but the element count that matters. To be consistent, the coder should develop his or her own grid of key words and what element those key words will be assigned. You will see, as you complete exercises for E & M cases in class and discuss them, that many students will use different elements. In the end, the element count usually will remain the same, thus arriving at the same level of service.

Information regarding past medical history, family history, or social history that is relevant to the chief complaint is also used to determine the appropriate level of service. Some providers overdocument, and, if the coder is not careful, he or she will assign a higher level of service as a result of taking all documentation into consideration. Make certain that the past medical history, social history, and family history are pertinent to the chief complaint.

For instance, a patient who is being seen for an ingrown toenail describes a past medical history of a deviated septum. That past medical history is not relevant to the chief complaint of an ingrown toenail. However, if the patient arrived for an ingrown toenail and indicated a past medical history of diabetes mellitus, that past medical history would be pertinent because patients with diabetes typically are susceptible to foot complications as a result of their disease. In some instances this will require some clinical knowledge or research on the coder's part to become more familiar with medical conditions, their signs, symptoms, and complications.

The **review of systems** is an inventory of systems related to the chief complaint. In the earlier example, the patient presented with an ingrown toenail. What related systems might the provider ask about in relation to the ingrown toenail? First decide what system the toenail belongs in (integumentary). If you were unsure, check the systems grid provided in Chapter 9. What other questions might the provider ask of this patient?

Have you had any fever or chills (signs of infection/constitutional)?

Have you had any difficulty bearing weight or walking (musculoskeletal)?

In this example, two additional systems have been identified: constitutional and musculoskeletal. Therefore this visit includes two additional reviews of systems.

STOP AND PRACTICE

Read the following scenarios and identify specific elements to determine whether they are review of systems, history of present illness, or past medical, social, or family history.

	History of Present Illness	Medical, Social, and Family History	Systems
EX: 1. Pain was severe.	Severity		
2. Patient complains of redness, tearing of eyes.	________	________	________
3. Patient complains of urinary frequency.	________	________	________
4. Patient complains of wheezing and coughing.	________	________	________
5. Patient complains of a 4-week history of severe ankle swelling.	________	________	________
6. Patient is a past cigarette smoker.	________	________	________
7. Patient's father is diabetic.	________	________	________
8. Patient denies dysphagia, heartburn, rectal bleeding, or hemorrhoids.	________	________	________
9. Patient reports a 2-week history of severe abdominal pain, mainly epigastric.	________	________	________
10. Patient's tetanus immunization is current.	________	________	________

TOOL 11-3

HISTORY GUIDELINES

History of Present Illness

Location	Where, radiation from-to
Quality	Sharp, burning, dull, productive, color
Severity	Scale 1-10, severe, mild, progressive
Associated signs and symptoms	Swelling, nausea, vomiting
Timing	Start, steady, intermittent, constant
Context	Activity at onset, causation
Duration	Length of time, time of presentation
Modifying factors	What helps, worsens, relieves

Medical History

Adult medical illnesses
Childhood illnesses
Trauma
Surgical history
Date of most recent medical exam and results
Age-appropriate feeding and dietary history

Family History

Marital status
Genetic diseases
Parents, children, siblings
Health status and/or cause of death of parents, siblings, children
Specific diseases related to chief complaint
Family history of chronic diseases such as hypertension, diabetes, cancer, heart disease, cardiovascular disease, psychiatric illness

Social History

Smoking
Alcohol
Caffeine
Drug use
Occupational history
Heterosexual, homosexual, bisexual
Place of birth, residence, education
Marital status, living arrangements
Level of education
Other relevant social factors

Allergies

Medications
Foods
Insects
Animals
Occupation related

Medications

Prescription
Over-the-counter medications
Doses, frequencies
Immunizations

Review of Systems

Constitutional	General appearance, vital signs, current state of health
Integumentary	Rash, color, sores, dryness
Eyes	Vision, cataracts, pain, redness, tearing, double/blurred vision
ENT/mouth	Ears: hearing, vertigo, earaches, infections, discharge Nose: colds, stuffiness, discharge, itching, nosebleeds Mouth and throat: teeth, gums, dentures, dry mouth, sore throat, hoarseness, bleeding
Cardiovascular	Shortness of breath, dizziness, hypertension, heart murmurs, chest pains, palpitations, dyspnea, orthopnea, rheumatic fever
Respiratory	Cough, sputum, wheezing, asthma, bronchitis, tuberculosis, emphysema, pneumonia
Gastrointestinal	Heartburn, appetite, vomiting, indigestion, frequency or change in bowel habits, gas, food intolerance, excessive bleeding, jaundice, hepatitis, gallbladder problems, weight differences
Genitourinary	Frequent urination, nocturia, hematuria, urgency Male specific: hernia, discharge, history of sexually transmitted diseases Female specific: age at menarche, menstrual history, pregnancies, history of sexually transmitted diseases
Musculoskeletal	Muscle or joint pain, arthritis, gout, backache
Neurologic	Fainting, seizures, weakness, paralysis, numbness, loss of sensation, tremors, blackouts
Hematologic and lymphatic	Anemia, bruising, bleeding, transfusion
Endocrine	Thyroid problems, heat or cold intolerance, diabetes
Psychiatric	Nervousness, tension, mood swings, panic, anxiety
Allergic/immunologic	Immunizations, allergies to medications, immune suppression, blood transfusion

STOP AND PRACTICE

Identify the key history elements in the following records.

1. Consultation

CONSULTATION

Indication for consultation:

Dear Dr. Jones:
Thank you for referring Mr. Smith for my evaluation of his low back pain and left sciatica.

History:

This is a 76-year-old man who has a long history of back problems dating back to his 40's. He does not recall a specific incident, however, remembers having to wear a back brace, the back pain continued to bother him. He had fusion of his lower back and then several months later, after slipping on some ice, had to have the procedure repeated. He had a disk that ruptured approximately 10 years ago that had to be removed at the same level as the fusion. Over the past year he has had increasing lower back pain with tendency that his pain had traveled down his left buttock and into his posterior thigh and down to the heel and buttocks on his left foot. His pain seems to mimic the pain he had prior to his fusion. He has not noticed any gross weakness in his leg. He has had no other problems with his bowels or bladder. His past history is otherwise significant for hypercholesterolemia and he apparently takes a cholesterol drug. He does not have any other specific medical problems that he reports to me. He denies problems with his heart or blood pressure.

Exam:

Examination:
He stands erect. He has limitation of motion of his lumbar spine in all directions. He is able to forward flex about 20 degrees and then has some discomfort. He has a well healed low back scar and left iliac crest scar no doubt from bone grafting. Straight leg raising is uncomfortable for him on the left and less so on the right. He has supple rotation of his hips. Muscle strength seems to be symmetrical both with regard to the plantar flexors and dorsal flexors of the ankles. Reflexes show asymmetry with decrease in his left knee jerk and an absent left knee jerk. He has good pedal pulses and adequate circulatory perfusion in his feet.

I reviewed the CT scan of his lumbar spine. He has significant lumbar stenosis at L3-4 and L4-5. The L5-S1 level looks less involved. He has evidence of an old laminectomy on the left at L5.

Diagnosis/assessment:

IMPRESSION:
Lumbar stenosis at L3-4 and L4-5.

PLAN:
My recommendation would be to get a MRI scan of his lumbar spine to further evaluate this. I think perhaps an epidural steroid injection would calm his symptoms.

Stacy Kraatt, MD

Patient name: ______

Date of service: ______

GODFREY MEDICAL ASSOCIATES
1532 Third Avenue, Suite 120 • Aldon, FL 77713 • (407) 555-4000

History Elements

Chief complaint ______

History of present illness ______

Review of systems ______

Past medical, family, social history ______

2. Outpatient office note

OFFICE NOTE

Chief complaint: ______

Date: ______

Vital signs: BP______ P______ R______

History:

The patient is a 74-year-old gentleman with history of NIDDM, HTN, CHF, anemia, atrial fib who was on hemodialysis due to acute or chronic renal insufficiency but regained some of his renal function. He has been off dialysis for the past three years. He presents today with urinary retention.

ALLERGIES: None
MEDICATION: See flow sheet
SOCIAL HISTORY: Currently lives with brother, wife deceased, denies smoking/alcohol
PAST MEDICAL: Diabetes, hypertension, congestive heart failure, chronic renal failure, anemia
PAST SURGERIES: Significant for below the knee amputation on left due to peripheral vascular disease due to diabetes.
FAMILY HISTORY: Diabetes and Hypertension

REVIEW OF SYSTEMS:
Denies any significant nausea, vomiting and his appetite is fine. Denies any chest pain, palpitations, shortness of breath. He does have some problems with urination, especially dysuria and urgency. He denied any black, tarry stools. His bowel movements are pretty much unchanged. The rest of the review of systems is essentially negative.

Exam:

PHYSICAL EXAMINATION:
Alert, oriented and stable and not in any kind of significant distress. BP 129/81, pulse 136. HEENT: Pupils equal and reactive to light. Slight pale conjunctiva. He has dry oral mucosa. Neck supple. Lungs, clear to auscultation. No lymphadenopathy. Chest, good air entry and clear to auscultation. Heart, S1 and S1 audible. Rhythm is regular with no S3 or murmur appreciated. Abdomen, soft, distended, positive bowel sounds, no mass, no organomegaly. Extremities, no edema, no rash, no pigmentation.

LABS:
WBC 8, hemoglobin 9.9, hematocrit 30.3, platelets 334. Urinalysis shows PH-5, 1+ protein, red blood cells 2-4, white blood cells 0-2. Chemistry shows sodium 132, potassium 4.2, chloride 96, CO2 21, BUN 106, creatinine 3.5, calcium 8.5. ECG shows atrial fibrillation.

Diagnosis/assessment:

ASSESSMENT:
History of multiple medical problems including:
1 NIDDM
2 Anemia which seems due to chronic renal failure
3 Chronic renal failure with high BUN/creatinine ratio
4 Atrial fibrillation
5 Hypothyroidism
6 Benign prostatic hypertrophy

I am starting him on Nephron FA 1 po qd and we see him again in 2 days.

Jay Corman MD

Patient name: ______

Date of service: ______

GODFREY MEDICAL ASSOCIATES
1532 Third Avenue, Suite 120 • Aldon, FL 77713 • (407) 555-4000

History Elements

Chief complaint ______

History of present illness ______

Review of systems ______

Past medical, family, social history ______

3. Emergency department record

EMERGENCY ROOM RECORD

Name:	**Age:** / **DOB:**	**ER physician:** Robert Rais, MD
Allergies/type of reaction:	**Usual medications/dosages:**	

Triage/presenting complaint: This is a 60-year-old female who comes to the ER after having a head injury. She stated she heard a "crunch" as she was walking up the stairs when she hit her head on an overhead beam directly above the stairs. This happened earlier today. She said she saw stars at that time and initially her neck and shoulders had some pain as well. She felt like she could feel pressure in her lower back and tailbone. She has not had any headache, nausea or vomiting but states she just does not feel herself. She has taken nothing for the pain.

Initial assessment:

Upon exam, this is a 60-year-old in no acute distress, vital signs are normal. Lungs are clear to auscultation. Heart, regular rate and rhythm. Normal leg raises and standing nor sitting seems to cause pain. We will get x-rays just to make sure, however, doesn't appear as anything significant is going on here.

Time	**T**	**P**	**R**	**BP**	**Other:**				

Medication orders:

Lab work:

X-Ray:

X-Ray, Cervical and Lumbar Spine were negative

Physician's report:

Patient was given Toradol IM with relief of her pain. She was instructed to take Ibuprofen 600 mg as needed up to three times per day for pain relief. If she has any increase in pain, numbness or tingling of the extremities, she should return to the ER or see her primary care physician as soon as possible.

Diagnosis:	**Physician sign/date**
	Robert Rai MD
Discharge **Transfer** **Admit** **Good** **Satisfactory** **Other:**	

GODFREY REGIONAL HOSPITAL
123 Main Street • Aldon, FL 77714 • (407) 555-1234

History Elements

Chief complaint ______________________

History of present illness ______________________

Review of systems ______________________

Past medical, family, social history ______________________

4. Office visit progress note

PROGRESS NOTE

Date/time
XX/XX/XX

S:

Patient is a 33-year-old who complains of pain, swelling and redness of the ear that started today. At the onset, the earlobe was symptomatic of swelling, redness and pain that has now extended to the helix. She has no earache, fevers, chills, nasal congestion, sore throat or cough.

O:

PHYSICAL EXAM:
There is marked erythema, swelling and warmth of the earlobe and this extends to the helix area. She has a small pustule of the earlobe close to two pierced areas. Tympanic membranes and pharynx are normal. Neck, supple without adenopathy. There is no pain of the TMJ areas.

A:

ASSESSMENT: Infected ear

P:

PLAN: Cephalexin 500 mg tid times five days. Apply warm packs and follow-up if symptoms do not resolve In five days.

Felix Washington MD

Patient ID

Patient name
Admit: XX/XX/XX
MR# XXXXXXX

PROGRESS NOTES

GODFREY REGIONAL HOSPITAL
123 Main Street • Aldon, FL 77714 • (407) 555-1234

History Elements

Chief complaint ______________________________

History of present illness ________________________

Review of systems ______________________________

Past medical, family, social history _________________

5. Emergency department record

EMERGENCY ROOM RECORD

Name:	Age: / DOB:	ER physician: Nancy Connelly, MD
Allergies/type of reaction:	**Usual medications/dosages:**	

Triage/presenting complaint: Patient comes to the ER with a laceration of her right lower leg. She was seen earlier today and had sutures removed from this area. She was doing fine yntil she was getting ready for bed and the wound came open. It has not bled significantly and she requests that the wound be closed again.

Initial assessment:

Laceration right left, upper calf

Time	T	P	R	BP	Other:

Medication orders:

Lab work:

X-Ray:

Physician's report:

Vitals signs normal.
Right lower extremity, there is an elliptical laceration over the right calf.

Plan:
Patient was advised that because sutures have already been placed to this area there is an increased risk of infection. Steri-strips were placed.

Diagnosis:

Physician sign/date

Nancy Connelly MD

Discharge **Transfer** **Admit** **Good** **Satisfactory** **Other:**

GODFREY REGIONAL HOSPITAL
123 Main Street • Aldon, FL 77714 • (407) 555-1234

History Elements

Chief complaint ______________________

History of present illness ______________________

Review of systems ______________________

Past medical, family, social history ______________________

Levels of History

Once the documentation has been reviewed and key components identified, that information will be used for determining the level of history provided during the encounter.

The levels of history are labeled problem focused, expanded problem focused, detailed, and comprehensive.

Problem-Focused History

- Chief complaint
- Brief history of present illness or problem

A problem-focused history focuses only on the chief complaint and the system that relates to that chief complaint. Because the problem-focused history typically does not involve an in-depth medical problem, a review of systems as well as past medical, family, and social history are not required for this level of history documentation.

An example would be a patient who presents for an earache. The problem-focused history might involve questions and information regarding the duration of the chief complaint and the severity of the earache only. This would be sufficient for the physician to complete the evaluation and management of the earache.

Expanded Problem-Focused History

- Chief complaint
- Brief history of present illness or problem(s)
- Problem-pertinent systems review

An expanded problem-focused history includes all the components of the problem-focused history with the addition of a relevant review of systems. Past medical, family, and social history is not required for this level.

The visit typically would involve the history of the present illness and "expand" into information regarding other systems that relate to the chief complaint.

An example would be a patient who presents with an earache and requires evaluation of the present illness as well as a review of relevant or related systems, such as the respiratory system.

Detailed History

- Chief complaint
- Extended history of present illness
- Problem-pertinent system review extended to include review of a limited number of additional systems
- Pertinent medical, family, and social history directly related to patient problem(s)

A detailed history would include an extended history of the present illness and a review of several systems. This level of history typically would be gathered when a patient's chief complaint requires evaluation of multiple systems. Medical, family, and social history would also be necessary if they relate or are pertinent to the patient's presenting problem or chief complaint.

An example would be a patient who presents for abdominal pain. The history of present illness might include information such as how severe the pain is, how long the pain has been present, whether it is associated with any particular incident or accident, and any additional signs and symptoms that may or may not be present. In addition, the patient and physician would provide information on additional systems, such as nausea or vomiting (gastrointestinal), dizziness (neurologic), weakness or fatigue (constitutional), urinary symptoms (urinary), shortness of breath (cardiovascular), and cough (respiratory).

Comprehensive History

- Chief complaint
- Extended history of present illness
- Review of systems directly related to problem(s) identified in history of present illness
- Review of all additional body systems
- Complete medical, family, and social history

A comprehensive history typically involves a complete history of present illness; review of systems; and a review of past medical, family, and social history. This level of service would usually be performed on a patient with multiple complaints that encompass multiple anatomic systems as well as a pertinent history that contributes to the nature of the chief complaint.

An example would be a patient who presents with a serious or life-threatening chief complaint, such as syncope. Although some patients presenting with syncope may be evaluated only on a more superficial level, such as expanded problem focused, the patient with multiple other medical problems and other contributing complaints may require a comprehensive history.

The comprehensive history would entail multiple elements of the history of present illness, such as that entered in the detailed history of patient illness; a complete review of systems, which involves the majority of systems; and a past medical, family, and social history. Again, the patient with syncope who simply "passed out" from lack of food or giving blood at the blood bank would probably not require an in-depth evaluation of his or her problem and therefore would not qualify for this level of history.

As you can see by many of the definitions given in CPT, there are a number of areas with vague guidelines. For instance, what is an "extended" history of present illness? How many elements does that involve?

Although CPT gives only the previously mentioned criteria for the level of history provided, third-party carriers typically use additional guidelines for determining the level of service. Use the history portion of Tool 11-2 to determine the appropriate level of service when assigning E & M codes to medical records.

INSTRUCTIONS ON USING AN E & M TOOL

Although many tools or processes are available for tracking or counting the elements of the E & M visit, this chapter will use the process shown in Tool 11-2. This tool is intended for use with any E & M service type that entails levels, such as office visits, consultation, hospital visits, and so forth. E & M services NOT based on levels are not included in the tool.

First, take the elements identified in question 1 in the Stop and Practice exercise on page 343 and "plot" them on the history portion of the grid.

History Elements

Chief complaint:	Lower back pain
History of present illness:	Duration (over the past year) Location (lower back pain) Quality (radiating) Signs or symptoms (not noticed any gross weakness)
Review of systems:	No problem with bowels (gastrointestinal system) No problem with bladder (genitourinary system)
Past medical, family, social history:	Past medical (history of back problems, other medical problems)

Discussion

Chief complaint:	Chief complaint as stated by the patient was "increasing lower back pain."
History of present illness:	Four elements were identified.
Level:	Detailed
Review of systems:	Two elements were identified.
Level:	Detailed
Past medical, family, and social history:	Past medical history was identified.
Level:	Detailed

Although a number of past medical history elements were identified, the past medical history requires only one element be identified and is only counted as "one" without regard for the number of elements identified.

When using the E & M tool, all elements must be met for the history portion. Therefore if one of the three components of history—history of present illness, review of systems, and past medical, family, and social history—is not met or meets a lower level, the level assigned will be lowered to the lowest element.

Note that "no history" or "no problem," known as *pertinent negatives,* counts as an element in this process. Despite the fact that information led to negative findings, the physician still reviewed the information; therefore the information is still given credit in this "counting" process.

In the selected example, all three history components qualify for a "detailed history." Because the patient was not documented as new versus established, the least significant visit type, established, would be assumed. Based on this information, it should be easy to fill out the relevant area of Tool 11-2, as shown below.

HISTORY	Final results for history (3 of 3 required)	Problem focused	Exp. problem focused	Detailed	Comprehensive
	HPI: ☒ Location ☐ Timing ☒ Quality ☒ Associated signs and symptoms ☐ Severity ☐ Modifying factors ☒ Duration ☐ Context	Brief (1-3) ☐	Brief (1-3) ☐	Extended (4 or more) ☐	Extended (4 or more) ☒
	ROS: ☐ Constitutional (wt. loss, etc.) ☐ Integumentary (skin, breast) ☐ Endocrine ☐ All/Immunology ☐ ENM and T ☐ Eyes ☐ Cardio/Vasc ☐ Respiratory ☒ GI ☒ GU ☐ Musculoskeletal ☐ Psychiatric ☐ Hem/Lymph ☐ Neurological ☐ "All others negative"	None ☐	Pertinent to problem (1 system) ☐	Extended (2-9 systems including pertinent system) ☒	Complete (10 or more systems or pertinent systems with the statement "all others negative") ☐
	PFSH (past medical, family, social history): ☒ Past Hx. (the pts. past experience with illness, operations, and treatments) ☐ Family Hx. (a review of medical events in the pts. family) ☐ Social Hx. (an age appropriate review of past and current activities)	None ☐	None ☐	Pertinent *(1 or 2 history area) ☒	Complete *(2 or 3 history areas) ☐

*Complete PFSH - 2 Hx areas a) Estab pts Office (Output) care; domiciliary care; home care; b) Emergency Dept. c) Subsequent nursing facility care
3 Hx areas a) New pt. Office (Outpt) care; domiciliary care; home care; b) Consultations c) Initial hospital care d) hospital observation e) Comprehensive nursing facility assessments

As you can see, the history level for this encounter is the same whether the CPT technique of determining history level is used or the 1995 guidelines are used. Each student will develop his or her own technique for identifying the correct information. As long as the answers are the same and the technique works for the individual coder, that technique is appropriate. Consistency is extremely important in coding. Therefore any tool that the coder can use to arrive at consistent answers is extremely helpful.

Considering that all three of the history elements must be met, what will be the history level for this chart?

STOP AND PRACTICE

Using exercises 2 through 5 from the previous Stop and Practice exercise beinning on p. 343, for which you identified the history components, complete the history portion of the E & M grid appropriately. Determine the history level for each exercise.

2. Outpatient office note

History Elements

Chief complaint ______________________________

History of present illness ______________________________

Review of systems ______________________________

Past medical, family, social history ______________________________

History level ______________________________

HISTORY	Final results for history (3 of 3 required)	Problem focused	Exp. problem focused	Detailed	Comprehensive
	HPI: ☐ Location ☐ Timing ☐ Quality ☐ Associated signs and symptoms ☐ Severity ☐ Modifying factors ☐ Duration ☐ Context	Brief (1-3) ☐	Brief (1-3) ☐	Extended (4 or more) ☐	Extended (4 or more) ☐
	ROS: ☐ Constitutional (wt. loss, etc.) ☐ Integumentary (skin, breast) ☐ Endocrine ☐ All/Immunology ☐ ENM and T ☐ Eyes ☐ Cardio/Vasc ☐ Respiratory ☐ GI ☐ GU ☐ Musculoskeletal ☐ Psychiatric ☐ Hem/Lymph ☐ Neurological ☐ "All others negative"	None ☐	Pertinent to problem (1 system) ☐	Extended (2-9 systems including pertinent system) ☐	Complete (10 or more systems or pertinent systems with the statement "all others negative") ☐
	PFSH (past medical, family, social history): Past Hx. (the pts. past experience with illness, operations, and treatments) Family Hx. (a review of medical events in the pts. family) Social Hx. (an age appropriate review of past and current activities)	None ☐	None ☐	Pertinent *(1 or 2 history area) ☐	Complete *(2 or 3 history areas) ☐

*Complete PFSH - 2 Hx areas a) Estab pts Office (Output) care; domiciliary care; home care; b) Emergency Dept. c) Subsequent nursing facility care
3 Hx areas a) New pt. Office (Outpt) care; domiciliary care; home care; b) Consultations c) Initial hospital care d) hospital observation e) Comprehensive nursing facility assessments

3. Emergency department record

History Elements

Chief complaint ______________________________

History of present illness ______________________________

Review of systems ______________________________

Past medical, family, social history ______________________________

History level ______________________________

HISTORY	Final results for history (3 of 3 required)	Problem focused	Exp. problem focused	Detailed	Comprehensive
	HPI: ☐ Location ☐ Timing ☐ Quality ☐ Associated signs and symptoms ☐ Severity ☐ Modifying factors ☐ Duration ☐ Context	Brief (1-3) ☐	Brief (1-3) ☐	Extended (4 or more) ☐	Extended (4 or more) ☐
	ROS: ☐ Constitutional (wt. loss, etc.) ☐ Integumentary (skin, breast) ☐ Endocrine ☐ All/Immunology ☐ ENM and T ☐ Eyes ☐ Cardio/Vasc ☐ Respiratory ☐ GI ☐ GU ☐ Musculoskeletal ☐ Psychiatric ☐ Hem/Lymph ☐ Neurological ☐ "All others negative"	None ☐	Pertinent to problem (1 system) ☐	Extended (2-9 systems including pertinent system) ☐	Complete (10 or more systems or pertinent systems with the statement "all others negative") ☐
	PFSH (past medical, family, social history): Past Hx. (the pts. past experience with illness, operations, and treatments) Family Hx. (a review of medical events in the pts. family) Social Hx. (an age appropriate review of past and current activities)	None ☐	None ☐	Pertinent *(1 or 2 history area) ☐	Complete *(2 or 3 history areas) ☐

*Complete PFSH - 2 Hx areas a) Estab pts Office (Output) care; domiciliary care; home care; b) Emergency Dept. c) Subsequent nursing facility care
3 Hx areas a) New pt. Office (Outpt) care; domiciliary care; home care; b) Consultations c) Initial hospital care d) hospital observation e) Comprehensive nursing facility assessments

STOP AND PRACTICE—cont'd

4. Office visit progress note

History Elements

Chief complaint ______________________________
History of present illness ______________________________
Review of systems ______________________________
Past medical, family, social history ______________________________
History level ______________________________

	Final results for history (3 of 3 required)	Problem focused	Exp. problem focused	Detailed	Comprehensive
HISTORY	HPI: ☐ Location ☐ Timing ☐ Quality ☐ Associated signs and symptoms ☐ Severity ☐ Modifying factors ☐ Duration ☐ Context	Brief (1-3) ☐	Brief (1-3) ☐	Extended (4 or more) ☐	Extended (4 or more) ☐
	ROS: ☐ Constitutional (wt. loss, etc.) ☐ Integumentary (skin, breast) ☐ Endocrine ☐ All/Immunology ☐ ENM and T ☐ Eyes ☐ Cardio/Vasc ☐ Respiratory ☐ GI ☐ GU ☐ Musculoskeletal ☐ Psychiatric ☐ Hem/Lymph ☐ Neurological ☐ "All others negative"	None ☐	Pertinent to problem (1 system) ☐	Extended (2-9 systems including pertinent system) ☐	Complete (10 or more systems or pertinent systems with the statement "all others negative") ☐
	PFSH (past medical, family, social history): Past Hx. (the pts. past experience with illness, operations, and treatments) Family Hx. (a review of medical events in the pts. family) Social Hx. (an age appropriate review of past and current activities)	None ☐	None ☐	Pertinent *(1 or 2 history area) ☐	Complete *(2 or 3 history areas) ☐

*Complete PFSH - 2 Hx areas a) Estab pts Office (Output) care; domiciliary care; home care; b) Emergency Dept. c) Subsequent nursing facility care
3 Hx areas a) New pt. Office (Outpt) care; domiciliary care; home care; b) Consultations c) Initial hospital care d) hospital observation e) Comprehensive nursing facility assessments

5. Emergency department record

History Elements

Chief complaint ______________________________
History of present illness ______________________________
Review of systems ______________________________
Past medical, family, social history ______________________________
History level ______________________________

	Final results for history (3 of 3 required)	Problem focused	Exp. problem focused	Detailed	Comprehensive
HISTORY	HPI: ☐ Location ☐ Timing ☐ Quality ☐ Associated signs and symptoms ☐ Severity ☐ Modifying factors ☐ Duration ☐ Context	Brief (1-3) ☐	Brief (1-3) ☐	Extended (4 or more) ☐	Extended (4 or more) ☐
	ROS: ☐ Constitutional (wt. loss, etc.) ☐ Integumentary (skin, breast) ☐ Endocrine ☐ All/Immunology ☐ ENM and T ☐ Eyes ☐ Cardio/Vasc ☐ Respiratory ☐ GI ☐ GU ☐ Musculoskeletal ☐ Psychiatric ☐ Hem/Lymph ☐ Neurological ☐ "All others negative"	None ☐	Pertinent to problem (1 system) ☐	Extended (2-9 systems including pertinent system) ☐	Complete (10 or more systems or pertinent systems with the statement "all others negative") ☐
	PFSH (past medical, family, social history): Past Hx. (the pts. past experience with illness, operations, and treatments) Family Hx. (a review of medical events in the pts. family) Social Hx. (an age appropriate review of past and current activities)	None ☐	None ☐	Pertinent *(1 or 2 history area) ☐	Complete *(2 or 3 history areas) ☐

*Complete PFSH - 2 Hx areas a) Estab pts Office (Output) care; domiciliary care; home care; b) Emergency Dept. c) Subsequent nursing facility care
3 Hx areas a) New pt. Office (Outpt) care; domiciliary care; home care; b) Consultations c) Initial hospital care d) hospital observation e) Comprehensive nursing facility assessments

PHYSICAL EXAMINATION

The physical examination, which reflects both the clinical judgment of the physician and the nature of the patient's complaints at the time of the examination, is based on a number of elements that are reviewed and documented during the course of the examination. These elements are defined by the number of organ systems or body areas that are examined on the basis of the complaint(s) and medical history.

Tool 11-4 demonstrates the elements included in the examination components.

The following *body areas* are recognized by CPT:

- Head
- Neck
- Chest (body area includes breasts, axillae)
- Abdomen
- Genitalia, groin, buttocks
- Back
- *Each* extremity

The following *organ systems* are recognized as physical examination elements:

- Eyes
- Ears, nose, mouth, throat
- Cardiovascular
- Respiratory
- Gastrointestinal
- Genitourinary
- Musculoskeletal
- Skin
- Neurologic
- Psychiatric
- Hematologic/lymphatic/immunologic

Keep in mind that the components for the examination portion of the E & M service are gathered as the result of the hands-on examination by the provider. The review of systems portion of the history consists of facts gathered from the patient. Care should be taken not to confuse these two E & M components.

The physical examination section is limited to the hands-on or visual examination of the patient. Questions asked of, and answers given by, the patient are included in the history elements. Also keep in mind that the body systems are those identified in Chapter 9 and that body areas are used when information may be vague and indeterminate regarding the specific system. For example, if the provider indicates "neck was normal," was the provider referring to the cervical lymph nodes in the neck, the musculoskeletal nature of the neck, or the thyroid? All three of these are different systems. Because determining which system is appropriate is not possible, one body area would be counted—the neck—for this exam. Keep in mind, however, that when completing a comprehensive physical examination, eight or more body systems are required, and therefore the coder should count body areas only when he or she is unable to identify specific organ systems.

Coders may use body areas or organ systems for each physical exam area but may not count both body area and organ system for one physical finding. In the previous example, coders could count body area/neck or body system/musculoskeletal, but not both.

STOP AND PRACTICE

For the following scenarios, identify whether they are history elements or physical examination elements and further define which of these elements they identify.

Scenario	History or Exam	Specific Element
1. Chest was unremarkable.	________	________
2. Auscultation of the chest was clear.	________	________
3. Patient denies difficulty swallowing.	________	________
4. Patient denies history of injury.	________	________
5. Patient dislocated left proximal phalange.	________	________
6. Patient takes Dilantin daily.	________	________
7. Patient appears in no acute distress.	________	________
8. Patient denies any acute distress.	________	________
9. Tympanic membranes are dull and inflamed.	________	________
10. Abdomen is unremarkable and reveals no tenderness, no guarding, and no organomegaly.	________	________

TOOL 11-4

EXAMINATION GUIDELINES

Constitutional	Measurement of certain number of vital signs with notation of abnormal findings General appearance of patient at time of exam
Eyes	Conjunctivae, lids, extraocular movement Reaction to light and accommodation Ophthalmic examination of retinal discs
ENT/teeth	External inspection of ears and nose Otoscopic exam of external auditory canals and tymphatic membranes Assessment of hearing Inspection of nasal mucosa, septum, turbinates Inspection of lips, teeth, gums Examination of oropharynx (salivary glands, palates, tongue, tonsils post-pharynx)
Neck	General exam of neck (masses, overall appearance) Exam of thyroid (enlargement, tenderness, mass)
Respiratory	Assessment of respiratory effort Percussion of chest (dullness, flatness) Palpation of chest Auscultation of lungs (breath sounds, rubs, clicks)
Cardiovascular	Palpation of heart Auscultation of heart Carotid arteries (pulse, amplitude, bruits) Abdominal arota (size, bruits) Femoral arteries (pulse, amplitude, bruits) Pedal pulses (pulse, amplitude) Exam of extremities for edema and varicosities
Chest	Inspection of breasts Palpatation of breasts and axillae (lumps, masses, tenderness)
Gastrointestinal*	Examination of abdomen (masses, tenderness) Examination of liver and spleen Examination for presence or absence of hernia
Genitourinary	Male: Examination of scrotal contents, examination of penis, digital rectal exam of prostate Female: Pelvic examination, exam of external genitalia, exam of urethra (masses, tenderness), exam of bladder (fullness, masses, tenderness), cervical exam (general appearance, discharge), exam of uterus (contour, mobility, tenderness), adnexa and parametria (masses, tenderness, nodularity)
Lymphatic	Palpation of lymph nodes of two or more areas: neck, axillae, groin, other
Musculoskeletal	Examination of gait/station Inspection of nails and digits (ischemia, infections, cyanosis) Assessment of stability of any dislocation Assessment of muscle strength and tone
Integumentary	Inspection of skin and subcutaneous tissue Palpation of skin and subcutaneous tissue
Neurologic	Test cranial nerves (note deficits) Examination of deep tendon reflexes Examination of sensation Examination of motor strength
Psychiatric	Evaluation of patient's judgment and insight Brief assessment of mental status to include (1) orientation to time, place, and person; (2) recent and remote memory; and (3) mood and affect. Review of former mental status

*Bowel sounds are not a physical examination element.

STOP AND PRACTICE

Take the Stop and Practice exercises you have already completed in your evaluation of the history component (see p. 343) and identify their physical examination elements.

1. Consultation
   Body areas ______
   Organ systems ______
2. Outpatient office note
   Body areas ______
   Organ systems ______
3. Emergency department record
   Body areas ______
   Organ systems ______
4. Office visit progress note
   Body areas ______
   Organ systems ______
5. Emergency department record
   Body areas ______
   Organ systems ______

Levels of Physical Examination

Now that the elements have been identified, let's discuss the different levels of physical examination as defined by CPT.

PROBLEM-FOCUSED EXAM Limited to part of body area or organ system affected; usually one area is identified.
EXPANDED PROBLEM-FOCUSED EXAM Limited examination of affected body area or organ systems and of other body area or organ systems that may contribute to the presenting complaint(s); two to four elements are required.
DETAILED EXAM Extensive examination of affected body areas and organ systems and of other body areas and organ systems that may contribute to the presenting complaint(s); five to seven elements are required.
COMPREHENSIVE EXAM Either a multisystem physical examination or complete examination of a single organ or body system; eight or more elements are required.

The counting process of the physical examination elements simply involves counting the number of body areas and organ systems that were identified. The following additional guidelines apply:

- Detailed examinations must include a detailed description of the affected system. Again, there is no definition provided for "detailed"; however, adjectives typically describe the examination of the affected body area or organ system as well as other systems. Only the affected system must be described in detail.
- A comprehensive examination must include a detailed examination as well.

For example, take the physical examination elements identified in question 1 of the previous Stop and Practice exercise (p. 350) and "plot" them on the examination portion of Tool 11-2.

EXAMINATION ELEMENTS
Body areas:
Organ systems: musculoskeletal, circulatory

		Problem focused	Exp. problem focused	Detailed	Comprehensive
E X A M	Body areas: ☐ Head, incl. face ☐ Chest, incl. breast and axillae ☐ Abdomen ☐ Neck ☐ Back, incl. spine ☐ Each extremity ☐ Genitalia, groin, buttocks Organ systems: ☐ Constitutional ☐ ENMT ☐ Respiratory ☐ Musculoskeletal ☐ Psych ☐ Eyes ☐ CV ☐ GI ☐ GU ☐ Skin ☐ Neurological ☐ Hem/lymph/imm	1 area or system ☐	2 to 4 areas or systems ☒	2 to 7 areas or systems MUST BE DETAILED ☐	8 or more systems or a complete exam of a single system ☐

Discussion

Although the musculoskeletal organ system is covered in depth, it counts as only one body system. The circulatory system is covered with the comments of "pedal pulses" and "adequate circulatory perfusion." Therefore, only two body areas or organ systems were identified in the physical examination component of this visit, qualifying for an expanded problem-focused examination.

You may count the examination of the spine under body area "spine" or as body system "musculoskeletal," but it may not be counted in both.

		Problem focused	Exp. problem focused	Detailed	Comprehensive
E X A M	Body areas: ☐ Head, incl. face ☐ Chest, incl. breast and axillae ☐ Abdomen ☐ Neck ☐ Back, incl. spine ☐ Each extremity ☐ Genitalia, groin, buttocks Organ systems: ☐ Constitutional ☐ ENMT ☐ Respiratory ☐ Musculoskeletal ☐ Psych ☐ Eyes ☐ CV ☐ GI ☐ GU ☐ Skin ☐ Neurological ☐ Hem/lymph/imm	1 area or system ☐	2 to 4 areas or systems ☐	2 to 7 areas or systems MUST BE DETAILED ☐	8 or more systems or a complete exam of a single system ☐

What will be the examination level for this sample exercise?

As you can see, the examination portion of Tool 11-2 is much simpler than the history component. Also, once an organ or body part that represents one system is identified, that system is already counted; therefore it is not necessary to count multiple organs or body areas in the same system. This will save time once you master this process.

STOP AND PRACTICE

Once again, take the exercises from the Stop and Practice on page 343 for which you identified the history elements and complete the examination portion of the E & M grid appropriately.

2. Outpatient office note

Examination Elements

Body areas ______________________________

Organ systems ______________________________

Exam level ______________________________

		Problem focused	Exp. problem focused	Detailed	Comprehensive
E X A M	Body areas: ☐ Head, incl. face ☐ Chest, incl. breast and axillae ☐ Abdomen ☐ Neck ☐ Back, incl. spine ☐ Each extremity ☐ Genitalia, groin, buttocks Organ systems: ☐ Constitutional ☐ ENMT ☐ Respiratory ☐ Musculoskeletal ☐ Psych ☐ Eyes ☐ CV ☐ GI ☐ GU ☐ Skin ☐ Neurological ☐ Hem/lymph/imm	1 area or system ☐	2 to 4 areas or systems ☐	2 to 7 areas or systems MUST BE DETAILED ☐	8 or more systems or a complete exam of a single system ☐

3. Emergency department record

Examination Elements

Body areas ______________________________

Organ systems ______________________________

Exam level ______________________________

		Problem focused	Exp. problem focused	Detailed	Comprehensive
E X A M	Body areas: ☐ Head, incl. face ☐ Chest, incl. breast and axillae ☐ Abdomen ☐ Neck ☐ Back, incl. spine ☐ Each extremity ☐ Genitalia, groin, buttocks Organ systems: ☐ Constitutional ☐ ENMT ☐ Respiratory ☐ Musculoskeletal ☐ Psych ☐ Eyes ☐ CV ☐ GI ☐ GU ☐ Skin ☐ Neurological ☐ Hem/lymph/imm	1 area or system ☐	2 to 4 areas or systems ☐	2 to 7 areas or systems MUST BE DETAILED ☐	8 or more systems or a complete exam of a single system ☐

STOP AND PRACTICE—cont'd

4. Office visit progress note

Examination Elements

Body areas ______________________

Organ systems ______________________

Exam level ______________________

EXAM		Problem focused	Exp. problem focused	Detailed	Comprehensive
E X A M	Body areas: ☐ Head, incl. face ☐ Chest, incl. breast and axillae ☐ Abdomen ☐ Neck ☐ Back, incl. spine ☐ Each extremity ☐ Genitalia, groin, buttocks Organ systems: ☐ Constitutional ☐ ENMT ☐ Respiratory ☐ Musculoskeletal ☐ Psych ☐ Eyes ☐ CV ☐ GI ☐ GU ☐ Skin ☐ Neurological ☐ Hem/lymph/imm	1 area or system ☐	2 to 4 areas or systems ☐	2 to 7 areas or systems MUST BE DETAILED ☐	8 or more systems or a complete exam of a single system ☐

5. Emergency department record

Examination Elements

Body areas ______________________

Organ systems ______________________

Exam level ______________________

EXAM		Problem focused	Exp. problem focused	Detailed	Comprehensive
E X A M	Body areas: ☐ Head, incl. face ☐ Chest, incl. breast and axillae ☐ Abdomen ☐ Neck ☐ Back, incl. spine ☐ Each extremity ☐ Genitalia, groin, buttocks Organ systems: ☐ Constitutional ☐ ENMT ☐ Respiratory ☐ Musculoskeletal ☐ Psych ☐ Eyes ☐ CV ☐ GI ☐ GU ☐ Skin ☐ Neurological ☐ Hem/lymph/imm	1 area or system ☐	2 to 4 areas or systems ☐	2 to 7 areas or systems MUST BE DETAILED ☐	8 or more systems or a complete exam of a single system ☐

MEDICAL DECISION MAKING

The third and final key component of levels of service determination is medical decision making. Within the medical decision-making component are three subcomponents, two of which must be met at the level assigned for medical decision making. These three subcomponents are (1) the number of diagnoses or management options, (2) the quantity and complexity of data, and (3) the risks of morbidity and mortality. Note that only two of these subcomponents must be met to assign the level for medical decision making.

Number of Diagnoses or Management Options

The number of diagnoses or presenting problems treated is considered in the overall evaluation of medical decision making. Documented differential diagnoses are essential in achieving the highest level of diagnosis or management options possible. These elements are defined as follows:

- Established problem, stable
- Established problem, worsening
- New problem, no additional workup planned
- New problem, additional workup planned

Quantity and Complexity of Data

The quantity and complexity of data attained are based on the tests ordered and interpreted as well as on medical records from, or discussion of results with, other health professionals.

Categories for data include:

- Laboratory
- Radiology
- Medicine
- Discussion of results with other medical professional
- Decision to request records
- Individual interpretation of data results
- Review of outside records

Risks of Morbidity and Mortality

The **risks of morbidity and mortality** are determined by the complexity of the presenting problems, treatments, and plan for additional treatment. For instance, treatment with over-the-counter medications would be considered low complexity, whereas the infusion of medications would increase patient risk.

Many elements help determine the level of risk of morbidity or mortality associated with the medical decision-making component. Tool 11-5 illustrates these key components. As opposed to the other components in the history, examination, and medical decision-making process, only one component of risk must be met (choose the highest level of risk associated with the visit).

STOP AND PRACTICE

For the following items, determine which medical decision-making element(s) have been identified.

	Number of Diagnoses or Management Options	Data	Risk
1. Review of lab data	________	________	________
2. Stable diabetes mellitus	________	________	________
3. Uncomplicated illness	________	________	________
4. Discussion of case with medical professional	________	________	________
5. Review of outside records	________	________	________
6. Review of radiologic studies	________	________	________
7. Rest, gargle	________	________	________
8. New patient, no additional workup	________	________	________
9. Individual interpretation of data results	________	________	________
10. Prescription drug management	________	________	________

STOP AND PRACTICE

Take the five records for which you have already assigned a level for history and examination and determine the medical decision-making elements. Identify the medical decision-making elements only in this exercise. We will plot them on the form shortly.

1. Consultation
   Diagnosis/management options ________________
   Quantity/complexity of data ________________
   Risk of morbidity/mortality ________________
2. Outpatient office visit
   Diagnosis/management options ________________
   Quantity/complexity of data ________________
   Risk of morbidity/mortality ________________
3. Emergency department record
   Diagnosis/management options ________________
   Quantity/complexity of data ________________
   Risk of morbidity/mortality ________________
4. Outpatient office progress note
   Diagnosis/management options ________________
   Quantity/complexity of data ________________
   Risk of morbidity/mortality ________________
5. Emergency department record
   Diagnosis/management options ________________
   Quantity/complexity of data ________________
   Risk of morbidity/mortality ________________

Levels of Medical Decision Making

Once the documentation has been reviewed and completed and the elements identified, it will be used to determine the level of medical decision making performed for the encounter. The levels of medical decision making are as follows:

Straightforward

- A minimum number of diagnosis or management options for the problem
- Minimal medical data to be reviewed and considered
- Minimal or no risk of morbidity or mortality

TOOL 11-5

RISK GRID (MEDICAL DECISION MAKING)

Level of Risk	Presenting Problem	Diagnostic Data	Management and Diagnostic Options
Minimal	One self-limited or minor problem	Lab test Chest x-rays ECG/EEG Ultrasound	Rest/gargle Elastic bandages Superficial dressings
Low	Two or more self-limited to minor problems One stable chronic illness Acute, uncomplicated illness/injury Physiologic tests not under stress	Noncardiovascular imaging study with contrast Superficial needle biopsies Lab tests requiring arterial puncture Skin biopsies	Over-the-counter drugs Physical therapy Occupational therapy IV fluids w/o additives Minor surgery with no risk
Moderate	One or more chronic illnesses with mild exacerbation Two or more stable chronic illnesses Undiagnosed new problem with uncertain prognosis Acute illness with systemic symptoms Acute complicated injury	Physiologic tests under stress Diagnostic endoscopies with no risk Deep needle or incisional biopsy Cardiovascular imaging with contrast, no identified risk Obtain fluid from body cavity	Minor surgery Elective major surgery Prescription drug management Therapeutic nuclear medicine Closed treatment of fracture or dislocation without manipulation
High	One or more chronic illnesses with severe exacerbation Acute or chronic illness or injury posing threat to life or bodily function Abrupt change in neurologic status	Cardiovascular imaging studies with contrast with identified risk Cardiac electrophysiologic test Diagnostic endoscopies with identified risk Discography	Elective major surgery Emergency major surgery Parenteral controlled substances Drug therapy requiring: Intensive monitoring Decision not to resuscitate *or* De-escalated care because of poor prognosis

ECG, Electrocardiogram; *EEG*, electroencephalogram; *w/o*, without.

DEFINE: Presenting problem typically does not need diagnostic workup or treatment that requires a physician to resolve symptoms.

EXAMPLE: Insect bite, abrasion

Low

- Limited diagnosis and options for management of the medical problem
- Limited data to be reviewed
- Low risk of morbidity or mortality

DEFINE: A minimal number of tests, minimal treatment, or both are necessary to resolve the symptoms or presenting complaint.

EXAMPLE: Ankle sprain with x-ray

Moderate

- Multiple diagnosis and medical management options
- Moderate complexity and volume of data to be reviewed
- Moderate risk of morbidity or mortality

DEFINE: Diagnostic workup is necessary, as is treatment by the provider, to resolve the symptoms or presenting complaint. Multiple medical problems are evaluated and treated, necessary to medically treat the condition, sign, or symptom by the physician.

EXAMPLE: Bronchitis with chest x-ray and prescription medication prescribed or given

High

- Extensive medical decision-making options for management of the medical problem
- Extensive review of data in terms of volume and complexity
- High risk of morbidity or mortality

DEFINE: Significant medical treatment and diagnostics are necessary. Typically the patient has significant risk for loss of life or limb.

EXAMPLE: Patient with severe exacerbation of a chronic, life-threatening disease

Once the elements have been identified, the elements should be plotted on the grid to determine the level of medical decision making for the encounter. Remember that only two of the three elements must be met for this element.

Take the elements identified in question 1 of the earlier Stop and Practice exercise (p. 343) and "plot" them on the medical decision-making portion of the grid tool.

Elements of Medical Decision Making

Diagnosis/management options:	New problem, additional workup planned
Quantity/complexity of data:	Radiology, CT (computed tomography) of the spine
Risk of morbidity/mortality:	Low; acute uncomplicated problem

Discussion

Diagnosis and management options would be considered a new problem. Although the problem was treated in the remote past, it would be considered a new problem if the treating physician feels the need to reevaluate the problem and obtain examination and data to determine whether the problem is the same or is another problem in addition to the previous problem.

Quantity and Complexity of Data

Magnetic resonance imaging (MRI) is planned but not performed; therefore it cannot be used.

Risk of Morbidity or Mortality

No prescription medications are prescribed, and the problem is not described as chronic.

Use the medical decision-making portion of Tool 11-2 to determine the appropriate level of service when assigning E & M codes to medical records.

Considering all this information, what would be the medical decision-making level for the sample exercise?

Box A: Number of diagnosis or management options (NxP=R)

MEDICAL	Problems to Exam Physician	Number	Points	Results
	Self-limited or minor (stable, improved or worsening)	Max=2	1	
	Est. problem; stable, improved		1	
	Est. problem; worsening		2	
	New problem; no additional workup planned	Max=1	3	
	New problem; additional workup planned		4	
	Bring total to line A Box D		TOTAL	3

Box B: Amount and/or complexity of data to be reviewed

DECISION		Points
	Review and/or order of clinical lab tests/procedures	1
	Review and/or order of tests/procedures in the radiology section of CPT	1
	Review and/or order of tests/procedures in the medicine section of CPT	1
	Discussion of diagnostic test results with performing physician	1
	Decision to obtain old records and/or obtain history from someone other than patient	1
	Review and summarization of old records and/or discussion of case with another health care provider	2
	Independent visualization of image, tracing, or specimen itself (not simply review of report)	2
	Bring total to line B Box D TOTAL	2

Box D: Final result for complexity of medical decision making (2 of 3 required)

MAKING						
	A	Number of diagnosis or management options	≤1 minimal	2 limited	3 multiple	≥4 extensive
	B	Amount and complexity of data to be reviewed	≤1 minimal	2 limited	3 moderate	≥4 extensive
	C	Risk of complications and/or morbidity or mortality	Minimal	Low	Moderate	High
		Type of decision making	Straight-forward	Low Complex	Moderate Complex	High Complex

Lowest of the two chosen determines the medical decision making

Box C: Risk of complication and/or morbidity or mortality

Risk level	Presenting problem(s)	Diagnostic procedure(s) ordered	Management options selected
MINIMAL	• One self-limited or minor problem (ex. cold, insect bite, tinea corporis)	• Lab tests requiring venipuncture • Chest x-ray • ECG/EEG • Urinalysis • Ultrasound/Echo • KOH prep	• Rest • Gargles • Elastic bandages • Superficial dressings
LOW	• Two or more self-limited or minor problems • One stable chronic illness (ex. HTN, DM) • Acute uncomplicated illness or injury (ex. sprain, cystitis, rhinitis)	• Physiological test not under stress (ex. PFT) • Non-cardiovascular imaging studies with contrast (ex. barium enema) • Superficial needle biopsy • Clinical lab tests requiring arterial puncture • Skin biopsy	• Over the counter drugs • Minor surgery w/ no identified risk • PT/OT • IV fluids without additives
MODERATE	• One or more chronic illnesses with mild exacerbation, progression, or side effects of treatment • Two or more stable chronic illnesses • Undiagnosed new problem with uncertain prognosis (ex. lump in breast) • Acute illness with systemic symptoms (ex. pneumonitis, colitis) • Acute complicated injury (ex. head injury with brief LOC)	• Physiologic tests under stress (ex. cardiac stress test, fetal contraction stress test) • Diagnostic endoscopies with no identified risk factors • Deep needle or incisional biopsy • Cardiovascular imaging studies with contrast and no identified risk factors (ex. arteriogram, cardiac catheterization) • Obtain fluid from body cavity (ex. LP, thoracentesis)	• Minor surgery w/ identified risk factors • Elective major surgery (open, percutaneous, or endoscopic) with no identified risk factors • Prescription drug management • Therapeutic nuclear medicine • IV fluids with additives • Closed treatment of fracture or dislocation without manipulation
HIGH	• One or more chronic illnesses with severe exacerbation, progression, or side effects of treatment • Acute or chronic illnesses or injuries that pose a threat to life or bodily function (ex. multiple trauma, acute MI, pulm embolus, severe resp distress, progressive severe rheumatoid arthritis, ARF, psychiatric illness with potential threat to self or others, peritonitis) • An abrupt change in neurological status (ex. seizure, TIA, weakness, or sensory loss)	• Cardiovascular imaging studies with contrast with identified risk factors • Cardiac electrophysiological tests • Diagnostic endoscopies with identified risk factors • Discography	• Elective major surgery (open, percutaneous, or endoscopic) with identified risk factors • Emergency major surgery (open, endoscopic, percutaneous) • Parenteral controlled substances • Drug therapy requiring intensive monitoring for toxicity • Decision not to resuscitate or to de-escalate care because of poor prognosis

Bring results to line C in Box D (use the highest level chosen)

There are a number of interpretations of some of the medical decision-making elements. Because CMS and many of the other insurance carriers interpret several of these elements differently (and, unfortunately, do not always provide a definitive interpretation), consistency is the most important factor in assigning the medical decision-making element. Many practices make decisions on how their practice will interpret these elements based on the best information available, and they commit those interpretations to their policy and procedure manuals. In addition, they often incorporate the input of the clinical staff to support their interpretations.

STOP AND PRACTICE

Take the four records previously used in the Stop and Practice exercise on page 343 for the history and exam components and identify the medical decision-making elements.

2. Outpatient office note

Medical Decision-Making Elements

Diagnosis/management options ______________________________

Quantity/complexity of data ______________________________

Risk of morbidity/mortality ______________________________

Medical decision-making level ______________________________

Box A: Number of diagnosis or management options (NxP=R)

MEDICAL	Problems to Exam Physician	Number	Points	Results
	Self-limited or minor (stable, improved or worsening)	Max=2	1	
	Est. problem; stable, improved		1	
	Est. problem; worsening		2	
	New problem; no additional workup planned	Max=1	3	
	New problem; additional workup planned		4	
	Bring total to line A Box D		TOTAL	

Box B: Amount and/or complexity of data to be reviewed

DECISION		Points
	Review and/or order of clinical lab tests/procedures	1
	Review and/or order of tests/procedures in the radiology section of CPT	1
	Review and/or order of tests/procedures in the medicine section of CPT	1
	Discussion of diagnostic test results with performing physician	1
	Decision to obtain old records and/or obtain history from someone other than patient	1
	Review and summarization of old records and/or discussion of case with another health care provider	2
	Independent visualization of image, tracing, or specimen itself (not simply review of report)	2
	Bring total to line B Box D	TOTAL

Box D: Final result for complexity of medical decision making (2 of 3 required)

MAKING						
	A	Number of diagnosis or management options	≤1 minimal	2 limited	3 multiple	≥4 extensive
	B	Amount and complexity of data to be reviewed	≤1 minimal	2 limited	3 moderate	≥4 extensive
	C	Risk of complications and/or morbidity or mortality	Minimal	Low	Moderate	High
		Type of decision making	Straight-forward	Low Complex	Moderate Complex	High Complex

Lowest of the two chosen determines the medical decision making

Box C: Risk of complication and/or morbidity or mortality

Risk level	Presenting problem(s)	Diagnostic procedure(s) ordered	Management options selected
MINIMAL	• One self-limited or minor problem (ex. cold, insect bite, tinea corporis)	• Lab tests requiring venipuncture • Chest x-ray • ECG/EEG • Urinalysis • Ultrasound/Echo • KOH prep	• Rest • Gargles • Elastic bandages • Superficial dressings
LOW	• Two or more self-limited or minor problems • One stable chronic illness (ex. HTN, DM) • Acute uncomplicated illness or injury (ex. sprain, cystitis, rhinitis)	• Physiological test not under stress (ex. PFT) • Non-cardiovascular imaging studies with contrast (ex. barium enema) • Superficial needle biopsy • Clinical lab tests requiring arterial puncture • Skin biopsy	• Over the counter drugs • Minor surgery w/ no identified risk • PT/OT • IV fluids without additives
MODERATE	• One or more chronic illnesses with mild exacerbation, progression, or side effects of treatment • Two or more stable chronic illnesses • Undiagnosed new problem with uncertain prognosis (ex. lump in breast) • Acute illness with systemic symptoms (ex. pneumonitis, colitis) • Acute complicated injury (ex. head injury with brief LOC)	• Physiologic tests under stress (ex. cardiac stress test, fetal contraction stress test) • Diagnostic endoscopies with no identified risk factors • Deep needle or incisional biopsy • Cardiovascular imaging studies with contrast and no identified risk factors (ex. arteriogram, cardiac catheterization) • Obtain fluid from body cavity (ex. LP, thoracentesis)	• Minor surgery w/ identified risk factors • Elective major surgery (open, percutaneous, or endoscopic) with no identified risk factors • Prescription drug management • Therapeutic nuclear medicine • IV fluids with additives • Closed treatment of fracture or dislocation without manipulation
HIGH	• One or more chronic illnesses with severe exacerbation, progression, or side effects of treatment • Acute or chronic illnesses or injuries that pose a threat to life or bodily function (ex. multiple trauma, acute MI, pulm embolus, severe resp distress, progressive severe rheumatoid arthritis, ARF, psychiatric illness with potential threat to self or others, peritonitis) • An abrupt change in neurological status (ex. seizure, TIA, weakness, or sensory loss)	• Cardiovascular imaging studies with contrast with identified risk factors • Cardiac electrophysiological tests • Diagnostic endoscopies with identified risk factors • Discography	• Elective major surgery (open, percutaneous, or endoscopic) with identified risk factors • Emergency major surgery (open, endoscopic, percutaneous) • Parenteral controlled substances • Drug therapy requiring intensive monitoring for toxicity • Decision not to resuscitate or to de-escalate care because of poor prognosis

Bring results to line C in Box D (use the highest level chosen)

STOP AND PRACTICE—cont'd

3. Emergency department record

Medical Decision-Making Elements

Diagnosis/management options ______________________

Quantity/complexity of data ______________________

Risk of morbidity/mortality ______________________

Medical decision-making level ______________________

Box A: Number of diagnosis or management options (NxP=R)

MEDICAL	Problems to Exam Physician	Number	Points	Results
	Self-limited or minor (stable, improved or worsening)	Max=2	1	
	Est. problem; stable, improved		1	
	Est. problem; worsening		2	
	New problem; no additional workup planned	Max=1	3	
	New problem; additional workup planned		4	
	Bring total to line A Box D		TOTAL	

Box B: Amount and/or complexity of data to be reviewed

DECISION		Points
	Review and/or order of clinical lab tests/procedures	1
	Review and/or order of tests/procedures in the radiology section of CPT	1
	Review and/or order of tests/procedures in the medicine section of CPT	1
	Discussion of diagnostic test results with performing physician	1
	Decision to obtain old records and/or obtain history from someone other than patient	1
	Review and summarization of old records and/or discussion of case with another health care provider	2
	Independent visualization of image, tracing, or specimen itself (not simply review of report)	2
	Bring total to line B Box D TOTAL	

Box D: Final result for complexity of medical decision making (2 of 3 required)

MAKING						
	A	Number of diagnosis or management options	≤1 minimal	2 limited	3 multiple	≥4 extensive
	B	Amount and complexity of data to be reviewed	≤1 minimal	2 limited	3 moderate	≥4 extensive
	C	Risk of complications and/or morbidity or mortality	Minimal	Low	Moderate	High
		Type of decision making	Straight-forward	Low Complex	Moderate Complex	High Complex

Lowest of the two chosen determines the medical decision making

Box C: Risk of complication and/or morbidity or mortality

Risk level	Presenting problem(s)	Diagnostic procedure(s) ordered	Management options selected
MINIMAL	• One self-limited or minor problem (ex. cold, insect bite, tinea corporis)	• Lab tests requiring venipuncture • Chest x-ray • ECG/EEG • Urinalysis • Ultrasound/Echo • KOH prep	• Rest • Gargles • Elastic bandages • Superficial dressings
LOW	• Two or more self-limited or minor problems • One stable chronic illness (ex. HTN, DM) • Acute uncomplicated illness or injury (ex. sprain, cystitis, rhinitis)	• Physiological test not under stress (ex. PFT) • Non-cardiovascular imaging studies with contrast (ex. barium enema) • Superficial needle biopsy • Clinical lab tests requiring arterial puncture • Skin biopsy	• Over the counter drugs • Minor surgery w/ no identified risk • PT/OT • IV fluids without additives
MODERATE	• One or more chronic illnesses with mild exacerbation, progression, or side effects of treatment • Two or more stable chronic illnesses • Undiagnosed new problem with uncertain prognosis (ex. lump in breast) • Acute illness with systemic symptoms (ex. pneumonitis, colitis) • Acute complicated injury (ex. head injury with brief LOC)	• Physiologic tests under stress (ex. cardiac stress test, fetal contraction stress test) • Diagnostic endoscopies with no identified risk factors • Deep needle or incisional biopsy • Cardiovascular imaging studies with contrast and no identified risk factors (ex. arteriogram, cardiac catheterization) • Obtain fluid from body cavity (ex. LP, thoracentesis)	• Minor surgery w/ identified risk factors • Elective major surgery (open, percutaneous, or endoscopic) with no identified risk factors • Prescription drug management • Therapeutic nuclear medicine • IV fluids with additives • Closed treatment of fracture or dislocation without manipulation
HIGH	• One or more chronic illnesses with severe exacerbation, progression, or side effects of treatment • Acute or chronic illnesses or injuries that pose a threat to life or bodily function (ex. multiple trauma, acute MI, pulm embolus, severe resp distress, progressive severe rheumatoid arthritis, ARF, psychiatric illness with potential threat to self or others, peritonitis) • An abrupt change in neurological status (ex. seizure, TIA, weakness, or sensory loss)	• Cardiovascular imaging studies with contrast with identified risk factors • Cardiac electrophysiological tests • Diagnostic endoscopies with identified risk factors • Discography	• Elective major surgery (open, percutaneous, or endoscopic) with identified risk factors • Emergency major surgery (open, endoscopic, percutaneous) • Parenteral controlled substances • Drug therapy requiring intensive monitoring for toxicity • Decision not to resuscitate or to de-escalate care because of poor prognosis

Bring results to line C in Box D (use the highest level chosen)

STOP AND PRACTICE—cont'd

4. Office visit progress note

Medical Decision-Making Elements

Diagnosis/management options ______________________________

Quantity/complexity of data ______________________________

Risk of morbidity/mortality ______________________________

Medical decision-making level ______________________________

Box A: Number of diagnosis or management options (NxP=R)

	Problems to Exam Physician	Number	Points	Results
MEDICAL	Self-limited or minor (stable, improved or worsening)	Max=2	1	
	Est. problem; stable, improved		1	
	Est. problem; worsening		2	
	New problem; no additional workup planned	Max=1	3	
	New problem; additional workup planned		4	
	Bring total to line A Box D		TOTAL	

	Box B: Amount and/or complexity of data to be reviewed	Points
DECISION	Review and/or order of clinical lab tests/procedures	1
	Review and/or order of tests/procedures in the radiology section of CPT	1
	Review and/or order of tests/procedures in the medicine section of CPT	1
	Discussion of diagnostic test results with performing physician	1
	Decision to obtain old records and/or obtain history from someone other than patient	1
	Review and summarization of old records and/or discussion of case with another health care provider	2
	Independent visualization of image, tracing, or specimen itself (not simply review of report)	2
	Bring total to line B Box D TOTAL	

Box D: Final result for complexity of medical decision making (2 of 3 required)

MAKING	A	Number of diagnosis or management options	≤1 minimal	2 limited	3 multiple	≥4 extensive
	B	Amount and complexity of data to be reviewed	≤1 minimal	2 limited	3 moderate	≥4 extensive
	C	Risk of complications and/or morbidity or mortality	Minimal	Low	Moderate	High
		Type of decision making	Straight-forward	Low Complex	Moderate Complex	High Complex

Lowest of the two chosen determines the medical decision making

Box C: Risk of complication and/or morbidity or mortality

Risk level	Presenting problem(s)	Diagnostic procedure(s) ordered	Management options selected
MINIMAL	• One self-limited or minor problem (ex. cold, insect bite, tinea corporis)	• Lab tests requiring venipuncture • Chest x-ray • ECG/EEG • Urinalysis • Ultrasound/Echo • KOH prep	• Rest • Gargles • Elastic bandages • Superficial dressings
LOW	• Two or more self-limited or minor problems • One stable chronic illness (ex. HTN, DM) • Acute uncomplicated illness or injury (ex. sprain, cystitis, rhinitis)	• Physiological test not under stress (ex. PFT) • Non-cardiovascular imaging studies with contrast (ex. barium enema) • Superficial needle biopsy • Clinical lab tests requiring arterial puncture • Skin biopsy	• Over the counter drugs • Minor surgery w/ no identified risk • PT/OT • IV fluids without additives
MODERATE	• One or more chronic illnesses with mild exacerbation, progression, or side effects of treatment • Two or more stable chronic illnesses • Undiagnosed new problem with uncertain prognosis (ex. lump in breast) • Acute illness with systemic symptoms (ex. pneumonitis, colitis) • Acute complicated injury (ex. head injury with brief LOC)	• Physiologic tests under stress (ex. cardiac stress test, fetal contraction stress test) • Diagnostic endoscopies with no identified risk factors • Deep needle or incisional biopsy • Cardiovascular imaging studies with contrast and no identified risk factors (ex. arteriogram, cardiac catheterization) • Obtain fluid from body cavity (ex. LP, thoracentesis)	• Minor surgery w/ identified risk factors • Elective major surgery (open, percutaneous, or endoscopic) with no identified risk factors • Prescription drug management • Therapeutic nuclear medicine • IV fluids with additives • Closed treatment of fracture or dislocation without manipulation
HIGH	• One or more chronic illnesses with severe exacerbation, progression, or side effects of treatment • Acute or chronic illnesses or injuries that pose a threat to life or bodily function (ex. multiple trauma, acute MI, pulm embolus, severe resp distress, progressive severe rheumatoid arthritis, ARF, psychiatric illness with potential threat to self or others, peritonitis) • An abrupt change in neurological status (ex. seizure, TIA, weakness, or sensory loss)	• Cardiovascular imaging studies with contrast with identified risk factors • Cardiac electrophysiological tests • Diagnostic endoscopies with identified risk factors • Discography	• Elective major surgery (open, percutaneous, or endoscopic) with identified risk factors • Emergency major surgery (open, endoscopic, percutaneous) • Parenteral controlled substances • Drug therapy requiring intensive monitoring for toxicity • Decision not to resuscitate or to de-escalate care because of poor prognosis

Bring results to line C in Box D (use the highest level chosen)

STOP AND PRACTICE—cont'd

5. Emergency department record

Medical Decision-Making Elements

Diagnosis/management options ____________________

Quantity/complexity of data ____________________

Risk of morbidity/mortality ____________________

Medical decision-making level ____________________

Box A: Number of diagnosis or management options (NxP=R)

	Problems to Exam Physician	Number	Points	Results
MEDICAL	Self-limited or minor (stable, improved or worsening)	Max=2	1	
	Est. problem; stable, improved		1	
	Est. problem; worsening		2	
	New problem; no additional workup planned	Max=1	3	
	New problem; additional workup planned		4	
	Bring total to line A Box D		TOTAL	

Box B: Amount and/or complexity of data to be reviewed

		Points
DECISION	Review and/or order of clinical lab tests/procedures	1
	Review and/or order of tests/procedures in the radiology section of CPT	1
	Review and/or order of tests/procedures in the medicine section of CPT	1
	Discussion of diagnostic test results with performing physician	1
	Decision to obtain old records and/or obtain history from someone other than patient	1
	Review and summarization of old records and/or discussion of case with another health care provider	2
	Independent visualization of image, tracing, or specimen itself (not simply review of report)	2
	Bring total to line B Box D TOTAL	

Box D: Final result for complexity of medical decision making (2 of 3 required)

MAKING	A	Number of diagnosis or management options	≤1 minimal	2 limited	3 multiple	≥4 extensive
	B	Amount and complexity of data to be reviewed	≤1 minimal	2 limited	3 moderate	≥4 extensive
	C	Risk of complications and/or morbidity or mortality	Minimal	Low	Moderate	High
		Type of decision making	Straight-forward	Low Complex	Moderate Complex	High Complex

Lowest of the two chosen determines the medical decision making

Box C: Risk of complication and/or morbidity or mortality

Risk level	Presenting problem(s)	Diagnostic procedure(s) ordered	Management options selected
MINIMAL	• One self-limited or minor problem (ex. cold, insect bite, tinea corporis)	• Lab tests requiring venipuncture • Chest x-ray • ECG/EEG • Urinalysis • Ultrasound/Echo • KOH prep	• Rest • Gargles • Elastic bandages • Superficial dressings
LOW	• Two or more self-limited or minor problems • One stable chronic illness (ex. HTN, DM) • Acute uncomplicated illness or injury (ex. sprain, cystitis, rhinitis)	• Physiological test not under stress (ex. PFT) • Non-cardiovascular imaging studies with contrast (ex. barium enema) • Superficial needle biopsy • Clinical lab tests requiring arterial puncture • Skin biopsy	• Over the counter drugs • Minor surgery w/ no identified risk • PT/OT • IV fluids without additives
MODERATE	• One or more chronic illnesses with mild exacerbation, progression, or side effects of treatment • Two or more stable chronic illnesses • Undiagnosed new problem with uncertain prognosis (ex. lump in breast) • Acute illness with systemic symptoms (ex. pneumonitis, colitis) • Acute complicated injury (ex. head injury with brief LOC)	• Physiologic tests under stress (ex. cardiac stress test, fetal contraction stress test) • Diagnostic endoscopies with no identified risk factors • Deep needle or incisional biopsy • Cardiovascular imaging studies with contrast and no identified risk factors (ex. arteriogram, cardiac catheterization) • Obtain fluid from body cavity (ex. LP, thoracentesis)	• Minor surgery w/ identified risk factors • Elective major surgery (open, percutaneous, or endoscopic) with no identified risk factors • Prescription drug management • Therapeutic nuclear medicine • IV fluids with additives • Closed treatment of fracture or dislocation without manipulation
HIGH	• One or more chronic illnesses with severe exacerbation, progression, or side effects of treatment • Acute or chronic illnesses or injuries that pose a threat to life or bodily function (ex. multiple trauma, acute MI, pulm embolus, severe resp distress, progressive severe rheumatoid arthritis, ARF, psychiatric illness with potential threat to self or others, peritonitis) • An abrupt change in neurological status (ex. seizure, TIA, weakness, or sensory loss)	• Cardiovascular imaging studies with contrast with identified risk factors • Cardiac electrophysiological tests • Diagnostic endoscopies with identified risk factors • Discography	• Elective major surgery (open, percutaneous, or endoscopic) with identified risk factors • Emergency major surgery (open, endoscopic, percutaneous) • Parenteral controlled substances • Drug therapy requiring intensive monitoring for toxicity • Decision not to resuscitate or to de-escalate care because of poor prognosis

Bring results to line C in Box D (use the highest level chosen)

OTHER ELEMENTS INFLUENCING THE ASSIGNMENT OF E & M LEVELS

Other elements that can be used to determine level of service in special circumstances include the following:

- Counseling
- Coordination of care
- Nature of presenting problem
- Time
- CMS "overarching" criteria

In instances in which counseling or coordination of care represents 50% or more of the time spent in completion of the visit or encounter, the provider may use the time element toward determining level of service. Again, the correct code will vary by location of service and new or established patient status. *Only in these instances does time become the controlling factor in determining level of service.*

As with all elements discussed so far, documentation is crucial to authenticating that the time element is the key factor in determining level of service. At a minimum, the amount of time spent in counseling or coordination of care must be documented, along with an explanation of the extent of that part of the service. **Counseling** may include such services as educating, instructing, or advising about care of the patient's condition or resolution of problem(s) presented. **Coordination of care** may include services such as setting up and monitoring home health care or making arrangements for other care to be provided outside the realm of the physician office visit.

After considering counseling and coordination of care, the level of service is ready to be assigned. If counseling, coordination of care, or both are determined to be the controlling factor, the level of service will be based solely on the time documented.

In addition to the additional factors contained in the CPT manual, CMS and other carriers who follow the CMS guidelines also consider Medicare Change Request 2321, which states:

> "Medical necessity of a service is the overarching criterion for payment in addition to the individual requirements of a CPT code. It would not be medically necessary or appropriate to bill a higher level of evaluation and management service when a lower level of service is warranted."

In other words, Medicare is stating that without regard to what level of service is attained based on identifying the history, physical examination, and medical decision-making components, the overriding component is whether the level of service assigned is medically necessary. For instance, if a patient presents for a dressing change and, based on the history, physical examination, and medical decision-making components the visit would be assigned a level 4 service, CMS states that this visit level should be downcoded to a level more in line with services that would be appropriate for a dressing change. As a result, the visit level would probably be reassigned as a level 1 or 2 service unless complications were involved that were evaluated at the time of the service.

Figure 11-3 is a complete grid from Tool 11-2 of elements of the case we have broken down thus far in this chapter in individual Stop and Practice exercises.

After determining the appropriate level of service (problem focused, expanded problem focused, detailed, or comprehensive) for each E & M visit, the type of service must be identified. These levels are based on the location of service and the status of the patient (i.e., new vs. established, initial vs. subsequent) discussed earlier.

In addition, there are a number of additional considerations for each type of service categories that need to be discussed before making a final E & M code selection.

Specific Types of E & M Service Categories

The following discussion details information regarding the types of E & M services listed in CPT. The second page of the E & M grid contains the information necessary to determine the actual CPT E & M code for the service provided.

OUTPATIENT OR OFFICE VISITS (99201-99215)

Outpatient or office visits should take place in the physician's office or outpatient setting. Remember that in the hospital setting the patient is still considered an outpatient until he or she is officially admitted. If the patient is admitted to the facility or hospital by the same physician during that day's encounter in the office or outpatient setting, hospital inpatient care codes or comprehensive nursing facility assessments should be used because these represent the more significant service performed by the physician.

New patient	99201-99205
Established patient	99211-99215

In the event both the office or outpatient visit and the initial hospital care visit are significant, the provider may incorporate the documentation from both visits to determine the level of service. Make certain, however, that the provider is aware of the necessity of documenting this information.

Completing the E & M Grid

After selecting the appropriate type of service, such as outpatient, inpatient, nursing facility, emergency room, and the patient's status, select the correct grid for assigning the actual E & M CPT code.

There are two grids for outpatient or office visit: one for new patients and one for established patients (Fig. 11-4). When there is no documentation to support a new patient visit, the least significant service is assumed. Therefore an established office or outpatient visit would be assigned in the

Evaluation and Management Leveling Sheet: 1995 Guidelines **GODFREY MEDICAL GROUP**

Patient Name/ID:__________ DOS:__________ Chief Complaint: lower back pain

	Final results for history (3 of 3 required)	Problem focused	Exp. problem focused	Detailed	Comprehensive
HISTORY	HPI: ☒ Location ☐ Timing ☒ Quality ☒ Associated signs and symptoms ☐ Severity ☐ Modifying factors ☒ Duration ☐ Context	Brief (1-3) ☐	Brief (1-3) ☐	Extended (4 or more) ☐	Extended (4 or more) ☒
	ROS: ☐ Constitutional (wt. loss, etc.) ☐ Integumentary (skin, breast) ☐ Endocrine ☐ All/Immunology ☐ ENM and T ☐ Eyes ☐ Cardio/Vasc ☐ Respiratory ☒ GI ☒ GU ☐ Musculoskeletal ☐ Psychiatric ☐ Hem/Lymph ☐ Neurological ☐ "All others negative"	None ☐	Pertinent to problem (1 system) ☐	Extended (2-9 systems including pertinent system) ☒	Complete (10 or more systems or pertinent systems with the statement "all others negative") ☐
	PFSH (past medical, family, social history): ☒ Past Hx. (the pts. past experience with illness, operations, and treatments) ☐ Family Hx. (a review of medical events in the pts. family) ☐ Social Hx. (an age appropriate review of past and current activities)	None ☐	None ☐	Pertinent *(1 or 2 history area) ☒	Complete *(2 or 3 history areas) ☐
EXAM	Body areas: ☒ Head, incl. face ☐ Chest, incl. breast and axillae ☐ Abdomen ☒ Neck ☐ Back, incl. spine ☒ Each extremity ☐ Genitalia, groin, buttocks Organ systems: ☒ Constitutional ☐ ENMT ☒ Respiratory ☐ Musculoskeletal ☐ Psych ☐ Eyes ☒ CV ☒ GI ☐ GU ☐ Skin ☒ Neurological ☐ Hem/lymph/imm	1 area or system ☐	2 to 4 areas or systems ☐	2 to 7 areas or systems MUST BE DETAILED ☐	8 or more systems or a complete exam of a single system ☒

*Complete PFSH - 2 Hx areas a) Estab pts Office (Output) care; domiciliary care; home care; b) Emergency Dept. c) Subsequent nursing facility care
3 Hx areas a) New pt. Office (Outpt) care; domiciliary care; home care; b) Consultations c) Initial hospital care d) hospital observation e) Comprehensive nursing facility assessments

Box A: Number of diagnosis or management options (NxP=R)

	Problems to Exam Physician	Number	Points	Results
MEDICAL	Self-limited or minor (stable, improved or worsening)	Max=2	1	
	Est. problem; stable, improved		1	
	Est. problem; worsening		2	
	New problem; no additional workup planned	Max=1	(3)	3
	New problem; additional workup planned		4	
	Bring total to line A Box D		TOTAL	3

Box B: Amount and/or complexity of data to be reviewed

		Points
DECISION	Review and/or order of clinical lab tests/procedures	(1)
	Review and/or order of tests/procedures in the radiology section of CPT	1
	Review and/or order of tests/procedures in the medicine section of CPT	(1)
	Discussion of diagnostic test results with performing physician	1
	Decision to obtain old records and/or obtain history from someone other than patient	1
	Review and summarization of old records and/or discussion of case with another health care provider	2
	Independent visualization of image, tracing, or specimen itself (not simply review of report)	2
	Bring total to line B Box D TOTAL	

Box C: Risk of complication and/or morbidity or mortality

Risk level	Presenting problem(s)	Diagnostic procedure(s) ordered	Management options selected
MINIMAL	• One self-limited or minor problem (ex. cold, insect bite, tinea corporis)	• Lab tests requiring venipuncture • Chest x-ray • EKG/EEG • Urinalysis • Ultrasound/Echo • KOH prep	• Rest • Gargles • Elastic bandages • Superficial dressings
LOW	• Two or more self-limited or minor problems • One stable chronic illness (ex. HTN, DM) • (Acute uncomplicated illness or injury) (ex. sprain, cystitis, rhinitis)	• Physiological test not under stress (ex. PFT) • Non-cardiovascular imaging studies with contrast (ex. barium enema) • Superficial needle biopsy • Clinical lab tests requiring arterial puncture • Skin biopsy	• Over the counter drugs • Minor surgery w/ no identified risk • PT/OT • IV fluids without additives
MODERATE	• One or more chronic illnesses with mild exacerbation, progression, or side effects of treatment • Two or more stable chronic illnesses • Undiagnosed new problem with uncertain prognosis (ex. lump in breast) • Acute illness with systemic symptoms (ex. pneumonitis, colitis) • Acute complicated injury (ex. head injury with brief LOC)	• Physiologic tests under stress (ex. cardiac stress test, fetal contraction stress test) • Diagnostic endoscopies with no identified risk factors • Deep needle or incisional biopsy • Cardiovascular imaging studies with contrast and no identified risk factors (ex. arteriogram, cardiac catheterization) • Obtain fluid from body cavity (ex. LP, thoracentesis)	• Minor surgery w/ identified risk factors • Elective major surgery (open, percutaneous, or endoscopic) with no identified risk factors • Prescription drug management • Therapeutic nuclear medicine • IV fluids with additives • Closed treatment of fracture or dislocation without manipulation
HIGH	• One or more chronic illnesses with severe exacerbation, progression, or side effects of treatment • Acute or chronic illnesses or injuries that pose a threat to life or bodily function (ex. multiple trauma, acute MI, pulm embolus, severe resp distress, progressive severe rheumatoid arthritis, ARF, psychiatric illness with potential threat to self or others, peritonitis) • An abrupt change in neurological status (ex. seizure, TIA, weakness,or sensory loss)	• Cardiovascular imaging studies with contrast with identified risk factors • Cardiac electrophysiological tests • Diagnostic endoscopies with identified risk factors • Discography	• Elective major surgery (open, percutaneous, or endoscopic) with identified risk factors • Emergency major surgery (open, endoscopic, percutaneous) • Parenteral controlled substances • Drug therapy requiring intensive monitoring for toxicity • Decision not to resuscitate or to de-escalate care because of poor prognosis

Bring results to line C in Box D (use the highest level chosen)

Box D: Final result for complexity of medical decision making (2 of 3 required)

MAKING	A	Number of diagnosis or management options	≤1 minimal	2 limited	(3 multiple)	≥4 extensive
	B	Amount and complexity of data to be reviewed	≤1 minimal	(2 limited)	3 moderate	≥4 extensive
	C	Risk of complications and/or morbidity or mortality	Minimal	(Low)	Moderate	High
		Type of decision making	Straight-forward	(Low Complex)	Moderate Complex	High Complex

Lowest of the two chosen determines the medical decision making

Hx Level: Detailed Exam Level: Expanded MDM Level: Low

FIGURE 11-3. Completed E & M grid for sample case.

OFFICE/OUTPATIENT VISIT, NEW PATIENT: 3 OF 3 REQUIRED

E and M CODE	HISTORY	EXAM	MEDICAL DEC MAKING	AVERAGE TIME
99201	F	F	S	10
99202	E	E	S	20
99203	D	D	L	30
99204	C	C	M	45
99205	C	C	H	60

OFFICE/OUTPATIENT VISIT, ESTABLISHED PATIENT: 2 OF 3 REQUIRED

E and M CODE	HISTORY	EXAM	MEDICAL DEC MAKING	AVERAGE TIME
99211	N/A	N/A	N/A	5
99212	F	F	S	10
99213	E	E	L	15
99214	D	D	M	25
99215	C	C	H	40

OFFICE CONSULT, NEW OR ESTABLISHED PATIENT: 3 OF 3 REQUIRED

E and M CODE	HISTORY	EXAM	MEDICAL DEC MAKING	AVERAGE TIME
99241	F	F	S	15
99242	E	E	S	30
99243	D	D	L	40
99244	C	C	M	60
99245	C	C	H	80

ED VISIT, NEW OR ESTABLISHED PATIENT: 3 OF 3 REQUIRED

E and M CODE	HISTORY	EXAM	MEDICAL DEC MAKING	AVERAGE TIME
99281	F	F	S	N/A
99282	E	E	L	N/A
99283	E	E	M	N/A
99284	D	D	M	N/A
99285	C	C	H	N/A

INITIAL HOSPITAL CARE: 3 OF 3 REQUIRED

E and M CODE	HISTORY	EXAM	MEDICAL DEC MAKING	AVERAGE TIME
99221	D/C	D/C	S/L	30
99222	C	C	M	50
99223	C	C	H	70

SUBSEQUENT HOSPITAL CARE: 2 OF 3 REQUIRED

E and M CODE	HISTORY	EXAM	MEDICAL DEC MAKING	AVERAGE TIME
99231	F	F	S/L	15
99232	E	E	M	25
99233	D	D	H	35

INITIAL INPATIENT CONSULT: 3 OF 3 REQUIRED

E and M CODE	HISTORY	EXAM	MEDICAL DEC MAKING	AVERAGE TIME
99251	F	F	S	20
99252	E	E	S	40
99253	D	D	L	55
99254	C	C	M	80
99255	C	C	H	110

INITIAL OBSERVATION CARE: 3 OF 3 REQUIRED

E and M CODE	HISTORY	EXAM	MEDICAL DEC MAKING	AVERAGE TIME
99218	D/C	D/C	S/L	
99219	C	C	M	
99220	C	C	H	

INITIAL OBS/INPT SAME DAY IN/OUT CARE: 3 OF 3 REQUIRED

E and M CODE	HISTORY	EXAM	MEDICAL DEC MAKING	AVERAGE TIME
99234	D/C	D/C	S/L	
99235	C	C	M	
99236	C	C	H	

Code assignment:

99241

Additional notes:

Hx = Prob focused
Ex = Comprehensive
MDM = Low
Consultation
All 3 elements required

F - Prob Focused **D - Detailed** **S - Straightforward**
M - Moderate **E - Exp Prob Focused** **C - Comprehensive**
L - Low **H - High**

INITIAL NURSING FACILITY CARE: 3 OF 3 REQUIRED

E and M CODE	HISTORY	EXAM	MEDICAL DEC MAKING	AVERAGE TIME
99304	D/C	D/C	S/L	25
99305	C	C	M	35
99306	C	C	H	45

SUBSEQUENT NURSING FACILITY CARE: 2 OF 3 REQUIRED

E and M CODE	HISTORY	EXAM	MEDICAL DEC MAKING	AVERAGE TIME
99307	F	F	S	10
99308	E	E	L	15
99309	D	D	M	25
99310	C	C	H	35

DOMICILARY, REST HOME, BOARDING CARE, NEW PT: 3 OF 3 REQUIRED

E and M CODE	HISTORY	EXAM	MEDICAL DEC MAKING	AVERAGE TIME
99324	F	F	S	20
99325	E	E	L	30
99326	D	D	M	45
99327	C	C	M	60
99328	C	C	H	75

DOMICILARY, REST HOME, BOARDING CARE, EST PT: 2 OF 3 REQUIRED

E and M CODE	HISTORY	EXAM	MEDICAL DEC MAKING	AVERAGE TIME
99334	F	F	S	15
99335	E	E	L	25
99336	D	D	M	40
99337	C	C	H	60

HOME VISIT, NEW PATIENT: 3 OF 3 REQUIRED

E and M CODE	HISTORY	EXAM	MEDICAL DEC MAKING	AVERAGE TIME
99341	F	F	S	20
99342	E	E	L	30
99343	D	D	M	45
99344	C	C	M	60
99345	C	C	H	75

HOME VISIT, ESTABLISHED PATIENT: 2 OF 3 REQUIRED

E and M CODE	HISTORY	EXAM	MEDICAL DEC MAKING	AVERAGE TIME
99347	F	F	S	15
99348	E	E	L	25
99349	D/I	D	M	40
99350	C/I	C	H	60

FIGURE 11-3, cont'd.

OFFICE/OUTPATIENT VISIT, NEW PATIENT: 3 OF 3 REQUIRED				
E and M CODE	HISTORY	EXAM	MEDICAL DEC MAKING	AVERAGE TIME
99201	F	F	S	10
99202	E	E	S	20
99203	D	D	L	30
99204	C	C	M	45
99205	C	C	H	60

OFFICE/OUTPATIENT VISIT, ESTABLISHED PATIENT: 2 OF 3 REQUIRED				
E and M CODE	HISTORY	EXAM	MEDICAL DEC MAKING	AVERAGE TIME
99211	N/A	N/A	N/A	5
99212	F	F	S	10
99213	E	E	L	15
99214	D	D	M	25
99215	C	C	H	40

FIGURE 11-4. Outpatient or office visit grids for new and established patients.

absence of medical documentation to support a new visit. Also remember that only documentation from the current visit may be used. Also, documentation that is not part of the medical record, such as financial documents, cannot be used to validate new patient status, so patient information forms—which are NOT medical documents—cannot be used. Coders must educate their physicians and clinical assistants to document this information in the encounter's medical documentation. There is a significant difference in the reimbursement for a new patient versus an established patient.

STOP AND PRACTICE

Take a sample office visit note (Fig. 11-5) and attempt to follow the whole process from beginning to end. Use the first page of Tool 11-2 and the outpatient or office visit/established patient grid as you go.

Step 1: Section/chapter of CPT would be Evaluation and Management.

Step 2: Determine type or location of service and choose the correct range of codes.

Step 3: Identify patient status (new or established) and determine appropriate gird.

Step 4: Identify history (history of present illness, review of systems) and past medical, family, and social history elements and grid accordingly.

Identify exam elements (body area or organ systems) and grid accordingly.

Identify medical decision-making elements (management/diagnosis options, data, risk of morbidity or mortality) and grid accordingly.

Step 5: Determine whether special circumstances necessitate assigning code by time.

Step 6: Assign appropriate E & M code.

Step 7: Place code(s) in appropriate order if applicable.

Step 8: Determine whether modifiers are needed.

OFFICE/OUTPATIENT VISIT, ESTABLISHED PATIENT: 2 OF 3 REQUIRED				
E and M CODE	HISTORY	EXAM	MEDICAL DEC MAKING	AVERAGE TIME
99211	N/A	N/A	N/A	5
99212	F	F	S	10
99213	E	E	L	15
99214	D	D	M	25
99215	C	C	H	40

The completed grid and E & M code assignment are shown in Figure 11-6.

HOSPITAL OBSERVATION SERVICES (99217-99220) (99234-99236)

Initial observation care	99218-99220
Observation discharge	99217
Observation/inpatient care/admit/ discharge same date	99234-99236

Patients must be designated as on "observation status" while they are in the hospital. Coding staff members may not choose to code observation status instead of inpatient visit simply because of reimbursement issues. This practice has been targeted by third-party audits for fraud and abuse. Only

OFFICE NOTE

Chief complaint: ____________________

Date: ____________

Vital signs: BP______P______R______

History:

The patient is a 19-year-old white female who has a rather long and complicated medical history. Since 16 years of age, the patient has had chronic fatigue, extreme exercise intolerance, episodes of anorexia nervosa, and recurrent syncopal episodes. She is not able to walk up a flight of stairs or walk more than a block due to fatigue and dyspnea with exertion.

Exam:

Patient was noted to have sinus bradycardia with heart rates in the 40s at time. She has had an Echocardiogram which showed mitral valve prolapse. ECG shows bradycardia, otherwise normal.

Diagnosis/assessment:

IMPRESSION:
Recurrent syncopal episode of unknown etiology. Patient has a history of sick sinus dysfunction. Possible sinus node dysfunction.

PLAN:
Follow-up with cardiology for additional workup. Continue meds as prescribed

Patient name: ____________________

Date of service: ____________

GODFREY MEDICAL ASSOCIATES
1532 Third Avenue, Suite 120 • Aldon, FL 77713 • (407) 555-4000

FIGURE 11-5. Sample office visit note.

Evaluation and Management Leveling Sheet: 1995 Guidelines **GODFREY MEDICAL GROUP**

Patient Name/ID:____________ DOS:____________ Chief Complaint: Chronic fatigue

	Final results for history (3 of 3 required)	Problem focused	Exp. problem focused	Detailed	Comprehensive
HISTORY	HPI: ☐ Location ☐ Timing ☐ Quality ☒ Associated signs and symptoms ☒ Severity ☒ Modifying factors ☒ Duration ☐ Context	Brief (1-3) ☐	Brief (1-3) ☐	Extended (4 or more) ☐	Extended (4 or more) ☒
	ROS: ☐ Constitutional (wt. loss, etc.) ☐ Integumentary (skin, breast) ☐ Endocrine ☐ All/Immunology ☐ ENM and T ☐ Eyes ☐ Cardio/Vasc ☐ Respiratory ☐ GI ☐ GU ☐ Musculoskeletal ☐ Psychiatric ☐ Hem/Lymph ☐ Neurological ☐ "All others negative"	None ☒	Pertinent to problem (1 system) ☐	Extended (2-9 systems including pertinent system) ☐	Complete (10 or more systems or pertinent systems with the statement "all others negative") ☐
	PFSH (past medical, family, social history): ☐ Past Hx. (the pts. past experience with illness, operations, and treatments) ☐ Family Hx. (a review of medical events in the pts. family) ☐ Social Hx. (an age appropriate review of past and current activities)	None ☐	None ☐	Pertinent *(1 or 2 history area) ☒	Complete *(2 or 3 history areas) ☐
EXAM	Body areas: ☐ Head, incl. face ☐ Chest, incl. breast and axillae ☐ Abdomen ☐ Neck ☐ Back, incl. spine ☐ Each extremity ☐ Genitalia, groin, buttocks Organ systems: ☐ Constitutional ☐ ENMT ☐ Respiratory ☐ Musculoskeletal ☐ Psych ☐ Eyes ☐ CV ☐ GI ☐ GU ☐ Skin ☐ Neurological ☐ Hem/lymph/imm	1 area or system ☒	2 to 4 areas or systems ☐	2 to 7 areas or systems MUST BE DETAILED ☐	8 or more systems or a complete exam of a single system ☐

*Complete PFSH - 2 Hx areas a) Estab pts Office (Output) care; domiciliary care; home care; b) Emergency Dept. c) Subsequent nursing facility care
3 Hx areas a) New pt. Office (Outpt) care; domiciliary care; home care; b) Consultations c) Initial hospital care d) hospital observation e) Comprehensive nursing facility assessments

Box A: Number of diagnosis or management options (NxP=R)

	Problems to Exam Physician	Number	Points	Results
MEDICAL	Self-limited or minor (stable, improved or worsening)	Max=2	1	
	Est. problem; stable, improved		1	
	Est. problem; worsening		(2)	2
	New problem; no additional workup planned	Max=1	3	
	New problem; additional workup planned		4	
	Bring total to line A Box D		TOTAL	

Box B: Amount and/or complexity of data to be reviewed

		Points
DECISION	Review and/or order of clinical lab tests/procedures	1
	Review and/or order of tests/procedures in the radiology section of CPT	(1)
	Review and/or order of tests/procedures in the medicine section of CPT	1
	Discussion of diagnostic test results with performing physician	1
	Decision to obtain old records and/or obtain history from someone other than patient	1
	Review and summarization of old records and/or discussion of case with another health care provider	2
	Independent visualization of image, tracing, or specimen itself (not simply review of report)	2
	Bring total to line B Box D TOTAL	1

Box D: Final result for complexity of medical decision making (2 of 3 required)

MAKING	A	Number of diagnosis or management options	≤1 minimal	(2 limited)	3 multiple	≥4 extensive
	B	Amount and complexity of data to be reviewed	(≤1 minimal)	2 limited	3 moderate	≥4 extensive
	C	Risk of complications and/or morbidity or mortality	Minimal	Low	(Moderate)	High
		Type of decision making	Straight-forward	Low Complex	Moderate Complex	High Complex

Lowest of the two chosen determines the medical decision making

Box C: Risk of complication and/or morbidity or mortality

Risk level	Presenting problem(s)	Diagnostic procedure(s) ordered	Management options selected
MINIMAL	• One self-limited or minor problem (ex. cold, insect bite, tinea corporis)	• Lab tests requiring venipuncture • Chest x-ray • EKG/EEG • Urinalysis • Ultrasound/Echo • KOH prep	• Rest • Gargles • Elastic bandages • Superficial dressings
LOW	• Two or more self-limited or minor problems • One stable chronic illness (ex. HTN, DM) • Acute uncomplicated illness or injury (ex. sprain, cystitis, rhinitis)	• Physiological test not under stress (ex. PFT) • Non-cardiovascular imaging studies with contrast (ex. barium enema) • Superficial needle biopsy • Clinical lab tests requiring arterial puncture • Skin biopsy	• Over the counter drugs • Minor surgery w/ no identified risk • PT/OT • IV fluids without additives
MODERATE	• (One or more chronic illnesses with mild exacerbation, progression, or side effects of treatment) • Two or more stable chronic illnesses • Undiagnosed new problem with uncertain prognosis (ex. lump in breast) • Acute illness with systemic symptoms (ex. pneumonitis, colitis) • Acute complicated injury (ex. head injury with brief LOC)	• Physiologic tests under stress (ex. cardiac stress test, fetal contraction stress test) • Diagnostic endoscopies with no identified risk factors • Deep needle or incisional biopsy • Cardiovascular imaging studies with contrast and no identified risk factors (ex. arteriogram, cardiac catheterization) • Obtain fluid from body cavity (ex. LP, thoracentesis)	• Minor surgery w/ identified risk factors • Elective major surgery (open, percutaneous, or endoscopic) with no identified risk factors • Prescription drug management • Therapeutic nuclear medicine • IV fluids with additives • Closed treatment of fracture or dislocation without manipulation
HIGH	• One or more chronic illnesses with severe exacerbation, progression, or side effects of treatment • Acute or chronic illnesses or injuries that pose a threat to life or bodily function (ex. multiple trauma, acute MI, pulm embolus, severe resp distress, progressive severe rheumatoid arthritis, ARF, psychiatric illness with potential threat to self or others, peritonitis) • An abrupt change in neurological status (ex. seizure, TIA, weakness, or sensory loss)	• Cardiovascular imaging studies with contrast with identified risk factors • Cardiac electrophysiological tests • Diagnostic endoscopies with identified risk factors • Discography	• Elective major surgery (open, percutaneous, or endoscopic) with identified risk factors • Emergency major surgery (open, endoscopic, percutaneous) • Parenteral controlled substances • Drug therapy requiring intensive monitoring for toxicity • Decision not to resuscitate or to de-escalate care because of poor prognosis

Bring results to line C in Box D (use the highest level chosen)

Hx Level: Problem focused Exam Level: Problem focused MDM Level: Limited

FIGURE 11-6. Completed E & M grid for the sample case shown in Figure 11-5.

OFFICE/OUTPATIENT VISIT, NEW PATIENT: 3 OF 3 REQUIRED

E and M CODE	HISTORY	EXAM	MEDICAL DEC MAKING	AVERAGE TIME
99201	F	F	S	10
99202	E	E	S	20
99203	D	D	L	30
99204	C	C	M	45
99205	C	C	H	60

OFFICE/OUTPATIENT VISIT, ESTABLISHED PATIENT: 2 OF 3 REQUIRED

E and M CODE	HISTORY	EXAM	MEDICAL DEC MAKING	AVERAGE TIME
99211	N/A	N/A	N/A	5
99212	F	F	S	10
99213	E	E	L	15
99214	D	D	M	25
99215	C	C	H	40

OFFICE CONSULT, NEW OR ESTABLISHED PATIENT: 3 OF 3 REQUIRED

E and M CODE	HISTORY	EXAM	MEDICAL DEC MAKING	AVERAGE TIME
99241	F	F	S	15
99242	E	E	S	30
99243	D	D	L	40
99244	C	C	M	60
99245	C	C	H	80

ED VISIT, NEW OR ESTABLISHED PATIENT: 3 OF 3 REQUIRED

E and M CODE	HISTORY	EXAM	MEDICAL DEC MAKING	AVERAGE TIME
99281	F	F	S	N/A
99282	E	E	L	N/A
99283	E	E	M	N/A
99284	D	D	M	N/A
99285	C	C	H	N/A

INITIAL HOSPITAL CARE: 3 OF 3 REQUIRED

E and M CODE	HISTORY	EXAM	MEDICAL DEC MAKING	AVERAGE TIME
99221	D/C	D/C	S/L	30
99222	C	C	M	50
99223	C	C	H	70

SUBSEQUENT HOSPITAL CARE: 2 OF 3 REQUIRED

E and M CODE	HISTORY	EXAM	MEDICAL DEC MAKING	AVERAGE TIME
99231	F	F	S/L	15
99232	E	E	M	25
99233	D	D	H	35

INITIAL INPATIENT CONSULT: 3 OF 3 REQUIRED

E and M CODE	HISTORY	EXAM	MEDICAL DEC MAKING	AVERAGE TIME
99251	F	F	S	20
99252	E	E	S	40
99253	D	D	L	55
99254	C	C	M	80
99255	C	C	H	110

INITIAL OBSERVATION CARE: 3 OF 3 REQUIRED

E and M CODE	HISTORY	EXAM	MEDICAL DEC MAKING	AVERAGE TIME
99218	D/C	D/C	S/L	
99219	C	C	M	
99220	C	C	H	

INITIAL OBS/INPT SAME DAY IN/OUT CARE: 3 OF 3 REQUIRED

E and M CODE	HISTORY	EXAM	MEDICAL DEC MAKING	AVERAGE TIME
99234	D/C	D/C	S/L	
99235	C	C	M	
99236	C	C	H	

Code assignment:

99212

Additional notes:

Hx = Prob focused
Exam = Prob focused
MDM = Limited
Office visit established
2/3 elements required

F - Prob Focused **D - Detailed** **S - Straightforward**
M - Moderate **E - Exp Prob Focused** **C - Comprehensive**
L - Low **H - High**

INITIAL NURSING FACILITY CARE: 3 OF 3 REQUIRED

E and M CODE	HISTORY	EXAM	MEDICAL DEC MAKING	AVERAGE TIME
99304	D/C	D/C	S/L	25
99305	C	C	M	35
99306	C	C	H	45

SUBSEQUENT NURSING FACILITY CARE: 2 OF 3 REQUIRED

E and M CODE	HISTORY	EXAM	MEDICAL DEC MAKING	AVERAGE TIME
99307	F	F	S	10
99308	E	E	L	15
99309	D	D	M	25
99310	C	C	H	35

DOMICILARY, REST HOME, BOARDING CARE, NEW PT: 3 OF 3 REQUIRED

E and M CODE	HISTORY	EXAM	MEDICAL DEC MAKING	AVERAGE TIME
99324	F	F	S	20
99325	E	E	L	30
99326	D	D	M	45
99327	C	C	M	60
99328	C	C	H	75

DOMICILARY, REST HOME, BOARDING CARE, EST PT: 2 OF 3 REQUIRED

E and M CODE	HISTORY	EXAM	MEDICAL DEC MAKING	AVERAGE TIME
99334	F	F	S	15
99335	E	E	L	25
99336	D	D	M	40
99337	C	C	H	60

HOME VISIT, NEW PATIENT: 3 OF 3 REQUIRED

E and M CODE	HISTORY	EXAM	MEDICAL DEC MAKING	AVERAGE TIME
99341	F	F	S	20
99342	E	E	L	30
99343	D	D	M	45
99344	C	C	M	60
99345	C	C	H	75

HOME VISIT, ESTABLISHED PATIENT: 2 OF 3 REQUIRED

E and M CODE	HISTORY	EXAM	MEDICAL DEC MAKING	AVERAGE TIME
99347	F	F	S	15
99348	E	E	L	25
99349	D/I	D	M	40
99350	C/I	C	H	60

FIGURE 11-6, cont'd.

the admitting physician for the observation may change the patient's status.

It is not necessary for the patient to be admitted to an observation area because one may not be available within the facility. It is only required that the patient's status be designated as "observation" in a specific area determined by the hospital.

Other than the admitting physician for observation status, physicians billing for E & M services should use outpatient codes. In many instances, other E & M services may have been performed on the same day. The following text shows which service should be billed when multiple E & M services are provided on the same day:

Admit and observation code	Bill Hospital Admit
Emergency department visit and observation code	Bill Observation Care
Office visit and observation code	Bill Observation Care
E & M services at site related to initiating observation status	Bill Observation Care

Three levels of initial observation care are delineated in the Initial Observation Care grid (Fig. 11-7) contained in the E & M coding grid. These are used when the patient is admitted to observation care and discharged on a subsequent date of service.

When subsequent days are provided in the observation unit, other than the initial observation day and the discharge day, these would be coded as office or outpatient visits because they are performed in the outpatient setting. Observation units in the hospital facility are considered to be outpatient in nature rather than inpatient.

HOSPITAL CARE (99221-99233)

Initial hospital care	99221-99223
Subsequent hospital care	99231-99233
Hospital discharge	99238-99239

Initial Hospital Care

Initial inpatient service codes may be assigned by the admitting physician for the first hospital visit whether the patient is established or new to that physician. When physicians other than the admitting physician initially see the patient, these encounters should be coded with consultation codes when requirements are met; if the consultation definitions are not met, subsequent visit codes should be used.

All services provided by the admitting physician on the same date, including those performed in another facility or setting, are included in the coding for initial inpatient hospital care. Three levels of initial hospital care are included in the Inpatient Hospital Visits part of the E & M coding grid (Fig. 11-8).

Subsequent Hospital Care

Subsequent inpatient hospital care codes are assigned by the admitting provider for additional inpatient visits occurring during the same admission on separate dates or for services of other consulting physicians when consultation guidelines have not been met.

Make certain that documentation is included in the hospital medical record for each day billed. Another focus of fraud and abuse investigation is the provider who bills multiple consecutive days of subsequent care when the provider may not have seen the patient on each of those days. Three levels of subsequent inpatient hospital care are included in the Subsequent Hospital Visits part of the coding grid (see Fig. 11-8).

Observation or Inpatient Care (Including Admission and Discharge Same Day)

These codes should be used when patients are admitted and discharged the same day from the inpatient on observation status. The term *same day* refers to the same calendar date. Do not bill by assigning individual discharge services or initial hospital care codes.

Discharge Services

Two codes may be used for coding and billing for the preparation of the patient for discharge: 99238 and 99239. These two codes are both time driven; therefore it is not necessary to determine the history, exam, and medical decision-making components for these services. However, when time is not

INITIAL OBSERVATION CARE: 3 OF 3 REQUIRED

E and M CODE	HISTORY	EXAM	MEDICAL DEC MAKING	AVERAGE TIME
99218	D/C	D/C	S/L	
99219	C	C	M	
99220	C	C	H	

INITIAL OBS/INPT SAME DAY IN/OUT CARE: 3 OF 3 REQUIRED

E and M CODE	HISTORY	EXAM	MEDICAL DEC MAKING	AVERAGE TIME
99234	D/C	D/C	S/L	
99235	C	C	M	
99236	C	C	H	

FIGURE 11-7. Observation grids for new and established patients.

INITIAL HOSPITAL CARE: 3 OF 3 REQUIRED

E and M CODE	HISTORY	EXAM	MEDICAL DEC MAKING	AVERAGE TIME
99221	D/C	D/C	S/L	30
99222	C	C	M	50
99223	C	C	H	70

SUBSEQUENT HOSPITAL CARE: 2 OF 3 REQUIRED

E and M CODE	HISTORY	EXAM	MEDICAL DEC MAKING	AVERAGE TIME
99231	F	F	S/L	15
99232	E	E	M	25
99233	D	D	H	35

FIGURE 11-8. Hospital care grids.

documented for the discharge services, the coder must assume the least significant service and assign 99238 for the discharge. Keep in mind that the attending physician is the only physician who may code or bill for the discharge because only one physician prepares the patient, signs the discharge papers, and arranges necessary follow-up.

CONSULTATIONS

Office consultations	99241-99245
Inpatient consultations	99251-99255

For an E & M service to be billed as a consultation, it must meet the following three criteria (referred to as the *3 R's*):

1. A documented ***r***equest for the consultation must be included in the patient record at both the consultant's office and the requesting physician's office.
2. The request should be submitted by a ***r***eferring provider or physician or a provider agency (e.g., Division of Blind Services, Vocational Rehabilitation) in which the requesting agency has a physician overseeing the requests.
3. A ***r***eport back to the requesting physician must also be a part of the medical documentation.

Although diagnostic and therapeutic services may be initiated by the consulting physician, the patient's care may not be assumed by the consulting physician. If, subsequent to the E & M service, the physician assumes management of the patient's care, consultation codes cannot be used.

"Patient-requested" consultations may not be billed with the outpatient and inpatient consultation codes but instead should be billed with the visit codes appropriate to the location of service. Types of consultations include office or outpatient, initial inpatient, and follow-up inpatient.

Beginning in 2006, in addition to the rules just mentioned, the written request must be documented in the referring physician's record as well. Failure to have this documentation may lead to consultations that may have to be coded or billed as visits, which carries a significant decrease in reimbursement.

Office or Outpatient Consultations

When consultations are performed in the office or outpatient location, codes from this subsection should be used. If, after the initial consultation, additional advice or specialty opinions are requested, these may be coded as office consultations as well.

Five levels of office or outpatient consultation are outlined in the Outpatient Consultation Codes part of the coding grid (Fig. 11-9).

Think back to the original chart that was reviewed at the beginning of the chapter. It was determined to be a consultation, based on the request by a referring physician for an expert opinion; it would therefore be assigned a code from this section. Because the consultation was performed on an outpatient basis, the code range 99241 to 99245 would be appropriate.

OFFICE CONSULT, NEW OR ESTABLISHED PATIENT: 3 OF 3 REQUIRED

E and M CODE	HISTORY	EXAM	MEDICAL DEC MAKING	AVERAGE TIME
99241	F	F	S	15
99242	E	E	S	30
99243	D	D	L	40
99244	C	C	M	60
99245	C	C	H	80

INITIAL INPATIENT CONSULT: 3 OF 3 REQUIRED

E and M CODE	HISTORY	EXAM	MEDICAL DEC MAKING	AVERAGE TIME
99251	F	F	S	20
99252	E	E	S	40
99253	D	D	L	55
99254	C	C	M	80
99255	C	C	H	110

FIGURE 11-9. Consultation grids.

Initial Inpatient Consultations

Because these codes specify "initial," only one initial consultation may be charged by each consultant per hospital admission. This code includes both the initial consultation, which is perhaps requested at the time of admission, or a later session during the hospitalization, in which the same physician is consulted. Only one of these visits would constitute a consult.

Five levels of initial inpatient consultation codes are included in the Initial Hospital Consultations part of the grid (see Fig. 11-9).

When additional consultative services are requested during the same hospitalization, codes from the subsequent hospital care range would be assigned.

Follow-up consultation codes and confirmatory consultations were deleted in the 2006 CPT code book.

It is often difficult to differentiate visits considered new or initial, which require all three key components to be met, from established or subsequent visits, which require only two of the three key components. Tool 11-1 contains those code ranges in each category for convenient reference.

EMERGENCY DEPARTMENT VISITS (99281-99285)

Each visit to the emergency department is considered new because the physician staff changes or presenting problems differ from visit to visit. Therefore all three key components must be met before a specific level of emergency department service can be billed.

To qualify as an emergency facility, the facility must be available 24 hours a day and must provide unscheduled episodic services to patients who present for immediate medical care. Five levels of emergency department services are out-

ED VISIT, NEW OR ESTABLISHED PATIENT: 3 OF 3 REQUIRED				
E and M CODE	HISTORY	EXAM	MEDICAL DEC MAKING	AVERAGE TIME
99281	F	F	S	N/A
99282	E	E	L	N/A
99283	E	E	M	N/A
99284	D	D	M	N/A
99285	C	C	H	N/A

FIGURE 11-10. Emergency department grids.

lined in the Emergency Department Visits part of the E & M coding grid (Fig. 11-10).

In addition to the usual levels of service documentation necessary with all E & M services, emergency department services for levels 4 and 5 require the following:

Level 4	Documentation of the necessity of urgent evaluation
Level 5	Documentation of the necessity of urgent treatment

This documentation may be implied. Keep in mind that the third-party auditing records must be able to identify clearly the presence of this documentation. The easiest way to meet this requirement is to make certain that the provider documents the information, either in dictation or somewhere on the emergency record.

Level 5 emergency room visits may also be assigned when the history and examination components cannot be met because of the patient's medical or psychiatric condition. Documentation should support that the patient was unable to provide the history or that a comprehensive examination was not possible because of the patient's condition, but the medical decision making still met high-complexity requirements.

In addition to the five levels of emergency department service, another code is used by the hospital emergency department. Code 99288, Direction of Emergency Medical Systems (EMS), is used when the physician directs personnel outside the facility, such as ambulance or paramedic personnel, by providing medical directives and instructions. Note that this code often is not reimbursed by third-party insurance carriers. Codeable services should be coded, however, whether or not they are reimbursable.

PEDIATRIC CRITICAL CARE PATIENT TRANSPORT (99289-99290)

Codes 99289 and 99290 are used for critical care services provided during transport from one facility to another for a critically ill or injured pediatric patient (24 months old or younger). These codes are assigned based on time, as follows:

99289	First 30 to 74 minutes
99290	Each additional 30 minutes

As with all time-driven codes, a minimum of one half of the time must be documented to assign the code. For instance, in code 99290, 15 minutes or more would have to be documented to code and bill for this service.

CRITICAL CARE SERVICES (99291-99292)

The critical care services category has been misused and abused by physicians throughout the United States for some time. In Pennsylvania, for example, one carrier banned the use of these codes because of the high volume of inappropriate usage by physicians. The coder should add these codes to the growing list of those watched closely for potential fraud and abuse.

Adult	99291-99292
Pediatric	99293-99294
Neonatal	99295-99296

Critical care services must meet ALL of the following guidelines:

- An unstable and/or critically ill patient
- Constant attention required from the provider for the time(s) coded and billed

Note that not all patients who are treated in the intensive care unit (ICU) of the hospital will qualify for critical care services. Care should be taken to make certain all requirements are met before these codes are used.

Critical care service is composed of several comprehensive services that make up the critical care charge. They include the following:

- Cardiac output measurement interpretation
- Chest x-rays
- Blood gases
- Use of computer-stored information
- Gastric intubation
- Temporary transcutaneous pacing
- Ventilation management
- Vascular access procedures

If additional services beyond those listed are provided, they may be billed along with the critical care code(s).

Because each code is based on the amount of time spent rendering critical care, this series of E & M codes may have more than one code billed per day. The documented time spent by the physician providing constant attention to unstable, critically ill, or injured patients is billed with these codes. The critical care time is calculated according to the total time spent with a patient on a specific date. It may include critical care time that is not continuous for the same calendar date.

For the criteria for each component of critical care to be met, a minimum of one half of the specified time element must be met. For instance, code 99291 is specified as the first hour of critical care provided on a given calendar date. If the time spent is less than 30 minutes (or less than one half of the total critical care time), it may not be billed as critical care code 99291. In this case, the appropriate level based on location of service would be billed, such as a hospital visit or an office visit.

The coder should also remember that critical care may be provided in ANY location as long as the requirements of constant attention for an unstable, critically ill or injured patient are met. The following example illustrates this concept.

> A patient arrives at the office in acute respiratory distress as the result of an acute asthmatic exacerbation. The patient is documented as unstable and critically ill and requires the constant attention of the physician for care. An ambulance is summoned, and the provider continues to provide constant care to the unstable, critically ill patient while en route to the hospital and in the emergency department.
>
> Total time: 2 hours, 15 minutes
> Office time: 30 minutes
> Ambulance: 1 hour
> Emergency department: 45 minutes

The following codes are used for billing critical care services:

99291	Critical care, first hour (at least 30 minutes up to 60 minutes)
99292	Critical care, each additional 30 minutes (at least 15 minutes up to 30 minutes)

These are all critical care services performed on the same calendar date. It is advisable that the provider document the time(s) spent with the patient, preferably by indicating start and stop times, or actual blocks of time (e.g., 3:10 PM to 3:55 PM). If additional clarification of time units for critical care visits is needed, the CPT manual has an excellent chart for reference purposes.

Make certain the physician understands the importance of documenting the unstable, critically ill or injured nature of the patient. Phrases such as "doing well," "stable," "without complaints," or "no acute distress" are not acceptable for documenting the critical care visit.

INPATIENT PEDIATRIC CRITICAL CARE AND NEONATAL INTENSIVE CARE (99468-99480)

Code 99471 and 99476 are used for pediatric critical care when provided on an inpatient basis. These codes are assigned on a "per day" basis, with 99293 for the initial day and code 99294 for each additional day. When codes are stated as "each, each additional," the services should be assigned codes based on units of service rather than each day as a separate line item. Consider the following example:

> Pediatric patient, age 4, admitted to pediatric ICU on 01/01/20xx and remained in pediatric ICU 01/02/20xx, 01/03/20xx, 01/04/20xx, and 01/05/20xx. These services would be assigned codes as follows:

01/01/20xx	Code 99475 X	1 unit
01/02 to 01/05/20xx	Code 99476 X	4 units

Codes 99468 through 99469 are the critical care codes for neonates. They may be used only for the critically ill or very low-birth-weight neonate. As with regular critical care codes, when the criteria for neonatal intensive care services can no longer be met, the appropriate location and level of service should be coded, such as a hospital visit.

Unlike the regular critical care codes, these neonatal codes should be reported only ONCE per calendar day, regardless of the amount of time or number of visits made per calendar day.

Neonatal intensive care services comprise a number of comprehensive medical services. They include the following:

- Monitoring and treatment of the patient
- Enteral or parenteral nutritional maintenance
- Metabolic or hematologic maintenance
- Pharmacologic control of the circulatory system
- Counseling of parents
- Case management services
- Personal direct supervision of health care team

All the following services are included in the charge for neonatal intensive care:

- Umbilical, central, or peripheral vessel catheterization
- Oral or nasogastric tube placement
- Endotracheal intubation
- Lumbar puncture
- Suprapubic bladder aspiration
- Bladder catheterization
- Initiation and management of mechanical ventilation of continuous positive airway pressure
- Surfactant administration
- Intravascular fluid administration
- Transfusion of blood components
- Vascular puncture
- Invasive or noninvasive electronic monitoring, including vital signs, bedside pulmonary function testing, and monitoring or interpretation of gases or oxygen saturation

Critically ill neonates are defined as requiring life support, such as respiratory or cardiac assistance, frequent or continuous vital sign monitoring, laboratory and blood gas interpretations, and frequent reevaluations by the provider (including constant observation by members of the health care team under the provider's supervision). The following two categories of codes are used for coding neonatal intensive care services.

Initial Neonatal Intensive Care (99477)

This code is used only for the initial date of admission of the critically ill neonate.

Subsequent Neonatal Intensive Care (99478-99480)

The neonate must remain critically ill and unstable for this code to be used. This code is assigned for EACH subsequent calendar day. In addition, codes exist for critically ill but stable neonatal visits and for low-birth-weight infant care.

These may be used as long as the neonatal intensive care requirements are met.

When the neonate no longer meets the guidelines for neonatal intensive care services but still remains hospitalized, regular inpatient hospital codes are appropriate.

NURSING FACILITY SERVICES (99301-99318)

When services are provided in nursing facilities, skilled nursing facilities, intermediate care facilities, and long-term care facilities, and when E & M services are provided in the psychiatric residential treatment facility, these codes are billed.

Initial nursing care	99304-99306
Subsequent nursing care	99307-99310
Nursing facility discharge	99315-99316
Other nursing facility	99318

Initial Nursing Care (New or Established Patient)

When comprehensive nursing facility assessment codes are billed, all other E & M services provided for the same day are included. In the case of nursing facility services, codes are assigned on the basis of the performance of a comprehensive nursing assessment or with subsequent nursing facility codes.

Comprehensive nursing facility assessment codes require the formulation or reformulation of a medical plan of care. One of the three levels of comprehensive nursing assessment codes may be used, as outlined in the comprehensive nursing facility assessment part of the coding grid (Fig. 11-11).

Subsequent Nursing Care

These codes are used to report services provided to patients in this type of facility when no further comprehensive assessment is required. This is an established visit code; only two of the three key components must be met for the particular level of service assigned. Three subsequent nursing facility codes are used, as outlined on the subsequent nursing facility care part of the coding grid (see Fig. 11-11).

Nursing Facility Discharge

These codes are used for services performed in conjunction with the final examination of the patient before discharge from the nursing facility. These services may include final examination of the patient; discussion of the nursing facility stay with the patient or patient's family; continuing care instructions provided to caregivers; discharge preparation; and final preparation of discharge records, prescriptions, and referral forms. This set of codes is time driven; therefore, when time is not documented, the least significant code, 99315, would be appropriate.

Nursing facility discharge 30 minutes or less	99315
Nursing facility discharge more than 30 minutes	99316

INITIAL NURSING FACILITY CARE: 3 OF 3 REQUIRED

E and M CODE	HISTORY	EXAM	MEDICAL DEC MAKING	AVERAGE TIME
99304	D/C	D/C	S/L	25
99305	C	C	M	35
99306	C	C	H	45

SUBSEQUENT NURSING FACILITY CARE: 2 OF 3 REQUIRED

E and M CODE	HISTORY	EXAM	MEDICAL DEC MAKING	AVERAGE TIME
99307	F	F	S	10
99308	E	E	L	15
99309	D	D	M	25
99310	C	C	H	35

FIGURE 11-11. Nursing facility service grids.

DOMICILIARY, REST HOME, AND CUSTODIAL SERVICES (99324-99337)

When services occur in a facility in which room, board, and other personal assistance services are provided, the codes from domiciliary, rest home, and custodial care services should be assigned. These facilities typically offer long-term care of the patient or boarder. New and established patient visit codes exist. As with other E & M codes, all three key elements must be met for new patients; only two of the three key elements must be met for established patients.

New patient	99324-99328
Established patient	99334-99337

Remember that the facility charges for the care and upkeep of the patient or boarder. This reimbursement billed by the facility does not include any medical services provided by the physician.

Domiciliary, rest home, and custodial care new and established services are outlined in the new and established domiciliary or rest home visits grids on the E & M coding grid (Fig. 11-12).

OVERSIGHT SERVICES, REST HOME, OR HOME CARE (99339-99340)

These codes are assigned when an individual physician supervises the care of a patient while the patient is residing in an assisted living facility. The codes are time based, and therefore documentation must state the time spent performing these services.

Code 99339 is assigned when 15 to 29 minutes is spent during one calendar month performing the oversight of the assisted living patient. These services may include revising care plans, writing reports of patient status, reviewing laboratory and other ancillary services, and discussing the patient's care.

Code 99340 would be assigned in those instances when the time spent in a given calendar month exceeds 30 minutes.

DOMICILARY, REST HOME, BOARDING CARE, NEW PT: 3 OF 3 REQUIRED				
E and M CODE	HISTORY	EXAM	MEDICAL DEC MAKING	AVERAGE TIME
99324	F	F	S	20
99325	E	E	L	30
99326	D	D	M	45
99327	C	C	M	60
99328	C	C	H	75
DOMICILARY, REST HOME, BOARDING CARE, EST PT: 2 OF 3 REQUIRED				
E and M CODE	HISTORY	EXAM	MEDICAL DEC MAKING	AVERAGE TIME
99334	F	F	S	15
99335	E	E	L	25
99336	D	D	M	40
99337	C	C	H	60

FIGURE 11-12. Domiciliary service grids.

HOME VISIT, NEW PATIENT: 3 OF 3 REQUIRED				
E and M CODE	HISTORY	EXAM	MEDICAL DEC MAKING	AVERAGE TIME
99341	F	F	S	20
99342	E	E	L	30
99343	D	D	M	45
99344	C	C	M	60
99345	C	C	H	75
HOME VISIT, ESTABLISHED PATIENT: 2 OF 3 REQUIRED				
E and M CODE	HISTORY	EXAM	MEDICAL DEC MAKING	AVERAGE TIME
99347	F	F	S	15
99348	E	E	L	25
99349	D/I	D	M	40
99350	C/I	C	H	60

FIGURE 11-13. Home service grids.

HOME SERVICES (99341-99350)

Home service codes are reserved for E & M services provided in the residential setting. These services do not have to be provided specifically in the patient's home, but merely in a residential setting. This could include a hotel or motel in which a patient is temporarily residing. Home services are outlined in the new and established home visits portion of the coding grid (Fig. 11-13).

New patient	99341-99345
Established patient	99347-99350

PROLONGED SERVICES (99354-99539)

When provider services are given over and above the usual E & M services outlined in the E & M section, they may be billed *with* face-to-face prolonged services or *without* face-to-face prolonged services.

Direct patient contact	99354-99357
Without direct patient contact	99358-99539

The difference between face-to-face and non–face-to-face services is the patient contact made during the face-to-face encounter. Non–face-to-face codes typically are used for services provided on behalf of the patient, without the presence of the patient (e.g., contact with health providers, arranging for health care outside the office or hospital setting, meeting with family members regarding the care of the patient).

Because these codes are based on time, rounding rules apply. To meet the stated criteria and bill for these services, the coder must document a minimum of one half of the stated time.

These codes are assigned according to cumulative time spent and documented on each calendar date; therefore the initial code is coded only once per day. Time does not need to be continuous but is correctly coded by the time spent per calendar date.

These codes are intended to be used in addition to the regular E & M services provided. Make certain to list the regular E & M services first because these indicate the most significant service and the chief reason for the encounter. In the event the prolonged service is not reimbursed, the primary E & M service is still considered for reimbursement.

NOTE: Many third-party carriers do not recognize these codes or do not reimburse for these services.

PHYSICIAN STANDBY SERVICES (99360)

In many instances, a provider may be requested to be available in the event services are needed. For example, in the case of a high-risk obstetric delivery, the neonatologist may be requested by the obstetrician to be available. This physician standby service code is intended for use ONLY when the physician ultimately does not provide any other service. As in the earlier case, if the neonatologist provides neonatal ICU services, the code for physician standby services is not applicable. In addition, the standby service physician may NOT provide services to other patients at the time the physician standby service is being billed. It is imperative that the provider coding and billing for this service makes certain that documentation by the requesting physician for this service is available and that the time of service is documented.

In the case of physician standby services, all the full 30 minutes must be provided before this service can be billed. Any standby services totaling less than a full 30 minutes may not be coded and billed. Code 99360 is the only code used for billing physician standby services.

Examples of physician standby services include operative standby, high-risk obstetric delivery, and standby for cesarean section. Remember that the physician standby service must be requested and documented.

Physician standby services may not be reimbursable by many third-party carriers, but they still should be coded and billed when appropriate.

CASE MANAGEMENT SERVICES (99363-99368)

When the provider is designated as responsible for coordinating, supervising, and initiating health care for the patient, the case management codes are used. Again, note that inclusion of these codes does not indicate guaranteed reimbursement for these services, even when they have been documented, coded, and billed correctly.

Anticoagulation management	99363-99364
Medical team conferences	99366-99368

Case management services are divided into two categories: anticoagulation management and medical team conferences.

Anticoagulation Management

New codes for 2007 identify anticoagulation management services. These codes are intended to be used only when provided by physicians, not nursing personnel. When patients begin anticoagulation therapy, it is common to perform prothrombin times on these patients regularly. In addition to the codes for initial 90 days and subsequent 90 days, the provider may also code and bill for the prothrombin study as well as the specimen handling when appropriate.

Team Conferences

Team conferences involve the participation of multiple health care providers in discussing, planning, and instituting the coordination, supervision, and initiation of health care services for a specified patient. The rounding factor may also apply here, according to the time, with one half of the time documented before the specific code can be used.

The following categories fall under team conference billing:

- Medical conference with interdisciplinary team, approximately 30 minutes
- Medical conference with interdisciplinary team, approximately 60 minutes

CARE PLAN OVERSIGHT SERVICES (99374-99380)

When a provider oversees the care of a patient requiring multiple services over a prolonged period, the care plan oversight codes should be considered. Typically, the provider is involved in the revision of care plans and the review of a number of reports, including laboratory and other studies. These services must be documented as extending over and above the usual services provided in the billed E & M services.

Caution should be used in coding these services: Only ONE physician may oversee the care of the patient using these codes ONLY when documentation that substantiates care beyond the usual services is provided. Infrequent service or lower levels of service are considered a part of the usual E & M services coded.

As with the other "times" recorded for E & M services, the coder must make certain the time is documented and the rounding rule is followed (one half of the amount of time specified must be documented before the code can be used).

The care plan oversight codes are subcategorized into locations of service: home health agency, hospice, and nursing facility. Coding and reimbursement for these services are based on the total cumulative time spent in supervision of the patient's care during a calendar month.

FRAUD ALERT: Specific Medicare regulations prohibit physicians who are medical directors of these facilities, or who are paid by the entity that owns them a specified dollar limit, from receiving compensation for care plan oversight services. Because these individuals have already been paid for direction of services, reimbursement of the care plan oversight services would represent duplication of payment.

Care plan oversight services are outlined as follows:

Home health agency patient	15 to 29 minutes per calendar month	99374
	30 minutes or more per calendar month	99375
Hospice patient	15 to 29 minutes per calendar month	99377
	30 minutes or more per calendar month	99378
Nursing facility patient	15 to 29 minutes per calendar month	99379
	30 minutes or more per calendar month	99381-99429

PREVENTIVE MEDICINE SERVICES

When medical care is provided for the purpose of preventive care of the patient, the preventive medicine service codes are appropriate. These codes are divided between new and established patient encounters and are further subdivided by age groups. Reimbursement varies according to the categories and subcategories because certain age group evaluations are considered more involved than others.

New patient	99381-99387
Established patient	99391-99397
Individual counseling	99401-99404
Group counseling	99411-99412
Other	99420-99429

Many third-party carriers abide by varying interpretations of the preventive medicine CPT codes. Some do not reimburse for any preventive care; others do not recognize the preventive medicine codes in CPT. Always check with specific carrier contracts to make certain of acceptable practice for coding these appropriately.

When a problem, complaint, or abnormality is noted during the course of the preventive medicine examination, it may be considered significant enough to warrant the coding of an additional E & M service code. These services are billed with modifier 25 to denote that significantly separate and distinct services have been performed. The diagnosis for the complaint, problem, or abnormality should be included in the other E & M service to further justify the request for reimbursement. Other insignificant services or E & M services for insignificant problems or complaints are not codeable or reimbursable in combination with the preventive medicine services already coded.

If immunizations, other separate services, or ancillary services are performed at the time of the preventive medicine service, these services are coded and billed as usual. In most instances, third-party consideration for reimbursement is made for these services, even when the third-party carrier may not reimburse for the actual preventive medicine service.

Preventive medicine services are outlined as follows:

New patients	Preventive medicine visit, under 1 year (infant)	99381
	Preventive medicine visit, early childhood (ages 1-4)	99382
	Preventive medicine visit, late childhood (ages 5-11)	99383
	Preventive medicine visit, adolescent (ages 12-17)	99384
	Preventive medicine visit, ages 18-39	99385
	Preventive medicine visit, ages 40-64	99386
	Preventive medicine visit, ages 65 and older	99387
Established patients	Preventive medicine, under 1 year (infant)	99391
	Preventive medicine, early childhood (ages 1-4)	99392
	Preventive medicine, late childhood (ages 5-11)	99393
	Preventive medicine, adolescent (ages 12-17)	99394
	Preventive medicine, ages 18-39	99395
	Preventive medicine, ages 40-64	99396
	Preventive medicine, ages 65 and older	99397

COUNSELING OR RISK FACTOR INTERVENTION (99401-99412)

These E & M codes are used ONLY for intervention purposes, not when patients have specific symptoms, problems, or complaints related to the risk factor. Counseling or risk factor intervention services are outlined as follows:

Individual counseling	15 minutes	99401
	30 minutes	99402
	45 minutes	99403
	60 minutes	99404
Group counseling	30 minutes	99411
	60 minutes	99412

NEWBORN CARE (99431-99440)

For care of the neonate, services are categorized by setting and type of service provided, as follows:

History and examination	Normal newborn infant, hospital and birthing room	99460
	Normal newborn infant, other than hospital or birthing room	99461
Subsequent newborn care	Normal newborn care, per subsequent day	99462
History, examination, discharge, and newborn care on same day	Normal newborn history, examination, discharge from hospital or birthing room, all on the same date	99463
Attendance at delivery	Initial attendance at delivery and stabilization of neonate (when documented and requested by delivering physician); may be reported also as 99431, normal newborn care	99464
Newborn resuscitation	Neonate requires chest compressions, positive-pressure ventilation, or other newborn resuscitation; when this service is billed, it is inappropriate to bill attendance at delivery (99436)	99465

NON–FACE-TO-FACE SERVICES (99441-99444)

Telephone Services	99441-99443
Online Medical Evaluation	99444

Telephone Calls

Telephone call services, as with all other services, must be documented. Documentation should include the date and time of the phone call, the content and complexity of the call, and the name of the person who spoke with the provider. These provider notes should be signed in the usual fashion. Telephone calls are categorized as follows:

5-10 minutes of medical discussion	99441
11-20 minutes of medical discussion	99442
21-30 minutes of medical discussion	99443

These codes may only be assigned when the telephone call does not originate from a related E & M service provided within the past 7 days or lead to an E & M service in the next 24 hours or soonest available appointment.

Online Medical Evaluation

When the physician corresponds with the patient online, code 99444 may be assigned. As with telephone services, the online medical evaluation may not be assigned if it is related to a E & M service provided in the past 7 days or lead to an E & M service in the next 24 hours or soonest available appointment.

SPECIAL EVALUATION AND MANAGEMENT SERVICES (99450-99456)

In response to the increasing demand for evaluative services other than for specific complaints or problems, evaluation codes were established for administrative evaluations. These evaluative services are used for establishing baseline information before the initiation of insurance policies or for approval of disability or workers' compensation benefits.

During the administration of these services, no medical management is instituted, nor is any modification made to the current treatment plan by the provider. These examinations are not intended to address the disability but simply to evaluate the progress or lack thereof and to make recommendations for further evaluation and treatment.

These services typically are billed to the requesting entity (e.g., disability insurance agency, life insurance company) rather than to the patient's current health insurance carrier. These services usually are requested by the entity and are authorized in advance.

Special E & M services are categorized as follows and include life and disability evaluation and work-related or medical disability.

Life/disability evaluation	Height, weight, blood pressure Medical history Blood sample or urinalysis following "chain of command" Completion of necessary forms/reports	99450
Work-related or medical disability (treating physician)	Completion of the medical history Examination commensurate with patient's condition Formulation of diagnosis, assessment of capabilities, calculation of impairment Development of future medical options Completion of necessary forms	99455
Work-related/ medical disability (other than treating physician)	Completion of the medical history Examination commensurate with patient's condition Formulation of diagnosis, assessment of capability, calculation of impairment Development of future medical options Completion of necessary forms	99456

This code is used ONLY by the consultant, not the treating physician. Code 99455 should be used by the treating physician.

OTHER EVALUATION AND MANAGEMENT SERVICES (99477-99499)

Unlisted E & M services are billed with code 99499. As with any unlisted procedure in CPT, this code must include a description of the service performed and a written report to accompany the claim to the insurance carrier.

STOP AND PRACTICE

Now that all the types of E & M service have been discussed, identify the history, examination, and medical decision-making components and determine what level of service should be coded in the following scenarios. Use the appropriate grid from Tool 11-2 (p. 339) for the location of service and the type of patient (new or established) and determine the correct level of service.

1. Office visit for an established patient who presents with new onset of left upper quadrant pain following a fall. Past medical history of gallbladder disease. Exam of the abdomen and pelvic exam were performed. Abdomen series negative. Diagnosis: Abdominal pain.

Step 1:	Evaluation and management	__________
Step 2:	Determine type or location	__________
Step 3:	Determine patient status (new or established)	__________
Step 4:	Determine correct range of codes/ appropriate grid	__________
Step 5:	Determine whether counseling or coordination of care	__________

STOP AND PRACTICE—cont'd

Step 6: Assign correct E & M code ____________
Step 7: Place in correct order (if applicable) ____________
Step 8: Determine whether modifier code(s) are applicable ____________
E & M code ____________

2. Office visit for follow-up for stable diabetes mellitus. Patient has multiple medical problems; however, all appear stable at this time. No complaints of diplopia; excessive thirst, or possible diabetic symptoms at this time. She notes that she has been symptom free except for some lower back pain in the last fewweeks. Exam completed of the back, heart, and lungs. Glucose level taken, which was normal. Assessment: type 2 diabetes.

Step 1: Evaluation and management ____________
Step 2: Determine type or location ____________
Step 3: Determine patient status (new or established) ____________
Step 4: Determine correct range of codes/ appropriate grid ____________
Step 5: Determine whether counseling or coordination of care ____________
Step 6: Assign correct E & M code ____________
Step 7: Place in correct order (if applicable) ____________
Step 8: Determine whether modifier code(s) is applicable ____________
E & M code ____________

3. Patient known to the physician is admitted to the inpatient hospital facility for possible stroke. History of right-sided numbness and weakness, 2 weeks' duration. No cough, no chest pain. Exam of respiratory, cardiovascular, and neurologic systems performed. CT of brain with contrast performed as well as labs, x-rays. Patient admitted for cardiovascular accident with neurologic symptoms.

Step 1: Evaluation and management ____________
Step 2: Determine type or location ____________
Step 3: Determine patient status (new or established) ____________
Step 4: Determine correct range of codes/ appropriate grid ____________
Step 5: Determine whether counseling or coordination of care ____________
Step 6: Assign correct E & M code ____________
Step 7: Place in correct order (if applicable) ____________
Step 8: Determine whether modifier code(s) is applicable ____________
E & M code ____________

4. Office visit for complaint of pain and swelling in knee. Patient presents with 2-week duration of red and painful swollen knee. No swelling or pain in other joints, no fever, no fatigue. Exam of both knees performed as well as neurologic exam. X-rays reveal osteoarthritis of both knee joints.

Step 1: Evaluation and management ____________
Step 2: Determine type or location ____________
Step 3: Determine patient status (new or established) ____________
Step 4: Determine correct range of codes/ appropriate grid ____________
Step 5: Determine whether counseling or coordination of care ____________
Step 6: Assign correct E & M code ____________
Step 7: Place in correct order (if applicable) ____________
Step 8: Determine whether modifier code(s) is applicable ____________
E & M code ____________

5. Office visit for patient with known diagnosis of hypertension who now presents with symptoms of fatigue and 2-week history of headaches. Past history of diabetes and CAD. Cardiovascular, respiratory, and neurologic exams are negative. Patient given new

STOP AND PRACTICE—cont'd

beta-blocker for hypertension and hypertension-associated headaches.

Step 1: Evaluation and management ______
Step 2: Determine type or location ______
Step 3: Determine patient status (new or established) ______
Step 4: Determine correct range of codes/ appropriate grid ______
Step 5: Determine whether counseling or coordination of care ______
Step 6: Assign correct E & M code ______
Step 7: Place in correct order (if applicable) ______
Step 8: Determine whether modifier code(s) is applicable ______

E & M code ______

6. 56-year-old patient with ear pain for the past 2 days after swimming over the weekend. Ear pain accompanied by fever, up to 102. No respiratory symptoms; however, patient has past history of extensive otitis media. Exams of ears, nose, and throat as well as chest are performed with a diagnosis of otitis media.

Step 1: Evaluation and management ______
Step 2: Determine type or location ______
Step 3: Determine patient status (new or established) ______
Step 4: Determine correct range of codes/ appropriate grid ______
Step 5: Determine whether counseling or coordination of care ______
Step 6: Assign correct E & M code ______
Step 7: Place in correct order (if applicable) ______
Step 8: Determine whether modifier code(s) is applicable ______

E & M code ______

7. 3-year-old patient with complaints of stomachache after dinner at home. Patient had spaghetti approximately 3-4 hours ago and began experiencing nausea and vomiting. No respiratory symptoms. No past history of abdominal problems; however, patient has bilateral ear tube placement. Exams of ENT, abdomen, and chest are performed. Abdomen series negative, labs negative. Patient prescribed Compazine for N/V, with diagnosis of food poisoning.

Step 1: Evaluation and management ______
Step 2: Determine type or location ______
Step 3: Determine patient status (new or established) ______
Step 4: Determine correct range of codes/ appropriate grid ______
Step 5: Determine whether counseling or coordination of care ______
Step 6: Assign correct E & M code ______
Step 7: Place in correct order (if applicable) ______
Step 8: Determine whether modifier code(s) is applicable ______

E & M code ______

8. 21-year-old patient seen in follow-up for otitis media after 10 days of antibiotic treatment. No complaints. ENT are clear. Resolved otitis media.

Step 1: Evaluation and management ______
Step 2: Determine type or location ______
Step 3: Determine patient status (new or established) ______
Step 4: Determine correct range of codes/ appropriate grid ______
Step 5: Determine whether counseling or coordination of care ______
Step 6: Assign correct E & M code ______
Step 7: Place in correct order (if applicable) ______

STOP AND PRACTICE—cont'd

Step 8: Determine whether modifier code(s) is applicable ______

E & M code ______

9. Office visit for a known asthmatic for regular follow-up. No complaints other than shortness of breath with exercise, resolving with nebulizer treatment ×2. No fatigue, chest pain. Exam includes respiratory, cardiovascular, ENT. Asthma controlled.

   Step 1: Evaluation and management ______
   Step 2: Determine type or location ______
   Step 3: Determine patient status (new or established) ______
   Step 4: Determine correct range of codes/appropriate grid ______
   Step 5: Determine whether counseling or coordination of care ______
   Step 6: Assign correct E & M code ______
   Step 7: Place in correct order (if applicable) ______
   Step 8: Determine whether modifier code(s) is applicable ______
   E & M code ______

10. 43-year-old patient with complaints of rash appeared approximately 2 to 3 days ago after trip to the country with her children. No other problems such as fatigue, joint pain. Exam reveals diffuse rash over the legs, arms, and back. Assessment: Rash of unknown etiology.

    Step 1: Evaluation and management ______
    Step 2: Determine type or location ______
    Step 3: Determine patient status (new or established) ______
    Step 4: Determine correct range of codes/appropriate grid ______
    Step 5: Determine whether counseling/coordination of care ______
    Step 6: Assign correct E & M code ______
    Step 7: Place in correct order (if applicable) ______
    Step 8: Determine whether modifier code(s) is applicable ______
    E & M code ______

Review of the E & M Coding Process

Briefly review the steps used in selecting correct codes from the E & M section:

Step 1: Determine Whether Service Is Evaluation and Management

Step 2: Determine Location of Service

Determine the location where service was performed and mark this on the E & M coding grid.

Step 3: Determine Patient Status (New or Established)

If it is not stated, the coder assumes the patient is established. Select the correct coding grid for determining level of service, which is based on location and patient status.

Step 4: Determine the Correct Level of Service

According to the components plotted on the E & M grid, determine the correct level of service.

Identify history, physical examination, and medical decision-making components and explain modifying circumstances.

Highlight or mark these components within the documentation and plot them on the E & M coding grid.

Step 5: Determine Whether Modifying Factors Are Key Elements

Determine whether history, physical examination, and medical decision-making components are the determining factors or whether modifying circumstances control the level of service.

If the five basic steps for coding E & M services are followed, regardless of the complexity of the services performed, E & M service coding is as simple as diagnostic coding. The idea is to keep basic guidelines in mind no matter how complicated the documentation or procedures appear to be. Using the step-by-step accumulation of only the needed components makes even the most complex and detailed case a simple one.

Step 6: Assign the Appropriate E & M Code

Step 7: Determine the Correct Order When More Than One Service Is Performed

Step 8: Determine Whether Modifier Code(s) Are Appropriate

Common Problems in Assigning E & M Codes

If you have trouble assigning a level of service that is too high or too low, some suggestions may help.

- Coding too high: After coding the service, attempt to code to the next lower level and see if the criteria there more accurately reflect the case.
- Coding too low: After coding the service, attempt to code to the next higher level. If the criteria for the higher level more accurately reflect the case presented, code higher. If the criteria do not reflect a higher level, the student coder can feel comfortable that the level selected is the most appropriate.

Other Common E & M Coding Errors

Examination criteria are NOT the same as a review of systems. Make sure to choose as physical examination criteria elements for which the physician actually performed an examination. Elements reviewed verbally or covered in a questionnaire format with the patient (typically before the examination) are review of systems components.

- Remember, new visits require three of three key elements for criteria to be met. Established visits require two of three key elements. Visits not specified as new are assumed to be established visits.
- Remember not to use chart notes indicating "probable," "possible," or other notations that are not definitive diagnoses.
- Only documented material may be used in the consideration of key factors.
- Codes involving time elements must be documented regarding the specific amount of time and the nature of the counseling or coordination of care.

Chapter in Review

Certification Review

- New patients have not visited the physician or physician group or specialty within the last 3 years. This includes all services provided to the patient regardless of location of service.
- "On call" or "covering" physicians assign E & M levels in the same manner as the physicians for whom they cover.
- Guidelines for each location of service and for levels of service are defined by the number of documented components required in the physician documentation.
- The *history* component is composed of history of present illness; chief complaint; review of systems; and past medical, social, and family history.
- The *physical examination* component is composed of body areas and organ systems as follows:
  Body areas: Head, neck, chest, abdomen, genitalia, back, each extremity
  Organ systems: Eyes; ears, nose, throat, mouth; cardiovascular, respiratory, gastrointestinal, genitourinary, musculoskeletal, neurologic, psychiatric, and hematologic/lymphatic/immunologic systems; skin
- The component *medical decision making* includes three elements, two of which must be met: diagnosis/management options, amount and complexity of data, risk of morbidity or mortality.
- Time is a factor in the determination of E & M levels of service only when more than 50% of the time is spent in counseling and coordination of care.
- Types of E & M services include the following:
  Outpatient/office visits
  Hospital observation services
  Hospital inpatient services
  Consultations (inpatient/outpatient)
  Emergency department services
  Critical care services
  Neonatal intensive care services
  Nursing facility services
  Domiciliary, rest home, custodial services
  Home services
  Prolonged services
  Physician standby services
  Case management services
  Care plan oversight services
  Preventive medicine services
  Counseling/risk factor intervention
  Newborn care services
  Special E & M services
- Basic steps for E & M coding are the following:
  Identify history, physical examination, and medical decision-making components.
  Determine location of service.

Determine patient status.
Determine level of service.
Determine whether modifying factors (e.g., time or modifier codes needed) are key elements.

Student Assignments

1. Study Chapter 11.
2. Review the Learning Objectives for Chapter 11.
3. Review the Certification Review for Chapter 11.
4. Complete the Stop and Practice exercises.
5. Complete the Chapter Review exercise to reinforce concepts learned in the chapter. Try the Practical Application exercises to apply all the concepts to actual medical documentation.
6. Complete the practice exercises on the companion Evolve site for reinforcement of E & M concepts.
7. Complete Chapter 11 Workbook exercises on procedure coding.

Chapter Review Exercise

For each of the following services, determine the location of service, determine new or established patient status, and list the range of codes that would be used for coding these services.

1. Initial nursing home visit
   Location ______
   New or established ______
   Range of codes 99304 – 99306
2. Visit to the outpatient clinic
   Location ______
   New or established ______
   Range of codes 99201-99215
3. Hospital consultation
   Location Consultation
   New or established ______
   Range of codes 99241 – 99255
4. Patient requested consult
   Location office
   New or established established
   Range of codes 99211-99215
5. Emergency department visit
   Location Emergency
   New or established ______
   Range of codes 99281 – 99288

For each of the following scenarios, assign the same information as above and the appropriate E & M code.

6. Office visit, established patient
   Problem-focused history
   Problem-focused examination
   Straightforward medical decision making
   Location ______
   New or established ______
   Range of codes ______
   Code selected ______
7. Emergency department visit
   Detailed history
   Expanded problem-focused examination
   Moderate medical decision making
   Location ______
   New or established ______
   Range of codes ______
   Code selected ______
8. Outpatient consultation, established patient
   Comprehensive history
   Comprehensive examination
   Moderate medical decision making
   Location ______
   New or established ______
   Range of codes ______
   Code selected ______
9. Hospital admit
   Comprehensive history
   Comprehensive examination
   High medical decision making
   Location ______
   New or established ______
   Range of codes ______
   Code selected ______
10. Hospital observation care
    Comprehensive history
    Detailed examination
    Moderate medical decision making
    Location ______
    New or established ______
    Range of codes ______
    Code selected ______

Practical Application

Review the following medical records and determine the appropriate type, location, and level of service and assign the appropriate E & M code(s). After determining the type or location of service, use Tool 11-2 to capture the history, physical examination, and medical decision-making components to determine the level of service and assign the appropriate E & M codes.

Check with your instructor to determine whether ICD-9-CM diagnostic code(s) should be assigned for these exercises for additional diagnostic coding practice.

1. Emergency department record

EMERGENCY ROOM RECORD

Name:	Age: / DOB:	ER physician: Robert Rais, MD
Allergies/type of reaction:	**Usual medications/dosages:**	
NKDA	Medications are listed on her medication flow sheet	

Triage/presenting complaint: SUBJECTIVE: This is a 54-year-old female who is a resident at a local Nursing home. She speaks Spanish and it is difficult to obtain a history from her. However, it is known from Nursing Home staff that she did fall today. They found her on the floor and since then she has been complaining of some back, shoulder and abdominal pain. She has ambulated down the stairs since falling. She does, however, still report some shoulder and back pain while here In the ER.

Initial assessment:

PAST MEDICAL HISTORY: Positive for diabetes, hiatal hernia, Status post cardiac surgery. She had aortic valve replacement, has a history of CAD, hypertension and has a history of suicidal ideation.

Time	T 97.0	P 88	R 22	BP128/74	Other:				

Medication orders:

Lab work: She was a little anemic with a hemoglobin of 11.0. Other labs were normal. Her INR was 2.0. Urinalysis was negative as was C-spine, lumbar spine and shoulder.

X-Ray:

Physician's report:

OBJECTIVE
Vital signs are stable. She is afebrile.
She is pleasant, alert and oriented and appears in no distress. She does complain of neck and back pain.
Lungs are clear to auscultation bilaterally. Abdomen is obese, soft, nondistended, nontender. Extremities show no brusing or swelling. No pedal edema is present. Neurological, nonfocal.

Diagnosis:

PLAN:
Patient will be sent back to Nursing Home. If she has worsening symptoms, she will return. Otherwise, continue present medication regimen.

Discharge **Transfer** **Admit** **Good** **Satisfactory** **Other:**

Physician sign/date

Robert Rai MD

GODFREY REGIONAL HOSPITAL
123 Main Street • Aldon, FL 77714 • (407) 555-1234

Step 1: Chapter or section of CPT — Evaluation and Management
Step 2: Type or location ____________
Step 3: Patient status ____________
Step 4: Level of history, exam, medical decision making ____________
Step 5: Counseling/coordination of care ____________
Step 6: Assign code ____________
Step 7: Assign correct order (if applicable) ____________
Step 8: Assign modifier code(s) when appropriate ____________
Evaluation and management code ____________
ICD-9-CM code(s) (optional) ____________

2. Outpatient office visit

OFFICE NOTE

Chief complaint: ______________________

Date: ______________

Vital signs: BP______ P______ R______

History:

32-year-old female with abdominal pain. Describes it as upper abdominal pain. She did vomit two times last evening. She tried some Darvocet, which did not provide any relief. States she has not been eating as her appetite has decreased significantly. No history of heartburns or ulcers, however, she does take TUMs on an occasional basis. She also has tried a heating pad on the area of her abdominal pain without relief. She does have her gallbladder. She had a C-Section approximately three weeks ago.

PAST MEDICAL HISTORY:
She has Factor V coagulopathy and protein S deficiency.

MEDICATIONS:
Coumadin 5 mg Monday, Wednesday and Friday, and 7.5 mg alternate days.

Exam:

LABORATORY AND IMAGING:
CBC and panel 20 were normal.

Diagnosis/assessment:

ASSESSMENT:
RUQ pain with radiation to back

PLAN:
This could be gallbladder or possible gallbladder associated pancreatitis. We will follow this closely and she will call immediately if symptoms worsen or fever develops. We will order gallbladder ultrasound, but this does not seem urgent at this time.

Patrick Olson MD

Patient name: ______________________

Date of service: ______________

GODFREY MEDICAL ASSOCIATES
1532 Third Avenue, Suite 120 • Aldon, FL 77713 • (407) 555-4000

Step 1: Chapter or section of CPT	Evaluation and Management
Step 2: Type or location	______________
Step 3: Patient status	______________
Step 4: Level of history, exam, medical decision making	______________
Step 5: Counseling/coordination of care	______________
Step 6: Assign code	______________
Step 7: Assign correct order (if applicable)	______________
Step 8: Assign modifier code(s) when appropriate	______________
Evaluation and management code	______________
ICD-9-CM code(s) (optional)	______________

3. Outpatient office visit

OFFICE NOTE

Chief complaint: ______

Date: ______

Vital signs: BP______P______R______

History:

Nine month old returns for recheck after recent treatment for ear infection. He does not appear to be in any distress per his parents. He has been eating OK, urinating and having regular bowel movements. NKDA

Exam:

Vital signs are stable. Weight is approximately 10 kg. Ears show erythematous TM's bilaterally. Neck reveals no lymphadenopathy, no masses. Eyes do show some green discharge of the left eye.

Diagnosis/assessment:

ASSESSMENT:
Recurrent otitis media

Patient placed on Augmentin 400 mg per 5 cc, 1/2 tsp bid for 8 days. Follow up in 10 days.

William Obert MD

Patient name: ______

Date of service: ______

GODFREY MEDICAL ASSOCIATES
1532 Third Avenue, Suite 120 • Aldon, FL 77713 • (407) 555-4000

Step 1: Chapter or section of CPT	Evaluation and Management
Step 2: Type or location	______
Step 3: Patient status	______
Step 4: Level of history, exam, medical decision making	______
Step 5: Counseling/coordination of care	______
Step 6: Assign code	______
Step 7: Assign correct order (if applicable)	______
Step 8: Assign modifier code(s) when appropriate	______
Evaluation and management code	______
ICD-9-CM code(s) (optional)	______

4. Outpatient office visit

OFFICE NOTE

Chief complaint: ______

Date: ______

Vital signs: BP_____ P_____ R_____

History:

This is an 8-month-old female who presents for her initial office visit. Parents report her nose has been stuffed up and she is now running a low-grade fever. She has been eating OK and her parents have been giving her Pedialyte as well. She has no history of ear infection. She did have some diarrhea earlier this week. She has had a cough as well. They have not noticed any rashes or difficulty breathing.

NKDA, currently on no medications

Exam:

She is afebrile, temperature is 97.7 axillary, respirations 28, weight approximately 10 kgs
Ears reveal erythematous TMs bilaterally, no discharge appreciated.
Eyes reveal some green discharge.
Nose reveals some green discharge present.
Neck exam reveals no adenopathy, no masses.
Lungs are clear to auscultation.
Cardiovascular is within normal limits.

Laboratory included RVS which was negative

Diagnosis/assessment:

ASSESSMENT:
Bilateral Otitis Media
Conjunctivitis

Patient was given 500 mg IV Rocephin now. Also prescribed Gentamicin ophthalmic ointment to apply to both eyes. If she is not better with 2-4 days, parents are to bring her back.

Felix Washington MD

Patient name: ______

Date of service: ______

GODFREY MEDICAL ASSOCIATES
1532 Third Avenue, Suite 120 • Aldon, FL 77713 • (407) 555-4000

Step 1: Chapter or section of CPT	Evaluation and Management
Step 2: Type or location	______
Step 3: Patient status	______
Step 4: Level of history, exam, medical decision making	______
Step 5: Counseling/coordination of care	______
Step 6: Assign code	______
Step 7: Assign correct order (if applicable)	______
Step 8: Assign modifier code(s) when appropriate	______
Evaluation and management code	______
ICD-9-CM code(s) (optional)	______

5. Emergency department note

EMERGENCY ROOM RECORD

Name:	Age:	ER physician:
	DOB:	Nancy Connelly, MD

Allergies/type of reaction:	Usual medications/dosages:
Allergies include Sulfa and Cefzil both which cause rash.	

Triage/presenting complaint: 1½-year-old who presents with his mother with complaints of fever for the past day. Mom states she has given him Tylenol several times but he seems to have worsened. She states he has had ear infections 2-3 times. States he has not been eating well, however voiding well, wetting diapers regularly. No diarrhea or problem with stools.

Initial assessment:

Vital signs are listed on ER sheet. Both right and left ears are erythematous. No abnormal discharge. Neck exam reveals no lymphadenopathy. Cardiovascular and pulmonary exam are normal.

Time	T	P	R	BP	Other:				

Medication orders:

Patient given Augmentin 400 mg per 5 cc, ¾ tsp for 10 days.

Lab work:

Strep pharyngitis test was negative

X-Ray:

Physician's report:

ASSESSMENT:
Bilateral otitis media

Diagnosis:	Physician sign/date
	Nancy Connelly MD
Discharge Transfer Admit Good Satisfactory Other:	

GODFREY REGIONAL HOSPITAL
123 Main Street • Aldon, FL 77714 • (407) 555-1234

Step 1: Chapter or section of CPT	Evaluation and Management
Step 2: Type or location	______________
Step 3: Patient status	______________
Step 4: Level of history, exam, medical decision making	______________
Step 5: Counseling/coordination of care	______________
Step 6: Assign code	______________
Step 7: Assign correct order (if applicable)	______________
Step 8: Assign modifier code(s) when appropriate	______________
Evaluation and management code	______________
ICD-9-CM code(s) (optional)	______________

6. Inpatient hospital history and physical examination

HISTORY AND PHYSICAL EXAMINATION

Godfrey Regional Hospital History and Physical
Admission: XX/XX/XX

Patient presented initially to the Emergency room after a chair she was sitting in fell and she fell backwards on her right shoulder. She was given Tylenol, however, she was still having extreme pain so her parents brought her to the ER. There was no head trauma, no LOC, denies chest pain or shortness of breath. No neck pain, no significant medical history.

Past medical history:

Family and social history:

Review of systems:

Physical exam:

She is awake, alert and in some distress from pain. HEENT: Head normocephalic. Pupils equal and reactive. Neck supple with good range of motion. The child had deformity at her right clavicle which was very tender. She had decreased range of motion at the elbow and wrist. Good radial pulse bilaterally. Chest clear, heart normal rate and rhythm. Abdomen positive bowel sounds, lower extremities showed good motor power.

Laboratory/radiology:

X-ray:

An x-ray in the ER demonstrated right shoulder revealed a compound fracture of the midclavicle.

Assessment:

Orthopedics was consulted and surgical reduction was recommended.

Plan:

She was admitted with surgery scheduled for tomorrow morning.
We will sedate patient with Morphine as needed for pain.
Patient to remain NPO in the event surgical intervention is necessary in the morning.

GODFREY REGIONAL HOSPITAL
123 Main Street • Aldon, FL 77714 • (407) 555-1234

Step 1: Chapter or section of CPT	Evaluation and Management
Step 2: Type or location	
Step 3: Patient status	
Step 4: Level of history, exam, medical decision making	
Step 5: Counseling/coordination of care	
Step 6: Assign code	
Step 7: Assign correct order (if applicable)	
Step 8: Assign modifier code(s) when appropriate	
Evaluation and management code	
ICD-9-CM code(s) (optional)	

7. Hospital visit

PROGRESS NOTE

Date/time
XX/XX/XX

S:

Patient was admitted approximately 24 hours ago with shortness of breath with a long history of chronic asthma and COPD. The patient had been running fevers with increasing cough and presented to the emergency room on the morning of the 5th.

O:

CXR on admission suggested right-sided infiltrate.
Repeat x-ray today shows no infiltrate or resolve infiltrate.

A:

P:

She has been on IV antibiotics since admission. We will switch to oral antibiotics for the next 24 hours and if she remains afebrile we discharge tomorrow on oral meds.

Jay Corman MD

Patient ID

Patient name
Admit: XX/XX/XX
MR# XXXXXXX

PROGRESS NOTES

GODFREY REGIONAL HOSPITAL
123 Main Street • Aldon, FL 77714 • (407) 555-1234

Step 1: Chapter or section of CPT	Evaluation and Management
Step 2: Type or location	______
Step 3: Patient status	______
Step 4: Level of history, exam, medical decision making	______
Step 5: Counseling/coordination of care	______
Step 6: Assign code	______
Step 7: Assign correct order (if applicable)	______
Step 8: Assign modifier code(s) when appropriate	______
Evaluation and management code	______
ICD-9-CM code(s) (optional)	______

8. History and physical

HISTORY AND PHYSICAL EXAMINATION

Godfrey Regional Hospital History and Physical
Admission: XX/XX/XX

This 64 year old who is para 4, was referred because of a large cystocele and uterine prolapse. The patient states that when she is on her feet, a bulge comes out her vagina between her legs. She was found to have a large cystocele and 2nd degree uterine prolapse. She does not have any significant problem with urinary control. She is admitted at this time for vaginal hysterectomy and A and P repair.

Past medical history:

Her general health is good, she is taking Lanoxin 0.25 mg, ½ tablet daily.

Family and social history:

Review of systems:

Physical exam:

Reveals a well-developed, well-nourished, slender, white female at 131 pounds. Blood pressure is 130/70, respirations 20, and pulse 78.

Ears:	Negative
Mouth:	Believe patient has dentures. Throat clear, tonsils are absent.
Neck:	Supple, no masses
Breasts:	Quite good turgor for her age, no masses felt
Lungs :	Clear to P and A
Heart:	Regular rate and rhythm, no murmurs
Abdomen:	Soft and nontender
Gyn:	When patient strains, bladder bulges down and out and the cervix comes our through the introitus.
Rectal:	Negative, moderate rectocele
Extremities:	No significant deformities noted, no edema, reflexes are physiologic.

Laboratory/radiology:

X-ray:

Assessment:

2nd degree uterine prolapse, cystocele with some rectocele.

Plan:

Vaginal hysterectomy, anterior repair and possibly posterior repair at the same time.

Rachel Perez MD

GODFREY REGIONAL HOSPITAL
123 Main Street • Aldon, FL 77714 • (407) 555-1234

Step 1: Chapter or section of CPT	Evaluation and Management
Step 2: Type or location	______________
Step 3: Patient status	______________
Step 4: Level of history, exam, medical decision making	______________
Step 5: Counseling/coordination of care	______________
Step 6: Assign code	______________
Step 7: Assign correct order (if applicable)	______________
Step 8: Assign modifier code(s) when appropriate	______________
Evaluation and management code	______________
ICD-9-CM code(s) (optional)	______________

9. Inpatient visit

PROGRESS NOTE

Date/time
XX/XX/XX

S:

This 73-year-old was admitted yesterday with mental status changes. At that time, the patient indicated he did not recall the events that led to his hospitalization.

O:

HEENT: Normal
Neck: Supple, no adenopathy
Chest: Reveals decreased breath sounds bilaterally, but no wheezing or rales
Heart: Normal
Abdomen: Normal
Neuro: Patient is alert and cooperative.

A:

IMPRESSION:
Mental status changes
Possible seizure disorder versus hypoglycemic reaction

P:

Will continue to monitor

Patient ID
Patient name
Admit: XX/XX/XX
MR# XXXXXXX

PROGRESS NOTES

GODFREY REGIONAL HOSPITAL
123 Main Street • Aldon, FL 77714 • (407) 555-1234

Step 1: Chapter or section of CPT	Evaluation and Management
Step 2: Type or location	______________
Step 3: Patient status	______________
Step 4: Level of history, exam, medical decision making	______________
Step 5: Counseling or coordination of care	______________
Step 6: Assign code	______________
Step 7: Assign correct order (if applicable)	______________
Step 8: Assign modifier code(s) when appropriate	______________
Evaluation and management code	______________
ICD-9-CM code(s): (optional)	______________

10. Consultation

CONSULTATION

Indication for consultation:

Patient is here on Dr. Smith's service. She has a diagnosis of acute respiratory failure, COPD, CHF, HTN, anemia and hypomagnesemia as well as Alzeheimer's and diabetes mellitus. I was asked to evaluate her hemorrhoids.

History:

Exam:

Examination was limited to primarily the anus. The patient is quite heavy and has edema of the skin of the lower extremities, back and buttocks. She has some early bed sores and possible early decubiti, however, I was not asked to evaluate these. She does have external hemorrhoidal tags which are not acutely thrombosed. There is some mild edema but it is not severe and on digital rectal exam I feel no palpable abnormalities.

Diagnosis/assessment:

IMPRESSION:
Mildly edematous external hemorrhoids

PLAN:
Anusol HC cream twice daily and after all stools.

Maurice Doater, MD

Patient name: ____________________

Date of service: ____________

GODFREY MEDICAL ASSOCIATES
1532 Third Avenue, Suite 120 • Aldon, FL 77713 • (407) 555-4000

Step 1: Chapter or section CPT	Evaluation and Management
Step 2: Type or location	__________
Step 3: Patient status	__________
Step 4: Level of history, exam, medical decision making	__________
Step 5: Counseling/coordination of care	__________
Step 6: Assign code	__________
Step 7: Assign correct order (if applicable)	__________
Step 8: Assign modifier code(s) when appropriate	__________
Evaluation and management code	__________
ICD-9-CM code(s) (optional)	__________

12

Anesthesia Services

LEARNING OBJECTIVES

After completing this chapter, the student will be able to:

- Comprehend the documentation used for anesthesia coding.
- Understand the types of anesthesia providers.
- Know the types of care provided by anesthesia providers.
- Understand and apply the principal elements of anesthesia coding.
- Comprehend the proper use of modifier codes for anesthesia services.
- Know the basic differences that make anesthesia coding unique.

CODING REFERENCE TOOLS

Tool 12-1
Anesthesia Coding Elements

KEY TERMS

American Society of Anesthesiologists
Anesthesia Assistant
Anesthesia Time Unit
Anesthesiologist
Base Unit
Certified Registered Nurse Anesthetist (CRNA)
General Anesthesia
Monitored Anesthesia Care (MAC)
Moribund
Patient-Controlled Analgesia
Physical Status Modifier
Qualifying Circumstance
Regional Anesthesia
Systemic Disease

Anesthesia Documentation and Coding Guidelines

ANESTHESIA SERVICES

Codes in the anesthesia section of CPT are arranged as outlined below. Note that the majority of subsections are by anatomic region, starting at the top of the body and progressing downward.

Head	00100-00222
Neck	00300-00352
Thorax (chest wall and shoulder girdle)	00400-00474
Intrathoracic	00500-00580
Spine and spinal cord	00600-00670
Upper abdomen	00700-00797
Lower abdomen	00800-00882
Perineum	00902-00952
Pelvis	01112-01190
Upper leg (except knee)	01200-01274
Knee and popliteal area	01320-01444
Lower leg (below knee, ankle, foot)	01462-01522
Shoulder and axilla	01610-01682
Upper arm and elbow	01710-01782
Forearm, wrist, and hand	01810-01860
Radiologic procedures	01916-01936
Burn excisions or debridement	01951-01953
Obstetric	01958-01969
Other procedures	01990-01999

The anesthesia record serves as the main document for information pertaining to services performed before, during, and after the administration of anesthesia. The procedure and documentation are usually provided by the health care professional and consist of the following information:

- Preanesthesia evaluation

A patient interview is conducted, including medical, anesthesia, and medication history. Also, an appropriate physical examination is usually performed before the administration of anesthesia. In addition, the provider will typically review any diagnostic data, such as x-rays, laboratory test results, and electrocardiograms. The plan for anesthesia care will be formulated and discussed with the patient or responsible party. At the conclusion of the evaluation, the provider will also assign a code to the physical status of the patient based on the information gathered and according to the procedures of the **American Society of Anesthesiologists**.

- Perianesthesia record

A record will be kept during the actual anesthesia administration and patient monitoring throughout the surgical procedure. The review immediately before anesthetic administration, patient monitoring by qualified anesthesia personnel, the patient's vital signs, amount of drugs and agents used, times given, technique, and patient status at the conclusion of the anesthetic event are all documented on the anesthesia record. Although anesthesia billing is usually by means of a billing card, codes that are assigned and billed must be substantiated by the anesthesia provider's documentation before, during, and after surgery.

- Postanesthesia record

After the completion of the surgical procedure, the anesthesia provider will continue to monitor the patient for vital signs, level of consciousness, additional drugs administered, all postanesthesia visits, and any prescribed follow-up.

All the aforementioned services are included in the code(s) assigned for anesthesia care.

Figure 12-1 represents an example of a preanesthesia evaluation record. Note that the anesthesia provider also obtains information such as review of systems and medical history (discussed in Chapter 11). Figure 12-2 represents an example of an anesthesia record, in which the provider documents the monitors, equipment, technique for anesthesia administration, start and stop times, vital signs, and other output measurements. Take a look at the first portion of the table that was reviewed in Chapter 10 of the steps or components needed for Current Procedural Terminology (CPT) coding, especially the anesthesia portion of that table.

CPT CODING STEPS: ANESTHESIA EXAMPLE

Step 1	
Identify chapter or section	General Regional Spinal
Range of codes	00100-01999 99100-99140
Step 2	
Determine type or location	Anatomic
Location	Head Upper Extremity
Step 3	
Specific type	Body area Eye Thyroid
Step 4	
Specific procedure information	Procedure Open Closed
Step 5	
Extent and specifics	Specifics Anesthesia time

Using the sample anesthesia record shown in Figure 12-2, evaluate it for documentation necessary to assign the correct anesthesia code(s) for the service(s) provided. In addition to capturing the actual procedure performed, capture the patient's medical status and any extenuating circumstances during this review.

History from: ☐ Patient ☐ Parent/guardian ☐ Significant other ☐ Chart ☐ Poor historian ☐ Language barrier

PRE-ANESTHESIA EVALUATION

☐ See previous anesthesia record dated ________ for information

Proposed procedure	Age	Sex	Height	Weight
P/E Tubes	5	☐ M ☒ F	in/cm	42 lb lb/kg

Pre-procedure vital signs
B/P: 120/80 P: 80 R: 18 T: 98^8 O_2 SAT %: 98

Current medications ☐ None
None

Previous anesthesia/operations ☐ None
n/a

Airway
☐ MP1 ☐ MP2 ☐ MP3 ☐ MP4
☐ Unrestricted neck ROM ☐ T-M distance = ________ ☐ Obesity ☐ ↓ neck ROM:
☐ ↓ mouth opening/TMJ ☐ Hx difficult airway ☐ Teeth poor repair ☐ Teeth chipped/loose:
☐ Edentulous ☐ Facial hair ☐ Short muscular neck

Family HX anes. problems

Allergies ☐ None

System	Comments	Diagnostic studies
☒ WNL **Respiratory** Asthma/RAD, Bronchiolitis, COPD, Emphysema, Bronchitis, Respiratory failure, Pleural effusion, Pulmonary embolism, Sinusitis/rhinitis, Environ. allergies, Chronic tonsillitis, Chronic OM, Recent URI, TB/+PPD, Pneumonia, Productive cough, SOB/dyspnea, OSA, Orthopnea, Wheezing	Tobacco use: ☐ Yes ☐ No ☐ Quit _____ Packs/Day for_____ Years *Pre-procedure* pulmonary assessment:	ECG Chest X-ray Pulmonary studies
☒ WNL **Cardiovascular** Hypertension, Hyperlipoproteinemia, CAD/cardiomyopathy, Angina, Stable/unstable, Myocardial infarction, CHF DOE PND, Peripheral vascular Dz, Exercise tolerance, Excellent/fair/poor, Abnormal ECG, Dysrhythmia, Hypovolemia, Chronic fatigue, Pacemaker/AICD, Murmur, Valvular Dz/MVP, Rheumatic fever, Endocarditis, Aneurysm	*Pre-procedure* cardiac assessment:	**Laboratory studies**
☒ WNL **Hepato/gastrointestinal** Obesity, Cirrhosis, Hepatitis/jaundice, Bowel obstruction, Ulcers, Hiatal hernia, GERD, N & V, Diarrhea, IBS, Pancreatitis, Gallbladder Dz, Diverticulum, Colon polyps	Ethanol use: ☐ Yes ☐ No ☐ Quit Frequency________ ☐ Hx ETOH abuse	
☒ WNL **Neuro/musculoskeletal** Arthritis/DJD, Back problems (LBP), CVA/TIA, Psychiatric disorder, Headaches, ↑ ICP/head injury, Loss of consciousness, Muscle weakness, Neuromuscular Dz, Paralysis, Paresthesia(s), Syncope, Seizures, Epilepsy		PT/PTT/INR: T&S/T&C: HCG: U/A: LMP:
☒ WNL **Renal/endocrine** Thyroid disease, Cushing's syndrome, Renal failure/dialysis, Renal insufficiency, Renal stones, Adrenocortical insuff., Prostate, BPH/CA, Diabetes mellitus, Type I/II/Gest., UTI, Pituitary disorder		**Other diagnostic tests**
☒ WNL **Other** Anemia, Bleeding disorder, Cancer, Chemotherapy, Radiation Tx, Dehydration, HIV/AIDS, Immunosuppressed, Sickle cell Dz/trait, Recent steroids, Transfusion Hx, Weight loss/gain, Herbal/OTC drug use, Illicit drug use		
☒ WNL **Pregnancy** TIUP, Pre-eclampsia, HELLP, SGA, LGA, PROM, Multiple gestation, VBAC, IUGR	☐ AROM ☐ SROM ☐ Pitocin drip ☐ Induction ☐ Mg drip ______gm/hr G: P: Weeks gest: EDC:	

Surgical diagnosis/problem list
SOM

Planned anesthesia/special monitors

Pre-anesthesia medications ordered
Fentanyl

Evaluator signature | **Date**

Physical status 1 2 3 4 5 E

Post-anesthesia care notes

Location | Time
B/P | O_2 Sat %
Pulse | Resp | Temp

☐ Awake ☐ Stable ☐ Mask O_2
☐ Somnolent ☐ Unstable ☐ NC O_2
☐ Unarousable ☐ Oral/nasal airway
Intubated - ☐ T-piece ☐ Ventilator
Regional - dermatome level:_____
☐ Continuous epidural analgesia
☐ Direct admit to hospital ward (PACU recovery not required)
☐ Recovery recorded on anes. form

Controlled medications			
Medication	Used	Destroyed	Returned

Provider | Witness

☐ No anesthesia related complications noted
☐ Satisfactory post anesthesia/analgesia recovery
☐ See progress notes for anesthesia related concerns

Provider | Date | Time

GODFREY REGIONAL HOSPITAL
123 Main Street • Aldon, FL 77714 • (407) 555-1234

FIGURE 12-1. Preanesthesia evaluation form.

Authorized for local reproduction

MEDICAL RECORD–ANESTHESIA	Procedure P/E Tubes	Item	Start	Stop
		Anesthesia	0700	0730
Date / OR no. / Page of / Surgeon(s)		Procedure	0710	0725

Pre-procedure
- ☒ Identified ☐ ID band ☐ Questioned
- ☒ Chart review ☐ Permit signed
- ☒ NPO since PM
- Pre-anesthetic state: ☐ Calm
- ☐ Awake ☐ Asleep
- ☒ Apprehensive ☐ Confused
- ☐ Uncooperative ☐ Unresponsive

Patient safety
- ☐ Anes. machine # ______ checked
- ☒ Safety belt on ☐ Axillary roll
- ☒ Arm restraints ☐ Arms tucked
- ☐ Pressure points checked and padded
- ☐ Eye care: ☐ Ointment ☐ Saline
- ☐ Taped ☐ Pads ☐ Goggles

Monitors and equipment
- ☒ Steth ☐ Esoph ☐ Precord ☐ Other
- ☐ Non-invasive B/P ☐ Nerve stimulator
- ☐ Continuous ECG ☒ V lead ECG
- ☐ Pulse oximeter ☐ Oxygen analyzer
- ☐ End tidal CO_2 ☐ Resp gas anlyzr
- ☐ Temp ______ ☐ EEG
- ☐ Warming blanket ☐ Fluid warmer
- ☐ Airway humidifier ☐ ______
- ☐ NG/OG tube ☐ Foley catheter
- ☐ Art line ______
- ☐ CVP ______
- ☐ PA line ______
- ☐ IV(s) ______
- ☐ ______

Anesthetic techniques
- Method: ☒ General ☐ Spinal
- ☐ Epidural ☐ Caudal ☐ Brachial
- ☐ Bier block ☐ Ankle blk ☐ M.A.C.
- General: ☐ Pre-O_2 ☐ L.T.A.
- ☐ Rapid sequence ☐ Cricoid pressure
- ☐ Intravenous ☐ Inhalation
- ☐ Intramuscular ☐ Rectal
- Regional: ☐ Position ______
- ☐ Prep ______ ☐ Local ______
- ☐ Needle ______
- ☐ Drug(s) ______
- ☐ Dose ______ ☐ Attempts x ______
- ☐ Site ______ ☐ Level ______
- ☐ Catheter ______ ☐ See remarks

Airway management
- ☐ Intubation ☐ Oral ☐ Nasal
- ☐ Direct vision ☐ Magill's ☐ Blind
- ☐ Diff. see rmks ☐ Fiber op ☐ Stylet
- ☐ Attemps x__ ☐ Blade ______
- ☐ Tube size__ ☐ Endobronchial
- ☐ Regular ☐ RAE ☐ Armored ☐ Laser
- ☐ Cuffed ☐ Min. occ. pres. ☐ Air ☐ NS
- ☐ Uncuffed, leaks at ____ cm H_2O
- ☐ Secured at ______ ☐ ET CO_2 present
- ☐ Breath sounds ______
- ☐ Circuit: ☐ Circle ☐ Non-rebreathing
- ☐ Airway: ☐ Oral ☐ Nasal ☐ Natural
- ☐ Mask case ☐ Via tracheostomy
- ☐ Nasal cannula ☐ Simple O_2 mask

Recovery room
- Time 755 B/P 120/80 O_2 Sat. 97
- ☒ PACU ☐ ICU ☐ L&D P 80 R 18 T 98.8
- ☐ Awake ☐ Spont resp ☐ Oral airway
- ☒ Asleep ☐ Ventilator ☐ Nasal airway
- ☐ Stable ☐ Extubated ☐ Face shield O_2
- ☐ Unstable ☐ Intubated ☐ T-piece O_2

Controlled drugs

Drug	Used	Destroyed	Returned
Provider		Witness	

Time:

		Totals
Agents	☐ Hal ☐ Enf ☐ Iso (%)	
	☐ N_2O ☐ Air (L/min)	
	Oxygen (L/min)	
	( )	
	( )	
	( )	
	( )	
	( )	
Fluids		
Monitors	Urine (ml)	
	EBL (ml)	
	ECG	
	% O_2 inspired (FIO_2)	
	O_2 saturation (SaO_2)	
	End Tidal CO_2	
	Temp: ☐ C ☐ F	
Vital signs	Baseline values; B/P; P; R	200, 180, 160, 140, 120, 100, 80, 60, 40, 20
Vent	Tidal vol. (ml)	
	Resp. rate	
	Peak pres. (cm H_2O)	
	PEEP (cm H_2O)	
Symbols for remarks		
Position		

Symbols
- x Anesthesia
- ⊙ Operation
- ∨ ∧ B/P cuff pressure
- ⊥ ⊤ Arterial line pressure
- △ Mean arterial pressure
- ● Pulse
- ○ Spontaneous resp
- ⌀ Assisted resp
- ⊗ Controlled resp
- T Tourniquet

Anesthesia provider(s)

Remarks:

Patient's identification *(For typed or written entries give: Name–last, first, middle: ID no. (SSN or other); hospital or medical facility.)*

Helen Smith

Anesthesia
Medical record
Optional form 517 (7–95)
Prescribed by GSA/ICMR,
FPMR (41 CFR) 101–11.203(b)(10)

GODFREY REGIONAL HOSPITAL
123 Main Street • Aldon, FL 77714 • (407) 555-1234

FIGURE 12-2. Anesthesia record.

CPT CODING STEPS

Procedure Coding Steps		Chart information
Step 1		
Identify CPT chapter or section	Anesthesia General Regional	Tympanostomy
Range of codes	00100-01999	General
Step 2		
Determine type or location	Anatomic location	Head
		Head Upper extremity
Step 3		
Specific type	Body area	Ear Eye Thyroid
Step 4		
Specific procedure	Tympanostomy	
Procedure Information	Open	
	Closed	
Step 5		
Extent/specifics	Specifics	Age 5, no medical problems Start time: 0800 Stop time: 0900
Step 6		
Assign code	Anesthesia section	Tympanostomy

At this point, the anesthesia section of the CPT book would be used to determine the appropriate code assignment of 00120, procedures on external, middle, or inner ear including biopsy; not otherwise specified. The only other code considerations would be 00124, otoscopy, or 00126, tympanotomy. Neither of these codes properly describes the procedure performed; therefore 00120 would be the only appropriate code for this procedure. Information regarding age, medical status, and time will be needed as the additional steps in anesthesia coding are learned.

Providers of Anesthesia Care

The administration and supervision of anesthesia services may be performed by an **anesthesiologist** or other qualified provider. The **certified registered nurse anesthetist (CRNA)**, or **anesthesia assistant** may perform or provide anesthesia care under the medical direction of the physician provider as long as the following criteria are met:

- Not more than four anesthesia procedures are performed concurrently.
- The physician is physically present.
- The physician does not perform anesthesia care while supervising the CRNA or anesthesia assistant. (The physician may perform some minimal services, including addressing an emergency for a short duration, providing periodic monitoring of an obstetrics patient, checking on postanesthesia patients, and completing paperwork for discharge.)

Reimbursement may be made for the medical direction of these nonphysician individuals in these circumstances when the physician does the following:

- Performs the preanesthetic examination and evaluation
- Prescribes the anesthesia plan
- Personally participates in the most demanding portions of the procedure
- Remains present and available for emergencies
- Performs the postanesthesia care

Types of Anesthesia Care

Anesthesia may be performed and coded as follows:

- General: Defined as a state of unconsciousness accomplished by the administration of drug(s) by inhalation or intramuscular, rectal, or intravenous injection.
- Regional: Administration of anesthesia to a specific region, such as spinal, epidural, or nerve blocks. Regional anesthetic interrupts the sensory nervous system, producing a block free of pain.
- Endotracheal: Anesthesia administered by insertion of a tube through which anesthetic drugs are administered.
- Epidural: Administration of an anesthetic substance into the vertebral spaces.
- Spinal: Any anesthesia administered in the spinal cord area.
- **Monitored anesthesia care** (MAC)

  MAC involves intraoperative monitoring of the patient's vital signs in anticipation of the need for administration of general anesthesia or an anesthetic agent or the possible development of an adverse reaction during the surgical procedure. For MAC to be considered reimbursable, the provider must perform the services listed previously, such as preevaluation and postevaluation, documentation throughout monitoring, and administration of anesthetic agents if medically necessary. MAC services must be considered medically necessary by documentation of the patient's condition. The medical condition must be significant enough to substantiate the need for MAC (e.g., present medications, patient's symptoms). A stable condition would not warrant the reimbursement of MAC.

  Anesthesia services that include MAC should always be reported with the use of an anesthetic modifier, QS, which is discussed later in this chapter.
- Conscious sedation

  Conscious sedation is often provided during some surgical procedures. During the administration of conscious sedation, a decreased level of consciousness is achieved, and the patient is still able to breathe on his or her own and respond to commands and stimuli. Assignment of these codes typically requires documentation to support that the patient was monitored. Other specific documentation requirements must be met and are outlined in the CPT book.

All the previously mentioned methods of anesthesia administration are codeable. In addition, local anesthesia may be performed, in which an anesthetic is applied dermally, intramuscularly, or subcutaneously.

In addition to administrating anesthesia during a surgical procedure, the anesthesia provider may also perform pain management services, either as part of the postoperative course of treatment or for surgical pain control. This therapy is typically provided by one of three methods:

- **Patient-controlled analgesia (PCA)**
  Patient-controlled analgesia allows self-administration of intravenous drugs through an infusion device. When this service is performed as part of postoperative care, the initial set-up time for patient-controlled analgesia may be included in the number of anesthesia time units only. No additional separate charge or code may be assigned for this service.
- Epidural analgesia
  This method involves the administration of a narcotic drug through an epidural catheter. Insertion of the catheter is coded from the nervous system subsection of the surgery chapter of CPT. Daily management of the epidural drug administration is coded from the anesthesia section.

  Epidural injection of a therapeutic agent in the treatment of a nonsurgical condition, usually performed on an outpatient basis, would also be coded and reported from the surgery/nervous section. The use of these codes is further considered when the surgery section of the CPT manual is covered in Chapter 13.
- Nerve blocks
  A nerve block is an injection of an anesthetic agent into or around a specific nerve to limit or alleviate pain of a body segment.

  Initial nerve blocks performed postoperatively may only add additional time units (as outlined for the epidural analgesic). Subsequent injections are considered part of the global anesthesia service and are not codeable, billable, or reimbursable in most cases.

  Nerve blocks performed nonsurgically are assigned codes from the surgery/nervous system section of CPT.

General Coding Guidelines

The coding and billing of anesthesia services, unfortunately, does not conform to many of the rules learned thus far for CPT evaluation and management services. If the student approaches coding for anesthesia services in the same manner as evaluation and management coding—that is, by following specific guidelines—then anesthesia services may be coded with ease.

GLOBAL COMPONENTS

Following are guidelines for anesthesia services. For the purposes of CPT coding, anesthesia services include:

- General anesthesia
- Regional anesthesia
- Supplementation of local anesthesia
- Other services that may be considered appropriate by the anesthesia provider during a procedure

Anesthesia services are considered a global component, with the following services included in the anesthesia charge:

- Preoperative and postoperative services
  In general, the anesthesia provider performs an examination before a surgical procedure. This is considered part of the preoperative care for the patient and is not separately reportable. If the surgery is cancelled, the anesthesia provider may be able to code and bill for an evaluation and management service.

  Postoperative care is also included in the anesthesia code and not separately codeable. If the anesthesia provider is involved in "significantly, separately identifiable" critical care services, those services may be coded and billed. In most instances the surgeon provides postoperative pain management. When medically necessary services during the postoperative period are required that cannot be rendered by the surgeon, some carriers will reimburse the anesthesia provider for these services.
- Anesthesia administration and care during the surgical procedure
  The National Correct Coding Initiative defines specific services that are considered integral to the administration of anesthesia and care provided during a surgical procedure. These services are not separately codeable and billable as a result. Examples include the following:
  - Transporting, positioning, prepping, draping patient
  - Placement of any external devices for monitoring purposes
  - Placement of peripheral intravenous lines of fluids or medications
  - Placement of airway
  - Laryngoscopy for placement of airway
  - Placement of nasogastric or orogastric tube
  - Intraoperative interpretation of functions monitored by external devices
  - Interpretation of laboratory determinations
  - Insertion of urinary bladder catheter
  - Blood specimens obtained from existing lines or venous or arterial puncture
  - Administration of medically required fluids and blood
  - Monitoring (e.g., electrocardiogram, temperature, blood pressure)

These services are considered bundled and may not be billed separately.

TOOL 12-1

ANESTHESIA CODING ELEMENTS

1. Anesthesia code for specified procedure
2. Physical status modifier
3. Qualifying circumstances (when applicable)
4. Modifier codes (when applicable)
5. Time units/relative value units

ANESTHESIA CODING ELEMENTS

Several components are considered in billing for anesthesia services (Tool 12-1). When gathering key elements for anesthesia coding, consider these components in the same manner that history, physical examination, medical decision making, and modifying circumstances were considered in the evaluation and management section of CPT (see Chapter 11).

STEPS TO ANESTHESIA CODING

Following are guidelines for coding anesthesia services.

Step 1: Determine Appropriate Chapter Within CPT

Keep in mind that the anesthesia provider may provide common services from the anesthesia section of CPT as well as other services such as nerve blocks from the nervous system subsection of the surgery chapter. Determination would be based on whether the service is definitive, restorative, or invasive in nature (surgery) or the administration of an analgesic (anesthesia).

Step 2: Determine the Anatomic Location of the Surgical Procedure

Codes in the anesthesia section are arranged in anatomic progression. In other words, codes start at the top of the body and end at the bottom of the body, with the exception of general areas such as obstetric.

A number of procedures may be assigned the same procedure codes because codes in the anesthesia section are general in nature. For instance, unlike the surgery section, where several codes are available for coding a mastectomy, only one code for mastectomy is available in the anesthesia section.

STOP AND PRACTICE

Determine the correct anatomic heading from the anesthesia section where the following procedures would be located.

Procedure	Anatomic Heading
1. Modified radical mastectomy	________
2. Inguinal hernia repair	________
3. Colonoscopy	________
4. Tympanostomy	________
5. Radical prostatectomy	________
6. Knee arthroscopy	________
7. Closed reduction tibia fracture	________
8. Arthroscopic rotator cuff repair	________
9. Radical orchiectomy	________
10. Excision malignant lesion, back	________

Step 3: Determine the Specific Body Part or Organ

Within the anesthesia anatomic heading, the specific body part or organ further defines where the correct CPT code assignment will be located.

STOP AND PRACTICE

Take the exercises begun in Step 2 and assign the specific body part or organ that would further refine the step-by-step process of identifying the appropriate CPT anesthesia code.

Procedure	Anatomic Heading	Body Part or Organ
1. Modified radical mastectomy	________	________
2. Inguinal hernia repair	________	________
3. Colonoscopy	________	________
4. Tympanostomy	________	________
5. Radical prostatectomy	________	________
6. Knee arthroscopy	________	________
7. Closed reduction tibia fracture	________	________
8. Arthroscopic rotator cuff repair	________	________
9. Radical orchiectomy	________	________
10. Excision malignant lesion, back	________	________

Step 4: Determine the Procedure(s) Performed

Determine the procedure(s) performed by analyzing information taken from the operative note or from the anesthesia record that reflects whether the procedure was incision, excision, repair, or reconstruction.

Step 5: Determine Specifics Regarding the Procedure

In addition to the anatomic system and specific body part, identify additional information that is specific to the procedure, such as open or closed, endoscopic or arthroscopic approach, and other information that further specifies the extent of procedure performed.

NEVER use a code from the surgery section for the administration of anesthesia by an anesthesia provider. As previously mentioned, using guidelines and modifiers that are specific to each section is imperative for correct CPT coding. When anesthesiologists perform surgical services, such as insertion of a Swan-Ganz catheter, they may assign codes from the surgery section as appropriate. Many medical and surgical services are eligible for additional payment when furnished in conjunction with the anesthesia services or when performed separately. Following are some examples:

- Swan-Ganz catheter
- Central venous pressure line insertion
- Intra-arterial lines
- Emergency intubation
- Critical care services
- Transesophageal echocardiogram

When these additional services are performed and codes are assigned, time units are not considered because they are not contained in the anesthesia section of CPT.

Make certain that coding from the anesthesiologist agrees with that of the surgeon because the insurance carrier will compare this information. If there are discrepancies between the information reported by the anesthesiologist and by the surgeon, payment may be denied or delayed for both providers. The anesthesia practice must establish a good working relationship between the anesthesiologist and the surgeon to avoid these problems.

If the student is unsure of the appropriate anatomic section from which the procedure should be coded, the CPT code of the surgeon and the anatomic portion of the surgery section can be checked as a guide.

Calculate Anesthesia Time Units

Time is always a factor in anesthesia coding. It is imperative that the anesthesia provider always document time accurately. An anesthesia record provided by the hospital usually allows for the recording of anesthesia time(s).

For purposes of coding and billing, *anesthesia time begins when the anesthesiologist or anesthesia provider begins the induction of anesthesia and ends when the provider completes the administration of anesthesia services.* As with all services provided, documentation plays a key role in coding and reimbursement for anesthesia.

Anesthesia time may be reported in 10-minute or 15-minute anesthesia time units, depending on the individual carrier. In coding for anesthesia services, one of the pieces of information to be gathered from third-party contracts is the proper time increment that individual carriers use. This information may be incorporated in the third-party contract worksheets, which are discussed in Chapter 22. Time units are calculated as follows:

- Total minutes/10-minute or 15-minute increments (whichever is applicable) × time units
- Time units less than 0.5 will be rounded down
- Time units equal to or greater than 0.5 will be rounded up

NOTE: For purposes of this text, assume that all time units are calculated based on 10 minutes per unit.

In addition to the time units, the **base unit** value of each procedure is also added to the total number of units on the claim form. For instance, the time units for the service may be calculated as four, with an additional two base units assigned for the value of the CPT anesthesia code, for a total of six units reported on the claim form. This information is reported on the health insurance claim form as illustrated in Figure 12-3. Reimbursement is based on the total units multiplied by a carrier-specific conversion factor that is agreed upon by the provider.

STOP AND PRACTICE

Practice calculating the time units for anesthesia services in the following examples.

1. Start time: 0900
   Stop time: 0945
   Basic units: 5
   Total units: ______________
2. Start time: 1000
   Stop time: 1020
   Basic units: 3
   Total units: ______________
3. Start time: 1145
   Stop time: 1245
   Basic units: 4
   Total units: ______________
4. Start time: 300
   Stop time: 345
   Basic units: 5
   Total units: ______________
5. Start time: 1045
   Stop time: 1115
   Basic units: 3
   Total units: ______________
6. Start time: 0900
   Stop time: 1030
   Basic units: 5
   Total units: ______________
7. Start time: 0800
   Stop time: 0850
   Basic units: 4
   Total units: ______________
8. Start time: 1000
   Stop time: 1115
   Basic units: 5
   Total units: ______________
9. Start time: 1115
   Stop time: 1240
   Basic units: 6
   Total units: ______________
10. Start time: 0900
    Stop time: 1015
    Basic units: 5
    Total units: ______________

Although some of the guidelines for anesthesia services are different from those applied to the rest of CPT procedural coding, all necessary information for payment consideration can be successfully communicated to the insurance carrier.

Let's summarize the steps covered thus far in this sample exercise:

Step 1		
Identify CPT chapter or section	Anesthesia	
Step 2		
Determine type or location	Anatomic location Head Upper extremity	Head
Step 3		
Specific type	Body area Ear Eye Thyroid	Ear
Step 4		
Specific procedure		Tympanostomy
Procedure information	Open/closed Incision	
Step 5		
Extent/specifics	Specifics Age Time	Age 5, no medical problems Start time: 0800 Stop time: 0900

1500

HEALTH INSURANCE CLAIM FORM

APPROVED BY NATIONAL UNIFORM CLAIM COMMITEE 08/05

PICA | PICA | CARRIER

1. MEDICARE (Medicare #) MEDICAID (Medicaid #) TRICARE CHAMPUS (Sponsor's SSN) CHAMPVA (Member ID#) GROUP HEALTH PLAN (SSN or ID) FECA BLK LUNG (SSN) OTHER (ID)

1a. INSURED'S I.D. NUMBER (For Program in Item 1)

2. PATIENT'S NAME (Last Name, First Name, Middle Initial)

3. PATIENT'S BIRTH DATE MM DD YY SEX M F

4. INSURED'S NAME (Last Name, First Name, Middle Initial)

5. PATIENT'S ADDRESS (No., Street)

6. PATIENT RELATIONSHIP TO INSURED Self Spouse Child Other

7. INSURED'S ADDRESS (No., Street)

CITY STATE

8. PATIENT STATUS Single Married Other

CITY STATE

ZIP CODE TELEPHONE (Include Area Code) ( )

Employed Full-Time Student Part-Time Student

ZIP CODE TELEPHONE (INCLUDE AREA CODE) ( )

9. OTHER INSURED'S NAME (Last Name, First Name, Middle Initial)

10. IS PATIENT'S CONDITION RELATED TO:

11. INSURED'S POLICY GROUP OR FECA NUMBER

a. OTHER INSURED'S POLICY OR GROUP NUMBER

a. EMPLOYMENT? (CURRENT OR PREVIOUS) YES NO

a. INSURED'S DATE OF BIRTH MM DD YY SEX M F

b. OTHER INSURED'S DATE OF BIRTH MM DD YY SEX M F

b. AUTO ACCIDENT? PLACE (State) YES NO

b. EMPLOYER'S NAME OR SCHOOL NAME

c. EMPLOYER'S NAME OR SCHOOL NAME

c. OTHER ACCIDENT? YES NO

c. INSURANCE PLAN NAME OR PROGRAM NAME

d. INSURANCE PLAN NAME OR PROGRAM NAME

10d. RESERVED FOR LOCAL USE

d. IS THERE ANOTHER HEALTH BENEFIT PLAN? YES NO *If yes*, return to and complete item 9 a-d.

READ BACK OF FORM BEFORE COMPLETING & SIGNING THIS FORM.

12. PATIENT'S OR AUTHORIZED PERSON'S SIGNATURE I authorize the release of any medical or other information necessary to process this claim. I also request payment of government benefits either to myself or to the party who accepts assignment below.

SIGNED ____ DATE ____

13. INSURED'S OR AUTHORIZED PERSON'S SIGNATURE I authorize payment of medical benefits to the undersigned physician or supplier for services described below.

SIGNED ____

PATIENT AND INSURED INFORMATION

14. DATE OF CURRENT: MM DD YY ILLNESS (First symptom) OR INJURY (Accident) OR PREGNANCY(LMP)

15. IF PATIENT HAS HAD SAME OR SIMILAR ILLNESS. GIVE FIRST DATE MM DD YY

16. DATES PATIENT UNABLE TO WORK IN CURRENT OCCUPATION MM DD YY FROM TO

17. NAME OF REFERRING PHYSICIAN OR OTHER SOURCE 17a. 17b. NPI

18. HOSPITALIZATION DATES RELATED TO CURRENT SERVICES MM DD YY FROM TO

19. RESERVED FOR LOCAL USE
Anesthesia: 1810 -2005 (115 minutes)

20. OUTSIDE LAB? YES NO $ CHARGES

21. DIAGNOSIS OR NATURE OF ILLNESS OR INJURY. (RELATE ITEMS 1,2,3 OR 4 TO ITEM 24E BY LINE)

1. 214 . 1 3. ___ . ___

2. ___ . ___ 4. ___ . ___

22. MEDICAID RESUBMISSION CODE ORIGINAL REF. NO.

23. PRIOR AUTHORIZATION NUMBER

	24. A. DATE(S) OF SERVICE From MM DD YY	To MM DD YY	B. PLACE OF SERVICE	C. EMG	D. PROCEDURES, SERVICES, OR SUPPLIES (Explain Unusual Circumstances) CPT/HCPCS	MODIFIER	E. DIAGNOSIS POINTER	F. $ CHARGES	G. DAYS OR UNITS	H. EPSDT Family Plan	I. ID. QUAL.	J. RENDERING PROVIDER ID. #
1	01 01 XX	01 01 XX	22		00300	P1		500 00	8		NPI	
2											NPI	
3											NPI	
4											NPI	
5											NPI	
6											NPI	

25. FEDERAL TAX I.D. NUMBER SSN EIN

26. PATIENT'S ACCOUNT NO.

27. ACCEPT ASSIGNMENT? (For govt. claims, see back) YES NO

28. TOTAL CHARGE $

29. AMOUNT PAID $

30. BALANCE DUE $

31. SIGNATURE OF PHYSICIAN OR SUPPLIER INCLUDING DEGREES OR CREDENTIALS (I certify that the statements on the reverse apply to this bill and are made a part thereof.)

SIGNED DATE

32. SERVICE FACILITY LOCATION INFORMATION a. b.

33. BILLING PROVIDER INFO & PH # ( ) a. b.

PHYSICIAN OR SUPPLIER INFORMATION

NUCC Instruction Manual available at: www.nucc.org **PLEASE PRINT OR TYPE** APPROVED OMB-0938-0999 FORM CMS-1500 (08-05)

FIGURE 12-3. Claim form illustrating placement of anesthesia units. Not all carriers will require claim completion as illustrated in the above claim. This sample is to demonstrate time units only.

STOP AND PRACTICE

Identify specifics regarding the procedures identified in the previous Stop and Practice exercises. Assume that time units are calculated in 10-minute increments. Remember that time units must be added to base units for the total unmber of units.

1. Modified radical mastectomy
   Start time: 0945 Stop time: 1145 Base units: 4
   Step 1: Identify CPT chapter/section: __________
   Step 2: Identify anatomic heading: __________
   Step 3: Identify body part or organ: __________
   Step 4: Determine procedure performed: __________
   Step 5: Determine procedure specifics: __________
   Total units: __________
2. Inguinal hernia repair
   Start time: 1000 Stop time: 1115 Base units: 3
   Step 1: Identify CPT chapter/section: __________
   Step 2: Identify anatomic heading: __________
   Step 3: Identify body part or organ: __________
   Step 4: Determine procedure performed: __________
   Step 5: Determine procedure specifics: __________
   Total units: __________
3. Colonoscopy
   Start time: 0900 Stop time: 0930 Base units: 3
   Step 1: Identify CPT chapter/section: __________
   Step 2: Identify anatomic heading: __________
   Step 3: Identify body part or organ: __________
   Step 4: Determine procedure performed: __________
   Step 5: Determine procedure specifics: __________
   Total units: __________
4. Tympanostomy
   Start time: 1100 Stop time: 1145 Base units: 3
   Step 1: Identify CPT chapter/section: __________
   Step 2: Identify anatomic heading: __________
   Step 3: Identify body part or organ: __________
   Step 4: Determine procedure performed: __________
   Step 5: Determine procedure specifics: __________
   Total units: __________
5. Radical prostatectomy
   Start time: 0100 Stop time: 0325 Base units: 5
   Step 1: Identify CPT chapter/section: __________
   Step 2: Identify anatomic heading: __________
   Step 3: Identify body part or organ: __________
   Step 4: Determine procedure performed: __________
   Step 5: Determine procedure specifics: __________
   Total units: __________
6. Knee arthroscopy
   Start time: 0315 Stop time: 0435 Base units: 3
   Step 1: Identify CPT chapter/section: __________
   Step 2: Identify anatomic heading: __________
   Step 3: Identify body part or organ: __________
   Step 4: Determine procedure performed: __________
   Step 5: Determine procedure specifics: __________
   Total units: __________
7. Closed reduction tibia fracture
   Start time: 0845 Stop time: 0950 Base units: 4
   Step 1: Identify CPT chapter/section: __________
   Step 2: Identify anatomic heading: __________
   Step 3: Identify body part or organ: __________
   Step 4: Determine procedure performed: __________
   Step 5: Determine procedure specifics: __________
   Total units: __________
8. Arthroscopic rotator cuff repair
   Start time: 0335 Stop time: 0510 Base units: 5
   Step 1: Identify CPT chapter/section: __________
   Step 2: Identify anatomic heading: __________
   Step 3: Identify body part or organ: __________
   Step 4: Determine procedure performed: __________
   Step 5: Determine procedure specifics: __________
   Total units: __________
9. Radical orchiectomy
   Start time: 0430 Stop time: 0615 Base units: 5
   Step 1: Identify CPT chapter/section: __________
   Step 2: Identify anatomic heading: __________
   Step 3: Identify body part or organ: __________
   Step 4: Determine procedure performed: __________
   Step 5: Determine procedure specifics: __________
   Total units: __________
10. Excision malignant lesion, back
    Start time: 0945 Stop time: 1115 Base units: 4
    Step 1: Identify CPT chapter/section: __________
    Step 2: Identify anatomic heading: __________
    Step 3: Identify body part or organ: __________
    Step 4: Determine procedure performed: __________
    Step 5: Determine procedure specifics: __________
    Total units: __________

Step 6: Assign CPT Code(s)

In addition to the CPT code(s) for the procedure performed, additional code assignments need to be considered.

Assign Qualifying Circumstance Codes (When Applicable)

Identify any **qualifying circumstances** for which these codes may be applicable. Not all anesthesia services have a qualifying circumstance. These are NOT modifier codes. If a qualifying circumstance is applicable, the following CPT codes would be used:

Anesthesia for extreme age, younger than 1 or more than 70 years	99100
Anesthesia complicated by total body hypothermia	99116
Anesthesia complicated by controlled hypotension	99135
Anesthesia complicated by emergency conditions (must specify)	99140

Keep in mind that "emergency" as conceptualized by the layperson does not constitute emergency in medical terms. Make certain that the procedure qualifies as a threat to life or limb when assigning code 99140. Patients scheduled for surgery and admitted on a specified date do not qualify as emergencies. Qualifying circumstances are billed in addition to the primary anesthesia services.

STOP AND PRACTICE

Consider the following procedures and assign CPT code(s) as appropriate, including qualifying circumstances when applicable.

	CPT Code(s)	Qualifying Circumstances (if Applicable)
1. Modified radical mastectomy, 76-year-old patient	________	________
2. Inguinal hernia repair, 37-year-old	________	________
3. Colonoscopy, 62-year-old	________	________
4. Tympanostomy, 6-month-old	________	________
5. Radical prostatectomy, emergency	________	________
6. Knee arthroscopy, 23-year-old	________	________
7. Closed reduction tibia fracture, 12-year-old	________	________
8. Arthroscopic rotator cuff repair, 45-year-old	________	________
9. Radical orchiectomy, 69-year-old	________	________
10. Excision malignant lesion, back, 34-year-old	________	________

Step 7: Assign Codes in Appropriate Order

Review the code assignments in the previous Stop and Practice exercise and determine, when applicable, if the order is appropriate. In many instances, as with Medicare, only one anesthesia code is reported for a surgical procedure unless the second anesthesia code is a secondary, or add-on, procedure. As will be discussed in later chapters, guidelines will vary by carrier. In the case of anesthesia coding and billing, one of the biggest dilemmas is the many different reporting requirements by individual carriers.

Step 8: Assign Modifier Codes(s) as Appropriate

Only six regular modifier codes are applicable for use with anesthesia services. These are discussed in the following paragraphs.

Modifier 22: Unusual Procedural Services

When services provided extend beyond the usual procedure and there is no procedure code to describe the service, modifier 22 may be appended to the procedure code to describe the complete services provided. A report documenting the additional services may be necessary for consideration of reimbursement.

Modifier 23: Unusual Anesthesia

When general anesthesia is used during procedures that typically do not require it, modifier 23 must be added to the procedure code. The procedure may be performed with the patient under local anesthesia or, in other circumstances, with no anesthesia.

Modifier 32: Mandated Services

Modifier 32 is used when services are requested by a third party or a peer review organization. As with other CPT modifiers, it is applicable to more than one section of CPT.

Modifier 51: Multiple Procedures

When multiple procedures are performed during the same anesthesia session, adding to patient risk and anesthesia time, each additional procedure should be listed using this modifier. Of note, this modifier should be listed on all subsequent procedures. The primary and most significant service should be billed, followed by subsequent procedures with the modifier 51 appended.

Reimbursement of subsequent procedures with the use of modifier 51 usually results in reduced reimbursement for these services. Because the preoperative, postoperative, and surgical procedures have been reimbursed already in the primary procedure, the reimbursement for subsequent procedures is reduced proportionately.

In the case of Medicare only one procedure is coded, with the total units of all procedures performed listed on the claim form for that procedure. Other carriers may also follow these guidelines. Therefore you will need to know the correct billing for carriers billed in your practice.

Modifier 53: Discontinued Procedure

When the anesthesiologist chooses to terminate the surgical or diagnostic procedure, the procedure code should have modifier 53 added. This modifier is NOT intended for use when the patient electively decides to terminate the procedure, nor is it appropriate for procedures that are terminated before they begin.

Modifier 59: Distinct Procedural Service

When multiple procedures are performed during the same surgical session but are independent from one another, they should be billed using modifier 59. Modifier 51 usually indicates that multiple procedures are performed through the same approach or at the same anatomic site. The use of modifier 59 defines procedures as independent of one another.

Modifier QS: Monitored Anesthesia Care

When MAC is provided rather than the induction of an anesthetic agent, modifier QS should be appended to the service along with any other appropriate modifier code(s). A modifier designating the provider of service should be assigned for anesthesia as follows:

- AA Performed by anesthesiologist
- AD Medically supervised by physician, more than four consecutive cases
- QK Medically supervised by physician, two to four cases
- QX CRNA with appropriate physician medical direction
- QY Medical direction of CRNA by anesthesiologist
- QZ CRNA without medical direction by anesthesiologist

In addition, modifier 47, anesthesia performed by surgeon, applies to this chapter as well. Although this modifier code is typically used by the surgeon, it may be used with anesthesia code when it is necessary for the surgeon to administer anesthesia.

In addition to regular modifier code(s), anesthesia services are also assigned a **physical status modifier**. This modifier describes the general health of the patient as a risk to anesthesia. Only one physical status modifier is assigned per patient case. All anesthesia services should have a physical status modifier. Some insurance carriers may not require a physical status modifier because they already have included this consideration in their basic reimbursement (e.g., Medicare). Services should always be coded according to CPT guidelines, however, unless the carrier specifies in writing that the provider should not use this modifier code.

As with other modifier codes, physical status modifiers provide additional information regarding requests for consideration for possible additional reimbursement based on the patient's condition. There are only six appropriate physical status modifiers:

- P1 Normal healthy patient with no risks
- P2 Patient with mild **systemic disease**
- P3 Patient with severe systemic disease
- P4 Patient with severe systemic disease considered to be a constant threat to life
- P5 Patient who is **moribund** (dying) and not expected to live without the surgical procedure
- P6 Patient who has been declared brain dead, organ removal for donor purposes

As previously discussed, the coder may code only for documented services and conditions. Remember that the patient with systemic disease may not be billed as such unless documentation from the treating provider (in this case, the anesthesiologist) supports this condition. Documentation by the surgeon may be used only if it has been reviewed and validated by the anesthesiologist.

In many instances the information needed to assign the appropriate physical status modifier will be found on the anesthesia billing card. The American Society of Anesthesiologists uses its own risk assignment, which coincides with the physical status modifier assignment. Although a large amount of information is obtained from this billing card (Fig. 12-4), the coder and biller should make certain documentation exists to substantiate services coded and billed. For instance, a normal, healthy patient, or physical status modifier P1, would sometimes be listed on the anesthesia billing card as ASA (American Society of Anesthesiologists) Risk Category 1.

ANESTHESIA BILLING RECORD

Patient information	**Facility information**
Patient name:	Facility name: Room #:
Demographics (see attached hospital facesheet)	Inpatient/outpatient/ER/ASC (please specify):

Procedure details:

Date of procedure:

ASA rating:

Surgery start: Surgery stop:

Anesthesia start: Anesthesia stop:

Time to PACU:

Procedure(s):

Diagnosis:

Type anesthesia:

Surgeon:

Anesthesiologist:

Anesthetist:

Supervising anethesiologist:

GODFREY MEDICAL ASSOCIATES
1532 Third Avenue, Suite 120 • Aldon, FL 77713 • (407) 555-4000

FIGURE 12-4. Sample anesthesia billing card.

STOP AND PRACTICE

Take the CPT code(s) assigned in the previous Stop and Practice exercise and add the appropriate modifier code(s), including the appropriate physical status modifier for each of the examples provided.

	CPT Code Assignment(s)	Modifier Code(s)	Physical Status Modifier(s)
1. Modified radical mastectomy, 76-year-old patient with severe chronic obstructive pulmonary disease	______	______	______
2. Inguinal hernia repair, 37-year-old	______	______	______
3. Colonoscopy, 62-year-old patient with controlled gastroesophageal reflux disease	______	______	______
4. Tympanostomy, 6-month-old	______	______	______
5. Radical prostatectomy, emergency patient with stage 3 prostate cancer and unstable angina	______	______	______
6. Knee arthroscopy, 23-year-old	______	______	______
7. Closed reduction tibia fracture, 12-year-old	______	______	______
8. Arthroscopic rotator cuff repair, 45-year-old with controlled hypertension and uncontrolled diabetes	______	______	______
9. Radical orchiectomy, 69-year-old	______	______	______
10. Excision malignant lesion, back, 34-year-old	______	______	______

Take another look at the chart or scenario for which a CPT anesthesia code was assigned earlier in the chapter. Capture the additional information needed to finish the code assignment(s) for this chart.

CPT CODING STEPS

Step 1		
Identify CPT chapter/section	Anesthesia	
General/general	regional/spinal	
00100-01999	00100-01999	
Step 2		
Determine type or location	Anatomic location	Head
	Head	Head
	Extremity	
Step 3		
Specific type	Body area	Ear
	Ear	
	Eye	
	Thyroid	
Step 4		
Specific procedure information	Procedure	Tympanostomy
	Open	
	Closed	
	Incision	
Step 5		
Extent/specifics	Specifics	Age 5, no medical problems
	Age	Start time: 0800
	Time	Stop time: 0900

Step 6
Assign CPT code(s) ______________________

Step 7
Place in correct coding order ______________________

Step 8
Assign modifier(s) as appropriate ______________________

It was determined that CPT code 00120 would be the appropriate code assignment for this chart. Additional code assignments must be made for physical status and qualifying circumstances (when applicable), and a calculation of time must also be made.

Take a look at Steps 5 through 8 in the coding process for anesthesia.

Step 5: Identify Specifics

Start time: 0800 Stop time: 0900

Assume the time unit being used by the carriers for this example is a 10-minute increment. The units would be calculated by taking the total number of minutes (60) and dividing them by 10. The sample chart has 6 time units.

Time units: 6 units
Base units: Available from resource-based relative value scale (RBRVS); for example, use 3 base units
Total units: 9 units

Step 6: Assign CPT Codes

As previously determined, those services would be appropriately assigned code 00120.

Assign qualifying circumstance codes (when applicable).

Because the child is older than 1 year and does not have any extenuating circumstances that complicate the procedure, a qualifying circumstance code in this case would not be appropriate.

Step 7: Place Codes in Correct Order

Most significant procedures should be listed first, followed by subsequent procedures.

Step 8: Assign Modifier Codes (as Applicable)

Assign the appropriate physical status modifier.

Because no medical conditions were documented and it appears that the patient is a healthy child, a physical status modifier of P1 would be appropriate. As indicated numerous times, when documentation does not support a higher coding level, the code with the least significance is assigned.

Chapter in Review

Certification Review

The elements of anesthesia coding include the following:

- Assignment of CPT codes
- Assignment of physical status modifiers
- Assignment of a qualifying circumstance code when appropriate
- Assignment of modifier codes as applicable
- Calculation of anesthesia time units
- Physical status modifiers describing the patient's presenting condition at the time of anesthesia
- Qualifying circumstance codes that indicate additional medical risks of morbidity and mortality, such as age, hypothermia, hypotension, or emergency surgery

Student Assignments

- Study Chapter 12.
- Review the Learning Objectives for Chapter 12.
- Review the Certification Review for Chapter 12.
- Complete the Chapter Review exercise to reinforce concepts learned in the chapter.
- Complete the Stop and Practice exercises in this chapter.

Chapter Review Exercise

Identify the correct anesthesia CPT codes for the following procedures.

Procedure	Anesthesia CPT Code
1. Cornea transplant	00144
2. Modified radical mastectomy	00404
3. Cesarean section	01961
4. Total hip replacement	01214
5. Femoral artery embolectomy	01274
6. Angioplasty	01920
7. Excision of cyst of humerus	01758
8. Knee arthroscopy	01382
9. Transurethral resection of the prostate	00914
10. Repair of hiatal hernia	00750
11. Excision benign lesion, face	00300
12. Reduction mammoplasty	00402
13. Repair deviated septum	00160
14. Cleft lip repair	00102
15. Esophagogastroduodenoscopy	00740
16. Liver transplant	00796
17. Lithotripsy	00872
18. Knee arthroplasty	01402
19. Tenodesis biceps tendon	01716
20. Closed reduction distal radial fixation	01820

Practical Application

Assign the correct CPT codes, all necessary modifiers, extenuating circumstances, and time units for coding the following services. Base units are typically assigned by the computerized billing system and therefore need not be calculated here.

1. An emergency appendectomy was performed on a 45-year-old patient with insulin-dependent diabetes that was not well controlled. The anesthesiologist began administration of general anesthesia at 10:00 AM and completed anesthesia services at 10:45 AM.

   Step 1: Identify CPT chapter/section __________

   Step 2: Identify anatomic heading __________

   Step 3: Identify body part or organ __________

   Step 4: Determine procedure performed __________

   Step 5: Determine procedure specifics __________

   Total time units __________

   Step 6: Assign modifier code(s) __________

   Step 7: Place in correct coding order __________

   Step 8: Assign modifier code(s) as appropriate __________

2. A 25-year-old patient was taken to the operating room for repair of a closed fracture to the radial shaft, which required manipulation by the orthopedic surgeon. Anesthesia administration began at 8:15 AM and was completed at 8:40 AM; surgical time was 25 minutes.

   Step 1: Identify CPT chapter/section __________

   Step 2: Identify anatomic heading __________

   Step 3: Identify body part or organ __________

   Step 4: Determine procedure performed __________

   Step 5: Determine procedure specifics __________

   Total time units __________

   Step 6: Assign modifier code(s) __________

   Step 7: Place in correct coding order __________

   Step 8: Assign modifier code(s) as appropriate __________

3. A 92-year-old female with the diagnosis of small bowel obstruction and severe systemic disease was taken to the operating room for repair and resection. Before completion of the resection, the patient became unstable as a result of her heart disease, and the procedure had to be terminated before completion. The abdomen was closed, and approximately 3 days later the patient was returned to the operation room for completion of the originally planned procedure.

   Original procedure anesthesia began at 7:00 AM and was terminated at 7:45 AM on 01/01/20xx. Completion of the procedure was performed on 01/04/20xx, with anesthesia administration beginning at 7:00 AM and concluding at 8:40 PM.

   Step 1: Identify CPT chapter/section __________

   Step 2: Identify anatomic heading __________

   Step 3: Identify body part or organ __________

   Step 4: Determine procedure performed __________

   Step 5: Determine procedure specifics __________

   Total time units __________

   Step 6: Assign modifier code(s) __________

   Step 7: Place in correct coding order __________

   Step 8: Assign modifier code(s) as appropriate __________

4. An 8-month-old child presented to the operating room for tonsillectomy and placement of PE tubes for tonsillitis and serous otitis media. The anesthesiologist arrived in the operating room suite at 7:00 AM; administration began at 7:10 AM and concluded at 7:55 AM.

   Step 1: Identify CPT chapter/section __________

   Step 2: Identify anatomic heading __________

   Step 3: Identify body part or organ __________

   Step 4: Determine procedure performed __________

   Step 5: Determine procedure specifics __________

Total time units: ______
Step 6: Assign modifier code(s) ______
Step 7: Place in correct coding order ______
Step 8: Assign modifier code(s) as appropriate ______

5. A 50-year-old male presented to the OR for repair of an incarcerated inguinal hernia. Induction of anesthesia began at 9:00 AM and ended at 9:45 AM.

Step 1: Identify CPT chapter/ section ______
Step 2: Identify anatomic heading ______
Step 3: Identify body part or organ ______
Step 4: Determine procedure performed ______
Step 5: Determine procedure specifics ______
Total time units: ______
Step 6: Assign modifier code(s) ______
Step 7: Place in correct coding order ______
Step 8: Assign modifier code(s) as appropriate ______

6. A 45-year-old female presented for diagnostic arthroscopic evaluation of the shoulder. On entering the shoulder compartment, the surgeon performed an arthroscopic rotator cuff repair. Anesthesia began at 10:00 AM and ended at 11:15 AM.

Step 1: Identify CPT chapter/ section ______
Step 2: Identify anatomic heading ______
Step 3: Identify body part or organ ______
Step 4: Determine procedure performed ______
Step 5: Determine procedure specifics ______
Total time units: ______
Step 6: Assign modifier code(s) ______
Step 7: Place in correct coding order ______
Step 8: Assign modifier code(s) as appropriate ______

7. A 75-year-old patient presented to the OR for an emergency laparoscopic cholecystectomy as a result of a ruptured gallbladder. The surgeon arrived at 8:00 AM, the anesthesiologist arrived at 8:15 AM, administration began at 8:30 AM, and the surgical procedure began at 8:45 AM with conclusion of both surgical and anesthetic services at 10:00 AM.

Step 1: Identify CPT chapter/ section ______
Step 2: Identify anatomic heading ______
Step 3: Identify body part or organ ______
Step 4: Determine procedure performed ______
Step 5: Determine procedure specifics ______
Total time units ______
Step 6: Assign modifier code(s) ______
Step 7: Place in correct coding order ______
Step 8: Assign modifier code(s) as appropriate ______

8. A patient arrived in the operative room with multiple injuries as the result of an automobile accident. An open reduction of a distal radial fracture was performed as well as open repair of a distal tibia–fibular fracture (patient is not Medicare).

Step 1: Identify CPT chapter/ section ______
Step 2: Identify anatomic heading ______
Step 3: Identify body part or organ ______
Step 4: Determine procedure performed ______
Step 5: Determine procedure specifics ______
Total time units ______
Step 6: Assign modifier code(s) ______
Step 7: Place in correct coding order ______
Step 8: Assign modifier code(s) as appropriate ______

9. A 79-year-old male presented to the operative suite for a cardiac catheterization with a balloon angioplasty performed. Anesthesia induction began at 7:00 AM and ended at 10:00 AM.

Step 1: Identify CPT chapter/section ______________

Step 2: Identify anatomic heading ______________

Step 3: Identify body part or organ ______________

Step 4: Determine procedure performed ______________

Step 5: Determine procedure specifics ______________

Total time units ______________

Step 6: Assign modifier code(s) ______________

Step 7: Place in correct coding order ______________

Step 8: Assign modifier code(s) as appropriate ______________

10. An 11-month-old child presented for insertion of ear tubes (tympanostomy). MAC was performed from 7:00 AM until 8:30 AM due to patient's age and history of seizures.

Step 1: Identify CPT chapter/section ______________

Step 2: Identify anatomic heading ______________

Step 3: Identify body part or organ ______________

Step 4: Determine procedure performed ______________

Step 5: Determine procedure specifics ______________

Total time units ______________

Step 6: Assign modifier code(s) ______________

Step 7: Place in correct coding order ______________

Step 8: Assign modifier code(s) as appropriate ______________

13

Surgery Services

LEARNING OBJECTIVES

After completing this chapter, the student will be able to:

- Know and apply the surgery coding guidelines.
- Understand and apply the bundled services guidelines for surgery coding.
- Comprehend the components of global surgery coding.
- Understand the medical complexity of specialty surgery services.
- Follow the usage and application of modifier codes in the surgery setting.
- Apply the surgery coding concepts to practical coding scenarios.

CODING REFERENCE TOOLS

Tool 13-1
Bundled Services Guidelines

Tool 13-2
Surgical Global Package Definitions

Tool 13-3
Surgery Coding Steps Process

Tool 13-4
Modifier 51/Modifier 59 Decision Tree

KEY TERMS

Only general surgical key terms are here. Specific medical terminology needed for each anatomic section is listed at the beginning of each review of systems.

-centesis

-ectomy

-orrhaphy

-ostomy

-otomy

-pexy

-plasty

Documentation Guidelines

SURGERY SERVICE CODES

Surgery documentation may represent the most complex part of *Current Procedural Terminology* (CPT) coding. In determining whether the services performed are indeed surgical in nature, the coder must review the procedure or operative note and decide whether the procedure was invasive, definitive, or restorative in nature. Many of the procedures contained in the surgery section would not, at first glance, appear to belong in there. Laypersons would think that only procedures performed in an operating room would be included. Procedures such as laceration repairs, lesion removals, application of casts or splints, colonoscopies, and other procedures, which would not appear significant, are also contained in the surgery section. Each of these procedures is invasive, definitive, or restorative in nature. For example, the application of a cast or splint is the prescribed medical protocol for a fracture and therefore would be considered the definitive procedure for the presenting problem.

General	10021-10022
Integumentary system	10040-19499
Musculoskeletal system	20000-29999
Respiratory system	30000-32999
Cardiovascular system	33010-37799
Hemic and lymphatic systems	38100-38999
Mediastinum and diaphragm	39000-39599
Digestive system	40490-49999
Urinary system	50010-53899
Male genital system	54000-55980
Female genital system	56405-58999
Maternity care and delivery	59000-59899
Endocrine system	60000-60699
Nervous system	61000-64999
Eye and ocular adnexa	65091-68899
Auditory system	69000-69990

Documentation for surgical procedures is often lengthy and contains many medical terms that must be interpreted to assign surgical codes correctly. For this reason, background or training in medical terminology will prove beneficial in the determination of exactly what procedures were performed as described in the operative report. In addition to the length and scope of the procedure reports, physicians often dictate the procedure they plan to perform at the beginning of the operative report; however, that is not necessarily indicative of the procedure(s) performed. The physician may include additional information in the operative report that may be coded in addition to the primary procedure. Descriptors often used by the physician in the operative note may not agree with coding principles that are applied in CPT code assignment.

For example, the surgeon dictates an operative report and indicates that a colonoscopy is performed. The operative note indicates that a colonoscopy was performed and two polyps were also removed by hot biopsy forceps during the procedure. If the coder assigns CPT codes based on the heading "colonoscopy," code 45378 would be assigned. It would be more appropriate to assign 45384, colonoscopy with removal of polyp(s), and would garner additional reimbursement for the surgeon or practice and facility. Another example would be the operative report that indicates a "complex closure" will be performed for a laceration of the arm. The term *complex* used by the surgeon, however, is not the standard for coding guidelines, which indicate *complex* must involve "more than a layered closure." The surgeon used the term *complex* perhaps because the laceration was large and required more time to suture. The code assignment should not be complex because the repair (CPT guidelines) is based on the following:

- Extent: simple, one layer; intermediate, two layers or one layer or debridement; complex, more than a layered closure
- Anatomic location
- Size (in centimeters)

In this instance, if the coder assigns CPT codes based on the physician's statement of "complex," the service would be coded too high and at audit the carrier would request money back.

Surgery coding is a perfect example of the many tasks of the office or surgical coder. As discussed in Chapter 1, the job of coder is not simply limited to reviewing reports and assigning codes. An integral part of any coder's job is education of the staff, including the physician or documenter(s) in the practice. Many physicians are not aware of the coding guidelines or the need for accurate and complete documentation so that appropriate codes for services may be assigned. Take the laceration example used previously; recall that one of the criteria for code assignment was size in centimeters. Note that the physician did not indicate the size in the opening header. In the event that size was not documented in the body of the operative note, the smallest size would have to be coded, thereby reducing the reimbursement significantly.

Adding to the complexity of interpreting the operative report is the fact that no physician dictates or documents in the same way. Even the same physician does not document identical procedures the same, so the coder must be equipped to read, interpret, query, and educate the physician AND assign the appropriate codes for correct reimbursement. The coder is integral to the success of a medical practice because he or she ensures correct reimbursement for services.

Look again at the surgery portion of Tool 9-1 (steps and components needed for CPT coding).

CPT CODING STEPS: SURGERY EXAMPLE

Step 1

Identify chapter	Definitive Restorative Invasive
Range of codes	10021-69990

Step 2

Determine type or location	Anatomic system Integumentary Respiratory

Step 3	
Specific type	Anatomic part Skin Finger
Step 4	
Specific procedure	Procedure information Excision Incision
Step 5	
Extent/specifics	Extent Size (in cm)

Steps 6 through 8 are discussed later.

A number of methods can be used to extract needed information from the operative report. The coder must be consistent; consistency in processing this information will make coding operative reports much easier.

Take a look at a sample operative report (Fig. 13-1) and decide what key words help determine the definitive, restorative, and invasive procedure(s) performed.

Some key guidelines need to be remembered when extracting key terms for this chart:

- Extract the key terms for the definitive, restorative, or invasive procedure only.
- Only other significant procedures that represent a significant additional procedure are coded.

CPT CODING STEPS

Type of Service	Surgery Examples	Chart Information
Step 1		
Identify chapter	Definitive Restorative Invasive	Definitive procedure(s) performed Chondroplasty
Range of codes	10021-69990	10021-69990
Step 2		
Determine type or location	Anatomic system Integumentary Respiratory	Musculoskeletal
Step 3		
Specific type	Anatomic part Skin Finger	Knee
Step 4		
Specific procedure information	Procedure Excision Incision	Arthroscopy
Step 5		
Extent/specifics	Extent arthroscopy, knee, diagnostic Size (in cm)	Arthroscopy, knee, chondroplasty

Keep in mind that many terms will be included in the operative report as well as significant information regarding the planned procedure, introduction of equipment, and the conclusion of the procedure. Most of this information will not be necessary for most surgical procedure coding. Until the student is comfortable with what to extract from the operative report, more than is necessary may be extracted and eliminated during the assignment of surgical procedure code(s).

Before attempting to review and extract key words from an operative report, a review of Chapter 1 may be appropriate. If you believe you need additional review of medical terms, acronyms, abbreviations, and other terms found in the operative reports, review Chapter 1 as appropriate.

Coding Guidelines

GLOBAL SERVICES

The global (package) concept of surgery was discussed in Chapter 9. A review of how this concept relates to surgical services is needed. Global surgical services represent the package concept, in which all preoperative, operative, and normal, uncomplicated, postoperative services are reimbursed under one CPT code.

It is imperative to keep this concept in mind when reading through the operative report. Remember that codes are assigned for definitive, restorative, and invasive procedures, not for the method of approach, anatomic structures that must be moved or incised, or anatomic structures that must be closed when the procedure is completed. Sometimes it will help to simply think about the procedure and what normally would occur to accomplish it.

For example, for a lesion to be excised (excision of lesion codes), it would be necessary to prepare the patient, cleanse the area, and make an incision (to excise the lesion). After the actual excision of the lesion, the incised area would require repair, possibly by suturing. All these services would be included in the excision of lesion code assignment. If it were necessary to perform additional services, such as a layered closure, however, that service would be codeable in addition to the excision of lesion code.

Individual guidelines for each subcategory in the surgery section are reviewed, and the guidelines are applied to some actual operative reports. Keep in mind that the operative reports contained in both the workbook and additional practice exercises are actual operative reports. In many cases, complete information has not been included, ambiguous statements are made, and there are discrepancies between the procedure in the top heading and the actual report. Unfortunately, this is why surgical coding can be challenging—there are few ideal operative reports. A good coder extracts the needed information, knows when to query (question) the physician, educates the documenter about information needed, and monitors the documentation process for needed improvements. This represents the difference between a satisfactory coder and an excellent asset to the practice.

OPERATIVE REPORT

Patient information:

Patient name:
DOB:
MR#:
Date of Procedure:

Preoperative diagnosis:

Internal derangement of left knee

Postoperative diagnosis:

Grade 4 chondromalacia medial femoral condyle
Chondromalacia of medial patellar facet grade 2

Procedure(s) performed:

Chondroplasty medial femoral condyle
Chondroplasty of patellofemoral joint

Chapter: Surgery Definitive/ Restorative
System: Musculoskeletal
Body part: Knee

Anesthesia:

General endotracheal

Assistant surgeon:

Specific Procedure: Arthroscopy

Description of procedure:

After induction of general anesthesia, the patient was prepped in the supine position, the extremity was prepped and draped in the usual manner. Through a lateral peripatellar stab wound, an arthroscope was inserted. A superior medial portal was made, and a medial parapatellar tendon portal was made for instrumentation. The retropatellar surfaces were significant for grade 2 chondromalacia which was debrided. The central ridge and lateral patellar facet were actually benign in appearance. The lateral compartment was intact. The meniscus was probed.

Repaired Cartilage: Chondroplasty

The medial compartment was significant for grade 4 chondromalacia with an open line undermined articular cartilage flap. This was debrided with shaver. There was no mensiscus tear. This comprised the majority of the weightbearing surfaces of the medial femoral condyle. After debriding this with a shaver, the instruments were removed. Wound was closed with Steri-strips, and compressive dressings were applied. Patient tolerated the procedure well and was taken to the recovery room in good condition.

Section: Surgery
System: Musculoskeletal
Body part: Knee
Procedure: Arthroscopy
Specific Procedure: Chondroplasty
29877

GODFREY REGIONAL HOSPITAL
123 Main Street • Aldon, FL 77714 • (407) 555-1234

FIGURE 13-1. Operative report for an arthroscopy.

SEPARATE PROCEDURE

CPT identifies some procedures as *separate procedure.* These codes should only be assigned when they are the only procedure performed on that anatomic site.

For instance, look at the operative report for the colonoscopy (Fig. 13-2). Assume that both a diagnostic colonoscopy (45378/separate procedure) and a colonoscopy with removal of polyp by snare (45385) were performed. Because there is a definitive procedure performed at the anatomic site (45385), code 45378 would not be used. The only time a separate procedure may be coded is when it is the only procedure. (A diagnostic colonoscopy with no definitive, invasive, or restorative procedures would be coded as 45378.)

ADD-ON PROCEDURES

Add-on codes are signified in CPT with the use of a plus sign (+). This symbol designates procedures performed in conjunction with a primary procedure. An add-on code without the primary procedure code should never be used.

EACH, EACH ADDITIONAL, PER PROCEDURES

When procedures are reported in CPT as "each," "each additional," or "per," multiple units of service should not be reported on several lines of the claim but should be calculated in units. For example, a split-thickness skin graft of the arm, 200 cm^2, would be coded as follows:

Code 15100	Split graft, trunk, arms, legs, first 100 sq cm or less
+Code 15101	Split graft, trunk, arms, legs, each additional 100 sq cm

Note the + add-on symbol in front of 15101; this code is "each additional" and would never be used without the code for the first 100 cm^2 (15100).

BUNDLED PROCEDURES

The other big challenge for surgery coders is determining whether services are included or bundled within the primary procedure. Procedures that are included or bundled are often referred to as *incidental procedures.* The complete description of the CPT manual often reveals this information. Some basic rules that the coder may follow when considering whether services are bundled are shown in Tool 13-1.

As previously mentioned, many excellent reference books and tools are available for determining bundled services. Check to see what coding books are available for specific specialties or general guidelines. In addition, review each third-party contract to determine guidelines regarding bundled services.

Correct Coding Initiative Guidelines

In addition to the guidelines outlined by CPT, additional guidelines further indicate what procedures are codeable and which are considered bundled. The following are general surgical guidelines for services that are considered bundled. Individual system guidelines are discussed later in this chapter.

BUNDLED SERVICES

- Administration of fluids or drugs during the operative period
- Anesthesia services (included in surgical procedure for Medicare)
- Biopsy performed after a procedure for evaluation
- Exposure and exploration of the surgical field
- Access through diseased tissue to the definitive surgical procedure
- Debridement of skin to repair a fracture
- Elimination of "incidental" other pathology in the removal, destruction, or other elimination of a lesion
- Excision or removal including incision or opening
- Procedure approach that fails (only the definitive or successful procedure may be reported)

SEPARATELY REPORTABLE SERVICES

- More invasive vascular access than usual administration of drugs or medicines
- Procedures such as insertion of central venous access devices
- Diagnostic biopsy when used to determine whether to proceed with another procedure
- When diagnostic endoscopy is used to determine whether to proceed with an open procedure, the endoscopic procedure is reportable if medical documentation substantiates the necessity for the diagnostic endoscopic procedure
- Treatment for underlying condition or an added course of treatment that is not part of the normal recovery from the surgical procedure
- Treatment for postoperative conditions that require return trips to the operating room

OPERATIVE REPORT

Patient information:

Patient name:
DOB:
MR#:
Date of Procedure: 01/04/XX
Surgeon: Dr. Smith

Preoperative diagnosis:

Screening colonoscopy

Postoperative diagnosis:

Diverticulosis of colon
Sigmoid polyp
Internal hemorrhoids

Procedure(s) performed:

Colonoscopy

Anesthesia:

RN sedation

Assistant surgeon:

Description of procedure:

The patient was brought to the Endoscopy suite and placed in the left lateral position. After he was connected to the ECG, blood pressure and pulse oximeter, IV sedation was given by IV Demerol and IV Versed. After adequate sedation was obtained, Xylocaine cream was used in the perirectal area. Rectal examination was performed.

Colonoscopy

The colonoscope was introduced through the rectum and passed all of the flexures into the cecum. Position in the cecum was identified by the ileocecal valve. The scope was withdrawn, visualizing all of the sites of the colon. The patient had some diverticulosis in the sigmoid colon. None of these were acutely inflamed. The patient had a small sessile polyp measuring 2–3 cm in the distal sigmoid. This was removed by snare technique. The scope was then retroflexed into the rectum. The patient had internal hemorrhoids and a small fibroepithelial polyp on the hemorrhoids. I did not remove it knowing that it was benign and I did not want to cause more bleeding from the hemorrhoids. The scope was withdrawn.

The patient tolerated the procedure well and was transferred to the Same Day Surgery Unit in stable condition.

Section: Surgery
System: Digestive disease
Body part: Rectum
Specific procedure: Endoscopy
Colonoscopy
Specifics: Polypectomy by snare
Code 45385

GODFREY REGIONAL HOSPITAL
123 Main Street • Aldon, FL 77714 • (407) 555-1234

FIGURE 13-2. Operative report for a colonoscopy.

TOOL 13-1

BUNDLED SERVICES GUIDELINES

1. Incidental procedures are considered *bundled.*

- If the procedure does not carry significant additional time, effort, and risk, the procedure is considered bundled. If the procedure does warrant additional consideration because of unusual circumstances, the use of a modifier is necessary along with an operative report explaining the additional complexities associated with the service that modified the service for additional consideration.

2 Surgical introduction/exploration performed in conjunction with a specified surgical procedure is considered bundled. For example, laparotomy performed in conjunction with the abdominal hysterectomy.

- In this example, the laparotomy is considered only the vehicle or approach by which the abdominal hysterectomy was performed. Therefore it is considered incidental or bundled, and may not be coded in addition to the primary procedure. However, when a laparotomy is performed independently for diagnostic purposes, the laparotomy may be coded and billed.
- A number of such procedures may be coded independently, but when used as the approach, they become bundled procedures.
- Before coding additional procedures through the same surgical incision, ask the question, "Is the procedure only the approach or vehicle by which the primary procedure was performed?"
- The rationale for "bundling" these services is that the third-party carrier should reimburse only once for the entire global procedure, which includes the pre-, post-, and operative procedures; that is, the preparation, incision, and repair or whatever services are performed during the operative session as a part of that reported service.

3 Normal supplies needed to perform the given procedure are included or bundled.

- When surgical procedures are performed in the provider's office, normal supply items are considered bundled. Hospital facilities bill according to their guidelines (discussed later).
- Surgical trays are allowed in addition to the procedure when billing certain procedures in the physician's office or outpatient setting as outlined by Centers for Medicare and Medicaid Services.

STOP AND PRACTICE

1. Develop a matrix of the most commonly performed procedures, services considered bundled, and what follow-up days are included so that surgical coding for services is consistent.
2. Develop such an outline specific to a particular practice and specialty (see Tool 13-1 for an example). This information will prove helpful in the coding of services.
3. It is also imperative to track the follow-up days in the practice for these procedures. After determining the appropriate number of follow-up days, post that information in a prominent place for the practice staff.

Many practices use a sticker on the front of the chart with the name of the procedure, the date of the procedure, and the time included for postoperative follow-up. Any procedures or services performed in this follow-up period will probably need a modifier to justify why they are NOT included in the global procedure.

Although the coder cannot expect the clerical and clinical staff to become coders, the inclusion of this information on the medical chart allows personnel to make certain that the coder is alerted to assign the appropriate modifier code. This is an excellent example of the staff education aspect of the coder's job.

Basic Layout

The surgery section of CPT is divided into anatomic sections in much the same way that ICD-9-CM is formatted. Within these subcategories the procedures are listed by anatomic site and by the performed procedure.

For example, in the integumentary subsection within the surgery section, the integumentary system is composed of skin and subcutaneous tissue, nails, and breasts. Different procedures within those sections may include incision, excision, introduction, repair, or reconstruction. Procedures vary from system to system. For instance, fractures and disloca-

TABLE 13-1 COMMON GLOBAL SURGICAL PROCEDURES

	Covered Assistant Surgeon Fee*		Global Follow-Up Days	
OBSTETRIC/GYNECOLOGIC PROCEDURE	**MEDICARE†**	**COMMERCIAL**	**MEDICARE**	**COMMERCIAL**
Laparotomy	Yes	No	90	45
Laparoscopy, diagnostic/with biopsy	Yes	Yes	10	15
Laparoscopy, other	Yes	No	90	15-45
Hysteroscopy	No	No	10	15
I/D Bartholin's	No	Yes	10	15
Excision Bartholin's cyst/gland	No	Yes	10	15
Vulvectomy	Yes	No	90	45
Colporrhaphy	Yes	No	90	15
Enterocele	Yes	No	90	15
D&C, nonobstetric	No	Yes	10	15
Total abdominal hysterectomy	Yes	No	90	90
Total abdominal hysterectomy with MMK	Yes	No	90	90
Vaginal hysterectomy	Yes	No	90	45
Ligation/transaction fallopian tube(s)	Yes	No	90	45
Salpingectomy	Yes	Yes	90	45
Treatment abortion	No	Yes	90	15

Intended as illustration only; verify and validate information for development of practice-specific specialty form(s).
*Assistant surgeon fee may be reimbursable when no qualified resident is available (specify).
†May also apply to third-party carriers following Medicare guidelines.
D&C, Dilation and curettage; *MMK,* Marshall-Marchetti-Krantz; *I/D,* incision and drainage.

tions is a category in the musculoskeletal system that would not be found in the integumentary system. Tool 13-3 outlines a detailed breakdown of the surgery chapter in the CPT book.

Keep in mind that the general layout of the CPT continues in the surgery section. Therefore when a code is listed flush with the left margin, all codes indented under that code pertain to part of all the definition of the main procedure.

Take a look at the knee arthroscopy codes, as follows:

29870	Arthroscopy, knee, diagnostic, with or without synovial biopsy (separate procedure)
29871	Arthroscopy, knee, surgical; for infection, lavage, and drainage
29873	with lateral release
29874	for removal of loose body or foreign body
29875	synovectomy, limited (separate procedure)
29876	synovectomy, major, two or more compartments

Code 29870 describes a diagnostic knee arthroscopy only. Synovial biopsy is considered incidental, or bundled, and therefore when performed in conjunction with a diagnostic knee arthroscopy, code 29870 would be assigned.

Note the "separate procedure" designation for 29870. As previously discussed, this indicator means that code 29870 would be assigned when only a diagnostic knee arthroscopy is performed. If surgical arthroscopic procedures are performed, the diagnostic arthroscopy would no longer be separate and therefore would be considered bundled.

When multiple procedures are performed that are not incidental or bundled, they would be reportable with a modifier 51 to indicate multiple procedures to the same anatomic site through the same approach.

EXAMPLE:
When arthroscopic lateral release of the knee is performed along with removal of a foreign body, the following code assignments would be appropriate:

29874-RT
29873-51-RT

Note that the modifier RT is also assigned to indicate the right knee. Also note that the procedures have been placed in the order of significance. In most instances, codes within the same subheading in the surgery section increase in significance. For instance, code 29874 is more significant than 29873. However, the coder should refer to the Resource-Based Relative Value Scale or other source for the actual value assigned to each code to make certain they are assigned in order of significance.

Modifiers

The surgery section of CPT has perhaps the most comprehensive listing of modifier codes describing the circumstances that fall outside the norm for global procedure concepts. The complex nature of surgery coding often requires appending

TOOL 13-2

SURGICAL GLOBAL PACKAGE DEFINITIONS

	CPT		MEDICARE	
Surgery category	Minor	Major (bundled)	Minor	Major (bundled)
	CPT surgical codes	All nonstarred CPT surgical codes	CPT Procedures and nonincision endoscopies	All nonstarred CPT surgical codes Except nonincision endoscopies
Preoperative care/ services	Visit allowed for new patients on same day or if significant services unrelated to surgery (use modifier[s])	Not defined	Not unless service is separately identifiable (use modifier)	Not allowed day of or day before surgery consultation or initial hospital care
Operative care/ surgery	Included	Included	Included	Included
Complications during surgery	Not defined	Not defined	Not defined	Not defined
Anesthetics (local, topical, digital)	Included	Included	Included	Included
Postoperative care/services	None, bill for follow-up visits	"Normal" only included	0-10 days (code-by-code basis)	90 days
Treatments for complications during postoperative period	Allowed	Allowed	Not allowed if code has 10-day follow-up and treatment during 10 days	Not allowed unless performed in *or*
Treatment-unrelated conditions during postoperative period	Billing allowed with use of proper modifiers	Billing allowed with use of proper modifiers	Billing allowed with use of proper modifiers	Billing allowed with use of proper modifiers

Definitions specifically for physician providing surgical services or other physicians providing a portion of the surgical global package.

more than one modifier code to the surgical procedure. In these instances it is important that the most significant modifier that affects reimbursement is listed first. Some carriers will allow up to two modifiers on the claim form, but others will only allow one. In those instances the code must assign modifier 99 with the procedure code, and then list the multiple modifiers in the correct order on the following line of the claim. A review of the modifiers applicable to the surgery section follows. These modifiers are applied to specific surgical cases throughout the chapter.

MODIFIER 22: UNUSUAL PROCEDURAL SERVICE

Modifier 22 describes the service as greater than that usually performed for the CPT code selected. A report is usually necessary to explain in detail the extensive service provided.

MODIFIER 26: PROFESSIONAL COMPONENT

Many services in the surgery, radiology, pathology, and medicine sections comprise two components for the total global procedure:

- Technical component—facility charge for equipment use, technician, supplies
- Professional component—charge for the professional interpretation and diagnosis of the service performed

When the physician supplies only the professional component of the global procedure, modifier 26 indicates that only this portion of service was provided and reimbursement is reduced. The facility providing the technical component bills for that service separately.

If the facility or provider codes this service incorrectly and the global component is reimbursed, the other provider receives a denial, indicating that reimbursement has already been made for this service.

TOOL 13-3

SURGERY CODING STEPS PROCESS

Step 1: Identify the Appropriate Chapter	
Surgery (definitive, restorative, invasive)	
Step 2: Identify Anatomic System	
Integumentary	10000-19999
Musculoskeletal	20000-29999
Respiratory	30000-32999
Cardiovascular	33000-39999
Digestive disease	40000-49999
Urinary system	50000-53999
Male genital	54000-55999
Female genital	56000-59999
Endocrine	60000-60699
Nervous	61000-64999
Eye/ocular adnexa	65000-68999
Auditory (ear)	69000-69999
Step 3: Identify Body Part	Code Range
(Example: Musculoskeletal/radius)	
Urinary/bladder	
Step 4: What Procedure	Code Range
Incision	
Introduction	
Amputation	
Scopy	
Excision	
Fracture/dislocation	
Arthrodesis	
Repair/reconstruction	
Identify key words:	
Step 5: Specific Information Regarding Procedure	Code Range
(Example: Musculoskeletal, radius, fracture, open, with, manipulation)	
Identify key words:	
Code assignment(s)/modifier(s):	

In addition, coding and billing for the global component when only the professional component was performed could be interpreted as fraud because the provider has billed and been paid for a service or a portion of a service that was not provided.

A good coding and billing technique is to identify services for which the provider does not have the ability to bill globally; this requires the use of modifier 26, which should be added to each of these procedure codes in the computerized billing system. This ensures that no one in the practice accidentally bills globally for professional services.

MODIFIER 32: MANDATED SERVICES

When surgical and diagnostic procedures listed in the surgery section are requested by a third party or a peer review organization, modifier 32 should be added. Reimbursement may not be considered in some instances without this modifier.

MODIFIER 47: ANESTHESIA BY SURGEON

When regional or general anesthesia is provided by the surgeon and not the anesthesiologist, modifier 47 should be added to the surgical procedure performed. The surgeon should use the codes in the surgery section. The anesthesiologist would not use this modifier or the surgery codes; the surgeon would not use the anesthesiology codes or modifiers.

MODIFIER 50: BILATERAL PROCEDURE

When procedures are performed bilaterally during the same operative session, modifier 50 should be added to the listing for this service. For this modifier to be used, the identical procedure must be performed on both the right and left sides. For instance, a closed fracture repair of the right distal radius is performed, and an open repair of the distal radius is performed on the left. Modifier 50 would not be appropriate because the exact procedure was NOT performed on both the left and right distal radii. Use of modifier 50 would also not be appropriate if the CPT descriptor is for more than one anatomic site, such as the repair of fractures of the right and left index fingers. The CPT descriptor is for phalanges and there are 10 fingers, so the use of the bilateral code would not be appropriate. In this instance, the level II modifiers FA to F9 from the Healthcare Common Procedure Coding System (HCPCS) would be used to identify the particular finger(s), but only if the carrier allows the use of HCPCS level II modifiers.

Two methods are used to attach the modifier to this service. In the first method, the surgical procedure code is listed alone and modifier 50 is added to the second procedure. In the second method, the code is listed only once with modifier 50 attached. The coder must determine which method is required by specific carriers.

Reimbursement for the second associated procedure is reduced because the preoperative and postoperative periods for both procedures have already been reimbursed in the primary procedure reimbursement.

MODIFIER 51: MULTIPLE PROCEDURES

Multiple procedures performed during the same operative session, typically through the same approach and in the same anatomic location, are coded with modifier 51. Make certain these additional procedures are not bundled or made a part of the global component of the primary procedure.

When subsequent procedures are billed with modifier 51, reduction is made on all subsequent procedures. Typically, the second procedure is reduced by 50%, with additional procedures reduced by 75%, to a maximum of four to six procedures reimbursed. CPT codes must be assigned correctly and listed in the correct order, with the most significant listed first.

Incorrect billing for these services has a dramatic effect on reimbursement. Look at the following scenario, which shows the correct and incorrect use of modifier 51.

Procedure code 58260	Charge $5000
Procedure code XXXXX	Charge $1500
Procedure code YYYYY	Charge $500

Correctly billed:

Code	Charge	Reimbursement
58260	$5000	$4000
XXXXX-51	$1500	$750 (reimbursed at ½)
YYYYY-51	$500	$125 (reimbursed at ¼)

Reimbursement amount: $4875

Incorrectly billed:

Code	Charged	Reimbursement
XXXXX	$1500	$1500
YYYYY-51	$500	$250 (reimbursed at ½)
58260-51	$5000 (¼)	$1250 (reimbursed at ¼)

Reimbursement amount: $3000

The total charge of the procedures is $7000. Correct coding results in a reimbursement of $4875 compared with the reimbursement of $3000 when procedures are incorrectly coded.

If multiple independent and distinct procedures are performed during the same operative session, they should be billed with modifier 59 instead.

MODIFIER 52: REDUCED SERVICES

When a portion of the usual service billed with the CPT code is eliminated or reduced, the coder must modify the surgical code with modifier 52. If the CPT descriptor is not met, it is necessary to assign an appropriate modifier to indicate why the global procedure was not performed. In some cases the facility may have performed only the technical component (as discussed with modifier 26) or the procedure was not completed according to the CPT descriptor. Modifier 52 would be appropriately appended to the CPT code. Reduction in reimbursement will probably result. A report may be requested to clarify the extent of services provided.

MODIFIER 53: DISCONTINUED PROCEDURE

When the physician decides to discontinue a procedure before completion, the coder must assign modifier 53. This modifier is *not* used for procedures that are electively cancelled before they are begun or that are terminated at the patient's request. Typically, this code is used for procedures that cannot be completed for medical reasons (e.g., a surgical procedure terminated because of the development of unstable blood pressure).

Make sure the physician reports all services performed, not just those completed. In the past, providers were not reimbursed for partial provision of service. Allowance is now made for that portion of the service completed before termination. Often, the most complex portion of the procedure may have been completed before termination, and the physician is reimbursed accordingly.

As previously discussed, a large number of the services listed in the surgical section of CPT are global package procedures that include both postoperative and preoperative periods. Because these services may encompass an extended period, circumstances arise in which the same physician does not provide the preoperative, postoperative, and surgical care. When this occurs, the following modifiers are appropriate.

MODIFIER 54: SURGICAL CARE ONLY

When only the surgical procedure itself is performed by the physician, that surgical procedure should be billed with modifier 54 appended. When these are global procedures, reimbursement is affected accordingly because other physicians will code and bill independently for the postoperative and preoperative components.

MODIFIER 55: POSTOPERATIVE MANAGEMENT ONLY

Modifier 55 is used when the physician provides only normal, uncomplicated postoperative care of the global surgical patient. This care is provided after a surgical procedure for a defined amount of time.

MODIFIER 56: PREOPERATIVE MANAGEMENT ONLY

Modifier 56 is used when the physician provides only preoperative care or services before the surgical procedure of the global package.

MODIFIER 57: DECISION FOR SURGERY

Modifier 57 is used primarily for evaluation and management services only, not for surgery services.

MODIFIER 58: STAGED OR RELATED PROCEDURE OR SERVICE BY SAME PHYSICIAN DURING POSTOPERATIVE GLOBAL PERIOD

For procedures to be considered as staged or related, they must meet the following criteria:

- Be planned at the time of the original procedure
- Be more extensive than the original procedure
- Provide therapy after diagnostic surgical procedure

An example of this is a simple fracture repair that must be repeated on a more complex level. Keep in mind that when a surgical procedure is performed, the insurance carrier will disallow additional payment for other services if it is unable to determine whether that service is "over and above" the usual postoperative care. Remember that most insurance claims are being scanned and interpreted by computer, and computers are not programmed to interpret medical care and standards of care. Without an appropriate modifier code, services performed during the postoperative period that should be given additional consideration may be disallowed or denied.

MODIFIER 59: DISTINCT PROCEDURAL SERVICE

When a procedure is performed on the same day as other surgical services but is independent and distinct, modifier 59 should be used. This modifier distinguishes the service as independently performed. An example is a surgical session in which repairs of a fractured wrist and fractured femur are performed. Two separate surgical approaches are necessary, requiring a complete and separate description of the medical complexity of two different operations on the same patient during a single surgical session.

Use of modifier 59 is distinct from that of modifier 51 (multiple procedures) in that the procedures are separate and are performed independently. Modifier 51 indicates multiple procedures have been performed by the same approach and in the same anatomic location. For this reason reimbursement for services coded with modifier 59 should be similar to that given when procedures are performed independently.

NOTE: CPT notes that modifier 59 should be used only when no other modifier is appropriate.

Modifiers 51 and 59 are perhaps the most difficult to distinguish from each other; Tool 13-4 represents a decision tree that may assist in the correct selection of these modifier codes.

MODIFIER 62: TWO SURGEONS

When one specific surgical procedure requires the expertise of two skilled surgeons, modifier 62 is attached to both claims by each of the surgeons. Typically, the two physicians have different skills, which are required for completion of the surgical procedure. Reimbursement to each participating physician is affected proportionately, with the sum of the reimbursements usually not exceeding 125% of the total usual allowance for the service.

Care should be taken to include this modifier when coding for services performed in cooperation with another surgeon. Without the proper use of this modifier, one surgeon will be reimbursed 100% of the allowance for services, and the other will receive denial for services because payment has already been made to another provider. For this error to be corrected, the original submission must be amended and a refund made to the carrier of the amount(s) paid so that each physician can be paid correctly. The two surgeons SHOULD NOT correct this error simply by "dividing" the reimbursement from the carrier because the tax records for the original submitting physician will reflect monies paid to him or her, and he or she will be taxed accordingly. For example, for cochlear implant surgery that requires both an ear-nose-throat and neurosurgeon skills, both physicians must use the same cochlear implant surgical code with modifier 62 on both claims.

MODIFIER 63: PROCEDURE PERFORMED ON INFANTS LESS THAN 4 KG

When surgical procedures are performed on infants weighing less than 4 kg, modifier 63 should be appended. This modifier applies only to procedures listed in the surgical section (10000-64999) and should not be appended to procedures on evaluation and management services in other sections of CPT.

TOOL 13-4

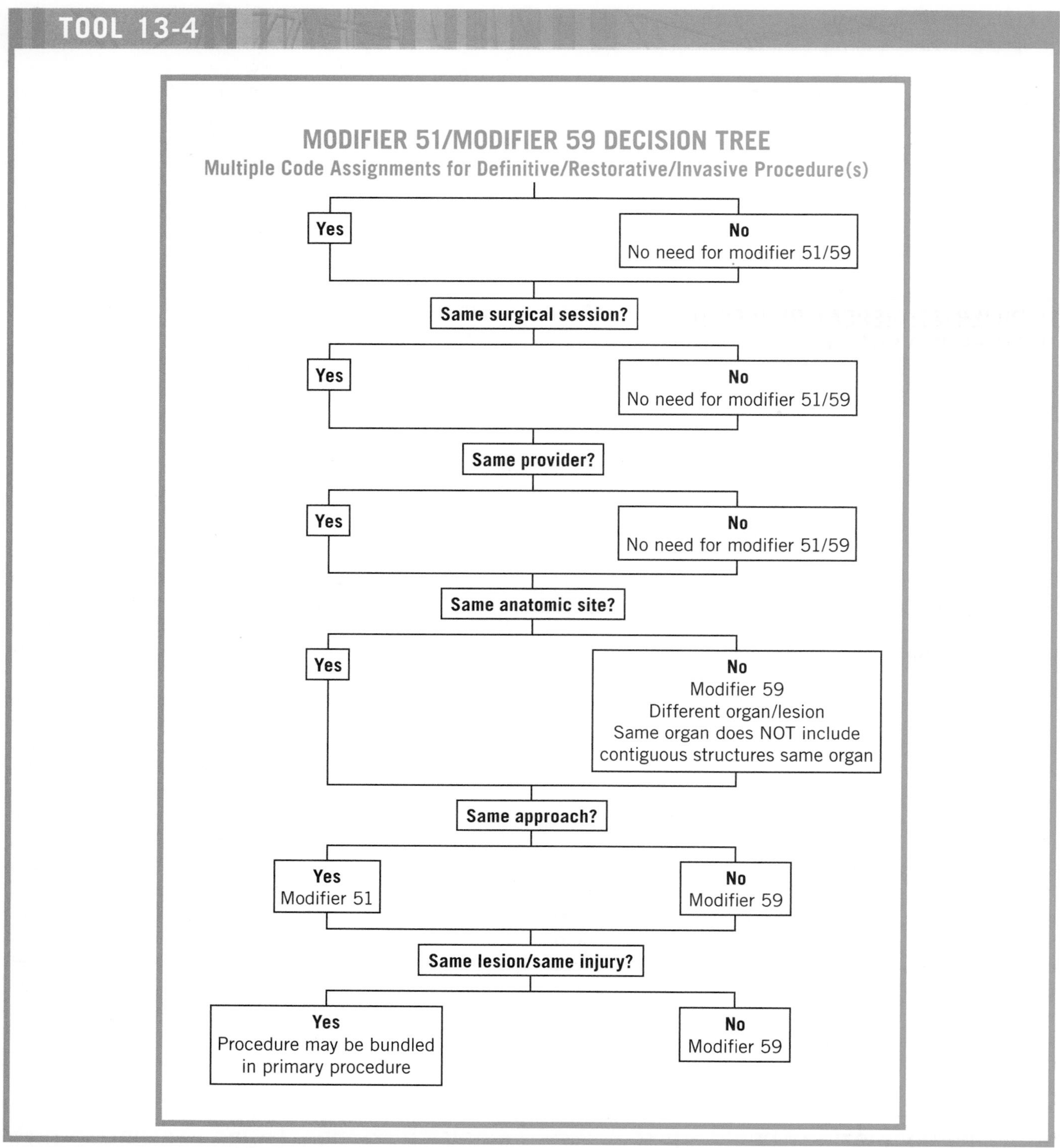

MODIFIER 66: SURGICAL TEAM

When the skills of multiple physicians (more than two) and the skills of highly technical personnel, as well as complex surgical equipment, are involved in a surgical procedure the services should be billed with modifier 66 attached (e.g., organ transplant requiring multiple surgeons for harvesting and transplanting and a multitude of personnel comprising the transplant team).

MODIFIER 76: REPEAT PROCEDURE, SAME PHYSICIAN

When procedures are repeated by the same physician, modifier 76 must be added to distinguish them from duplicate or misbilled items. For example, multiple electrocardiograms (ECGs) on the same day are required for a patient with a cardiac disorder to determine the progression or resolution of the problem. If these multiple ECGs are billed without the use of modifier 76 on subsequent ECGs, they will be denied as duplicate services.

MODIFIER 77: REPEAT PROCEDURE, ANOTHER PHYSICIAN

When procedures are repeated by another physician, subsequent services must be submitted with modifier 77 attached.

MODIFIER 78: RETURN TO THE OPERATING ROOM FOR RELATED PROCEDURE DURING POSTOPERATIVE GLOBAL PERIOD

When it is necessary for a patient to return to surgery during the global postoperative period for a procedure related to the original procedure, those subsequent procedure(s) must be billed with modifier 78 attached. Make certain when assigning this modifier code that the original procedure was performed in the operating room and that the subsequent procedure falls within the postoperative period.

MODIFIER 79: UNRELATED PROCEDURE OR SERVICE, SAME PHYSICIAN DURING GLOBAL OR POSTOPERATIVE PERIOD

When a patient is in the normal, uncomplicated postoperative follow-up period and an additional service or procedure that is found in the surgery section of CPT is needed, modifier 79 should be appended to that service. An example is the patient who has had a fracture reduction and now requires repair of a hernia. The same general surgeon performs both operations. Modifier 79 is appended to the second procedure to signify to the carrier that the two procedures are unrelated and should be considered independently. Keep in mind that the use of modifiers to indicate unrelated, related, or staged care during the postoperative period apply only to the original surgeon and practice. Other physicians not associated with the surgeon or surgeon's practice are not excluded from payment during the postoperative period for services performed, and these modifiers should be appended for payment consideration.

When an assistant surgeon is required for the performance of a surgical service, one of the following modifiers should be attached to the assistant surgeon's service. Assistant surgeon fees are reimbursed at a significantly lower amount than those of the primary surgeon. Typically, insurance carriers reimburse this service at an average of 10% to 20% of the original allowance.

Insurance carriers differ regarding criteria for the medical necessity of an assistant surgeon in certain procedures. The coder may want to gather this information from the various carriers with whom the provider contracts and incorporate it into the third-party contract worksheet (discussed later).

MODIFIER 80: ASSISTANT SURGEON

When an assistant surgeon bills for services, the same surgical procedure submitted by the primary surgeon should be used. Care should be taken to distinguish between two surgeons and assistant surgeons services. When the second surgeon provides skilled services specific to his or her specialty, these services are coded as two surgeons. A second surgeon who provides no additional skills but simply assists would be coded as an assistant surgeon.

In many instances the second surgeon may be requested to "stand by" in the event that his or her skills are needed. If those specialty skills are not needed and that surgeon chooses, or is requested, to participate in the operation, the services must be coded as assistant surgeon.

There is a significant difference in the reimbursement of assistant surgeon services and two surgeon services. Typically, the reimbursement for assistant surgery codes is approximately 10% to 20% of the allowance for the primary surgical charge. Reimbursement for two surgeons is approximately 50% to 65% for each physician of the allowance for the specified surgery code.

MODIFIER 81: MINIMUM ASSISTANT SURGEON

When minimal services are required from the assistant surgeon, the use of modifier 81 is appropriate. Many insurance carriers do not recognize modifier 81 and request that if an assistant surgeon is necessary, then modifier 80 (assistant surgeon) or 82 (assistant surgeon when qualified resident surgeon not available) should be used. Each third-party carrier should have this information available. The coder may wish to incorporate this information into the third-party contract coding worksheet, discussed in Chapter 19.

MODIFIER 82: ASSISTANT SURGEON WHEN QUALIFIED RESIDENT SURGEON IS NOT AVAILABLE

When the participation of an assistant surgeon is necessary because a qualified resident surgeon is not available, the use of modifier 82 is appropriate. This may occur at facilities in which residents are not available or are available only during certain hours. Because the third-party carrier is not aware of the circumstances or availability of residents at facilities, this information (lack of qualified residents) should be documented in the operative records of both the assistant surgeon and the primary surgeon.

MODIFIER 90: REFERENCE (OUTSIDE LABORATORY)

When laboratory procedures are billed and reported but are performed by another party, such as a clinical laboratory facility, the service must be coded with modifier 90 attached. Note that laboratory services may not be billed to Medicare intermediaries unless the billing entity also provides those services; therefore modifier 90 is not appropriate for any laboratory services for Medicare patients.

The purpose of this modifier is to declare that the provider is billing for services even though financial arrangement has been made with a third-party laboratory that will perform these services. In the event the third-party laboratory erroneously bills for these services as well, modifier 90 indicates what the financial arrangement is and that the provider should be paid for the services.

MODIFIER 99: MULTIPLE MODIFIERS

When two or more modifiers are necessary to adequately describe provided services, the use of modifier 99 is attached to the billed CPT code. This is followed by a list of the multiple modifiers applicable for that service. It may be accomplished on the face of the claim form or by attachment of an explanation to the claim.

Modifier 99 is frequently necessary in billing appropriately for surgical services because many of these services require the use of multiple modifiers to describe unusual procedural circumstances. For example, a surgeon performs a secondary procedure that requires the use of modifier 51, and the surgeon discontinues it because of a problem with the stabilization of the patient, which requires modifier 53. The secondary procedure should be billed with the attachment of modifier 99 to indicate that multiple unusual circumstances occurred and must be considered for payment. These multiple circumstances may be described on an attachment as with the modifiers 51 and 53, or they may be listed on the face of the claim.

NOTE: Medicare allows coding with a maximum of two modifiers without the use of modifier 99. These would be listed following the CPT code as follows:

CPT code-modifier 1/modifier 2

58260-51/80

Now that the general guidelines and principles for coding surgical services have been discussed and surgical modifier codes have been reviewed, basic rules for coding surgical procedures with CPT codes should be reviewed. These rules follow many of the same guidelines presented in previous chapters of this text but they also encompass some specific guidelines for surgery.

Because these modifiers are so crucial to correct payment for surgical services, take a minute to identify the correct modifier code(s) needed for the following scenarios. If none is needed, indicate "None." Surgical codes at this point have not yet been reviewed, so it is not necessary to assign the appropriate CPT code.

STOP AND PRACTICE

Assign modifiers as appropriate.

Surgical Scenario	Modifier(s)
1. Patient presents for hernia repair and removal of lesion of the face.	________
2. Patient presents for knee arthroscopy and shoulder arthroscopy.	________
3. Patient presents for multiple laceration repairs.	________
4. Patient presents for esophagogastroduodenoscopy (EGD); the scope cannot be advanced to the duodenum.	________
5. Patient has repair or removal of nail due to ingrown nail.	________
6. Patient has knee arthroscopy with arthroscopic lateral release and medial and lateral meniscectomy.	________
7. Patient had fracture repair with application of cast previously and now returns for replacement cast.	________
8. Patient has fracture of femur with preoperative and surgical care provided by surgeon at local hospital. Returns home for postoperative care only.	________
9. Closed reduction of tibia/fibular fracture was performed; however, it was necessary for the patient to return to the operating room and for the physician to perform an additional procedure to correct the defect.	________
10. Closed reduction of a distal radius fracture with application of cast was performed in the emergency department. Patient now returns for additional surgical intervention. The patient is taken to the operating room where an open reduction of the same fracture is performed.	________

Now that all the general concepts, layout, and steps in identifying components of the operative report have been discussed, it is time to take a look at the remaining steps of the coding process for the surgery section.

Steps in Coding from the Surgery Section

A basic review of the steps for coding surgical procedures is found in Tool 13-3. Details of these steps follow.

The coder should have the surgical (operative or procedure) report available for review. If the physician provides vague or inaccurate information, it may be billed incorrectly and the coder, provider, and others involved may be liable for services billed and not performed. The physician may indicate on the billing card or information sheet only performed services that he or she believes should be billable. When the coder reviews the surgical or operative report, he or she may often find additional billable and codeable services.

Step 1: Identify Chapter or Section of CPT

All the procedures discussed in this chapter are from the surgery section of the CPT. They are defined as definitive, restorative, or invasive (or all three) in nature.

Step 2: Identify the System

- Integumentary
- Musculoskeletal
- Respiratory
- Cardiovascular
- Hematologic and lymphatic
- Digestive
- Urinary
- Male genital
- Female genital
- Maternity care and delivery
- Endocrine
- Nervous
- Eye and ocular adnexa
- Auditory system

By identifying the appropriate system on which the procedure was performed, the coder has eliminated a large portion of codes from the surgery section of the CPT. Background or training in medical terminology and anatomy and physiology is important in determining this information. Refer to Table 9-1, which identifies body systems and specific components of each system if necessary.

STOP AND PRACTICE

Identify the appropriate system for each of the following surgical procedures.

Surgical Procedure	Anatomic System
1. Excision malignant lesion	________
2. Arthroscopic knee meniscectomy	________
3. Modified radical mastectomy	________
4. Transurethral resection of the prostates (TURP)	________
5. Vasectomy	________
6. Open reduction internal fixation (ORIF), distal radius	________
7. Laceration repair	________
8. Three-vessel coronary artery bypass graft (CABG)	________
9. Endoscopic ethmoidectomy	________
10. Vaginal hysterectomy	________

Step 3: Identify the Anatomic Site

After identifying the anatomic system, the coder must determine the anatomic site or part the procedure is being performed on. Keep in mind that the coding process is a "breaking down" process. With the procedure identified as invasive, restorative, or definitive, the other chapters of the CPT book have been eliminated. When the system has been identified, the code has eliminated all the other subsections in the surgery section. Care should be taken so that when the correct categories or breakdowns are chosen, the codes are found only in that section. Once the coder ventures outside the categories determined as appropriate, the codes will probably be incorrect. When using this process, the coder will often find that the breakdown process takes one and only one code—*the right code.*

STOP AND PRACTICE

Take the same surgical procedures as in the previous Stop and Practice exercise and determine step 3 for each procedure.

	Anatomic System	Anatomic Site
1. Excision malignant lesion	________	________
2. Arthroscopic knee meniscectomy	________	________
3. Modified radical mastectomy	________	________
4. TURP	________	________
5. Vasectomy	________	________
6. ORIF, distal radius	________	________
7. Laceration repair	________	________
8. Three-vessel CABG	________	________
9. Endoscopic ethmoidectomy	________	________
10. Vaginal hysterectomy	________	________

Step 4: Identify the Approach or Procedure Performed

From the operative report, the coder must determine whether the definitive, restorative, or invasive procedure was incision, excision, introduction, manipulation, repair, reconstruction, fracture repair, or correction of dislocation. Just because the procedure required an incision does not mean the code will come from the incision category. If the procedure is an excision of a lesion, for instance, the approach is the incision. The definitive procedure is "excision," so the code is located in the excision section.

If a scope such as an arthroscope is inserted for diagnostic purposes and before the conclusion of the case, a surgical intervention is performed and the diagnostic scope will not be assigned a code.

STOP AND PRACTICE

For each surgical procedure provided, list the anatomic system, part, and approach or procedure. Refer to the list of body systems used previously and feel free to review some of the headings (e.g., incision, excision, arthrodesis, repair, fracture) that appear in the surgery section of CPT.

Surgical Procedure	Anatomic System	Anatomic Part	Approach or Procedure
1. Excision malignant lesion	________	________	________
2. Arthroscopic knee meniscectomy	________	________	________
3. Modified radical mastectomy	________	________	________
4. TURP	________	________	________
5. Vasectomy	________	________	________
6. ORIF, distal radius	________	________	________
7. Laceration repair	________	________	________
8. Three-vessel CABG	________	________	________
9. Endoscopic ethmoidectomy	________	________	________
10. Vaginal hysterectomy	________	________	________

Step 5: Determine Extent and Specifics of Procedure

The surgical or operative report should indicate the extent of the procedure, such as whether the procedure was simple, complex, closed, or open. If this is not documented, the assumption must be made of minimal service for that procedure. Consider the following example:

Laceration repair, thumb

If the extent is not documented, then the example would be billed as a "simple" repair, less than 2.5 cm. Infact, the services may be complex and involve a 5.0-cm laceration, a substantial difference in the amount of reimbursement.

STOP AND PRACTICE

Take the following excerpts from actual surgical reports and extract the information that will be needed to correctly assign CPT codes for the services performed. These same exercises will be used to complete the coding process below.

Following is an example:

1. PREOPERATIVE DIAGNOSIS: Bilateral heel decubiti
   POSTOPERATIVE DIAGNOSIS: Bilateral heel decubiti
   PROCEDURE: Debridement of bilateral heel decubiti to muscle
   ANESTHESIA: None
   BLOOD LOSS: Minimal

   CLINICAL HISTORY: The patient is an 89-year-old white female who presents with bilateral heel decubiti. She continues to have some necrotic debris and nonviable tissue. She presents for elective debridement.

   DESCRIPTION OF PROCEDURE: She was brought to ambulatory care and placed in the right lateral decubitus position. Both heels were sprayed with Betadine and sterilely draped. We excised all the nonviable tissue underneath with good bleeding. We had to go down to muscle. She tolerated the procedure well. Plan is to continue the collagenase dressing and follow up in 2 weeks.

   Step 1: Identify chapter or section of CPT: Surgery
   Step 2: Identify anatomic system: integumentary

   Debridement was performed to the skin, down to the muscle

   Step 3: Identify anatomic part: skin
   Step 4: Identify procedure or approach: debridement, skin
   Step 5: Identify additional specifics regarding procedure: Performed to both heels, down to muscle

   Provide the information needed to code the remaining scenarios as well.

2. PREOPERATIVE DIAGNOSIS: Right breast cancer
   POSTOPERATIVE DIAGNOSIS: Right breast cancer
   OPERATION: Right simple mastectomy
   ANESTHESIA: General endotracheal
   ANESTHESIOLOGIST: Dr. X
   FINDINGS: A 2-cm mass a 2 o'clock

   PROCEDURE: Patient was placed on the operating room table in the supine position. After general anesthesia was induced, the patient was prepped and draped in routine sterile fashion. An elliptical transverse incision was made around the right breast, including the nipple, to the level of the anterior ancillary line. Both superior and inferior skin flaps were raised with sharp dissection. Hemostasis was achieved with 3-0 and 2-0 silk ties.

   After the flaps were raised, the breast was then taken off the pectoralis muscles, including the pectoralis fascia. After the breast was completely removed from medial to lateral, hemostasis was again achieved with 2-0 and 3-0 silk sutures. Two Jackson–Pratt drains were placed beneath the skin flaps, and the skin flaps were anchored down to the chest wall using 2-0 chromic sutures.

   The Jackson–Pratt drains were then brought out through separate stab wounds in the inferolateral aspect of the wound. The skin edges were then approximated with 3-0 silk interrupted sutures. A dry sterile dressing was placed, and the patient was taken to the recovery room in stable condition.

   Step 1: Identify chapter or section of CPT: Surgery
   Step 2: Identify anatomic system: ________________
   Step 3: Identify anatomic part: ________________
   Step 4: Identify procedure: ________________
   Step 5: Identify additional specifics or approach regarding procedure: ________________

3. PREOPERATIVE DIAGNOSIS: Radius and ulnar shaft fracture
   POSTOPERATIVE DIAGNOSIS: Same
   PROCEDURE: Closed manipulative reduction, percutaneous pin fixation

   INDICATIONS: The patient is a 12-year-old who sustained left forearm fractures in both bones 3 days ago. A grade I open fracture was treated with superficial debridement and oral antibiotics. Radiographs confirmed transverse fracture mid shaft, radius, and ulna with significant angulation.

   PROCEDURE: With the patient adequately anesthetized under general anesthesia, the left upper extremities were prepped and draped in a sterile manner. Image intensifier was used to visualize the unreduced fracture. A small longitudinal incision was made over the radial aspect of the radial styloid just proximal to the growth plate. Soft tissue was retracted, and a drill hole was placed with a 3.2 drill bit through the radial aspect of the cortex. The drill was then directed proximally to elongate the entry hole. A

STOP AND PRACTICE—cont'd

Synthes flexible titanium nail was contoured and then inserted; this was driven proximally across the fracture site as reduction was performed. This was left about a centimeter short of final resting place. The second incision was made over the more radial aspect of the olecranon. Drill hole was then placed in the olecranon and a flexible titanium nail was introduced and driven proximal, as the fracture was reduced. The nail was ultimately advanced across the fracture and left about 1 cm short of its desired final resting place. Both pins were clipped near the skin surface and a driver used to advance them proximally 1 cm to the final resting point. Image intensification revealed anatomic alignment and position, with pins at the appropriate length. It was definitively ascertained that the radial pin was indeed proximal to the growth plate. The wounds were closed with interrupted suture of 4-0 nylon, sterile bulky dressing, and a well-padded long arm splint was applied. The patient tolerated the procedure well and was stable on transport to the recovery room.

Step 1: Identify chapter or section of CPT: Surgery
Step 2: Identify anatomic system: ______________
Step 3: Identify anatomic part: ______________
Step 4: Identify procedure: ______________
Step 5: Identify additional specifics/approach regarding procedure: ______________

4. PREOPERATIVE DIAGNOSIS: Left shoulder pain with possible biceps tendon tear
POSTOPERATIVE DIAGNOSIS: Biceps tendon tear, degenerative labral tear, rotator cuff tear
OPERATIVE PROCEDURES: Diagnostic arthroscopy, shoulder; biceps tenotomy; debridement labral tearing; arthroscopic rotator cuff repair; subacromia decompression/acromioplasty
PROCEDURE: Patient is taken to the operating room and after general anesthesia the left upper extremity is examined. The portal sites as well the subacromial bursa were injected with Marcaine. Standard diagnostic arthroscopy was performed. Posterior labrum and superior labrum were noted to have significant degenerative fraying and tearing. Rotator cuff was noted as torn. The undersurface was debrided back with arthroscopic shaver. Bursa was resected and cuff tear was identified. A 5-mm Arthrex corkscrew suture anchor was placed with two suture arms attached. Viper suture retriever was used to put both arms through the cuff and retractor held cuff in position while sutures were tied.
Subsequent acromioplasty was performed. No evidence of impingement was noted. Patient's shoulder was irrigated copiously and drained. Wounds were closed with Biosyn and Steri-Strips.
Step 1: Identify chapter or section of CPT: Surgery
Step 2: Identify anatomic system: ______________
Step 3: Identify anatomic part: ______________
Step 4: Identify procedure: ______________
Step 5: Identify additional specifics/approach regarding procedure: ______________

5. PREOPERATIVE DIAGNOSIS: Presyncope with intermittent junctional bradycardia
POSTOPERATIVE DIANOGSIS: Same
OPERATION: Dual-chamber DDD transvenous pacemaker placement
PACEMAKER GENERATOR Pacesetter Model 2010T
SETTINGS: Bipolar leads: Atrial: pulse width 0.6 msec. Sensitivity 1 mV. Pulse amplitude 4 volts. Refractory period 275 msec.
Ventricular bipolar lead: Pulse width 0.6 msec. Sensitivity 2 mV. Pulse amplitude 4 volts. Refractory period 250 msec.
Pacemaker mode: DDD. Rate 70 pulses per minute. AV delay: 155 msec.
Lead threshold: Atrial lead model P452PBV. Threshold 0.45 volts at 0.6 mA. Pulse width 0.6 msec. P-wave amplitude 3 mV. Lead impedance 490 ohm.
Ventricular lead: Bipolar lead model 10167. Threshold 0.7 volts with 0.8 mA at pulse width of 0.6 msec. R-wave amplitude 14.5 mV. Lead impedance 750 ohm.
OPERATION: The patient was prepped and draped in the usual manner. Using sedation and 1% Xylocaine anesthesia, an infraclavicular incision was made. The pocket was carried down to the fascia and placed subfascially. Then the subclavian vein was located with a needle and a guide wire placed into the vein. Two introducers were placed over this wire, and the atrial and ventricular leads were placed into the superior vena cava. Then the atrial lead was put into place and the leads screwed in. The ventricular lead was placed in the ventricular apex.
Thresholds were measured as obtained and found to be adequate. The lead was checked for length on fluoroscopy and then attached into the pocket around a collar with a 2-0 silk suture. Then the leads and generator were connected together and the pacemaker placed into the pocket.
Step 1: Identify chapter or section of CPT: Surgery
Step 2: Identify anatomic system: ______________

STOP AND PRACTICE—cont'd

Step 3: Identify anatomic part: ________________
Step 4: Identify procedure: ________________
Step 5: Identify additional specifics/approach regarding procedure: ________________

6. PREOPERATIVE DIAGNOSIS: Status post–multiple endoscopic polypectomies
POSTOPERATIVE DIAGNOSIS: Internal and external hemorrhoids, sigmoid diverticulosis, multiple benign sigmoid polyps
PROCEDURE: Flexible colonoscopy with multiple electrocauterization polypectomies
Patient, under sedation, was placed on the table in left lateral position. Fiberoptic flexible video colonoscopy was introduced through the anal canal. There was a minimal degree of prolapsed hemorrhoids. Scope was passed through the rectum into the sigmoid colon. At the proximal rectum and distal sigmoid colon, multiple tiny benign-appearing polyps were detected. These were biopsied and then electrocauterized to totally remove them. Scope was then passed through the sigmoid into the descending colon, splenic flexure, transverse colon, hepatic flexure, ascending colon, and cecum. Bowel prep was excellent. No additional polyps were identified during the procedure.
The scope was removed, and the patient tolerated the procedure well.
Step 1: Identify chapter or section of CPT: Surgery
Step 2: Identify anatomic system: ________________
Step 3: Identify anatomic part: ________________
Step 4: Identify procedure: ________________
Step 5: Identify additional specifics/approach regarding procedure: ________________

7. PREOPERATIVE DIAGNOSIS: Bilateral inguinal hernias and umbilical hernia
POSTOPERATIVE DIAGNOSIS: Bilateral inguinal hernias and umbilical hernia
PROCEDURE PERFORMED: Laparoscopic repair of bilateral inguinal hernias with mesh, open umbilical hernia repair
INDICATION FOR PROCEDURE: The patient is a 64-year-old white male who was referred to my clinic for evaluation and treatment of bilateral inguinal hernias. At that time he was found to have an umbilical hernia. The procedure for repair was explained to the patient with risks and benefits, questions were answered, and consents were signed.
FINDINGS AND CHIEF COMPONENTS: The patient was taken to the operating room prepped and draped in the usual sterile fashion and placed in the supine position with the arm extended. General anesthesia and endotracheal intubation was provided as per the anesthesiology department. A Foley catheter was placed sterilely.
A 1-cm infraumbilical semilunar incision was made, and dissection was carried down to the level of the anterior rectus fascia using Bovie cautery. The fascia was grasped on either side using Kochers and a number 0 Vicryl stitch was placed on either side. The fascia was opened sharply. A Kelly clamp was run through the pubic symphysis without any difficulty. The balloon dilator was placed and inflated to the appropriate level bilaterally. There was minimal bleeding. The balloon was removed, and the scope was introduced. Insufflation was obtained to the appropriate level.
The right inguinal hernia was addressed first. There was a large direct component and a small indirect component to a pantaloon hernia. These were taken down without any disruption of the peritoneal cavity. A Bard medium right mesh was placed without difficulty and tacked minimally to the anterior abdominal wall using the superior edge of the mesh only. The hernia sac was placed on top of the mesh and held in place.
The left inguinal hernia was addressed. The patient was found to have a very large indirect hernia, which was reduced without difficulty. The hernia sac was taken down without difficulty. A Bard medium left mesh was placed without any difficulty. Again, it was tacked in a similar fashion as the right side. Holding the hernias on top of the mesh, the preperitoneal space was deflated without difficulty. The testicles were palpated and found to be in the appropriate area.
The umbilical hernia was then addressed. This was done in an open fashion. The hernia sac was dissected free of the surrounding tissue, excised, and sent for specimen. A small defect was found in the midline just below the umbilicus. This was cleaned up, and a 0 Vicryl suture was run approximately three times and tied off. The umbilicus was reconnected to the anterior abdominal wall using a 3-0 Vicryl single stitch. The stay sutures on the anterior rectus fascia from the laparoscopic procedure were then closed without any difficulty. The skin was closed with a 4-0 running subcuticular stitch, Steri-Strips, and Band-Aid. All incisions were anesthetized with approximately 3 mL of 0.5% Marcaine in total.

STOP AND PRACTICE—cont'd

The patient tolerated the procedure well. The Foley catheter was removed without difficulty. The patient had clear yellow urine with no change in characteristic throughout the procedure. He was extubated and sent to the recovery room in good condition. He is expected to make an uneventful recovery. He will be discharged and followed up in my clinic within the next week or two.

Step 1: Identify chapter or section of CPT: Surgery
Step 2: Identify anatomic system: ______________
Step 3: Identify anatomic part: ______________
Step 4: Identify procedure: ______________
Step 5: Identify additional specifics/approach regarding procedure: ______________

8. PREOPERATIVE DIAGNOSIS: Mature, white hand motions cortical cataract; pseudoexfoliation with poorly dilating pupil; glaucoma, controlled on one medicine
POSTOPERATIVE DIAGNOSIS: Same
OPERATION: Complex cataract extraction, right eye
ANESTHESIA: Local, retrobulbar with a modified lid block
ESTIMATED BLOOD LOSS: Less than 0.1 mL
COMPLICATIONS: None

INDICATIONS: This 70-year-old patient complains of a marked decline in vision in his right eye. He has been treated for glaucoma. The risks and benefits of this complex cataract extraction were discussed with the patient. His preoperative vision was hand motions. I had no view of his fundus. He only dilated to 45 mm, and mechanical stretching will be used during this case.

PROCEDURE: Patient was given intravenous (IV) sedation before retrobulbar and a lid block. The eye was massaged for 5 minutes by the surgeon. He was prepped and draped. The eyelashes were taped off of the field. A speculum was placed. A peritomy was made. The cautery was used. A 3-mm incision was made and tunneled into the clear cornea superiorly. Second site was made at the 2 o'clock position. This chamber was entered with the keratome. The chamber was deepened with Viscoat. The iris was stretched using Viscoat and a mechanical technique. A continuous tear capsulotomy was made. The nucleus was hydrodissected. Phacoemulsification was done using extra Viscoat and a Dodick cracker. The nucleus was extremely hard. One minute and 55 seconds of ultrasound and an estimated phacoemulsification time of 1 minute, 6 seconds were used. The cortex was removed with the automated hand piece. The capsular band was carefully polished. An 18.5 diopter AMOSI40NB implant was inserted into the capsular bag and dialed into the 3 and 9 o'clock position. Miostat was used to bring the pupil to a small round size. All the residual Viscoat and Provisc was removed. The conjunctiva was sutured with an 8-0 Vicryl. The patient received TobraDex ointment and Pilocarpine drops. His eye was patched. He received an inferior injection of gentamicin as well as Celestone. The patient will be followed in the outpatient clinic. He will be followed very closely for glaucoma and will receive Diamox 500 mg as a sequel now and also at bedtime. He developed some heart arrhythmias, and this will be checked out by a family practice physician.

Step 1: Identify chapter or section of CPT: Surgery
Step 2: Identify anatomic system: ______________
Step 3: Identify anatomic part: ______________
Step 4: Identify procedure: ______________
Step 5: Identify additional specifics/approach regarding procedure: ______________

9. PREOPERATIVE DIAGNOSIS: Bilateral carpal tunnel syndrome, status–post right carpal tunnel release
OPERATIVE PROCEDURE PERFORMED: Left carpal tunnel release with median nerve decompression
OPERATIVE ANESTHESIA: IV regional

OPERATIVE TECHNIQUE: The patient was brought to the operating room and placed under IV regional anesthetic without episode. The left upper extremity was thoroughly prepped and draped in the usual sterile fashion from the tourniquet level distally. A gently curvilinear incision was carried out across the volar aspect of the left wrist, through the skin and subcutaneous tissue. Meticulous sharp and blunt dissection was then carried down, dissecting down to and exposing the transverse carpal ligament's proximal border. The median nerve was identified and protected. The transverse carpal ligament divided completely, taking care to protect the underlying median nerve. The motor branch of the median nerve was then visualized and demonstrated to be intact and unencumbered. There were no masses or loose bodies or significant synovitis within the carpal tunnel. Hemostasis was obtained by individual electrocautery of individual bleeding points. No deep tissue sutures were placed after copious irrigation of the wound. The skin was closed using interrupted simple sutures of 4-0 nylon. Sterile Adaptic gauze, sterile 4 × 4, and a

STOP AND PRACTICE—cont'd

sterile soft roll cast padding was applied, followed by application of the Ace bandage. The tourniquet was gradually released without episode. The patient subsequently was returned to same-day surgery in good condition, having tolerated the procedure without apparent incident. He'll be followed up in the orthopedic outpatient clinic as scheduled unless any untoward events happen requiring evaluation before his scheduled visit.

Step 1: Identify chapter or section of CPT: Surgery
Step 2: Identify anatomic system: ________________
Step 3: Identify anatomic part: ________________
Step 4: Identify procedure: ________________
Step 5: Identify additional specifics/approach regarding procedure: ________________

10. PREOPERATIVE DIAGNOSIS: Right ureterolithiasis, nephrolithiasis
POSTOPERATIVE DIAGNOSIS: Same
PROCEDURE: Ureteroscopy with laser lithotripsy of ureteral stone; laser lithotripsy and basketing of right renal stones
OPERATIVE TECHNIQUE: Patient was taken to the operating room where he was placed in the dorsal lithotomy position. Groin area was prepped and draped in the usual sterile fashion.
A 21 French cystoscope was inserted and urethra and bladder were examined and found within normal limits. The ureteroscope was advanced up the right ureter. A stone was found in the proximal portion of the ureter. A 400 micro-holmium laser fiber was used to break the stone into several pieces and a stone basket was used to remove the pieces.
Scope was reintroduced and advanced up into the kidney. Several small stones were identified and also fragmented with the laser. We fragmented at least three more stones in the kidney using the flexible ureteroscopy.
The scope was removed, a guide wire was placed, and a stent was placed over the top of the guide wire. Patient was awakened, extubated, and transferred to the postoperative recovery room in stable condition.

Step 1: Identify chapter or section of CPT: Surgery
Step 2: Identify anatomic system: ________________
Step 3: Identify anatomic part: ________________
Step 4: Identify procedure: ________________
Step 5: Identify additional specifics/approach regarding procedure: ________________

STOP AND PRACTICE

Using the breakdown of information for each of the surgical procedures, look up the CPT code(s) for the scenarios previously reviewed.

The example uses the sample scenario from the previous Stop and Practice exercise and walks through the process of assigning CPT codes from the information gathered thus far.

1. PREOPERATIVE DIAGNOSIS: Bilateral heel decubiti
POSTOPERATIVE DIAGNOSIS: Bilateral heel decubiti
PROCEDURE: Debridement of bilateral heel decubiti to muscle
ANESTHESIA: None
BLOOD LOSS: Minimal
CLINICAL HISTORY: The patient is an 89-year-old white female who presents with bilateral heel decubiti. She continues to have some necrotic debris and nonviable tissue. She presents for elective debridement. Her wound is overall improved and mostly contains granulation tissue.
DESCRIPTION OF PROCEDURE: She was brought to ambulatory care and placed in the right lateral decubitus position. Both heels were sprayed with Betadine and sterilely draped. We excised all the nonviable tissue underneath with good bleeding. We had to go down to muscle. She tolerated the procedure well. Plan is to continue the collagenase dressing and follow up in 2 weeks.

Step 1: Identify chapter or section of CPT: Surgery
Step 2: Identify anatomic system: Integumentary

Debridement was performed to the skin, down to the muscle

STOP AND PRACTICE—cont'd

Step 3: Identify anatomic part: Skin
Step 4: Identify procedure or approach: Debridement, skin
Step 5: Identify additional specifics regarding procedure: Performed to both heels, down to muscle
Step 6: Assign CPT code(s)
Code will be located in:
Surgery chapter
Integumentary system
Skin
Excisional debridement section
Code range 11040-11044 for skin debridement. Stated as "down to muscle"; therefore code 11042 would be appropriate.

2. Step 1: Identify chapter or section of CPT: Surgery
   Step 2: Identify anatomic system: ______________
   Step 3: Identify anatomic part: ______________
   Step 4: Identify procedure: ______________
   Step 5: Identify additional specifics/approach regarding procedure: ______________
   Step 6: CPT code(s) assignments: ______________
3. Step 1: Identify chapter or section of CPT: Surgery
   Step 2: Identify anatomic system: ______________
   Step 3: Identify anatomic part: ______________
   Step 4: Identify procedure: ______________
   Step 5: Identify additional specifics/approach regarding procedure: ______________
   Step 6: CPT code(s) assignments: ______________
4. Step 1: Identify chapter or section of CPT: Surgery
   Step 2: Identify anatomic system: ______________
   Step 3: Identify anatomic part: ______________
   Step 4: Identify procedure: ______________
   Step 5: Identify additional specifics/approach regarding procedure: ______________
   Step 6: CPT code(s) assignments: ______________
5. Step 1: Identify chapter or section of CPT: Surgery
   Step 2: Identify anatomic system: ______________
   Step 3: Identify anatomic part: ______________
   Step 4: Identify procedure: ______________
   Step 5: Identify additional specifics/approach regarding procedure: ______________
   Step 6: CPT code(s) assignments: ______________
6. Step 1: Identify chapter or section of CPT: Surgery
   Step 2: Identify anatomic system: ______________
   Step 3: Identify anatomic part: ______________
   Step 4: Identify procedure: ______________
   Step 5: Identify additional specifics/approach regarding procedure: ______________
   Step 6: CPT code(s) assignments: ______________
7. Step 1: Identify chapter or section of CPT: Surgery
   Step 2: Identify anatomic system: ______________
   Step 3: Identify anatomic part: ______________
   Step 4: Identify procedure: ______________
   Step 5: Identify additional specifics/approach regarding procedure: ______________
   Step 6: CPT code(s) assignments: ______________
8. Step 1: Identify chapter or section of CPT: Surgery
   Step 2: Identify anatomic system: ______________
   Step 3: Identify anatomic part: ______________
   Step 4: Identify procedure: ______________
   Step 5: Identify additional specifics/approach regarding procedure: ______________
   Step 6: CPT code(s) assignments: ______________
9. Step 1: Identify chapter or section of CPT: Surgery
   Step 2: Identify anatomic system: ______________
   Step 3: Identify anatomic part: ______________
   Step 4: Identify procedure: ______________
   Step 5: Identify additional specifics/approach regarding procedure: ______________
   Step 6: CPT code(s) assignments: ______________
10. Step 1: Identify chapter or section of CPT: Surgery
    Step 2: Identify anatomic system: ______________
    Step 3: Identify anatomic part: ______________
    Step 4: Identify procedure: ______________
    Step 5: Identify additional specifics/approach regarding procedure: ______________
    Step 6: CPT code(s) assignments: ______________

Now that we have gathered all the information necessary for assigning the appropriate CPT code(s), we will look at the steps in assigning the proper codes, sequence, and modifier code(s) when appropriate.

Step 6: Assign CPT Code(s) as Appropriate

Step 7: Put Codes in Appropriate Order and Make Certain the Code Used Is Inclusive of All Services Provided

Read the notes in the CPT manual carefully. The most common inclusions and exclusions are listed. Coding references, such as surgery bundling books and cross-coding references, are helpful in determining whether services are considered bundled. In addition, Medicare uses a list of bundled codes in the National Correct Coding Initiative, which is updated annually.

SUGGESTION: Begin organizing your own listings of bundled and unbundled services. The *Coder's Resource Handbook* uses a number of tools contained in this book as a basis; use this resource or other resources you have available or begin one of your own. Being prepared and able to assign codes efficiently represents the signs of a good coder.

STOP AND PRACTICE

Using the scenarios in the earlier Stop and Practice exercises in this chapter, take the CPT code(s) assigned in the previous Stop and Practice exercise (Step 6) and determine whether they are already in appropriate order. If not, place in order.

Step 8: Select the Appropriate Modifier Code(s) When Applicable

If the procedure code typically is not billed in addition to the global surgical code already listed, the coder must substantiate the reason for requesting reimbursement by the use of the appropriate surgery section modifier.

Operative report documentation is similar to other physician or provider documentation already reviewed. Many coders, however, find the review of operative report documentation and the coding of operative reports to be more overwhelming.

The deluge of medical terms found in medical records is not cause for alarm because many of these have little importance in coding for services. The use of a medical dictionary may be helpful in reviewing reports if knowledge of medical terminology for a particular specialty is minimal.

As in the evaluation and management section, successful surgical coding involves selecting only the components necessary for coding the surgical procedure(s). The important part of reading and coding the operative or surgical report is to identify and mark (e.g., circle, highlight, underline) ONLY the coding components needed. For instance, the anesthesia administered, the position of the patient, the number of sutures, and the sponge count may not be important in coding surgical services. Learn to filter out the nonessential components; then the operative report will not be as complicated as it appears.

STOP AND PRACTICE

Using the scenarios in the previous Stop and Practice exercises, take the CPT code(s) assigned, place in the appropriate order, and add modifier code(s) where appropriate for the surgery scenarios.

1. Step 6: CPT code(s) assignment: ____________________
   Step 7: Assign in appropriate order: ____________________
   Step 8: Assign modifier code(s) as appropriate: ____________________
2. Step 6: CPT code(s) assignment: ____________________
   Step 7: Assign in appropriate order: ____________________
   Step 8: Assign modifier code(s) as appropriate: ____________________
3. Step 6: CPT code(s) assignment: ____________________
   Step 7: Assign in appropriate order: ____________________
   Step 8: Assign modifier code(s) as appropriate: ____________________
4. Step 6: CPT code(s) assignment: ____________________
   Step 7: Assign in appropriate order: ____________________
   Step 8: Assign modifier code(s) as appropriate: ____________________
5. Step 6: CPT code(s) assignment: ____________________
   Step 7: Assign in appropriate order: ____________________
   Step 8: Assign modifier code(s) as appropriate: ____________________
6. Step 6: CPT code(s) assignment: ____________________
   Step 7: Assign in appropriate order: ____________________
   Step 8: Assign modifier code(s) as appropriate: ____________________
7. Step 6: CPT code(s) assignment: ____________________
   Step 7: Assign in appropriate order: ____________________
   Step 8: Assign modifier code(s) as appropriate: ____________________
8. Step 6: CPT code(s) assignment: ____________________
   Step 7: Assign in appropriate order: ____________________
   Step 8: Assign modifier code(s) as appropriate: ____________________

STOP AND PRACTICE—cont'd

9. Step 6: CPT code(s) assignment: ____
   Step 7: Assign in appropriate order: ____
   Step 8: Assign modifier code(s) as appropriate: ____
10. Step 6: CPT code(s) assignment: ____
    Step 7: Assign in appropriate order: ____
    Step 8: Assign modifier code(s) as appropriate: ____

Determine the appropriate breakdown and code(s) for the following procedures.
EXAMPLE: Removal of skin foreign body by incision
SYSTEM: Integumentary system
ANATOMIC LOCATION: Skin
PROCEDURE: Incision
SPECIFICS: Removal of foreign body
Code Choice(s):
10120 Incision and removal foreign body, subcutaneous tissue, simple
10121 Incision and removal foreign body, subcutaneous tissue, complicated

Because the operative report is not available and no further information is provided, documentation is not present to support the complicated code. Therefore the code assignment will be as follows:
10120 No modifier is necessary

Procedure	System	Anatomic Site	Anatomic Approach Specifics Code(s)	Extent Specifics	CPT Codes
1. Removal tumor, bone, finger					
2. Arthroscopy, knee, diagnostic					
3. Colonoscopy with polyp removal, two by snare					
4. Repair, laceration, arm, 3.5 cm, simple					
5. Full-thickness skin graft, arm, 10 cm^2					
6. Excision malignant lesion, 4.0 cm, arm					
7. Cystectomy, partial					
8. Coronary artery bypass graft, venous, two grafts					
9. Closed reduction, distal radial fracture					
10. Tonsillectomy and adenoidectomy, age 10					
11. Abdominal hysterectomy					
12. Salpingectomy, unilateral					
13. Vasectomy					
14. Extracapsular cataract removal with lens implant					
15. Removal foreign body from the external ear					
16. Prostatectomy, radical, with limited pelvic lymphadenectomy					

STOP AND PRACTICE—cont'd

Procedure	System	Anatomic Site	Anatomic Approach Specifics Code(s)	Extent Specifics	CPT Codes
17. Laparoscopic appendectomy	______	______	______	______	______
18. Bronchoscopy with brushings	______	______	______	______	______
19. Thoracentesis	______	______	______	______	______
20. Closed treatment of metacarpal fracture, with manipulation	______	______	______	______	______

The exercises above should have seemed simple if the breakdown method discussed earlier in the chapter was used. By using those same principles in an actual operative report—extracting only the information needed for the coding assignment—the coder will be able to identify those procedures performed. However, before attempting this process, it may help to view an actual procedure being performed and what typically is included in that procedure. Using the practice activities on the Evolve site that accompanies this text, view a colonoscopy being performed. As you watch the procedure being performed, make your list of key terms. If you are not familiar with all the sections in the surgery chapter, you may wish to locate the general area from which the code will be obtained and identify key elements in the report. Keep in mind that some of the information will not be relevant to the assignment of CPT or ICD-9-CM codes, so that information may be eliminated.

Now take a look at the colonoscopy report on the Evolve site and make a preliminary list of key words or elements extracted from the operative report without concern about whether this information may or may not be needed for coding purposes. Later, you will begin to recognize only the necessary key words.

Your key words list may look similar to this:

Colonoscopy was introduced through the rectum
Passed into the cecum (represented a full colonoscopy)
Diverticulosis in sigmoid colon
Sessile polyp in distal sigmoid
Removed by snare
Internal hemorrhoids
Small fibroepithelial polyp

Separate the key words by procedure(s) or diagnoses, such as the following:

- Procedure(s)
  Colonoscopy through rectum/into cecum
  Polyp removed by snare
- Diagnosis
  Diverticulosis in sigmoid colon
  Sessile polyp in distal sigmoid
  Internal hemorrhoids

Apply the key procedure words identified above into the information needed to code the operative report:

Procedure:	Colonoscopy
Identify system:	Digestive
Anatomic part:	Rectum
Procedure:	Scope, specifically colonoscopy; codes start with 45378
Specifics:	Colonoscopy with removal of polyp by snare
Code(s):	45385

Surgical coding presents a challenge to many coders. Pinpointing and working with only the components needed significantly simplifies the review of operative and surgical reports.

STOP AND PRACTICE

For the following operative reports, use the same process as previous exercises and extract the key elements needed to assign CPT codes and modifier code(s) when necessary.

1. Operative report

OPERATIVE REPORT

Patient information:

Patient name:
DOB:
MR#:

Preoperative diagnosis:

Breast mass, left breast, 2 o'clock radius, microcalcifications and also symptomatic cholelithiasis

Postoperative diagnosis:

Same

Procedure(s) performed:

Lumpectomy. Frozen section on breast benign.

CONDITION: Stable

PROGNOSIS: Excellent

Anesthesia:

Assistant surgeon:

Description of procedure:

The patient was brought to the operating room and placed on the table in the supine position. After general anesthesia was achieved she was prepped and draped over the left breast. Curvilinear incision was made in the skin lines over the palpable breast mass. Underlying breast tissue was excised, excising a portion of breast about 5 x 7 x 4 cm, constituting a partial mastectomy in the upper outer quadrant area in about the 2 o'clock radius. This contained the palpable abnormality. This was sent to pathology for frozen section and the pathologist did not find a discreet mass, just dense fibrous tissue and on frozen section found dense fibrous scarring as well as some cysts and lots of microcalcifications present.

Adam Westgate MD

GODFREY REGIONAL HOSPITAL
123 Main Street • Aldon, FL 77714 • (407) 555-1234

Step 1: Identify chapter or section of CPT: Surgery
Step 2: Identify anatomic system: ______________
Step 3: Identify anatomic part: ______________
Step 4: Identify procedure/approach: ______________
Step 5: Identify additional specifics regarding procedure: ______________
Step 6: Assign CPT code(s): ______________
Step 7: Place in appropriate order: ______________
Step 8: Assign modifier code(s) as appropriate: ______________

2. Emergency department record

EMERGENCY ROOM RECORD

Name:	Age:	ER physician:
	DOB:	

Allergies/type of reaction:	Usual medications/dosages:
No known drug allergies	Not provided

Triage/presenting complaint: Fall

Initial assessment: History of Present Illness: 92-year-old male apparently sitting in a chair at the nursing home, fell asleep, and fell forward onto his head. He has no complaints of head or neck pain, just the laceration on his forehead. Did not lose consciousness. He has a couple of small skin tears on his hands as well. No other specific complaints. He is moving his extremities without difficulty.

Time	T 97.5	P 72	R 20	BP 166/85	Other:					

Medication orders:

Lab work:

X-Ray:

Physician's report: Past Medical History: Significant for hypothyroidism, osteoarthritis, hypertension, GI bleeding, vascular disease

Social History: Living In a nursing home

Review of Systems: Not presently ambulatory. He is hard of hearing and wears hearing aids. He has a lot of bleeding from the forehead wound. He denies neck pain, nausea or vomiting. Denies any chest pain or palpitations. Denies any numbness or weakness in his extremities. He has a skin tear on both hands.

Physical Exam: Alert, cooperative and pleasant. HEENT: Pupils round, equal and reactive to light. External ocular movements intact. Rest of HEENT normal. Neck is supple. No cervical spine tenderness. Full range of motion without elicited pain. Upper and lower extremities within normal limits. Skin: He has a 4-5 cm laceration on the left upper portion of the forehead. Skin tears on both hands, however, moves his hands without difficulty. There is no vascular or tendon Injury noted.

ER Course: Area of forehead wound was injected with 1% Lidocaine with epinephrine. Sutures were placed, however one area continued to ooze so a pressure dressing was applied. He was taken to CT scan, which indicated some areas of encephalomalacia but no evidence of any acute process. No evidence of a hematoma. He was given a tetanus booster before discharge.

Diagnosis:	Physician sign/date
	Robert Rai MD
Discharge Transfer Admit Good Satisfactory Other:	

GODFREY REGIONAL HOSPITAL
123 Main Street • Aldon, FL 77714 • (407) 555-1234

Step 1: Identify chapter or section of CPT: Surgery
Step 2: Identify anatomic system: ________________
Step 3: Identify anatomic part: ________________
Step 4: Identify procedure/approach: ____________
Step 5: Identify additional specifics regarding procedure: ________________
Step 6: Assign CPT code(s): ________________
Step 7: Place in appropriate order: ____________
Step 8: Assign modifier code(s) as appropriate: ________________

3. Operative note

OPERATIVE REPORT

Patient information:

Patient name:
DOB:
MR#:

Preoperative diagnosis:

Left knee degenerative meniscus tear

Postoperative diagnosis:

Same

Procedure(s) performed:

Partial Medial Meniscectomy

Anesthesia:

Assistant surgeon:

Description of procedure:

Patient was brought to the OR, placed on the operating table in supine position. Anesthesia was induced without complication and lower extremity was draped in standard sterile fashion. The suprapatellar pouch and medial and lateral gutters showed no abnormality. The undersurface of the patella showed Grade II and Grade III cartilage changes.

The medial compartment was inspected and showed complex posterior horn medial meniscus tear. Remaining meniscus tissue after partial meniscectomy showed good stability. The lateral meniscus was inspected and appeared to be without defects or tears. The posterior cruciate ligament was intact. Knee was irrigated, portals closed with Vicryl sutures. Sterile dressing was applied and patient taken to post anesthesia recovery area in stable condition.

GODFREY REGIONAL HOSPITAL
123 Main Street • Aldon, FL 77714 • (407) 555-1234

Step 1: Identify chapter or section of CPT: Surgery
Step 2: Identify anatomic system: ____________
Step 3: Identify anatomic part: ____________
Step 4: Identify procedure/approach: ____________
Step 5: Identify additional specifics regarding procedure: ____________
Step 6: Assign CPT code(s): ____________
Step 7: Place in appropriate order: ____________
Step 8: Assign modifier code(s) as appropriate: ____________

4. Operative report

OPERATIVE REPORT

Patient information:

Patient name:
DOB:
MR#:

Preoperative diagnosis:

Soft tissue swelling on the dorsum of right foot.

Postoperative diagnosis:

Same

Procedure(s) performed:

Excision of soft tissue swelling on the dorsum of right foot.

INDICATION:

The patient is a 93-year-old Caucasian female who referred from the Regional Nursing Home for a chronic exophytic growth on the dorsum of the right foot. She is in the nursing home for rehabilitation from hip surgery. The patient had a partial hip replacement done in early November of this year. Subsequent to that, she recovered and was sent to the nursing home for further rehab. The patient has noticed a small swelling of the dorsum of the right foot which has been there prior to her hip surgery. This has since grown in size and is painful now. The pain is aggravated by the use of special footwear that she needs to wear at this time. As a result, she sought medical treatment for the same.

EXAM:

On examination, an exophytic growth about 1.5 x 1.5 cm. is seen on the dorsum of the right foot just over the ankle joint. The surrounding skin appears to be a little inflamed. There is no discharge from the swelling. The surface of the swelling appears to be somewhat ulcerated. There is no similar lesion seen anywhere else on the foot. A stage II decubitus ulcer can be seen over the heel of the right foot. The foot itself appears to be well profused and distal pulses are intact.

Description of procedure:

The patient was brought into the OR and laid out on the stretcher in a supine position. The entire foot and the lower leg was prepped and draped using the usual aseptic precautions. Local anesthesia in the form of 1% Lidocaine and 0.25% Marcaine was used to infiltrate the skin all around the swelling. Next, using a marking pin, an elliptical shaped area was marked out all around the swelling. After ensuring that this area was sufficiently anesthetized, a 15 blade was used to make an elliptical incision encompassing the entire swelling with some skin margin on each side. The incision was deepened using a pair of Metzenbaum scissors. Holding 1 end of the incision by a pair of forceps, the Metzenbaum scissors was used to excise the swelling from the subcutaneous tissue. This was carried out from 1 end to the other and the entire swelling was removed in 1 piece. This was then sent to Pathology for histopathological examination. The operative site was then examined and hemostasis was achieved using the Bovie. An attempt was made to then approximate the skin edges. Given the location of the surgery and the fact that the skin appeared to be fairly stretched all around, the skin edges were then undermined with the Metzenbaum scissors so as to achieve greater purchase. The wound was then closed using single 3-0 vertical mattress sutures of 3-0 Ethilon. This was able to achieve satisfactory approximation of the wound edges. Betadine ointment was then applied over the incision and a dry dressing was then given. The healed decubitus was then dressed separately using a clear Tagaderm dressing. The patient tolerated the procedure well and remained hemodynamically stable throughout. She was then wheeled out of the OR to the Recovery Room in stable condition accompanied by the surgeon and the anesthetist.

Rachel Perez MD

GODFREY REGIONAL HOSPITAL
123 Main Street • Aldon, FL 77714 • (407) 555-1234

Step 1: Identify chapter or section of CPT: Surgery
Step 2: Identify anatomic system: ____________
Step 3: Identify anatomic part: ____________
Step 4: Identify procedure/approach: ____________
Step 5: Identify additional specifics regarding procedure: ____________
Step 6: Assign CPT code(s): ____________
Step 7: Place in appropriate order: ____________
Step 8: Assign modifier code(s) as appropriate: ____________

5. Operative report

OPERATIVE REPORT

Patient information:

Patient name:
DOB:
MR#:

Preoperative diagnosis:

Impacted angulated left distal radius fracture.

Postoperative diagnosis:

Impacted angulated left distal radius fracture.

Procedure(s) performed:

Open reduction and internal fixation of the left distal radius fracture.

Anesthesia:

Assistant surgeon:

Description of procedure:

After adequate anesthesia was obtained, the left upper extremity was prepped and draped in usual sterile fashion. Next, a volar incision was made and dissection was carefully carried down to the fracture which was reduced. Then, utilizing a Hand Innovations plate with the aid of K-wires holding the fracture reduced, the plate was applied and secured with multiple screws distal and proximal to the fracture. Hardware placement was confirmed on AP and lateral fluoroscopy. The DIEJ was stressed and intact. After hardware was placed, the fracture was stressed and appeared to have good stability under fluoroscopy. Tourniquet deflated, hemostasis obtained. A layered closure was performed. Sterile dressing with volar splint were applied. There were no intraoperative complications.

GODFREY REGIONAL HOSPITAL
123 Main Street • Aldon, FL 77714 • (407) 555-1234

Step 1: Identify chapter or section of CPT: Surgery
Step 2: Identify anatomic system: ________________
Step 3: Identify anatomic part: ________________
Step 4: Identify procedure/approach: ______________
Step 5: Identify additional specifics regarding procedure: ________________________

Step 6: Assign CPT code(s): ____________________
Step 7: Place in appropriate order: ______________
Step 8: Assign modifier code(s) as appropriate: ________________________________

6. Operative report

OPERATIVE REPORT

Patient information:

Patient name:
DOB:
MR#:

Preoperative diagnosis:

Crohn's disease requiring central venous access for hyperalimentation.

Postoperative diagnosis:

Crohn's disease requiring central venous access for hyperalimentation.

Procedure(s) performed:

Insertion of left-sided subclavian double-lumen central venous catheter.

Anesthesia:

1% lidocaine.

Assistant surgeon:

Description of procedure:

The patient was placed in the supine position with the neck extended to the right side. The left side of the chest was prepared and draped in the usual manner using Betadine solution. The subclavian vein on the left side was percutaneously and easily entered, and the guide wire was advanced into the superior vena cava. The double-lumen central venous catheter with VitaCuff was placed through the guide wire into the superior vena cava. Good blood flow was obtained. The catheter was sutured to the skin using 2-0 silk sutures and connected to IV solution. A dry sterile dressing was applied.

The patient tolerated the procedure well.

GODFREY REGIONAL HOSPITAL
123 Main Street • Aldon, FL 77714 • (407) 555-1234

Step 1: Identify chapter or section of CPT: Surgery
Step 2: Identify anatomic system: ____________
Step 3: Identify anatomic part: ____________
Step 4: Identify procedure/approach: ____________
Step 5: Identify additional specifics regarding procedure: ____________
Step 6: Assign CPT code(s): ____________
Step 7: Place in appropriate order: ____________
Step 8: Assign modifier code(s) as appropriate: ____________

7. Operative report

OPERATIVE REPORT

Patient information:

Patient name:
DOB:
MR#:

Preoperative diagnosis:

History of abdominal bloating.

Postoperative diagnosis:

1) Two small diverticula in the ascending colon.
2) A 4 mm polyp, which was snared, cauterized and removed from 25 cm from the rectal opening.
3) Hyfrecation of six dominative polyps in the rectal vault.

Procedure(s) performed:

COLONOSCOPY SEDATIVE: The procedure, risks, and possible consequences (including hemorrhage/perforation/ operation/etc.) were explained to and understood and accepted by the patient.

Anesthesia:

Fentanyl 150 mcg, Versed 8 mg

Assistant surgeon:

Description of procedure:

With the patient in the left lateral recumbent position, anoscopic examination was performed. This was unremarkable. The videocolonoscope was introduced, and after gentle manipulation, examination was carried out to the appendiceal orifice. The scope was slowly withdrawn, and colonic mucosa was closely inspected. In the ascending colon near the hepatic flexure there were two small diverticula encountered. At 25 cm from the rectal opening a 4 mm polyp was encountered. This was snared and cauterized at the base. It was removed and sent for pathology. In the rectal vault there were six small dominative polyps. These were just hyfrecated. The scope was retroflexed and this was unremarkable.

IMPRESSION: 1) Two small diverticula, ascending colon. 2) A 4 mm polyp at 25 cm, which was removed and sent for pathology. 3) Six dominative polyps in the rectal vault. COMMENTS: The patient tolerated the procedure well. 02 saturation and blood pressure remained stable throughout the procedure.

Picture #1: Diverticula in ascending colon.
Picture #2: Cecum.
Picture #3: Polyp at 25 cm.
Picture #4: Retroflexion of scope in rectal vault.

Adam Westz MD

GODFREY REGIONAL HOSPITAL
123 Main Street • Aldon, FL 77714 • (407) 555-1234

Step 1: Identify chapter or section of CPT: Surgery
Step 2: Identify anatomic system: ________________
Step 3: Identify anatomic part: ________________
Step 4: Identify procedure/approach: ________________
Step 5: Identify additional specifics regarding procedure: ________________
Step 6: Assign CPT code(s): ________________
Step 7: Place in appropriate order: ________________
Step 8: Assign modifier code(s) as appropriate: ________________

8. Operative report

OPERATIVE REPORT

Patient information:

Patient name:
DOB:
MR#:

Preoperative diagnosis:

Acute biliary colic.

Postoperative diagnosis:

Acute biliary colic.

Procedure(s) performed:

Laparoscopic cholecystectomy with operative cholangiogram.

Anesthesia:

Assistant surgeon:

Description of procedure:

The patient was prepped in the usual manner and under general anesthesia, an elliptical incision was made in the infraumbilical fold and the abdomen was entered through a mini-laparotomy. A 10 mm blunt trocar was inserted into the abdomen. Pneumoperitoneum was produced with 4 liters of C02. The scope was inserted. A second 10 mm trocar was inserted into the epigastrium and two 5 mm trocars were inserted into the right flank under direct vision. The gallbladder was identified and grasped with graspers and retracted superiorly over the liver. Exposing the triangle of Calot, the cystic artery was identified, doubly clipped, and divided. The cystic duct was identified and clipped distally. A rent was made in the duct and a cholangiocatheter was inserted and cholangiogram was obtained. This was normal. The cholangiocatheter was removed. The cystic duct was doubly clipped and divided. The remaining portion of the gallbladder was removed from the gallbladder bed using hook cautery dissection. Hemostasis was secured with electrocautery. The right upper quadrant was irrigated with saline. After a final check for hemostasis, the gallbladder was delivered from the infraumbilical wound. Pneumoperitoneum was reduced, trocar sheaths were removed. The fascia was closed in the midline using O-PDS, and the skin was closed with 4-0 Monopril subcuticular suture. Sterile dressings were applied.

Blood loss was minimal. Sponge and instrument counts were correct. The patient was awake and stable at the end of the procedure.

Rachel Perez MD

GODFREY REGIONAL HOSPITAL
123 Main Street • Aldon, FL 77714 • (407) 555-1234

Step 1: Identify chapter or section of CPT: Surgery
Step 2: Identify anatomic system: ____________
Step 3: Identify anatomic part: ____________
Step 4: Identify procedure/approach: ____________
Step 5: Identify additional specifics regarding procedure: ____________
Step 6: Assign CPT code(s): ____________
Step 7: Place in appropriate order: ____________
Step 8: Assign modifier code(s) as appropriate: ____________

9. Operative report

OPERATIVE REPORT

Patient information:

Patient name:
DOB:
MR#:

Preoperative diagnosis:

Left carpal tunnel syndrome.

Postoperative diagnosis:

Left carpal tunnel syndrome.

Procedure(s) performed:

Left open carpal tunnel release.

Anesthesia:

Assistant surgeon:

Description of procedure:

Ms. Olson was brought to the operative suite and transferred with care to the operative table. After the induction of Bier block anesthesia her left upper extremity was prepped and draped in the usual sterile fashion. A 2.5 cm mid palmar incision was made and dissection carried carefully down to expose the palmar fascia. The palmar fascia was incised and the transverse carpal ligament exposed. A rent in the ligament was created sharply and a curved hemostat placed under the ligament to protect the median nerve. The ligament was then divided in its entirety distally.

Attention was turned proximally and under direct vision the median nerve, the volar floor and fascia were split a short distance in the forearm. The wound was copiously irrigated. The skin was closed with interrupted Nylon. A sterile hand bandage with plaster was applied. Ms. Olson tolerated the procedure well. She transferred to the PARR stable.

GODFREY REGIONAL HOSPITAL
123 Main Street • Aldon, FL 77714 • (407) 555-1234

Step 1: Identify chapter or section of CPT: Surgery
Step 2: Identify anatomic system: ______________
Step 3: Identify anatomic part: ______________
Step 4: Identify procedure/approach: ______________
Step 5: Identify additional specifics regarding procedure: ______________
Step 6: Assign CPT code(s): ______________
Step 7: Place in appropriate order: ______________
Step 8: Assign modifier code(s) as appropriate: ______________

10. Operative report

OPERATIVE REPORT

Patient information:

Patient name:
DOB:
MR#:

Preoperative diagnosis:

Perimenopausal Bleeding

Postoperative diagnosis:

Same

Procedure(s) performed:

Fractional D & C and cervical biopsy

Anesthesia:

Assistant surgeon:

Description of procedure:

Field was prepped and draped In the usual manner. With the patient In the lithotomy position, examination was done. Uterus was found to be slightly enlarged. Cervix Is hypertrophied, closed. Weighted speculum was applied. Anterior lip of cervix was grasped with a tenaculum. Endocervical curettage was done. A small amount of end cervical curretting was performed. Cervix was further dilated with Hanks dilator. Endocervical curettage was done with a small sharp curette. Moderate amount of polypoid-like tissue was obtained.

Rachel Perez MD

GODFREY REGIONAL HOSPITAL
123 Main Street • Aldon, FL 77714 • (407) 555-1234

Step 1: Identify chapter or section of CPT: Surgery
Step 2: Identify anatomic system: ____________
Step 3: Identify anatomic part: ____________
Step 4: Identify procedure/approach: ____________
Step 5: Identify additional specifics regarding procedure: ____________
Step 6: Assign CPT code(s): ____________
Step 7: Place in appropriate order: ____________
Step 8: Assign modifier code(s) as appropriate: ____________

Chapter in Review

Certification Review

- Global surgical services include the preoperative care, surgery, and normal uncomplicated postoperative follow-up.
- Bundled procedures apply to services considered global services.
- Incidental procedures are services considered insignificant and therefore are included in the global surgery component.
- Fracture repairs are classified as open or closed procedures, and they do not necessarily correlate with the injury description of open or closed.
- The proper use of modifier codes for surgery services often determines whether services typically included in the global component should be considered for payment.
- When a diagnostic approach is undertaken followed by a definitive surgery procedure, the diagnostic approach is considered incidental or bundled in the major surgery procedure.

Student Assignments

- Study Chapter 13.
- Review the Learning Objectives for Chapter 13.
- Complete the Stop and Practice exercises.
- Review the Certification Review for Chapter 13.
- Complete the Chapter Review exercise, assigning the appropriate CPT codes and modifiers.
- Complete the practice exercises on the Evolve site to reinforce of the concepts contained in Chapter 13.
- Complete the Practical Application exercises for Chapter 13.
- Complete the Workbook exercises for Chapter 13 as assigned by your instructor.

Chapter Review Exercises

Use the steps learned in Chapter 13 for assigning the correct CPT code(s) to the following scenarios.

1. Patient presented for excision of multiple lesions of the back, face, and arms. Several of these lesions are suspected to be malignant in nature, so we will biopsy them and send to pathology.

   Patient was prepped and draped in the usual sterile fashion. Excision of a 2-cm lesion was made from the lower back area with 0.5-cm margins, as it was suspected this lesion was malignant. Simple repair was made. Another lesion was excised from the face, 0.5 cm, which was also closed. Two lesions on the arm, both approximately 1.2 cm in size, were also excised and closed appropriately.

   Surgical pathology indicated that the lower back and both arms lesions were, in fact, malignant. The face lesion reported back as benign.

   CPT procedure codes: ______________________

2. Patient presents for excisional breast biopsy. The patient is prepped and draped in the usual sterile manner. An incision is made around the whole lesion, and the lesion is removed in toto. Lesion appeared to be approximately 2 cm in diameter, and it was sent to surgical pathology for evaluation. The wound was copiously irrigated and closed appropriately.

   CPT procedure codes: ______________________

3. The patient presents with a lesion on the face area that is approximately 4.0 cm in size. Due to the size of the lesion and its location, it was decided to perform this procedure under general anesthesia, as a skin graft might be necessary for closure.

   The area was prepped and draped in the usual sterile fashion. Excision of the lesion was carried out in the usual fashion and sent to surgical pathology. To close the skin defect, a split-thickness skin graft approximately 2 × 2 cm was obtained from the thigh area and applied to the defect area on the cheek, which measured approximately 3.5 cm × 4.0 cm. Dressings were placed on both the donor site and the recipient site.

   CPT procedure codes: ______________________

4. Patient presents for closure of a 6.5-cm laceration to the forehead. Apparently, the patient was involved in an automobile accident earlier in the day and suffered a laceration to the forehead when her head hit the windshield. She was initially seen in the emergency department, and plastic surgery was called to close this head laceration. The patient was prepped in the usual sterile fashion, and the wound was repaired in two layers. Dressing was applied, and the patient was discharged in satisfactory condition.

   CPT procedure codes: ______________________

5. Patient presents for removal of splinter from finger. Patient was playing with a wooden broomstick and apparently ran his hand over the broom handle. On examination, there appears to be a small wooden splint directly beneath the skin. An incision was made after probing, and the splinter was removed. Wound was closed with Steri-Strips, and dressing was applied.

   CPT procedure codes: ____________________

6. Patient presents with pain in the lower leg after falling from a ladder this morning while repairing his house. X-rays indicate a possible hairline fracture of the tibial–fibula area, and the patient will be placed in a walking cast in the likelihood of a fracture and for convenience.

   CPT procedure codes: ____________________

7. Patient presents for knee arthroscopy after several months of knee pain and "catching" knee joint. Patient is prepped and knee area is prepared in the usual sterile fashion. The arthroscope is introduced, and the patellofemoral joint appears to be normal. The lateral compartment appears to be intact; however, the medial joint has some synovium that was excised as well as meniscus that needed to be shaved; this was performed.

   The patient is returned to the recovery room in satisfactory condition.

   CPT procedure codes: ____________________

8. Patient presents for status post–pin removal after open reduction and internal fixation of a bimalleolar ankle fracture approximately 2 years ago. Apparently, one of the pins has dislodged and can be manipulated under the skin and now the patient complains of pain and irritation in that area. The pin is removed, the area is closed with sutures, and the patient is returned to the recovery room in satisfactory condition.

   CPT procedure codes: ____________________

9. Patient presents for knee injection complaining of returning pain to the knee joint after strenuous exercise this weekend. We have treated the patient conservatively with a knee joint injection in the past and that has been successful. The patient was prepped in the usual manner, Marcaine was used to inject the knee joint, and the patient will return on a PRN (as-needed) basis.

   CPT procedure codes: ____________________

10. Patient presents with painful wrist after an automobile accident. Range of motion is limited by pain and swelling, and x-rays revealed that the distal radius has been fractured in two locations. The patient is prepped and draped in the usual sterile manner. An incision is made, and the distal radius is identified and manipulated into place. Two pins are placed for alignment purposes, and the incision is closed appropriately. A short arm cast is applied, and the patient is to follow up in 2 weeks.

    CPT procedure codes: ____________________

11. Patient presents for admission for replacement of pacemaker for dysrhythmia due to battery life. The patient has had satisfactory results from the pacemaker, and the pulse generator needs to be replaced. An incision is made, the pacemaker pocket is entered, and the pulse generator is disconnected from the leads. Pulse generator is changed for a serial number 252XX, model number AI-4465; leads are reconnected as they were intact; and the pacemaker pocket is closed appropriately with sutures. The patient tolerated the procedure well.

    CPT procedure codes: ____________________

12. This 45-year-old patient presents for placement of a central line for chemotherapy administration. Patient was recently diagnosed with breast carcinoma with poor venous access, so her physician has requested a central line be placed. The catheter was inserted into the subclavian and advanced appropriately. No tunneling was necessary. X-rays indicated the catheter was appropriately positioned in the subclavian, and the patient was sent to the recovery area in satisfactory condition.

    CPT procedure codes: ____________________

13. This 65-year-old presents for removal of a tunneled peripheral central venous catheter that was placed approximately 3 weeks ago for IV antibiotic therapy. The patient's condition has improved significantly, and there is no longer a need for the central line. The patient is prepped, and the catheter is removed with no problems encountered.

    CPT procedure codes: ____________________

14. Bronchoscopy; diagnostic with biopsy
    This 45-year-old patient presented for diagnostic bronchoscope for possible lung nodule. The patient was prepped and draped, and the scope was introduced through to the right upper lobe. The scope was advanced into the right middle and lower lobe, where a biopsy was obtained of a

suspicious nodule. The scope also examined the left upper and lower lobe. At this point, the scope was withdrawn.

CPT procedure codes: 31625

15. Thoracentesis
The patient was prepped and draped in the usual fashion at which time a catheter was placed into the thorax, 0.5 liter of mucous fluid was obtained from the bronchus, and the catheter was left in place for further drainage before removal.

CPT procedure codes: 34422

16. Septoplasty
The patient presents for repair of a deviated septum after an altercation with her boyfriend. The patient was prepped and draped and an incision was made into the septum, at which time the nasal septum was outfractured, roughened areas were smoothed, an internal splint was placed, and the patient was sent to the recovery room in satisfactory condition.

CPT procedure codes: 30520

17. EGD
The patient presents for an upper gastrointestinal endoscopy for possible esophageal dilation and polyps. The scope was introduced into the esophagus, visualizing two esophageal polyps that were excised using snare technique. At the gastroesophageal junction, an extreme narrowing occurred and we were unable to advance the scope further. At this point, the scope was removed. The patient was given further analgesics and a guide wire was placed, over which dilation of the esophagus was successfully performed.

CPT procedure codes: 43253, 43251-M51

18. Colonoscopy
The patient presented for a screening colonoscopy. He is positive for a pertinent past family history of colon cancer, so it has been suggested that he undergo a screening colonoscopy for preventive measurements. The patient was prepped and the scope was introduced through the rectum. The cecum was identified and the scope was slowly withdrawn, observing a number of diverticula as well as a polyp at the rectosigmoid junction that was fulgurated. Two polyps in the sigmoid colon were also visible, and they were excised using snare technique. An additional lesion in the sigmoid colon was also biopsied but not removed.

CPT procedure codes: 45385
45383-M51, 45380-M51

19. Ear tubes
A 4-year-old with history of serous otitis media presents for insertion of pressure-equalization (PE) tubes bilaterally. Patient was taken to operating room and, after adequate general anesthesia was obtained, draped in appropriate manner. With an ear speculum, the external ear canal was cleaned of impacted cerumen. A myringotomy incision was placed in the right ear, and serous effusion was present and suctioned free. A tympanostomy tube was then placed without difficulty. Cortisporin otic suspension and cotton ball were placed, and an identical procedure was then performed on the left ear. Patient was awakened and taken to the recovery room in satisfactory condition.

CPT procedure codes: 69436-M50

20. Cataract extraction
Patient taken to the operating room where viscous lidocaine was placed in the left eye. Patient was then administered IV sedation and prepared for the procedure. Blade was used to make a stab incision at approximately the 3 o'clock position. Unpreserved 1% lidocaine was then irrigated into the chamber and then filled with Vitrax. Keratome was advanced into the anterior chamber. Stab capsulotomy was made and forceps used to complete the capsulorrhexis. Nucleus of the lens was hydrodissected and phacoemulsification of the nucleus of the lens was carried out. Residual cortex was aspirated and the posterior capsule was polished. Lens was introduced and placed into the capsular bag, and the patient was taken to the recovery room in satisfactory condition.

CPT procedure codes: 66984-LT
↑ modifier

Practical Application

Take the following case scenarios and apply CPT code(s), modifiers, and ICD-9-CM codes as appropriate. Make certain to place diagnostic codes as well as CPT code(s) in the appropriate order.

1. Operative report

OPERATIVE REPORT

Patient information:

Patient name:
DOB:
MR#:

Date:
Surgeon:
Anesthetist:

Preoperative diagnosis:

Mass right breast

Postoperative diagnosis:

Infiltrating ductal carcinoma

Procedure(s) performed:

Excisional biopsy of right breast with frozen section, followed by lumpectomy and axillary node dissection

Anesthesia:

Assistant surgeon:

Description of procedure:

The patient was placed in the operating room on the operating table in the supine position. After induction of general anesthesia, the right breast and axilla were prepped with DuraPrep and draped in the usual manner. The patient had a palpable lump in the upper right breast, correlating with the normal mammogram and sonogram. A transverse incision of about 5 cm was made. This was deepened through subcutaneous tissue. Bleeders were cauterized. The palpable mass was felt and excision was carried around this lesion down to the deeper layer. The lesion was about 2 inches above the areola. The specimen was removed and x-rayed, and this confirmed that the lesion was removed. This was then sent to Pathology for frozen section. The results were infiltrating ductal carcinoma less than 1 cm in diameter with adequate margin, the closest margin being 6 mm from the tumor. While we were waiting for the frozen section, the incision was closed. The decision was made to proceed with lumpectomy and axillary node dissection; this had been agreed to by the patient earlier.

The skin was then marked, and an elliptical incision was made at least 2 cm from each edge of the incision. An elliptical incision was made, and the incision was carried down to the pectoralis fascia. The previous biopsy site was not entered. The specimen was completely removed. The wound was irrigated and packed with wet saline gauze. We then proceeded with the axillary node dissection, which was made through a separate axillary incision about 6 cm in length. This was deepened through subcutaneous tissue. The axilla was entered. The axillary vein was identified. Palpable nodes were noted. A few were enlarged and suspicious, about 1–2 cm in diameter. The long thoracic nerve and thoracodorsal nerve were seen and preserved. The veins in the lymphatics were hemoclipped and divided, and the axilla was cleared between the two nerves, and the thoracodorsal vessels were preserved. There was no evidence of any lymph nodes adherent to the nerves or the axillary vein, and the apex of the axilla was clear. The dissection was completed and submitted for pathology. The wound was irrigated. A Jackson-Pratt was placed in the wound in the axilla through a separate stab wound and was secured with 2-0 silk. After irrigation, the incisions were closed with interrupted 2-0 Vicryl. Then another layer of running 3-0 Vicryl on the dermis and the skin with subcuticular 4-0 Dexon was used. Neosporin and dressings were applied. The breast was covered with an Ace bandage on the chest for compression. Blood loss was about 100 cc.

Adm Westy MD

GODFREY REGIONAL HOSPITAL
123 Main Street • Aldon, FL 77714 • (407) 555-1234

CPT code(s) ____________________

ICD-9-CM code(s) ____________________

2. Operative report

OPERATIVE REPORT

Patient information:

Patient name:
DOB:
MR#:

Date:
Surgeon:
Anesthetist:

Preoperative diagnosis:

Right gynecomastia, skin tag

Postoperative diagnosis:

Same

Procedure(s) performed:

OPERATIVE PROCEDURE: Right subcutaneous mastectomy; excision of skin tag, right groin
INDICATIONS: The patient is a 75-year-old gentleman who has had enlargement and tenderness in the right breast for about six months. His sonogram and mammogram show changes consistent with gynecomastia.
OPERATIVE FINDINGS: Beneath the right areola there was a 4 × 3 cm condensation of fibrous breast tissue. There was no clinical evidence of malignancy. The pathologic examination is pending at this time.

Anesthesia:

Assistant surgeon:

Description of procedure:

TEXT OF NOTE:
The patient was brought to the operating room and identified by myself as Andrew Smith for the purpose of the above stated procedure. Intravenous sedation was administered. The right breast was sterilely prepped and draped. Under a satisfactory level of sedation, I inscribed a circumareolar incision oriented in the lower outer quadrant. The dermis and subcutaneous breast tissue were infiltrated with 1% lidocaine with epinephrine. The incision was made with the 15 blade. The areola was elevated off of the breast tissue using the scalpel and electrocautery. The lesion was circumferentially excised with the electrocautery and removed. Some minor bleeding points were cauterized. The wound was irrigated with antibiotic solution and sponged dry. Satisfactory hemostasis was observed. The wound was closed with interrupted 3-0 Monocryl and running 4-0 subcuticular Monocryl. Mastisol, Steri-strips, and an Opsite dressing were applied.
The right groin was exposed and prepped with Betadine. The dermis at the base of the skin tag was infiltrated with lidocaine with epinephrine and the skin tag was removed by shave excision. The base was cauterized. A bandage dressing was applied. The final instrument, sponge, and needle counts were correct. Estimated blood loss was minimal. The patient tolerated the procedure well and was returned to the recovery room in satisfactory condition.

Adm Westy MD

GODFREY REGIONAL HOSPITAL
123 Main Street • Aldon, FL 77714 • (407) 555-1234

CPT code(s)

____

____

ICD-9-CM code(s)

____

____

3. Operative report

OPERATIVE REPORT

Patient information:

Patient name:
DOB:
MR#:

Date:
Surgeon:
Anesthetist:

Preoperative diagnosis:

Suspicion of torn rotator cuff, left shoulder

Postoperative diagnosis:

Torn rotator cuff, left shoulder

Procedure(s) performed:

Diagnostic arthroscopy, left shoulder with arthroscopic subacromial decompression; open repair of torn rotator cuff; placement of infusion catheter

Anesthesia:

Assistant surgeon:

Description of procedure:

The patient was placed supine on the operating room table on the beach chair attachment and a satisfactory general anesthetic was given. Preoperative intravenous cephalosporin antibiotic was given. Bilateral pneumatic compression sleeves were on the calves and were operative throughout the procedure. The patient was placed in the modified beach chair position. The left shoulder was widely prepped sterilely with DuraPrep times two including the lateral neck, anterolateral, posterior torso, axilla, arm, and down to the hand. The left shoulder was draped in the usual sterile fashion.

Arthroscope cannula was introduced via a standard posterior portal into the glenohumeral joint. Inflow to the joint was via the arthroscopy pump. Normal saline was delivered in this fashion. Outflow was from the cannula to suction. A flow of irrigation was maintained for purposes of visualization and removal of debris.

Arthroscope was placed. The biceps tendon was intact without evidence of stretching or tearing of its fibers or hemorrhage on its surface. Its attachment to the glenoid was intact. The anterior and posterior labrum structures were intact without evidence of thinning or detachment. The articular surfaces of the humeral head and glenoid were intact without evidence of fibrillation or cartilaginous cracking or tears. No subchondral bone was exposed. The anterior, posterior, and inferior recesses were of normal size with no evidence of loose body. The anterior ligamentous structures were intact without evidence of pathology. The rotator cuff showed some fraying at its water-shed area. It was followed out to its attachment site and showed some detachment and retraction. Decision was made to perform an arthroscopy acromioplasty.

The arthroscope was replaced through the same posterior portal into the subacromial space. A separate standard lateral portal was then made. A rotary shaver was used to perform a bursectomy, with debris produced removed via suction attached to a rotary shaver. A rotary burr was then used to perform an anterior inferior acromioplasty, with debris produced removed via suction attached to the burr. The undersurface of the distal clavicle was not prominent and did not require resection.

Because of the location of the tear and the extreme difficulty it would cause to try to repair this arthroscopically, the decision was made to perform this open.

Skin incision was made along the skin lines, roughly halfway between the acromioclavicular joint and the lateral tip of the acromion. The incision was carried through subcutaneous tissue. Hemostasis was achieved as necessary. Full-thickness skin flaps were raised. The deltoid fascia was incised perpendicularly to its fibers. The rotator cuff was identified and the detachment was identified. Two Ultra Fix suture anchors were then placed at appropriate locations and weaved into the edge of the rotator cuff tendon. The tendon was then brought to its normal attachment site without tension. The elbow was at the patient's side. A strong repair was obtained.

The wound was copiously irrigated with normal saline antibiotic solution. An 18-gauge spinal needle was placed percutaneously through the deltoid muscle into the subacromial space, followed by placement through the needle of an epidural type catheter. The tip of the catheter remained in the subacromial space as the needle was withdrawn. The catheter was taped to the patient's skin with sterile tape. The acromioplasty was noted to be quite sufficient as the tip of the index finger could easily be placed between the rotator cuff and remaining acromion. The deltoid fascia was reapproximated with interrupted figure-of-8 sutures of 0 Ethibond. The subcutaneous tissue was copiously irrigated with normal saline antibiotic solution. The subcutaneous tissue was closed with interrupted inverted sutures of 2-0 Vicryl, followed by closure of the skin with staples. The subcutaneous tissue, prior to closure, was infiltrated with 0.5% Marcaine with epinephrine. This was also injected into the subacromial space. The portals were closed with staples. The end of the epidural type catheter was connected to an infusion pump filled with 100 ccs of 2% lidocaine without epinephrine at delivery rate of 2 ccs per hour.

Dry sterile dressings were applied to the incision and catheter sites and held in place during the removal of the drapes. Dressings were taped into place. Shoulder immobilizer was applied.

The patient tolerated the procedure well. There were no complications. She was awakened in the operating room and transported to the PACU in satisfactory condition.

GODFREY REGIONAL HOSPITAL
123 Main Street • Aldon, FL 77714 • (407) 555-1234

CPT code(s)

ICD-9-CM code(s)

4. Operative report

OPERATIVE REPORT

Patient information:

Patient name:
DOB:
MR#:

Date:
Surgeon:
Anesthetist:

Preoperative diagnosis:

Medial meniscal tear, left knee

Postoperative diagnosis:

Complex posterior horn tear, medial meniscus, left knee; complete ACL tear (previous partial tear) and synovitis of the notch and medial compartment

Procedure(s) performed:

Left knee arthroscopy and partial arthroscopic medial meniscectomy

Anesthesia:

Assistant surgeon:

Description of procedure:

After suitable general anesthesia had been achieved, the patient's left knee was prepped and draped in the usual manner. Prior to prepping, thigh tourniquet was applied, and after draping, inflated to 300 mm of mercury. No inflow cannula was used. Arthroscope was inserted through an anterior medial porthole. The lateral compartment was examined first. There was noted to be stable intact lateral meniscus. Examination of the notch revealed what appeared to be an old partial ACL tear, which had been recently completed to a complete ACL tear. There was torn ACL tissue that was being impinged and was excised. There was noted to be marked synovitis of the notch. Using the radiofrequency probe, synovial bleeders were cauterized. Examination of the medial compartment revealed synovitis along the medial gutter. Using the cautery, this was cauterized. There was noted to be a complex tear of the posterior horn of the medial meniscus with a lot of large meniscal flaps. Using combination punch and shaver, the meniscus that was unstable was excised, excising pretty much the entire posterior horn. Remainder of the meniscus was contoured, and the articular surfaces medially looked in good shape. Articular surface laterally looked in good shape. The patellofemoral joint was examined, and there was noted to be some diffuse mild grade II changes on the patella with minimal articular cartilage flaps. The trochlea also showed some very mild superficial wear with no flaps. The knee joint was then thoroughly irrigated and the arthroscope removed. Stab wounds were closed with 4-0 nylon. The patient's knee was then instilled with 80 mg of Kenalog and 20 cc of 0.5% Marcaine. Dressing was then applied. Tourniquet was released. Following tourniquet release, good circulation was noted to return to the foot.

The patient tolerated the procedure well and returned to the recovery room in stable condition.

GODFREY REGIONAL HOSPITAL
123 Main Street • Aldon, FL 77714 • (407) 555-1234

CPT code(s) ____________________

ICD-9-CM code(s) ____________________

5. Operative report

OPERATIVE REPORT

Patient information:

Patient name:
DOB:
MR#:

Date:
Surgeon:
Anesthetist:

Preoperative diagnosis:

Displaced fracture, distal left radius and ulna
This is a 15-year-old white male who came to the emergency room with a displaced fracture of his distal left radius and ulna that was attempted to be reduced with Versed and morphine in the emergency room, but was unable to have good reduction and subsequently was brought back to the operating room for general anesthesia reduction.

Postoperative diagnosis:

Same

Procedure(s) performed:

Closed reduction of distal left radius and ulna

Anesthesia:

Assistant surgeon:

Description of procedure:

With the patient under general anesthesia, traction made on his distal radius and ulna, and countertraction placed into his upper arm; finally after the fifth attempt, satisfactory reduction was achieved after manipulating the fracture with the thumbs pushing the distal fragment palmarly and ulnarly. Subsequently, the fracture then showed satisfactory reduction. The arm was then wrapped with a Webril and then a plaster cast sufficient enough to hold it in position. The arm was placed in mild pronation and slight ulnar deviation with some mild flexion to the wrist. A significant flexion was not done, because previously when this was tried when he was awake, he would get numbness along the distribution of the median nerve.

The patient tolerated this procedure well. He will be kept overnight to watch the neurovascular status, and if there is any compromise, he may need to have the cast split, but this will be watched quite closely.

GODFREY REGIONAL HOSPITAL
123 Main Street • Aldon, FL 77714 • (407) 555-1234

CPT code(s) __________

ICD-9-CM code(s) __________

6. Operative report

OPERATIVE REPORT

Patient information:

Patient name:
DOB:
MR#:

CONSENT:
Informed consent obtained from the patient after full disclosure of risks and indications to the patient.

Preoperative diagnosis:

Hematochezia with weight loss

Postoperative diagnosis:

See findings below.

Procedure(s) performed:

Colonoscopy with biopsies

Anesthesia:

Assistant surgeon:

Description of procedure:

After obtaining informed consent, the patient was brought into the OR and put in the left lateral position. IV line maintained. IV sedation was given and vitals were monitored throughout the procedure, which included pulse, pulse oximetry, blood pressure, level of consciousness, and ECG monitoring. First digital rectal examination was done, and then Olympus 140 colonoscope was introduced into the rectum and advanced all the way up to the cecum, identified by the ileocecal valve and appendical orifice. There were lots of areas of pockets of stools, solid stools, which were washed away. Examination was fair; prep was fair. In the cecum there was an abnormal area of cecal fold that was biopsied; appeared to be inflamed, no polyps. The rest of the examination essentially was within normal limits. In the rectal area there was one abnormal-appearing fold with polypoid appearance to it, a flat lesion with shiny mucosa. It was hot-biopsied, and ulceration was seen. There are no masses, no tumors, and no AV malformation. She does have a moderate-sized internal hemorrhoid. Scope was taken out.

FINDINGS:
1. Abnormal cecal fold; biopsies taken to rule out IBD.
2. Normal-appearing rectal fold with some polypoid flat lesion on biopsies taken; sent for histopathology.
3. Moderate-sized internal hemorrhoid.

PLAN:
Follow up with biopsy results.

Patrick Adams MD

GODFREY REGIONAL HOSPITAL
123 Main Street • Aldon, FL 77714 • (407) 555-1234

CPT code(s) ______________________

ICD-9-CM code(s) ______________________

7. Operative report

OPERATIVE REPORT

Patient information:

Patient name:
DOB:
MR#:

Preoperative diagnosis:

Foreign body (quarter) stuck in esophagus

Postoperative diagnosis:

Same

Procedure(s) performed:

Upper gastrointestinal endoscopy and foreign object removal

Anesthesia:

Assistant surgeon:

Description of procedure:

Patient is a 3-year-old who swallowed a quarter. X-ray confirms position in the high esophagus. The patient was brought to the endoscopy suite where continuous oximetry, blood pressure, and ECG monitoring were placed. Anesthesia administered (inhalation anesthesia—see their notes). Following this, oral airway was placed. The Olympus flexible fiberoptic endoscope was introduced through the pharynx without difficulty. Immediately upon entering the esophagus, the coin was noted. This was grasped with a tooth tenaculum and then pulled intact from the esophagus.
Patient tolerated the procedure well.

IMPRESSION:
Foreign object, 25-cent piece in esophagus, removed

Patrick Olson MD

GODFREY REGIONAL HOSPITAL
123 Main Street • Aldon, FL 77714 • (407) 555-1234

CPT code(s) ____________________ ____________________

ICD-9-CM code(s) ____________________ ____________________

8. Operative report

OPERATIVE REPORT

Patient information:

Patient name:
DOB:
MR#:

Preoperative diagnosis:

Chronic cholecystitis with cholelithiasis

Postoperative diagnosis:

Same

Procedure(s) performed:

Laparoscopic cholecystectomy

Anesthesia:

Assistant surgeon:

Description of procedure:

The abdomen was prepped and draped in a routine manner. An incision was made in the umbilicus, Veress needle placed and the abdomen insufflated with 3.2 liters of carbon dioxide. A 5-mm trocar was placed and a 10-mm trocar was also placed. It was then possible to grasp the gallbladder and push it laterally toward and above the liver. The cystic duct and cystic artery were identified. The gallbladder was removed in its entirity using cautery. The gallbladder was pulled out and multiple stones also pulled out. The area was irrigated well, the abdomen insufflated. The incisions were closed with figure of eight sutures of 2-0 Vicryl and Steri-strips applied.

GODFREY REGIONAL HOSPITAL
123 Main Street • Aldon, FL 77714 • (407) 555-1234

CPT code(s)

____

____

ICD-9-CM code(s)

____

____

9. Operative report

OPERATIVE REPORT

Patient information:

Patient name:
DOB:
MR#:

Date:
Surgeon:
Anesthetist:

Preoperative diagnosis:

Bladder neck infection

Postoperative diagnosis:

Same

Procedure(s) performed:

Incision of bladder neck infection

Anesthesia:

General

Assistant surgeon:

Description of procedure:

After the patient was prepped and draped in the lithotomy position, using the resectoscope, the urethra and bladder were inspected. He had about a ten French bladder neck contraction. Guidewire was inserted through the contraction, and then using the Collins knife cutting at the two, ten, seven, and five o'clock positions, the bladder neck was opened. Electrical cautery was used to obtain hemostasis.
Patient tolerated procedure well.

Rachel Perez MD

GODFREY REGIONAL HOSPITAL
123 Main Street • Aldon, FL 77714 • (407) 555-1234

CPT code(s)

ICD-9-CM code(s)

10. Operative report

OPERATIVE REPORT

Patient information:

Patient name:
DOB:
MR#:

Date:
Surgeon:
Anesthetist:

Preoperative diagnosis:

Postoperative diagnosis:

Procedure(s) performed:

Caudal epidural steroid injection

Anesthesia:

Assistant surgeon:

Description of procedure:

In the prone position, after sterile prep and drape and localization of the skin using a 22-gauge 3.5-inch spinal needle, the tip of the needle is placed into the epidural space caudally and confirmed with 2 cc of Isovue M-300, which is seen to spread into the sacral space. After a negative aspiration, 15 cc of 1/8% bupivacaine with a total of 80 mg of Depo-Medrol was injected without difficulty.

The patient tolerated the injection well. There were no complications.

ASSESSMENT: Chronic low back pain with radiculopathy.

PLAN: The patient received his second epidural steroid injection today via the caudal route without complications. The patient states that the first epidural steroid injection did not help him with his low back pain. Therefore we decided to go ahead and deliver the epidural steroid injection from the caudal route to see if this could give us any benefit in his chronic pain. Will go ahead and have him follow up in ten days, and if he does not notice any benefit from the second epidural steroid injection, then will go ahead and proceed with diagnostic lumbar facet blocks, since some of his low back pain may be secondary to facet disease. The patient was given a prescription for hydrocodone last year, but the patient states that the hydrocodone made him feel sick. Therefore he was given a prescription for Dilaudid, but he states that he did not feel as though the Dilaudid was helping him very much. So therefore he has discontinued his current medications. He is still taking Mobic without complications.

Rachel Perez MD

GODFREY REGIONAL HOSPITAL
123 Main Street • Aldon, FL 77714 • (407) 555-1234

CPT code(s) ________________

ICD-9-CM code(s) ________________

14

Coding Complexities of Surgical Procedures

LEARNING OBJECTIVES

After completing this chapter, the student will be able to:

- Understand the application of the surgical coding concepts learned in Chapter 13 to specific anatomic systems.
- Know the intricacies of coding integumentary procedures such as lesion removals, wound repairs, and breast procedures.
- Comprehend the use of fracture repair codes in the musculoskeletal section of Current Procedural Terminology (CPT).
- Understand the difference between open procedures and those performed endoscopically.
- Apply bundling and unbundling concepts to surgical coding.
- Understand and apply National Correct Coding Initiative (NCCI) guidelines for coding surgical procedures.
- Apply CPT coding guidelines for procedure coding to practical coding scenarios.

Anatomy in the Surgery Section

Within the surgery section of CPT are specific rules for several anatomic sites. These are also included in the summary information of the CPT manual. It is imperative to refer to the selected CPT code and to review all guidelines, inclusions, and exclusions, in much the same way as is required for *International Classification of Diseases, 9th Revision, Clinical Modification* (ICD-9-CM) diagnostic coding. Presented in this chapter is a list of key medical terms that apply to the divisions in the CPT book. This list is not inclusive and does not replace a medical terminology or anatomy and physiology course. It should, however, help the coder select the appropriate code(s). Use the review of medical terminology and anatomy from Chapter 1 when necessary for coding surgical procedures, or begin to accumulate key words and abbreviations necessary for surgical coding.

It is recommended that every coder possess a current CPT manual. This allows for notations specific to coding guidelines, reminders, hints, and other information needed to code for specific procedures to be recorded. One suggestion would be to take each breakdown discussed in the individual surgical procedures section and list the bulleted items needed to code for those services.

For instance, to code for excision of a lesion, the student would locate the code(s) in the integumentary section, skin, and excision of lesions. Additional elements needed for this specific coding are discussed. The complete breakdown would look something like the following example. The bulleted items would be placed right above the lesion section and would include the following:

- Method (destruction, excision, shaving)
- Nature (malignant, benign)
- Anatomic site
- Size (in cm)

NOTES: Cannot be combined

Simple closure included, complicated closures may be coded

From this brief bulleted format, the student can identify from the operative report that codes for lesions will be assigned. The student could turn to the integumentary section, lesions, read the list of needed information, and identify what information to gather from the operative report.

Integumentary System (10040-19499)

INTEGUMENTARY SERVICES

Skin, Subcutaneous, and Accessory Structures

Incision and drainage	10040-10180
Excision or debridement	11000-11044
Paring or cutting	11055-11057
Biopsy	11100-11101
Removal of skin tags	11200-11201
Shaving of epidermal or dermal lesions	11300-11313
Excision-benign lesions	11400-11471
Excision-malignant lesions	11600-11646
Nails	11719-11765
Pilonidal cyst	11770-11772
Introduction	11900-11983
Repair (closure)	
Repair-simple	12001-12021
Repair-intermediate	12031-12057
Repair-complex	13100-13160
Adjacent tissue transfer or rearrangement	14000-14350
Skin replacement surgery and skin substitutes	15002-15431
Flaps (skin and/or deep tissues)	15570-15738
Other flaps and grafts	15740-15879
Pressure ulcers	15920-15999
Burns, local treatment destruction	16000-16036
Benign or premalignant lesions	17000-17250
Malignant lesions, any method	17260-17286
Mohs' micrographic surgery	17311-17315

Breast

Incision	19000-19030
Excision	19100-19272
Introduction	19290-19298
Mastectomy procedures	19300-19307
Repair and/or reconstruction	19316-19396
Other procedures	19499

SKIN, SUBCUTANEOUS, AND ACCESSORY STRUCTURES

Key Medical Terms

Adjacent tissue transfer
Allograft
Biopsy
Centimeters (cm)
Debridement
Donor site
Full-thickness skin graft (FTSG)
Homograft
Lesion
Mastectomy
Pinch skin graft
Recipient site
Split-thickness skin graft (STSG)
Square centimeters
W plasty, X plasty, Z plasty
Xenograft

The integumentary system subsection includes the skin and the subcutaneous and accessory structures, which include the nails and breasts (Figs. 14-1 and 14-2). It consists of services such as the following:

- Incision and drainage
- Excision, debridement
- Biopsies
- Shaving of epidermal and dermal lesions

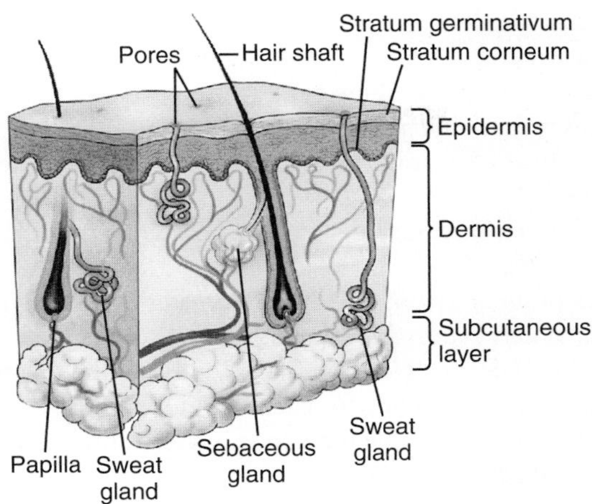

FIGURE 14-1. Diagram of skin.

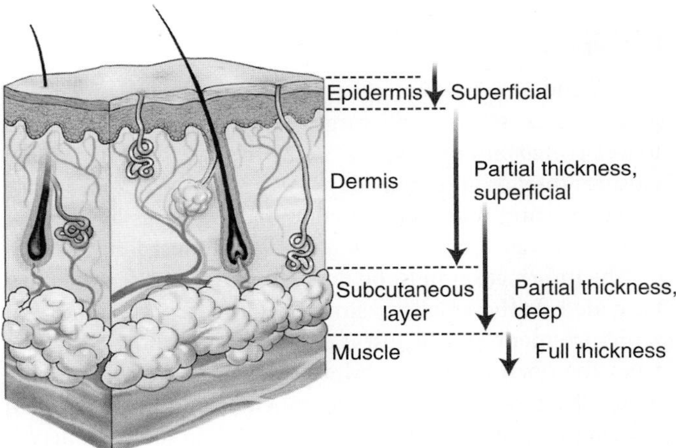

FIGURE 14-2. Degree of burn and depth of tissue involvement.

- Excision, benign lesions
- Excision, malignant lesions
- Nails
- Repairs
- Tissue transfers
- Skin grafts
- Skin flaps
- Burns, treatment
- Destruction, lesions
- Breast procedures

Specific guidelines for this subsection follow.

Incision and Drainage

Incision and drainage typically involve cutaneous or subcutaneous drainage of cysts, infections, hematomas, abscesses, seromas, or other fluid collections from the skin. When it becomes necessary to incise and drain lesions that are not confined within the integumentary system, codes from other sections of the CPT book would be appropriate.

NCCI edits indicate that when it is necessary to incise and drain a lesion as part of another procedure, it is not separately reportable.

Excision, Debridement

Debridement is defined as the cleaning of an area or skin or wound. This may be accomplished by saline washing or by the excising or cutting away of tissue with scissors or scalpel. The process of debridement cleans the surface of the skin and removes any dead, or necrotic, tissue.

Codes in this section further define the debridement based on the extent. Codes 11000 and 11001, for instance, are assigned based on the percentage of skin area treated. Codes 10040 through 11044 are based on the depth of the excisional debridement as follows:

Skin, partial thickness	11040
Skin, full thickness	11041
Skin and subcutaneous tissue	11042
Skin, subcutaneous tissue, and muscle	11043
Skin, subcutaneous tissue, muscle, and bone	11044

Biopsy

Biopsy codes are only used when a sampling or specimen of skin is excised for further evaluation. When an entire lesion is removed, the biopsy code would not be appropriate.

Each biopsy site may be coded separately as long as the sites are not contiguous, or adjoining. When multiple biopsies are obtained through the same incision site, only one biopsy code would be assigned.

Code 11100 is for biopsy of the first lesion, and code 11101 would be assigned for each additional biopsy site of another lesion. Keep in mind the coding guideline of "each" and "each additional" discussed in Chapter 9.

For instance, if biopsy were performed to four separate lesions, the coding would be assigned as follows:

11100 (1 unit)
11101 (3 units)

It would not be appropriate to list each biopsy separately.

Lesions

This is the same section used for demonstrating the breakdown method to locate CPT codes. A lesion is defined as any pathologic change in tissue. It may be determined malignant (cancerous) or benign (noncancerous). In addition, it may be removed by a number of methods, including the following:

- Surgical instrumentation used to remove or excise a lesion.
- Lesion is destroyed, leaving none available for biopsy; can be accomplished by a several methods, including laser, chemicals, or electrocautery.

- Paring or cutting: A small instrument known as a *curette* is used to peel or scrape away lesion.
- Shaving: Using a scalpel or sharp instrument, the lesion is extracted or removed horizontally.

These procedure codes include simple closure (the provider uses the incision as the "approach" by which the lesion excision is performed). A closure other than simple may be billed, as long as the provider has documented the reason why a more complicated closure was medically necessary. The exception is any lesion less than 0.5 cm cannot be assigned a closure code regardless of the extent.

Excision codes are assigned according to the diameter in centimeters of the excised lesion plus margins, *not* according to the size of the incision necessary to remove the lesion. The size stated in the surgical pathology report is not appropriate to use for coding; CPT states it should be indicated by the surgeon at the time of excision. In addition, many specimens may shrink after excision because of the solution in which they are placed. The lesion size is the lesion at its greatest measurement plus the minimal margins required as determined by the surgeon. CPT uses metric measurements throughout; therefore lesions are measured in centimeters. In the case that an operative report indicates size in inches, the conversion is the following:

1 inch = approximately 2.54 cm

For example:

If a lesion is excised measures 4 cm × 2 cm × 1 cm plus 1-cm margins, the lesion excision would be as follows:

Largest lesion measurement: 4 cm
Margins: 1 cm on each side of lesion
Therefore the final size would be 4 cm + 1 cm + 1 cm = 6-cm lesion excision

Multiple lesion removals require multiple codes and should not be combined. When multiple excisions are performed, modifier 51 should be appended to all subsequent excisions when they are assigned different CPT codes. However, when multiple lesions are removed that would be assigned the same CPT code, modifier 59 should be appended to indicate the lesions are distinct, from a different anatomic site.

Keep in mind that lesion codes, such as destruction of lesion codes, are coded by the number of lesions, and these codes would not warrant modifier 51 assignment for subsequent excisions. Destruction of lesions, rather than excision, involves the ablation or destruction by electrosurgery, cryosurgery, laser, or chemicals. When benign or premalignant lesions are destroyed, codes are assigned as follows:

Destruction of 10 lesions:
First lesion 17000
Second through fourteenth lesions 17003

Key elements would again be the following:

- Method (destruction, excision, shaving, paring, cutting)
- Nature (malignant, benign)
- Anatomic site
- Size (in cm)

NOTES: Cannot be combined

Reexcision same session, code final excision only

Reexcision separate session day, code procedure with modifier 58

Simple closure included, intermediate/complex closures are codeable

Exception is lesions 0.5 cm in diameter or less, which are not separately reportable

Additional directives from NCCI indicate the following:

- Assign only one code for each lesion removed.
- When more than one technique is used, only the successful procedure is reported.
- Any tissue or biopsy obtained during the excision of the lesion is not separately reportable.
- If multiple lesions are excised through the same incision, only one lesion code is reportable.

WOUND AND LACERATION REPAIRS

Repair codes may be assigned for wounds repaired with surgical sutures, staples, and surgical glue (commonly referred to as *Dermabond*) only. When Steri-Strips are used for wound closure, they are not considered as repairs. An appropriate evaluation and management code may be necessary for the level of history, examination, and medical decision making.

The information must be documented or the service must be coded as the smallest, simple wound repair. Significant reimbursement may be lost if needed information is missing from the documentation. Educate documenters on missing or needed information. If the documenter supplies the needed information, an addendum to information in the documentation must be made before coding may be revised.

Multiple wound repairs of the same anatomic grouping and extent may be combined and reported as a single code. For example, an intermediate repair of the trunk (2.5 cm) and an intermediate repair of the arm (2.5 cm) may be combined and coded as follows:

2.5 cm trunk + 2.5 cm arm = 5.0 cm intermediate repair
Intermediate repair of the trunk and/or extremities 2.6 to 7.5 cm = 12032

In cases in which multiple complexities or anatomic groupings are involved, the most significant service or most complicated repair would be listed first and the remainder in descending order of significance. Facial laceration repairs are considered more significant than nonfacial codes due to the nature of the repair.

Repair complexities are defined as follows:

- Simple: Single-layer closure, without extensive debridement. This usually includes repair of the dermis or epidermis only. Note that different types of sutures may be used for different areas; however, this does not constitute "layered" closure.

- Intermediate: Layered closure or single-layer closure with extensive debridement (must be documented). This repair usually involves closure of the "deep" layer with sutures, followed by closure of the "skin" with another layer of sutures. However, it may also consist of a single-layer closure with appropriate documentation that extensive debridement has been performed. Preprocedural "cleansing" would not be considered extensive debridement.
- Complex: More than layered closure (e.g., scar revisions, traumatic lacerations, creation of defects, W/X/Y/Z plasty [e.g., reshaping the wound in the shape of a "W," "X," "Y," "Z" to ensure appropriate closure]). This repair typically involves both a layered closure as described in the intermediate wound repair as well as additional work that must be performed either before or after the actual repair. In these instances the wound may need to be "re-created," or modified in some manner before closure. This may be represented in the form of a W-, X-, Y- or Z-plasty, which may involve additional incisions or extension of existing wounds so that a more repairable area is created.

Simple debridement is considered an integral part of wound or laceration repair. Only when the wound requires extensive cleaning or debridement may the services be coded according to a higher level of service.

The bulleted list would appear as follows:

- Extent of repair (simple, intermediate, complex)
- Anatomic site
- Size of repair (always in centimeters)

NOTES: Can be combined when same extent or same anatomic grouping

Staples and adhesive glues may be coded; adhesive strips may not be coded

Not coded when performed as part of incisional repair

Skin Replacement Surgery and Skin Substitutes

When a closure or repair is not possible, skin grafts or tissue transfers or rearrangements may be performed.

To code skin grafts correctly, the coder must identify the type of graft being performed. They are categorized as follows:

- Adjacent tissue transfers or rearrangement

  Not a free skin graft, the tissue is not completely removed but is incised on two of three sides and rotated, or advanced, into position. The advantage of adjacent tissue transfers is that the vasculature is still attached and the transfer stands an increased chance of success.
- Pinch skin graft

  A small amount of tissue, a "pinch," is removed from the original location (donor site) and placed on the new site (recipient site). Codes are assigned based on the recipient site(s) only for all graft codes.
- Split-thickness skin graft (STSG)

  Only the top layer of skin is obtained from the donor site and transferred to the recipient site. The recipient site may still have some viable skin tissue and only the top layer of skin is necessary for repair.
- Full-thickness skin graft (FTSG)

  The full thickness of skin (all three layers) is harvested from the donor site and transferred to the recipient site. This procedure is used for more extensive wounds and burns.

A number of additional skin graft codes were added to CPT in the 2006 edition to incorporate the many new skin-grafting techniques recently developed. New definitions of some of these techniques are as follows:

- Skin replacement: Tissue or graft that permanently replaces lost skin with healthy skin.
- Skin substitute: Biomaterial, engineered tissue or materials, cells, or tissue substituted for skin autograft or allograft.
- Temporary wound covering: Temporary skin surface providing only temporary coverage.
- Tissue-cultured skin: Small portion of tissue is taken and cultured in the laboratory to increase its size. These are typically performed when the patient does not have sufficient skin to obtain a suitable autograft.
- Acellular dermal replacement grafts: These grafts involve synthetic replacement where the dermal layer is permanent but the epidermal layer is composed of a temporary, usually silicone, substance that needs to be replaced at a later time.
- Tissue-cultured allogeneic skin substitute: Skin substitute cultured in the laboratory, containing both the dermal and the epidermal layer.

The size of the graft is measured in square centimeters. For this measurement to be obtained, the calculation is as follows:

$$\text{Width} \times \text{Length of graft} = \text{cm}^2$$

Adjacent tissue transfers or rearrangements such as rotational flaps, advancement flaps, and W- or Z-plasty procedures include the excision of a lesion in conjunction with advancement or rotational flap. These grafts are used to preserve the integrity of the vessels and adjoining structures. When codes from the adjacent tissue tranfer/rearrangement code section are used, they include the excision of any lesion as a part of the procedure and therefore would not be separately reportable.

Codes from the 15002 to 15005 series (preparation of graft site) may be used only when extensive preparation of the site is necessary. It may not be used for debridement or cleaning, but it requires the excision of necrotic tissue to prepare the recipient site for the graft.

Grafts may be obtained from a source other than the patient, such as in the case of allografts (grafts obtained from a healthy donor [usually a cadaver]) or xenografts (biologic graft or porcine [pig] graft).

Location of the appropriate code(s) from this section would be as follows:

- Type of graft (adjacent or free)
- Extent (pinch, split, full, allograft, xenograft), temporary wound covering, tissue-cultured skin, acellular dermal replacement grafts, tissue-cultured allogeneic skin substitute

- Anatomic location
- Size (cm^2)

NOTES: Recipient site only coded
Measurements in square centimeters only
"Each additional" reported in units

Other tissue flaps and grafts are also performed, usually of deeper tissue or with neurovascular or other components still intact. Some of the most common are as follows:

- Delayed flap graft: Portion of skin is lifted off the tissue below, usually keeping blood vasculature intact.
- Island pedicle flap: Contains an artery and vein in the tissue removed, with removal of fat and subcutaneous tissue before implantation.
- Neurovascular pedicle flap: Contains an artery, vein, and nerve; used when sensation needs to be restored.

Many of these procedures involve extensive immobilization efforts, which are not included in the graft code(s). Therefore additional code(s) for the immobilization may be assigned.

MISCELLANEOUS INTEGUMENTARY PROCEDURES

A number of integumentary procedures that represent a wide variety of services not covered in the individual headings of the integumentary system are covered under the heading "Other Procedures." Some of the most common are as follows:

- Dermabrasion: The skin area to be treated is frozen with a chemical and the area is sanded with motorized equipment with a brush.
- Chemical peels: A chemical is applied to the face that causes the skin to shed its outer layer.
- Blepharoplasty: Removal or repair of the excess skin of the eyelid. Usually performed for cosmetic purposes, this procedure is sometimes performed for medical reasons as well.
- Lipectomy: Liposuction is typically performed to remove excess lipedematous tissue from the body. Codes are arranged in order of area treatment.

TREATMENT OF BURNS

Burn treatment typically involves a series of treatments for the affected areas. Documentation should reflect the degree of burn as well as whether the treatment is initial or subsequent. Burns are typically categorized as follows:

- Superficial: Painful reddened skin, involving only the epidermis (outer layer of skin)
- Partial thickness: Resulting in blisters and erythema, involving the dermis of the skin
- Superficial partial thickness: Resulting in loss of the epidermis, involvement of the full-thickness skin
- Full thickness: Extends beyond the skin into muscle, bone, or both

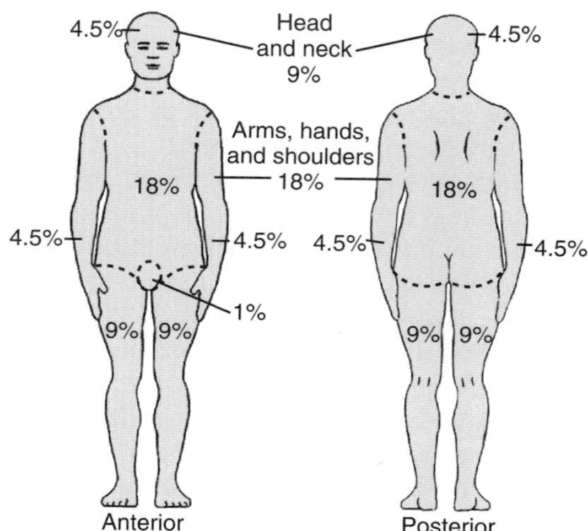

FIGURE 14-3. Rule of nines estimating extent of burns.

Figure 14-3 illustrates the rule of nines, which is the standard calculation for body surface area affected by the burn.

MOHS' MICROGRAPHIC SURGERY

When Mohs' micrographic surgical technique is used for removing a lesion, the surgeon serves as both surgeon and surgical pathologist. The lesion is excised down to the level of tissue where malignant cells are no longer detectible. This typically involves excision, examining tissue under the microscope, with additional excision as deemed necessary until all malignant tissue has been eradicated.

BREAST PROCEDURES

Incisions, excisions, and reconstructive procedures are included within the anatomic grouping for breast procedures. When reviewing the operative report, identify the extent of the breast excision. When only a sampling of a cyst or lesion is removed, the procedure is considered a *biopsy.* Removal of an entire cyst or lesion may be coded on the basis of whether the lesion or cyst is identified by a preoperative marker or clip or is simply excised. Additional codes may be assigned if the preoperative marker or clip is used to identify the cyst or lesion.

Mastectomies are classified according to the extent of the breast removal. Lumpectomies or simple mastectomies encompass removal of only part of the breast and surrounding tissue; a complete mastectomy may involve removal of the breast as well as excision of specific lymph nodes (identified with individual codes). In addition to codes for the extent of the mastectomy, additional codes may be assigned for the implantation of a breast prosthesis (either at the time of the mastectomy or later).

NCCI guidelines specify the following stipulations in assigning codes for breast procedures:

- Mastectomy codes encompass all removal of lesion codes when performed on the same site and during the same surgical session.
- Diagnostic biopsies or breast excision procedures performed before the mastectomy for purposes of determining the need for a mastectomy are separately reportable. Modifier 58 may be appropriate to indicate the procedures were staged.
- Diagnostic biopsies are not separately reportable if preoperative diagnosis already exists.
- Sentinel node biopsy is separately reportable if performed before excision of breast lesion or mastectomy.

Categories for the breast section that the coder may wish to note in the CPT manual are as follows:

- Type of procedure (incision, excision, repair, reconstruction)
- Extent and method (needle, open)
- Procedure (biopsy, removal)
- Specifics (e.g., mastectomy level)

NOTE: Watch biopsy code techniques.

A radiologic marker must be placed by the surgeon for surgeon coding. Always keep in mind what physician or provider you are coding for. If you are coding for the surgeon, for instance, and he or she does not perform the placement of the radiologic marker or does not document such, you would not assign a code for the placement of the radiologic marker.

STOP AND PRACTICE

Try these integumentary coding exercises for practice in applying the coding guidelines learned in this section. Remember to assign code(s) and modifier(s) and place multiple codes in the appropriate sequence (order).

	Anatomic Site	Procedure and Technique	Specifics	Code(s)
1. Excision malignant lesion, face, 2.0 cm				11642
2. Excision malignant lesion, arm, 2.0 cm				19100
Excision malignant lesion, face, 2.5 cm				
3. Breast biopsy, percutaneous needle				
4. Laceration repair, 2.0 cm, face				
5. Laceration repairs as follows:				
Face, 2.0 cm, simple				12011
Face, 3.0 cm, intermediate				12052
Hand, 2.0 cm, simple				12001
Arm, 2.0 cm, simple				12001
Code assignment(s):				
6. Destruction malignant lesion, 2.0 cm, face				
Excision malignant lesion, 1.5 cm, face				
Excision benign lesion, 2.5 cm, arm				
Code assignment(s):				
7. Excision malignant lesion, face, 2.0 cm with 0.5 cm margins				
8. Split-thickness skin graft from thigh to cheek, 2 × 3 cm				
9. Repair of nail bed				
10. Adjacent tissue transfer, arm, 20 cm^2 with removal of malignant lesion, arm, 16 cm^2				

STOP AND PRACTICE

Assign CPT codes for the following operative reports. Make sure you continue to use the technique of breaking down the information needed to code. Follow the guidelines listed previously for each subcategory of the integumentary system. You may wish to add the bullets discussed for each section to your CPT book so those guidelines will be readily available as you search for the appropriate code(s).

1. Operative report

OPERATIVE REPORT

Patient information:

Patient name:
DOB:
MR#:

Date:
Surgeon:
Anesthetist:

Preoperative diagnosis:

Lesion right forehead.

Postoperative diagnosis:

Same.

Procedure(s) performed:

Excision lesion right forehead.

Anesthesia:

Assistant surgeon:

Description of procedure:

The patient was admitted for excision of this lesion, which appeared suddenly over the past 2-3 weeks. We had planned to do this last week but the patient developed a temperature, which aborted the procedure until today. The procedure was to be done under general anesthesia because it was clear we could not do this with local; the patient was screaming and yelling and would probably jump out of the bed.

This patient was brought to surgery. General anesthesia, light, was provided using a mask and inhalation of agents. She was properly positioned. The right temple lesion was clearly evident measuring 1 × 1 cm, pigmented, mole-type lesion. The reason we were excising it was because of the sudden history and sudden appearance. The area was cleaned with saline, infiltrated with 2% Xylocaine, then excised completely and submitted for pathology. Hemostasis was achieved using the hand-held cautery device, and then wound reconstituted primarily with sutures of 5-0 Prolene.

Antibiotic ointment applied. The patient was discharged back to parents to followup in a week's time for wound check and suture removal and review and discussion of pathology findings at that time.

Rachel Perez MD

GODFREY REGIONAL HOSPITAL
123 Main Street • Aldon, FL 77714 • (407) 555-1234

Step 1: Identify CPT chapter or section: Surgery
Step 2: Identify anatomic system: ________
Step 3: Identify anatomic site: ________
Step 4: Identify procedure/technique: ________
Step 5: Identify additional specifics: ________
Step 6: Assign CPT code(s): ________
Step 7: Place code(s) in appropriate order: ________
Step 8: Assign modifier code(s) as appropriate: ________

2. Operative report

OPERATIVE REPORT

Patient information:

Patient name:
DOB:
MR#:

Date:
Surgeon:
Anesthetist:

Preoperative diagnosis:

1. Intraoral tumor.
2. Right nasal ala skin lesion.

Postoperative diagnosis:

1. Intraoral tumor.
2. Right nasal ala basal cell carcinoma measuring 0.9 cm.

Procedure(s) performed:

Excision of intraoral tumor, excision of right nasal ala basal cell carcinoma with bilobe flap reconstruction.

Anesthesia:

Assistant surgeon:

Description of procedure:

INDICATIONS FOR SURGERY: The patient is a 70-year-old white female who presents with an intraoral lesion that has been slowly growing for the past several months, as well as a lesion on her nose over the right alar dome. She now presents for elective excision and treatment of these lesions.

DESCRIPTION OF OPERATIVE PROCEDURE: The patient was brought to the Operating Room and placed supine on the operating room table. After adequate general anesthesia and endotracheal intubation, the patient was prepped and draped in the usual sterile fashion. Using 1% Lidocaine with epinephrine, the skin and subcutaneous tissue around the lesion of the right alar dome was anesthetized. After adequate local anesthesia and epinephrine effect, a shave biopsy was performed of this basal cell carcinoma which measured 0.9 cm in size. The specimen was sent to pathology and came back positive for basal cell carcinoma all margins involved. The patient then had a 3 mm margin excision and sent to pathology with sutured orienting the pathologist. Frozen section of this excision was negative for any tumor at the margins. A bilobe flap was outlined along the right nasal side wall. Using skin hooks, the bilobed flap was undermined widely in the submuscular plane. Once this myocutaneous flap was adequately mobilized the remaining wound edges were also mobilized to allow for closure without tension. The flap was then in-set using 5-0 Vicryl suture for the deep layer and a combination of 5-0 and 6-0 nylon suture for the skin. Please note that during flap transfer, the skin, subcutaneous tissue and nasal muscle was transferred together with the flap.

Using separate instruments, separate syringe and needles, the intraoral lesion was anesthetized with 1% Lidocaine with epinephrine for the epinephrine effect. After adequate time had elapsed, the lesion was excised with a number 15 blade scalpel. The cheek was retracted with a small intraoral retractor and the specimen was sent to pathology for permanent sections. Hemostasis was achieved with electrocautery. The mucosa was then closed with running and locking 2-0 chromic suture. At the end of the procedure, the patient was successfully extubated in the Operating Room. Her face had been cleaned and the suture line was covered with Bacitracin ointment. At the end of the procedure, the patient was taken to PACU for recovery in stable condition.

GODFREY REGIONAL HOSPITAL
123 Main Street • Aldon, FL 77714 • (407) 555-1234

Step 1: Identify CPT chapter or section: Surgery
Step 2: Identify anatomic system: ______________
Step 3: Identify anatomic site: ______________
Step 4: Identify procedure/technique: ______________
Step 5: Identify additional specifics: ______________
Step 6: Assign CPT code(s): ______________
Step 7: Place code(s) in appropriate order: ______________
Step 8: Assign modifier code(s) as appropriate: ______________

3. Operative report

OPERATIVE REPORT

Patient information:

Patient name:
DOB:
MR#:

Date:
Surgeon:
Anesthetist:

Preoperative diagnosis:

Bilateral upper extremity lesions.

Postoperative diagnosis:

Bilateral upper extremity lesions.

Procedure(s) performed:

Excision biopsy left upper extremity lesions × 3 (lipomas), right extremity lesion × 1 (lipoma).

Anesthesia:

IV Sedation, local anesthesia.

Assistant surgeon:

Description of procedure:

INDICATIONS FOR PROCEDURE: Ms. Frye is a 70 year-old female who had multiple lesions of both upper extremities causing her discomfort and she wished them removed. She understood the risks including bleeding, infection, scarring and agreed.

DESCRIPTION OF PROCEDURE: The patient was taken to the Operating Room and both upper extremities were prepped and draped in sterile fashion. IV sedation and local anesthesia was used. An incision was made over each of the lesions. There were three in the left upper extremity essentially on the exterior aspect of the left forearm and one on the external aspect of the right forearm. A 15 blade knife was used to make an incision approximately l cm over each of these lesions and they were each removed in their entirety. They all appeared to be lipomas.

The wounds were closed with 5-0 Vicryl. They were sent to Pathology for evaluation individually.

The patient tolerated the procedure well.

Maurice Doater, MD

GODFREY REGIONAL HOSPITAL
123 Main Street • Aldon, FL 77714 • (407) 555-1234

Step 1: Identify CPT chapter or section: Surgery
Step 2: Identify anatomic system: ____________
Step 3: Identify anatomic site: ____________
Step 4: Identify procedure/technique: ____________
Step 5: Identify additional specifics: ____________
Step 6: Assign CPT code(s): ____________
Step 7: Place code(s) in appropriate order: ____________
Step 8: Assign modifier code(s) as appropriate: ____________

4. Operative report

OPERATIVE REPORT

Patient information:

Patient name:
DOB:
MR#:

Date:
Surgeon:
Anesthetist:

Preoperative diagnosis:

Microcalcifications left breast. Rule out carcinoma.

Postoperative diagnosis:

Benign microcalcifications with fibrocystic changes.

Procedure(s) performed:

Needle localization with excision biopsy of microcalcifications of left breast.

Anesthesia:

Assistant surgeon:

Description of procedure:

She was brought to surgery this morning. I had met her in the office and discussed the mammographic findings that were of concern. I advised her as to what the next steps were going to be. With her consent, she was admitted this morning for the same.

On admission an IV line was started. She was taken to the X-ray Suite where needle localization was successfully performed to the area of microcalcifications in the left breast. She was then brought to surgery for the definitive procedure. At surgery, pre-op on call, she received 1 gram of Ancef. She was then brought to surgery. Procedure was to be done under monitored anesthesia, IV sedation and local infiltration. She was placed on the OR table. Her left breast, left chest wall and left arm were cleaned with Duraprep and draped and the operation started. The needle entry point was in the upper outer quadrant of the left breast. Following prepping and draping, the operation started. Using my usual anesthetic mix, the planned circular incision site was infiltrated with the mix until adequate anesthesia was obtained and the circular incision was made encompassing the needle entry point for about 2 inches. Going through skin and subcutaneous tissue, breast substance was entered into. Then I followed the course of the wire all the way until the hook was reached. At this point, all tissue contained within the curve of the hook was excised. With needle in continuity, all was submitted for specific mammography. J was advised that all of the affected tissues had been removed. Subsequently this was submitted for frozen section exam which showed that these were benign microcalcifications or fibrocystic breast changes, benign. The operation terminated at this point. Hemostasis achieved. Breast was reconstructed with 2-0 chromic for the subcu, skin 4-0 nylon. Appropriate dressings applied. The patient taken from surgery to the recovery room in satisfactory condition where J did meet with patient and her husband and advised them as to my findings, much to their relief. She will be discharged home later this morning. I will see her in the office a week from today.

Rachel Perez MD

GODFREY REGIONAL HOSPITAL
123 Main Street • Aldon, FL 77714 • (407) 555-1234

Step 1: Identify CPT chapter or section: Surgery
Step 2: Identify anatomic system: ____________
Step 3: Identify anatomic site: ____________
Step 4: Identify procedure/technique: ____________
Step 5: Identify additional specifics: ____________
Step 6: Assign CPT code(s): ____________
Step 7: Place code(s) in appropriate order: ____________
Step 8: Assign modifier code(s) as appropriate: ____________

5. Operative report

OPERATIVE REPORT

Patient information:

Patient name:
DOB:
MR#:

Date:
Surgeon:
Anesthetist:

Preoperative diagnosis:

Deflated reconstructive breast implant

Postoperative diagnosis:

Same.

Procedure(s) performed:

Replacement of implant

Anesthesia:

Assistant surgeon:

Description of procedure:

INDICATION: This 69-year-old white female had undergone a right breast reconstruction post mastectomy using a tissue expander and implant technique. Shortly after tattooing her nipple-areolar complex, she noted that her implant was increasingly soft and smaller. On examination, it was apparent that her implant was deflating.

FINDINGS: A pinpoint hole on the posterior aspect of the implant. The only explanation for this is that it seems reasonable is that the implant may have been flipped over at the time of the tattooing when local anesthetic was infiltrated beneath the areola. The new implant set in the existing pocket very nicely and no further modifications to the pocket were necessary.

PROCEDURE: The patient was brought to the Operating Room where uncomplicated general anesthesia was induced. The surgical site was prepped with Duraprep and routine sterile drapes applied. The existing inframammary incision was reopened sharply and extended the electrocautery to the implant capsule.The only defect in the implant appeared to be a pinpoint hole on the posterior aspect of the implant.

The wound was irrigated with dilute Betadine solution and a new breast implant was selected. This was a McGhann Style 363LF saline filled textured breast implant reference Number 27-363140LF, Serial Number 2638, Lot Number 56977I. The implant was inspected and prepared and inserted using a no touch technique and inflated with normal saline to 450 cc's. The implant sat nicely in the existing pocket and the size seemed to be appropriate. Accordingly, the wound was closed with running 3-0 Vicryl for the implant capsule and muscular fascia. Buried interrupted 4-0 Biosyn for the buried dermal closure and running 5-0 plain gut for the skin. Steri-strips were used to cover the wound followed by a sterile dressing. The patient was awakened and transported to the Recovery Room in excellent condition having tolerated the procedure well with minimal blood loss.

Adam Westy MD

GODFREY REGIONAL HOSPITAL
123 Main Street • Aldon, FL 77714 • (407) 555-1234

Step 1: Identify CPT chapter or section: Surgery
Step 2: Identify anatomic system: ________
Step 3: Identify anatomic site: ________
Step 4: Identify procedure/technique: ________
Step 5: Identify additional specifics: ________
Step 6: Assign CPT code(s): ________
Step 7: Place code(s) in appropriate order: ________
Step 8: Assign modifier code(s) as appropriate: ________

Musculoskeletal System (20000-29909)

MUSCULOSKELETAL SYSTEM SERVICES

General	20000-20999
Head	21010-21499
Neck (soft tissue) and thorax	21501-21899
Back and flank	21920-21935
Spine/vertebral column	22010-22899
Abdomen	22900-22999
Shoulder	23000-23929
Humerus (upper arm) and elbow	23930-24999
Forearm and wrist	25000-25999
Hand and fingers	26010-26989
Pelvis and hip joint	26990-27299
Femur (thigh region) and knee joint	27301-27599
Leg (tibia and fibula) and ankle	27600-27899
Foot and toes	28001-28899
Application of casts and strapping	29000-29799
Endoscopy/arthroscopy	29800-29999

Key Medical Terms

Cervical
Closed treatment
Fascia
Internal or external fixation
Manipulation
Open reduction and internal fixation (ORIF)
Open treatment
Percutaneous skeletal fixation
Vertebral interspace
Vertebral segment
Thoracic

This section encompasses the repair or revision of the musculoskeletal system (Fig. 14-4). Keep in mind that the services in this subcategory are global and thus include both preoperative and postoperative care. Subsections are anatomic sites such as the following:

- General
- Head
- Neck
- Back/flank
- Spine
- Shoulder
- Humerus, elbow
- Forearm, wrist
- Hand, fingers
- Pelvis, hip joint
- Femur, knee joint
- Leg, ankle joint
- Foot, toes
- Casts, strapping, splinting
- Endoscopy, arthroscopy

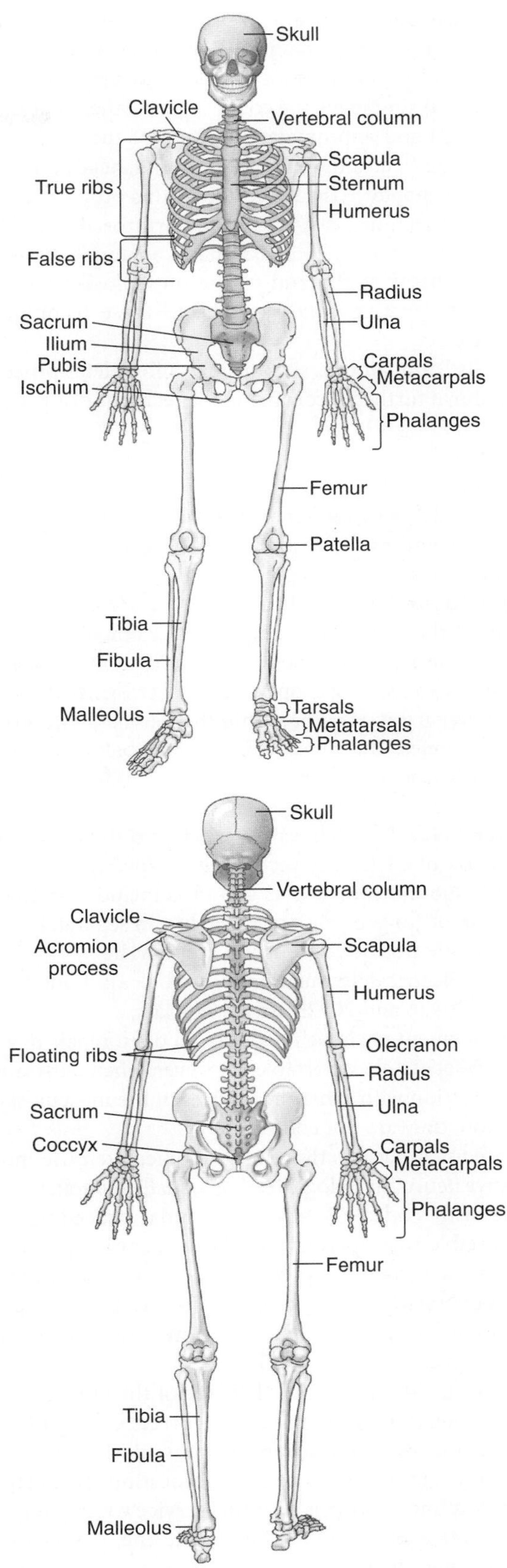

FIGURE 14-4. Axial and appendicular skeleton.

Note that the subsections of the musculoskeletal section are in anatomic progression. The anatomic sections start at the head and progress down the body to the feet and toes. This makes it simple for the coder to know the section (musculoskeletal) and approximate location of the anatomic site in the section (feet at the end of the chapter, head at the beginning of the chapter). The exception to this progression is the last two subsections: cast/splints and arthroscopies. Because these two sections encompass many anatomic parts, they have been listed at the end of the musculoskeletal section for ease in locating codes specific to these techniques or procedures.

The list of anatomic sites of musculoskeletal procedures breaks down further according to the technique or procedure performed:

- Incision
- Excision
- Repair, revision, and reconstruction
- Fracture and/or dislocation
- Manipulation (where applicable)
- Arthrodesis (when applicable)

One of the most confusing coding elements pertains to excision of lesions and biopsies. The student must determine whether the excision or biopsy is being performed on the skin (integumentary system) or within the muscles, tendons, ligaments, or bones. This must be determined before locating the appropriate code(s) because they are in different anatomic systems.

Several NCCI guidelines are specific to the musculoskeletal section of CPT. They include the following:

- If a tissue transfer such as a graft is included in the code descriptor for the primary procedure, a separately reportable tissue transfer code is not appropriate.
- When electrical stimulation is used to aid bone healing, codes 20974 and 20975 are appropriate.
- Debridement of tissue related to an open repair of a fracture is separately reportable. However, when performed in conjunction with other procedures in the musculoskeletal section, they are not codeable.
- Procedures, such as those of the spine, often use intraoperative neurophysiologic testing. Usually separately reportable with code 95920, an additional procedure is not reportable when performed by the operating physician.
- Spinal arthrodesis, exploration, and instrumentation include manipulation of the spine as an integral part of these procedures and therefore are not separately reportable.
- Modifiers 50, LT, and RT (left side of the body, right side of the body) are essential to the correct coding of a large number of procedures from the musculoskeletal system.
- If a physician treats a fracture, dislocation, or injury with a cast, splint, or strip as an initial service without any other definitive procedure or treatment, the physician may report an evaluation and management service as appropriate and the appropriate casting/splint code(s).
- Codes for removal of internal fixation are not reportable when they are a necessary integral part of another procedure.
- If a closed reduction of a fracture fails and it is converted to an open procedure, only the more extensive procedure should be reported.

INJECTIONS (UNDER INTRODUCTION/REMOVAL)

Trigger point injections are included in the "General" heading of the musculoskeletal system because these injections can be performed at multiple sites. Note that the trigger point injection codes are assigned not by the number of injections but by the number of trigger points and number of muscles.

Joint injections (arthrocentesis) are also included in the general section of musculoskeletal as well. These codes are assigned on the basis of the size of the joint being injected: small (fingers, toes), medium (temporomandibular joint [TMJ], wrist, elbow, ankle, olecranon bursa, acromioclavicular), and major (shoulder, hip, knee, subacromial bursa).

Removal of hardware codes are also located in this general section. When difficulties are encountered with previously placed wires, pins, or rods, and it becomes necessary to remove these devices, codes from 20670 to 20680 are used. If the removal is performed during the postoperative period of the original fracture or surgical procedure, modifier 58 (staged or related procedure) would be appended to this secondary procedure. Most hardware removals, however, occur long after the postoperative period and do not require a modifier. Diagnostic statements would typically be from the V54 series, attention to surgical hardware, as the primary diagnosis.

BONE GRAFTS

Bone graft harvesting may be billed separately only when it is not listed as part of the primary procedure already billed.

SPINE (VERTEBRAL COLUMN) CODING ASSIGNMENT

Within the spine section, bone grafting and instrumentation codes are usually assigned in addition to the main surgical procedure. Bone grafts are often necessary to replace diseased bone or bone that has been removed as part of the surgical procedure, and are reported with codes from the bone graft section (20900-20938). Note that all these codes carry a relatively new symbol (Ø) that has not been seen up to this point. This symbol indicates that modifier 51 does not need to be assigned to this series of codes even when multiple procedures are performed. CPT guidelines assume that codes from the bone graft section are often used in conjunction with other codes and does require modifier 51 for these procedures.

Many of the codes in this section will require the use of multiple units for services because a number of the codes are assigned on the basis of "each vertebral segment." For instance, 22600 is explained as "Arthrodesis, posterior or posterolateral technique, single level; cervical below C2 segment." If an arthrodesis is performed on C2-C3, C3-C4, and C4-C5, for instance, code 22614 would be assigned with multiple days or units of three rather than as three separate line items on the claim form for three segments. A vertebral segment is defined as the basic constituent part into which the spine is divided. A vertebral interspace is the compartment between two adjacent vertebral bodies. One vertebral interspace (C2-C3, for example) would be described as one space, the space between the second and third vertebral segments.

Cervical vertebrae are located in the region from the base of the skull to the top of the back (Fig. 14-5). The thoracic spine includes the vertebrae from the base of the neck to just above the small of the back. The lumbar spine includes the vertebrae in the lower back and terminates just above the top of the buttocks.

For codes from the spine section to be assigned, the following breakdown should be used:

- Procedure performed (excision, fracture, manipulation)
- Anatomic site (intervertebral space or vertebral segment, cervical [C], thoracic [T], or lumbar [L] area of spine)
- Number of vertebral spaces or segments

NOTES: Arthrodesis may be coded in addition to surgical procedure.

Instrumental may be coded in addition to surgical procedure.

Modifier 62 should be used when two surgeons work together, each as primary surgeon, on spinal procedures.

FRACTURES AND DISLOCATIONS

Caution should be applied in reading the descriptions of services. Care must be taken to determine the type of procedure and extent of treatment already included in the service, such as closed, open, with or without manipulation, or with traction (Figs. 14-6 and 14-7).

Fractures and dislocations occupy probably the largest section and number of codes of any section in the CPT manual. These services are perhaps the easiest to code with the following breakdown of services performed.

- Anatomic site
- Specific site (distal, proximal, shaft)
- Open or closed
- With or without manipulation
- With or without fixation (internal or external)

NOTES: Fracture/dislocation care includes application of initial cast.

Refractures or reductions require modifier code(s).

Keep in mind the definitions of fractures to assign correct code(s) for services:

- Closed treatment: Surgical procedure does not involve surgically opening the site of the fracture for the purpose of repair.
- Open treatment: Procedure involves surgical opening of the site and visualization of the fracture for repair and treatment. Open treatment may also include a remote opening to place an intramedullary nail or rod at the fracture site even though the fracture is not visualized.

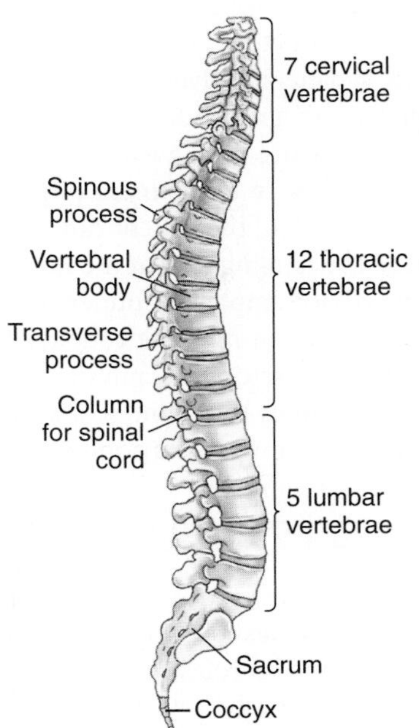

FIGURE 14-5. Spine.

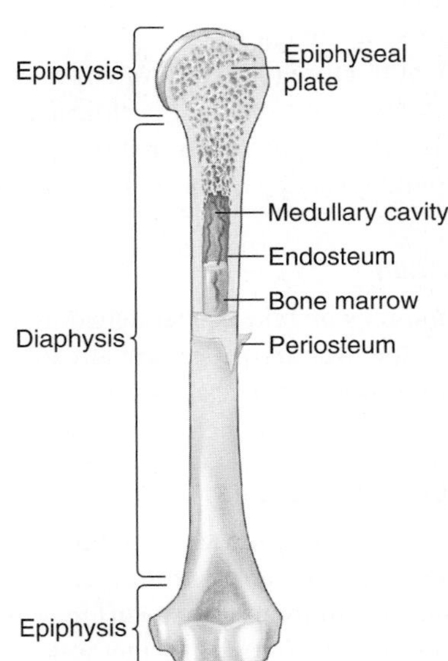

FIGURE 14-6. Long bones.

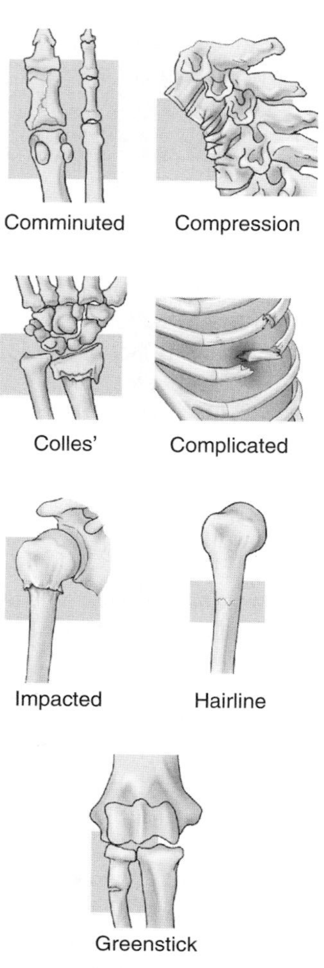

FIGURE 14-7. Fractures.

- Percutaneous skeletal fixation: Fixation device or appliance is placed across the fracture site, usually with the assistance of x-ray imaging.

NOTE: The type of fracture (closed or open) may have no correlation with the type of treatment performed. For example, a closed fracture may require open treatment or skeletal fixation, and it should be coded accordingly.

External Fixation

External fixation may be billed separately only when it is not listed as part of the primary procedure already billed. External fixation is the use of external skeletal pins and wires to treat a fracture or other bone deformity.

Fracture Repeat Reductions

When it is necessary to reduce a fracture a second time, exactly as performed previously, modifier 76 (same physician) or modifier 77 (different physician) may be used. If the fracture must be reduced by another method (e.g., closed the first time, open the second; no manipulation the first time, manipulation required the second time) modifiers 76 and 77 would not be appropriate. In this case, modifier 58 would be appropriate (if the first and second procedure were both performed outside the operating room).

BUNION PROCEDURES

Hallux valgus (bunion) is a deformity of the first metatarsophalangeal joint. A number of techniques are used for the repair of bunions. All the codes for bunion repairs, codes 28290-28299, include the following:

- Capsulotomy
- Arthrotomy
- Synovial biopsy or synovectomy
- Neuroplasty
- Tendon release
- Tenotomy
- Tenolysis
- Excision of medial eminence
- Excision of associated osteophytes
- Placement of internal fixations

APPLICATION OF CASTS OR SPLINTS

When musculoskeletal definitive, restorative, or invasive procedures are performed to realign fractures, the application and removal of the cast or splint that immobilized that fracture or dislocation are included in the surgical code. This is considered part of the surgical procedure. If the treating provider does not provide the restorative, definitive care for the fracture or dislocation but perhaps only stabilizes the fracture until another provider gives treatment, the first provider may code for the history, examination, and medical decision making (an evaluation and management code) and for the application of the cast or splint by the provider or a licensed employee under the provider's supervision.

For example, a patient arrives at the emergency department and is given a diagnosis of misaligned fracture of the distal radius. The fracture repair will require surgical intervention, so the emergency department physician orders the application of a splint until the patient can see the orthopedic surgeon. Because the nursing staff at the hospital applied the splint and they are not employees under the supervision of the provider, the physician may not code for the application of the splint. In the office setting, the physician or his employed representative would apply the splint, so assignment of a code for the splint application would be appropriate.

ARTHROSCOPIC PROCEDURES

In addition to the surgical procedures outlined in the musculoskeletal section, the last subsection is arthroscopic procedures, those performed through a scope for visualization of a joint. Operative reports for arthroscopic procedures used indicate that a scope was inserted, as well as trocars, sheaths, or both. Again, watching for key words will assist in the proper assignment of procedure codes. If the procedure(s) is performed arthroscopically, only those codes from this section may be used. Once it has been established the procedure was performed arthroscopically, the coder should stay within this section when assigning codes (unless other open procedures are performed as well).

Watch a video of an arthroscopic procedure that is available on the companion Evolve site so you may envision the completion of an arthroscopic procedure.

As with the other surgical sections, the codes are listed in anatomic order starting at the temporomandibular joint and ending at the foot.

When arthroscopic procedures are coded, the following guidelines should be applied:

1. When surgery is performed arthroscopically, the diagnostic arthroscopic procedure is included and should not be coded (the term *separate procedure* is included).
2. Multiple arthroscopic procedures on the same anatomic site should have the modifier 51 appended to indicate multiple procedures.
3. When arthroscopic procedures are followed by a portion of the open surgery performed, both codes may be used. If no surgical intervention is performed through an arthroscopic procedure, a diagnostic arthroscopic code may be assigned in addition to the appropriate open surgical codes. Modifier 51 should be assigned to the least significant procedure(s).
4. In the case of knee arthroscopies (Fig. 14-8) according to CPT guidelines, the three compartments of the knee (medial, lateral, and femoropatellar) are considered distinct. When different procedures are performed on different compartments of the knee, they may be coded (e.g., if a meniscectomy is performed to the lateral compartment and a synovectomy is performed to the femoropatellar joint, both procedures may be coded). NCCI edits indicate that chondroplasty performed at the same time as other arthroscopic procedures is not reimbursable. The coder will need to check with the specific carriers to determine appropriate coding in these instances.

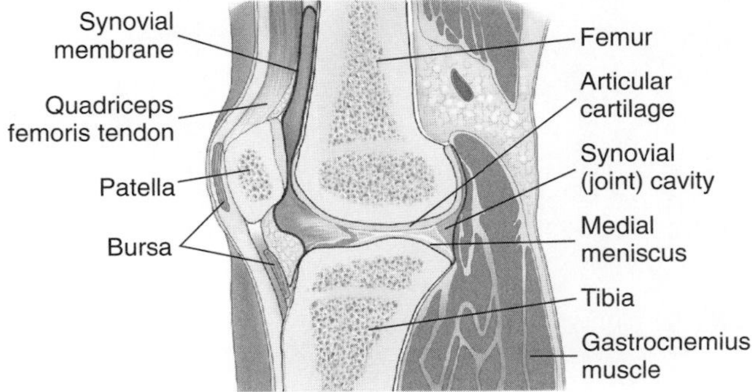

FIGURE 14-8. Knee joint.

Codes for arthroscopic procedures would be broken down as follows:

- Technique (arthroscopic rather than open or closed)
- Anatomic site
- Procedures performed (e.g., meniscectomy, release, repair)

NOTES: Multiple procedures require the use of modifier 51 when performed in the same anatomic location.

Procedures converted from arthroscopic to open need modifier 51.

Anatomic modifiers RT and LT would be appropriate in many instances.

Note that NCCI edits indicate that procedures converted from arthroscopic to open should only be coded to the most significant service, whereas CPT indicates they are both codeable and billable. Coders will, once again, need to check with the specific carriers to determine the appropriate coding in these instances.

ANATOMIC MODIFIERS

Caution should be used in the musculoskeletal section because many codes will require the inclusion of modifier code(s) to the procedure. The use of anatomic modifiers, however, is often misunderstood, and codes are assigned incorrectly. Keep in mind that the anatomic modifier(s) RT (right side of body) and LT (left side of body) should only be assigned to codes that are specific to anatomic sites that have only two sites. For instance, consider the following example:

> Excision of extensor tendon, with implantation of synthetic rod for delayed tendon graft, hand or finger, each rod an RT/LT modifier or an FA to F9 modifier could not be appended because the code refers to both fingers and hands. Code 26415

In this example—code 25800 arthrodesis, wrist, complete without bone graft—only the wrist is referred to; therefore because one has only a right and left wrist, the application of either an RT or an LT modifier would be appropriate.

Although the addition or omission of this anatomic modifier may not seem significant, it may result in payment denial for services, or the carrier may return the claim with a notation such as "not valid modifier for this service." Both outcomes result in nonpayment or delay in payment for services.

STOP AND PRACTICE

Determine the appropriate breakdown and code(s) for the following procedures.

	Anatomic Site	Procedure and Technique	Specifics	Code(s)
1. Removal of displaced pin from fracture site				
2. Closed repair, distal radius fracture				25600
3. Shoulder capsulorrhaphy				
4. Rotator cuff repair				
5. Incision and drainage, deep abscess, forearm				
6. Removal of foreign body, musculature, thigh				
7. Right shoulder arthroscopy with claviculectomy				
8. Diagnostic right knee arthroscopy with medial/ lateral meniscectomy				
9. Repair of left calcaneus fracture with cast application				
10. Arthroscopic TMJ repair				

STOP AND PRACTICE

Take the following operative reports and assign CPT codes appropriately. Make sure you continue to utilize the technique of breaking down the information needed to code. Utilize the guidelines listed earlier for each subcategory of the musculoskeletal system. You may wish to add the "bullets" we discussed for each section to your CPT book so those guidelines will be readily available as you search for the appropriate code(s).

1. Operative report

OPERATIVE REPORT

Patient information:

Patient name:
DOB:
MR#:

Date:
Surgeon:
Anesthetist:

Preoperative diagnosis:

Lateral patellar facet syndrome, left knee

Postoperative diagnosis:

Same

Procedure(s) performed:

Arthroscopy, left knee with open lateral retinacular release

Anesthesia:

Assistant surgeon:

Description of procedure:

The patient was placed supine on the operating room table and a satisfactory general anesthetic was given. Preoperative intravenous cephalosporin antibiotic was given. Pneumatic tourniquet was placed high about the left thigh. No leg holder was used. The left knee was shaved in the proposed incisional location. The leg was prepped sterilely with DuraPrep from the tourniquet to the foot, and the left knee was draped in the usual sterile fashion. Tourniquet was inflated to 350 mm of mercury. Arthroscope cannula was introduced via an anteromedial portal at the joint line, followed by the arthroscope. Inflow to the knee from the arthroscopy pump to the cannula at a setting of 15 mm of mercury. The knee was distended with normal saline in this fashion. Outflow from the cannula to suction. A flow of irrigation was maintained for purposes of visualization and removal of debris. There was no pathology or loose body in the medial gutter. The cartilaginous surfaces of the medial femoral condyle and medial tibial plateau were intact without evidence of fibrillation or breakdown. The medial meniscus showed no evidence of intrasubstance tear or peripheral detachment. The intercondylar notch showed no evidence of pathology. The visualized portions of the anterior and posterior cruciate ligaments were intact without evidence of stretching or tearing of their fibers or hemorrhage on their surfaces. The cartilaginous surfaces of the lateral femoral condyle and lateral tibial plateau were intact without evidence of fibrillation or breakdown. The lateral meniscus showed no evidence of intrasubstance tear or peripheral detachment except for the usual detachment in the region of the popliteus tendon, which was not elongated. The lateral gutter showed no evidence of pathology or loose body. There was no pathology or loose body in the suprapatellar area. The medial plica showed no evidence of pathology or damage. The cartilaginous surface of the patella, as well as the intracondylar notch, showed no evidence of fibrillation, breakdown, or pathology. There was a tight lateral retinaculum noted through a range of motion of the knee. A longitudinal skin incision was made laterally adjacent to the patella. The incision was carried through subcutaneous tissue. Hemostasis was achieved as necessary. Full-thickness skin flaps were raised. A nick was made in the lateral patellar retinaculum and a lateral patella release was performed in its entirety. This freed up the lateral aspect of the patella as visualized arthroscopically, which allowed better lift-off and enhanced medial glide of the patella. The knee was copiously irrigated with normal saline antibiotic solution from the arthroscopy pump during the procedure. As much fluid as possible was suctioned from the knee at the conclusion of the procedure. The arthroscope portal was closed with a single simple suture of 3-0 Ethilon. The lateral release incision was closed with interrupted vertical mattress sutures of 3-0 Ethilon. A total of 30 ccs of a combination of 0.5% Marcaine with epinephrine plus 5 mgs of morphine was injected into the knee. Dry sterile dressings were applied, followed by sterile circumferential cast padding. Tourniquet was deflated. All drapes were removed, including the tourniquet. Ace bandage was applied about the knee area. The patient tolerated the procedure well. There were no complications. He was awakened in the operating room and transported to the recovery room in stable condition.

GODFREY REGIONAL HOSPITAL
123 Main Street • Aldon, FL 77714 • (407) 555-1234

Step 1: Identify chapter or section of CPT: Surgery
Step 2: Identify anatomic system: ____________
Step 3: Identify anatomic site: ____________
Step 4: Identify procedure/technique: ____________
Step 5: Identify additional specifics: ____________
Step 6: Assign CPT code(s): ____________
Step 7: Place code(s) in appropriate order: ____________
Step 8: Assign modifier code(s) as appropriate: ____________

2. Operative report

OPERATIVE REPORT

Patient information:

Patient name:
DOB:
MR#:

Date:
Surgeon:
Anesthetist:

Preoperative diagnosis:

Chondromalacia patella, left knee, and possible medial meniscal tear, left knee

Postoperative diagnosis:

Chondromalacia patella and diffuse grade IV; chondromalacia medial femoral condyle from 0 to 80° and synovitis of the notch

Procedure(s) performed:

Left knee arthroscopy, synovectomy of the notch, chondroplasty patella and medial femoral condyle

Anesthesia:

Assistant surgeon:

Description of procedure:

After suitable general anesthesia had been achieved, the patient's left knee was prepped and draped in the usual manner. Prior to prepping, thigh tourniquet was applied, and after draping, inflated to 300 mm of mercury. Arthroscope was inserted through an anterior medial portal. The patient was noted to have marked synovitis of the notch. Thickened synovial tissue was excised with the shaver, and synovial bleeders were cauterized using the radiofrequency probe. Lateral compartment revealed intact articular surfaces and a stable intact lateral meniscus. Examination of the medial compartment revealed a lot of flakes of loose articular cartilage floating free inside the knee. Medial meniscus was intact and stable with probing. There was noted to be diffuse grade IV changes, 80% of the medial femoral condyle from 0–80°. Articular cartilage flaps were smoothed with the shaver. Examination of the patellofemoral joint revealed diffuse grade IV changes, but minimal articular cartilage flaps except at the inferior pole of the patella where there was a substantial cluster of articular cartilage flaps. These were smoothed with the shaver. Synovial bleeders were cauterized with the radiofrequency probe after excision of a thickened medial plica. Knee joint was then thoroughly irrigated, and the arthroscope was removed. Stab wounds were closed with 4-0 nylon. Dressing was then applied. Tourniquet was released. Following tourniquet release, good circulation was noted to return to the foot.
Patient tolerated the procedure well and returned to the recovery room in stable condition.

GODFREY REGIONAL HOSPITAL
123 Main Street • Aldon, FL 77714 • (407) 555-1234

Step 1: Identify chapter or section of CPT: Surgery
Step 2: Identify anatomic system: ____________
Step 3: Identify anatomic site: ____________
Step 4: Identify procedure/technique: ____________
Step 5: Identify additional specifics: ____________
Step 6: Assign CPT code(s): ____________
Step 7: Place code(s) in appropriate order: ____________
Step 8: Assign modifier code(s) as appropriate: ____________

3. Operative report

OPERATIVE REPORT

Patient information:

Patient name:
DOB:
MR#:

Date:
Surgeon:
Anesthetist:

Preoperative diagnosis:

Dupuytren contractures, both hands

Postoperative diagnosis:

Dupuytren contractures, both hands

Procedure(s) performed:

OPERATION SUMMARY: Release Dupuytren contractures, both hands
OPERATIVE FINDINGS: Dupuytren contractures, both hands
TISSUE REMOVED: Dupuytren contractures

Anesthesia:

Assistant surgeon:

Description of procedure:

Under adequate regional anesthetic, patient was prepped and draped in a sterile manner, and the left hand was released first. Incision was made over the palm. The 4th and 5th fingers were the ones that were tight, and these were carefully released, dissecting down, removing the thickened fascia scar layer of Dupuytren. This was completed while carefully preserving all neurovascular structures, both of the fingers were released so they would extend nicely without any tension and were quite free. Once release was completed and meticulous hemostasis was obtained, the incision was closed with Proline sutures. Dressings were applied. Attention was then turned to the opposite, that is, the right hand. On this hand the thumb was quite tight and this had to be released. Incision was made over the contracture and it was carefully dissected off and removed completely. This freed the thumb completely and it moved well and easily. Following this, then the 5th finger was released as well. However, there was ankylosis of the joint, that is the proximal interphalangeal joint, and this could not be freed. The contracture portion was freed so that the MP joint would move well, but with the ankylosed joint this could not be released. Upon release of these while carefully protecting all neurovascular structures and with meticulous hemostasis being obtained, these incisions as well were closed with Proline sutures. Dressings were applied and the patient was discharged to recovery in a stable condition. Patient tolerated this procedure well. Estimated blood loss, 25 cc. Sponge and needle count report is correct.

POSTOPERATIVE PLAN: He will follow up Saturday for dressing changes and next week for reexamination and dressing change.

GODFREY REGIONAL HOSPITAL
123 Main Street • Aldon, FL 77714 • (407) 555-1234

Step 1: Identify chapter or section of CPT: Surgery
Step 2: Identify anatomic system: ______
Step 3: Identify anatomic site: ______
Step 4: Identify procedure/technique: ______
Step 5: Identify additional specifics: ______
Step 6: Assign CPT code(s): ______
Step 7: Place code(s) in appropriate order: ______
Step 8: Assign modifier code(s) as appropriate: ______

4. Operative report

OPERATIVE REPORT

Patient information:

Patient name:
DOB:
MR#:

Date:
Surgeon:
Anesthetist:

Preoperative diagnosis:

Malposition of right both-bone forearm fracture
INDICATIONS FOR PROCEDURE: This is a 10-year-old female who sustained a both-bone forearm fracture and was treated with closed reduction and casting initially. She had gone on to malposition, despite appropriate casting, and the patient states that she had been wrestling with her brother, hitting her brother on top of the head with her cast. After discussion of the options, risks, and benefits of the surgical procedure, all questions were answered and consents were signed. The patient was taken to the operating room.

Postoperative diagnosis:

Malposition of right both-bone forearm fracture

Procedure(s) performed:

Closed reduction, intermedullary nailing radius

Anesthesia:

General

Assistant surgeon:

Description of procedure:

COMPLICATIONS: None
TOURNIQUET TIME: 36 minutes
The patient was taken to the operating room and placed supine on the operating room table. General anesthesia was obtained. The cast was then removed from the upper extremity. Obvious deformity was identified. Closed reduction was then able to be obtained with C-arm to verify adequacy of reduction. We then made a 1-cm incision over the area of Lister's tubercle, just proximal to the distal growth plate. We placed a 2.0-mm titanium flexible rod into the intermedullary canal with a radius and passed this past the fracture site. It was then bent and cut off. This was then sewed up with 3-0 Monocryl after irrigation with Bacitracin saline solution. The patient was placed into a well-padded long-arm cast after dressing it with Xeroform and 4 × 4s and sterile Webril. She was then extubated in the operating room, transferred from the operating room to her bed, and taken to the postanesthesia recovery room in stable condition.

GODFREY REGIONAL HOSPITAL
123 Main Street • Aldon, FL 77714 • (407) 555-1234

Step 1: Identify chapter or section of CPT: Surgery
Step 2: Identify anatomic system: ______
Step 3: Identify anatomic site: ______
Step 4: Identify procedure/technique: ______
Step 5: Identify additional specifics: ______
Step 6: Assign CPT code(s): ______
Step 7: Place code(s) in appropriate order: ______
Step 8: Assign modifier code(s) as appropriate: ______

5. Operative report

OPERATIVE REPORT

Patient information:

Patient name:
DOB:
MR#:

Date:
Surgeon:
Anesthetist:

Preoperative diagnosis:

1. Grade 2 open fracture of left distal radius and ulnar shafts
2. Fracture of left radial head

INDICATIONS FOR OPERATION: This 7-year-old young man fell out of a box on the back of a 4-wheeler. The patient fell on his left outstretched arm. He had pain around the wrist and elbow with deformity of the wrist. X-rays revealed a rather significantly displaced radial head fracture at the elbow, and a rather significantly displaced distal forearm fracture with the radius overriding in the ulna 45° angulated volarly. There was an open wound in the distal forearm that was initially thought to be greater than 1 cm in length, but at the time of surgery was found to be less than 1 cm in length. Probably the spike of the radius came through this. The patient was taken to the operating room for treatment of his fractures. Please see my History and Physical for the considerations discussed with the parents.

Postoperative diagnosis:

1. Grade 1 open fracture of left distal radius and ulnar shafts
2. Fracture of left radial head

Procedure(s) performed:

1. Open treatment of left distal radius and ulnar shaft fractures with debridement, irrigation, and closed reduction of radius and ulna
2. Closed reduction (closed treatment with manipulation), left radial head
3. Application of long-arm cast

Anesthesia:

Assistant surgeon:

Description of procedure:

The patient was taken to the operating room and placed supine on the operating table. General anesthesia was administered and achieved and he was intubated. Initially, traction was applied to the left forearm through the flexed elbow, and manipulation of the radial head was carried out through the skin, and actually, a fairly good reduction of this was carried out. It was not felt that open treatment of that would improve that significantly enough to warrant it. A majority of the translation and angulation was corrected. It was felt that there was acceptable position. Traction was further applied and a closed reduction of the distal radius and ulna was obtainable.

At this point the left upper extremity was scrubbed, prepped, and draped free and in standard fashion. No tourniquet was used. The open wound in the distal forearm measured about 1 cm or slightly less in width. It was extended both radially and ulnarly and the soft tissues were bluntly dissected. The wound went down to the radius. The entire area was copiously irrigated with antibiotic saline solution. A small portion of the skin edge was debrided. There was no gross contamination of the wound. I did not explore for the median nerve.

Fluoroscopic visualization of both fractures was satisfactory. The forearm wound was closed with interrupted 4-0 nylon sutures and a sterile dressing was applied. At this point the patient was placed in finger trap traction and further traction was carried out to reduce as close as possible the radial head and the distal radius and ulna. A well-padded long-arm cast was applied, with the forearm in some pronation and the elbow flexed to 90 degrees.

There were no complications and the patient tolerated the procedure well. He was awakened in the operating room and transported to Recovery in good condition.

GODFREY REGIONAL HOSPITAL
123 Main Street • Aldon, FL 77714 • (407) 555-1234

Step 1: Identify chapter or section of CPT: Surgery
Step 2: Identify anatomic system: ______
Step 3: Identify anatomic site: ______
Step 4: Identify procedure/technique: ______
Step 5: Identify additional specifics: ______
Step 6: Assign CPT code(s): ______
Step 7: Place code(s) in appropriate order: ______
Step 8: Assign modifier code(s) as appropriate: ______

Respiratory System (30000-32999)

RESPIRATORY SYSTEM SERVICES

Nose	30000-30999
Accessory sinuses	31000-31299
Larynx	31300-31599
Trachea and bronchi	31600-31899
Lungs and pleura	32035-32999

Key Medical Terms

Atelectasis
Broncho
Chronic obstructive pulmonary disease (COPD)
Dyspnea
Hemoptysis
Orthopnea
Rhino
Septo
Thoracentesis
Transbronchial
Upper respiratory infection (URI)

This system, similar to the musculoskeletal system, follows the anatomic progression of the body. The system starts with the nose, where air is breathed, through the sinuses, the larynx, down the trachea, and into the lungs (Figs. 14-9 and 14-10). Locating the right subsection within the respiratory system section is straightforward.

Subsections of the respiratory system section include the following:

- Nose
- Accessory sinuses
- Larynx
- Trachea, bronchi
- Lungs, pleura

Some general coding guidelines apply to the respiratory section. Many of these are incorporated in the NCCI guidelines and specifically address issues regarding bundling. They are as follows:

- When a diagnostic or surgical endoscopy is performed, a separate CPT code should not be reported for the diagnostic procedure to evaluate the access regions.
- When it is medically necessary, two endoscopic procedures performed on two regions of the respiratory system through two different scopes are separately reportable.
- If findings from a diagnostic endoscopy lead to the performance of a nonendoscopic surgical procedure during the same patient encounter, the diagnostic procedure may

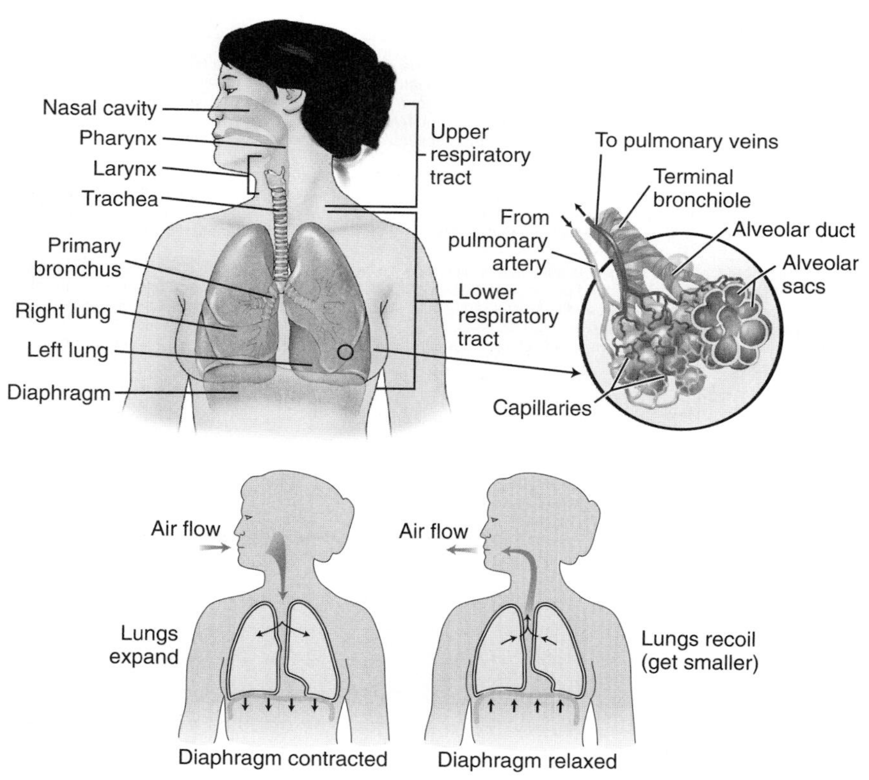

FIGURE 14-9. The respiratory system showing a bronchial tree.

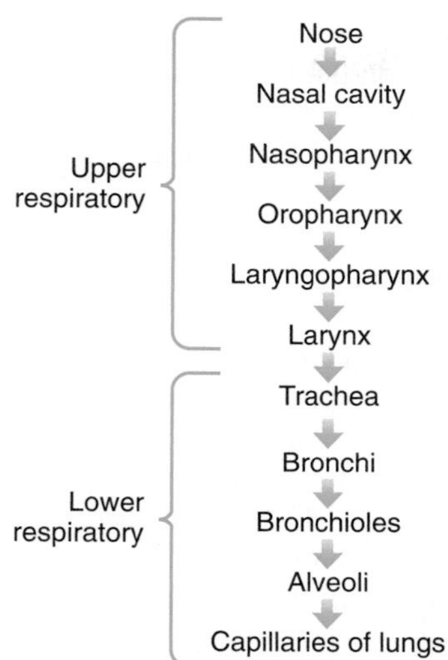

FIGURE 14-10. Schematic of the order in which air passes through the upper respiratory and into the lower respiratory system.

be separately reportable. However, this does not include scout endoscopic procedures performed solely to evaluate the surgical field.

- A diagnostic endoscopy is not separately reportable with a surgical endoscopic procedure performed on the same area.
- In line with the scopy procedure converted to an open procedure, if a sinusotomy is performed in conjunction with a sinus endoscopy, only one service would be reported.
- Any control of bleeding performed during an endoscopic procedure is not separately reportable.
- When laryngoscopy is required for placement of a tracheostomy, the laryngoscopy is not separately reportable.

NASAL REPAIR PROCEDURES

Care should be taken to distinguish between the open repair procedures performed on the nose and procedures performed endoscopically. Rhinoplasty, or surgical repair of the nose, differs from the septoplasty codes, in which the primary purpose is to repair or reconstruct only the septum of the nasal column. This is commonly performed to correct a deviated septum, which may have occurred as the result of an insult or injury to the nose. When the repair of a deviated septum is performed solely for cosmetic purposes, the procedure is typically not covered by insurance carriers. However, often a deviated septum results in nasal obstruction, or difficulty with breathing, which, in most instances would be considered medically necessary to correct and would be covered by insurance. When these types of procedures are performed, it is wise to contact the insurance carrier involved to get preauthorization to perform these procedures to clarify for both the patient and the provider whether the service will be paid by the carrier.

ACCESSORY SINUS PROCEDURES

Most of these procedures are performed endoscopically (31231-31294). In many instances, multiple procedures will be performed (modifier 51), often bilaterally (modifier 50). Keep in mind that there are three sets of sinus cavities (ethmoid, maxillary, and sphenoid), and each set has right and left sides. Once the procedure is identified as a sinus endoscopy, the following information should be gathered from the operative report:

- Sinus cavity(ies) procedures performed
- Specific procedure(s) performed

NOTES: Watch for separate procedure code(s).

Apply multiple modifiers appropriately (most significant to reimbursement first).

LARYNGOSCOPY PROCEDURES

Laryngoscopic procedures may be direct or indirect and sometimes are identified as microdirect or microindirect, indicating that some type of operating microscope may have been used to successfully complete the procedure(s). Separate codes are assigned when procedures are performed with an operating microscope. Make certain that magnifying loupes are not used in these instances.

Laryngoscopies should be coded with the following information:

- Diagnostic or operative
- Direct or indirect
- With or without operating microscopy
- Specific procedure(s) performed

NOTES: Diagnostic laryngoscopy included in surgical interventions

Modifier 51 for multiple procedures

Laryngoscopic procedures are performed either indirectly, with the use of a mirror to image the larynx, or directly, with the larynx directly visualized. In some instances a diagnostic laryngoscope will be performed, or a biopsy. However, if a definitive surgical procedure would be performed to the same area that is biopsied, only the definitive procedure would be coded.

BRONCHOSCOPY

Bronchoscopy is performed by an endoscopic approach for the purpose of visualizing the trachea, vocal cords, and bronchi. Brushings, biopsies, and other interventional procedures may be performed at the time of a diagnostic bronchoscopy. The "separate procedure" rule applies, and diagnostic bronchoscopy would NOT be coded when a surgical bronchoscopic procedure was performed. Careful attention should be made to the biopsy codes because the approach is different (transbronchial or bronchial) as are the number of site(s). For instance, code 31628 is for bronchoscopic transbronchial biopsy(ies) of a single lobe, without regard to the number of biopsies performed to that one lobe. Additional biopsy(ies) can be coded in this instance only when they are taken from another lobe.

Breakdown for this section is as follows:

- Diagnostic or surgical
- Biopsy(ies)/site(s)
- Procedure(s) performed

NOTE: Modifier 51 when multiple procedures are performed endoscopically

Bronchoscopy codes (31622-32640) are inherently bilateral procedures; therefore it is not appropriate to code a bronchoscopic code more than once when performed on both the right and the left side. All bronchoscopy codes also include any fluoroscopic guidance that may be performed.

THORACENTESIS AND THORACOSTOMY

When a puncture is made for the purpose of inserting a chest tube for drainage of air or fluid from the pleural space so a collapsed lung may be expanded, the procedure is known as a *tube thoracostomy.* When a puncture is made for the sole purpose of removing fluid or air, such a procedure would be coded to the *thoracentesis* code 32421. When, however, the tube is inserted and left in place, code 32422 would be appropriate.

TRACHEOSTOMY

As you have probably already become aware, a number of procedures in the respiratory system appear very similar; these are thoracostomy, thoracotomy, tracheotomy, tracheostomy, laryngectomy, and laryngotomy. One must watch carefully to make certain that the correct procedure is being assigned the correct code.

Tracheostomy is one of the most common procedures performed on the trachea. The procedure involves making an incision and creating an artificial opening for breathing or prolonged ventilation. The procedure may be performed as a planned procedure (31600-31601) or on an emergency basis (31603-31605).

STOP AND PRACTICE

Determine the appropriate breakdown and code(s) for the following procedures.

Procedure	Anatomic Site	Procedure and Technique	Specifics	Code(s)
1. Bronchoscopy, diagnostic	______	______	______	______
2. Tracheostomy	______	______	______	______
3. Tracheotomy	______	______	______	______
4. Thoracentesis with tube placement	______	______	______	______
5. Endoscopic ethmoidectomy, bilateral	______	______	______	______
Right maxillary antrostomy	______	______	______	______
Concha bullosa resection	______	______	______	______
6. Endoscopic sphenoidotomy with tissue removal	______	______	______	______
7. Laryngoscopy with foreign body removal	______	______	______	______
8. Emergency endotracheal intubation	______	______	______	______
9. Bronchoscopy with washings	______	______	______	______
10. Bronchoscopic transbronchial lung biopsy, lower left lung	______	______	______	______
Bronchoscopic transbronchial lung biopsy, right upper lung	______	______	______	______

STOP AND PRACTICE

Take the following operative reports and assign CPT codes appropriately. Make sure you continue to use the technique of breaking down the information needed to code. Use the guidelines listed earlier for each subcategory of the respiratory system. You may wish to add the "bullets" discussed for each section to your CPT book so those guidelines will be readily available as you search for the appropriate code(s).

1. Operative report

OPERATIVE REPORT

Patient information:

Patient name:
DOB:
MR#:

Date:
Surgeon:
Anesthetist:

Preoperative diagnosis:

Chronic left maxillary and ethmoid sinusitis, left middle turbinate hypertrophy

CLINICAL NOTE:
The patient is a 54-year-old white female with chronic left maxillary and ethmoid sinusitis, not responding to conservative medical treatment. Preoperatively on CT scan, post treatment she was found to have complete opacification. The patient had opacification of the left maxillary sinus and left chronic ethmoid sinusitis.

Postoperative diagnosis:

Chronic left maxillary and ethmoid sinusitis, left middle turbinate hypertrophy

OPERATIVE FINDINGS:
There is chronic mucosal thickening of the left maxillary sinuses. Right middle turbinate was partially removed to prevent postoperative synechia/scarring and obstruction of the ostiomeatal complex, which was opened surgically.

Procedure(s) performed:

Endoscopic left total ethmoidectomy. Left middle meatal enterostomy. Left partial middle turbinectomy.

Anesthesia:

General

Assistant surgeon:

Description of procedure:

The patient was brought to the operating room and placed in the supine position. General endotracheal anesthesia was administered. The nose was vasoconstricted with topical Afrin and injected with 6 cc 1% lidocaine with 1:100,000 parts of epinephrine into the left middle turbinate and lateral nasal wall mucosa.

Using a two-view monitor for visualization, the 0 degree sinus endoscope was placed in the left nasal cavity and the left middle turbinate was lateralized with a Freer elevator. Using the sharp edge of the Freer, the anterior ethmoid air cells were entered and bone and mucosa were removed with straight and upbiting Blakesley forceps. The left maxillary sinus ostia was identified and an enterostomy, approximately 1 cm in diameter, was made with the upbiting forceps and power microdebrider. The left maxillary sinus cavity was examined with a 30- and 70-degree sinus endoscope and it showed chronic, thickened mucosa with no evidence of fungus or mucopurulent discharge. The left total ethmoidectomy was completed with Blakesley forceps and the power microdebrider. The specimen was sent to Pathology for permanent section. An anterior inferior portion of the left middle turbinate was incised with turbinate scissors.

Upon completion of the procedures, the left ethmoid sinus cavity was packed with MeroGel and two Kennedy nasal tampons. A 9-cm standard tampon was placed along the floor of the nose, which was impregnated with Bacitracin ointment. The sutures of the tampon were tied together, and a nasal turbinate pad was placed. The oropharynx was suctioned. There was adequate hemostasis present. The patient was awakened from general anesthesia, extubated, and brought to the recovery room in stable condition, having tolerated the procedure well.

ESTIMATED BLOOD LOSS: Less than 10 cc

Maurice Doater, MD

GODFREY REGIONAL HOSPITAL
123 Main Street • Aldon, FL 77714 • (407) 555-1234

Step 1: Identify chapter or section of CPT: Surgery
Step 2: Identify anatomic system: ______
Step 3: Identify anatomic site: ______
Step 4: Identify procedure/technique: ______
Step 5: Identify additional specifics: ______
Step 6: Assign CPT code(s): ______
Step 7: Place code(s) in appropriate order: ______
Step 8: Assign modifier code(s) as appropriate: ______

2. Operative report

OPERATIVE REPORT

Patient information:

Patient name:
DOB:
MR#:

Date:
Surgeon:
Anesthetist:

Preoperative diagnosis:

Postoperative diagnosis:

Procedure(s) performed:

Anesthesia:

Assistant surgeon:

Description of procedure:

Doyle splints were placed in the nose. An Aquaplast splint was placed on the dorsum of the nose.

The patient tolerated both procedures well and there were no complications. The patient was thus removed directly to recovery room in stable condition.

ESTIMATED BLOOD LOSS: 50 cc

COMPLICATIONS: None. Instrument count correct at the end of the procedure.

Maurice Doater, MD

GODFREY REGIONAL HOSPITAL
123 Main Street • Aldon, FL 77714 • (407) 555-1234

Step 1: Identify chapter or section of CPT: Surgery
Step 2: Identify anatomic system: ______
Step 3: Identify anatomic site: ______
Step 4: Identify procedure/technique: ______
Step 5: Identify additional specifics: ______
Step 6: Assign CPT code(s): ______
Step 7: Place code(s) in appropriate order: ______
Step 8: Assign modifier code(s) as appropriate: ______

3. Operative report

PROCEDURE NOTE

Patient information:

Patient name:
DOB:
MR#:

Date:
Surgeon:
Anesthetist:

Preoperative diagnosis:

INDICATION:
Shortness of breath, recurrent right pleural effusion, history of bronchogenic carcinoma

The patient was identified by name bracelet prior to procedure. The Pharmaseal thoracentesis kit with catheter was used, sterile technique. 1% local lidocaine and Betadine scrub were used.

Postoperative diagnosis:

Procedure(s) performed:

Thoracentesis

Anesthesia:

Assistant surgeon:

Description of procedure:

FINDINGS:
The right posterior chest was prepped with Betadine, sterile technique. A Pharmaseal catheter was instilled into the right posterior clavicular line, 200 spaces below the scapula, and 1.2 liters of serosanguineous fluid was removed without difficulty. The patient had decreased shortness of breath prior to procedure. The patient tolerated the procedure well. Will check chest x-ray.

Maurice Doate MD

GODFREY REGIONAL HOSPITAL
123 Main Street • Aldon, FL 77714 • (407) 555-1234

Step 1: Identify chapter or section of CPT: Surgery
Step 2: Identify anatomic system: ____________
Step 3: Identify anatomic site: ____________
Step 4: Identify procedure/technique: ____________
Step 5: Identify additional specifics: ____________
Step 6: Assign CPT code(s): ____________
Step 7: Place code(s) in appropriate order: ____________
Step 8: Assign modifier code(s) as appropriate: ____________

4. Operative report

PROCEDURE NOTE

Patient information:

Patient name:
DOB:
MR#:

Date:
Surgeon:
Anesthetist:

Preoperative diagnosis:

INDICATION:
Rule out recurrent bronchogenic carcinoma
Patient was identified by name bracelet prior to procedure. Patient had topical lidocaine via the nares and oropharynx prior to procedure. A total of 8 mg of IV Versed was given in 1 mg titrations. Video Olympus bronchoscope was used.

Postoperative diagnosis:

CONCLUSIONS:
1. No endobronchial lesions
2. Transbronchial biopsies and brushings obtained in the right upper lobe density

Procedure(s) performed:

Bronchoscopy

Anesthesia:

Assistant surgeon:

Description of procedure:

FINDINGS:
The bronchoscope was passed via the left naris without difficulty. The epiglottis and aryepiglottic folds were normal in appearance and color. The vocal cords moved equally and approximated with phonation. Bronchoscope was passed into the tracheobronchial tree. Right upper lobe, right middle lobe, and right lower lobe were all patent with no endobronchial lesions seen. Significant mucus was cleared. Left lower lobe and left upper lobe were also patent with no endobronchial lesions seen.
The bronchoscope was taken through the right upper lobe. Then with fluoroscopic guidance, brushings and biopsies were obtained of the density in the right upper lobe. Bleeding stopped spontaneously. The patient tolerated the procedure well.

Maurice Doater, MD

GODFREY REGIONAL HOSPITAL
123 Main Street • Aldon, FL 77714 • (407) 555-1234

Step 1: Identify chapter or section of CPT: Surgery
Step 2: Identify anatomic system: ______
Step 3: Identify anatomic site: ______
Step 4: Identify procedure/technique: ______
Step 5: Identify additional specifics: ______
Step 6: Assign CPT code(s): ______
Step 7: Place code(s) in appropriate order: ______
Step 8: Assign modifier code(s) as appropriate: ______

5. Operative report

PROCEDURE NOTE

Patient information:

Patient name:
DOB:
MR#:

Date:
Surgeon:
Anesthetist:

Preoperative diagnosis:

HISTORY:
Right lower lobe mass

Postoperative diagnosis:

IMPRESSION:
CT guided biopsy of right lower lung mass

Procedure(s) performed:

CT guided lung biopsy

Anesthesia:

Assistant surgeon:

Description of procedure:

TECHNIQUE:
The patient was positioned supine and an appropriate area of puncture was made over the lower portion of the chest. An appropriate area was cleansed and anesthetized with 3 ccs of 1% Xylocaine. An 18-gauge spring-loaded needle was inserted approximately 4 cm to the right of the midline into a 6 × 5 cm mass in the right base medially. Three cores of tissue were removed using the co-axial spring-loaded 18-gauge biopsy needle. No bleeding could be seen in the chest after the study and there was no pneumothorax identified. The patient received 1 mg of Versed intravenously for sedation.

Maurice Doater, MD

GODFREY REGIONAL HOSPITAL
123 Main Street • Aldon, FL 77714 • (407) 555-1234

Step 1: Identify chapter or section of CPT: Surgery
Step 2: Identify anatomic system: ______________
Step 3: Identify anatomic site: ______________
Step 4: Identify procedure/technique: ______________
Step 5: Identify additional specifics: ______________
Step 6: Assign CPT code(s): ______________
Step 7: Place code(s) in appropriate order: ______________
Step 8: Assign modifier code(s) as appropriate: ______________

Cardiovascular System (33010-37799)

CARDIOVASCULAR SYSTEM SERVICES

Heart and pericardium	30010-33999
Arteries and veins	34001-37799

Key Medical Terms

Abdominal aortic aneurysm (AAA)
Anastomosis
Aneurysm
Angioplasty
Atherectomy
Atrioventricular leads
Bypass graft
Catheterization
Central venous access device
Coronary artery bypass graft (CABG)
Defibrillator
Endarterectomy
Pacemaker
Pacemaker battery
Percutaneous transluminal coronary angioplasty (PTCA)
Pulse generator
Thrombectomy
Thromboendarterectomy

Subcategories of the cardiovascular system (Figs. 14-11, 14-12, and 14-13) section include the following:

- Heart and pericardium
- Arteries and veins

When coding for cardiology services, the coder will find the appropriate codes in several sections within the CPT coding manual. Cardiovascular surgical procedures are located in the surgery section, whereas nonsurgical cardiovascular services are located in the medicine section. In addition, a number of diagnostic studies and radiologic imaging codes will be located in the radiology section.

Note that heart catheterization, coronary angioplasty, stents, and atherectomies are not included in the cardiovascular surgery section because they are considered noninvasive in nature. They are located in the medicine section of CPT and are discussed in Chapter 17. The cardiovascular section encompasses surgical intervention for cardiovascular disease.

PACEMAKER AND DEFIBRILLATOR SYSTEMS

A number of assist devices are placed in the cardiovascular system to help regulate heart rhythm. A pacemaker is implanted for the purpose of regulating an irregular heartbeat, and a defibrillator is usually implanted when the heart has stopped beating or the rhythm is extremely slow (bradycardia). A number of factors must be considered when coding for pacemakers and defibrillators, outlined as follows:

- Permanent, replacement, temporary, removal, repair, conversion
- Pacemaker or defibrillator
- Approach for procedure
- With or without replacement of electrodes
- Electrode(s) replaced (atrial/ventricular)

NOTE: The pulse generator is the "battery" of the pacemaker.

When the pulse generator, or battery, is being replaced, it is appropriate to assign the code for removing the old battery as well as the insertion of the new battery. This is only one of two areas in CPT where the removal and replacement for services may be reported separately. In most instances removal to accommodate replacement would not be reported.

When additional electrodes are being inserted for pacing, the use of code 33244 or 33225 is appropriate when two leads are placed with the assist device—one is placed in the atrium and one in the ventricle to regulate the heart into regular rhythm. These devices can be placed through an epicardial approach, which involves entering the chest cavity and placing

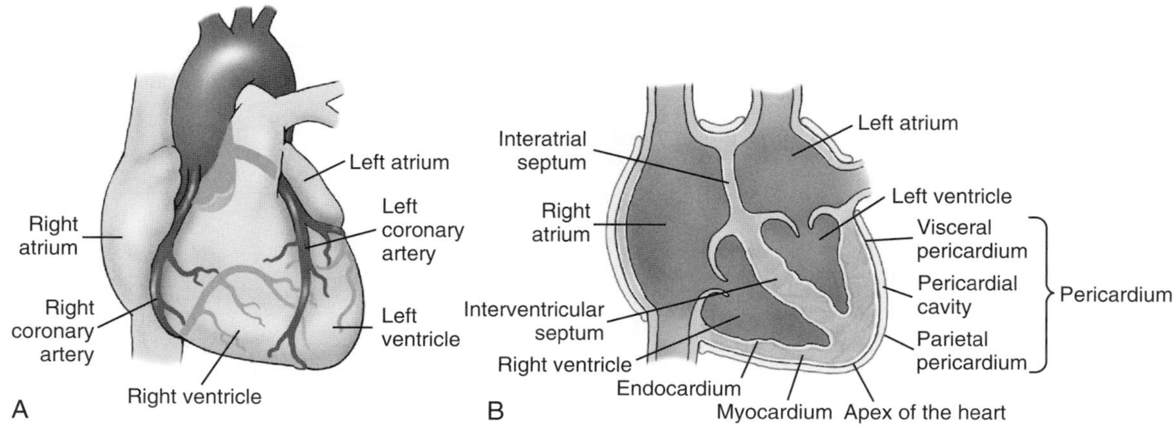

FIGURE 14-11. **A,** Location of the coronary arteries. **B,** Chambers of the heart.

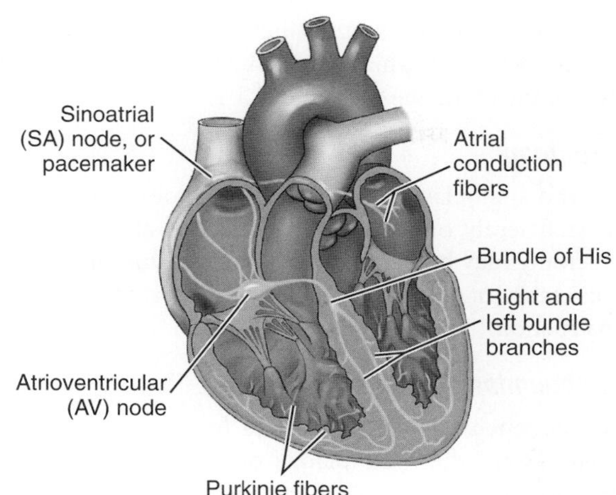

FIGURE 14-12. Electrical conduction patterns of the heart.

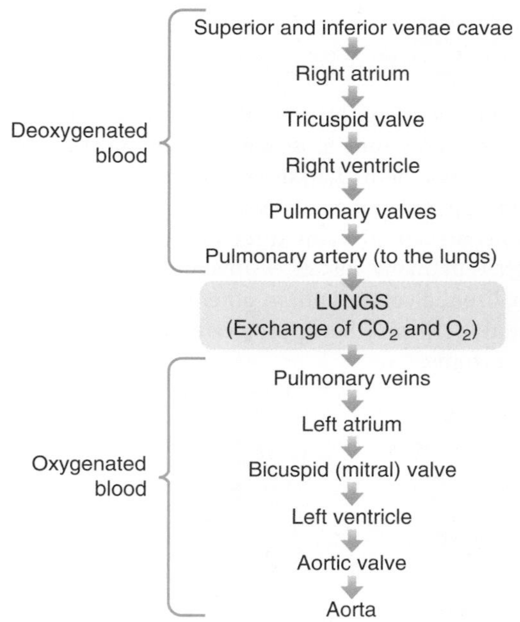

FIGURE 14-13. Oxygenated/deoxygenated status of blood.

the lead on the epicardial sac of the heart. When the device is placed through a transvenous approach, the device is placed within a pocket.

ELECTROPHYSIOLOGIC PROCEDURES

This section of codes within the cardiovascular surgery section contains codes for the surgical treatment of supraventricular dysrhythmias or irregular rhythms of the heart. A number of methods such as tissue ablation, disruption, and reconstruction may be used for correcting the dysrhythmia. The procedures typically involve making an incision, exposing the heart, and then performing the corrective method of resolving the dysrhythmia.

Patient-Activated Event Recorders

These devices are typically implanted so that the patient can signal when cardiac events occur in order to assist in a rhythm problem that has been difficult to diagnose.

ARTERIAL GRAFTING FOR CORONARY ARTERY BYPASS

When arteriovenous grafting associated with coronary artery bypass is reported, the following codes are appropriate:

Arterial graft	33533-33536
Combined arterial-venous graft	33517-33523

COMBINED ARTERIOVENOUS GRAFTING FOR CORONARY BYPASS

When arteriovenous grafting for coronary bypass procedure is reported, the following services are also coded and billed:

Combined arterial-venous graft	33517-33523
Arterial graft	33533-33536

To code coronary bypass grafts correctly, the coder must determine the following:

- Venous or arterial or venous *and* arterial grafting
- Number of grafts
- Procurement of grafts (upper extremity, 35500; femoropopliteal, 35572), separately codeable

SELECTIVE OR NONSELECTIVE PLACEMENT OF CATHETERS

A variety of codes in the cardiovascular section involve the placement of catheters. When these catheters are used for imaging, the coding assignment involves the determination of whether the placement is selective or nonselective.

When nonselective placement of catheters is performed, it indicates that the catheter was placed directly into a vessel without manipulation into vessels other than the one accessed. Selective placement means that the catheter must be further manipulated into other parts or branches of the vascular system than the original entry vessel. When it is necessary to access additional branches of the arterial and venous system, these are referred to as the *first order, second order,* and *third order* of the vascular family. Appendix L, located in the back of the CPT manual, designates these first-, second-, and third-order families when the assumption is made that the site of original access is the aorta. Appendix L will prove helpful in assigning codes for vascular services.

VENOUS ACCESS DEVICES

Venous access devices and catheters are also included in the cardiovascular section of surgery. The coder must determine the type of device being placed to assign the correct codes for these procedures. A central venous catheter is placed temporarily, usually for short periods (10 to 14 days) to supplement intravenous infusion. Venous access devices involve the placement of a permanently implanted catheter under the skin, and in some cases include an implanted reservoir. These devices are implanted for long periods and are completely hidden beneath the skin. For the venous access devices to be coded correctly, the following information should be extracted from the operative report:

- Introduction, removal, revision of venous catheter
- Venous or peripheral placement
- Tunneled or nontunneled catheter
- Age of patient
- Placement of pump or port in addition to catheter

CARDIOVASCULAR REPAIR CODES

A number of repair codes are in the surgical cardiovascular section.

Aneurysm

Aneurysm repair may involve excision of the area of the vessel that has been dilated, repair or bypass of the area when necessary, or both. In addition to code assignments based on the surgical technique, aneurysm repair codes are also assigned based on the location of the aneurysm.

Angioplasty

Repair of the vessel involves the placement of a balloon inside the vessel for purposes of dilation of the vessel in the area of an obstruction. Note that the angioplasty codes located in the surgical cardiovascular section include locations other than the coronary vessels, which are included in the cardiography section of the medicine section of CPT.

Atherectomy

When the angioplasty technique alone does not dilate the vessel sufficiently, or the area obstructs even after dilation, an atherectomy may be performed. This procedure involves the surgical excision of plaque that has accumulated and resulted in obstruction.

Thromboendarterectomy

A thromboendarterectomy involves incision to expose the affected vessel, where the plaque or thrombus creating the obstruction and the lining of the vessel are removed. After this portion of the procedure is performed, sutures are usually placed to secure the diameter of the vessel to ensure patency of the vessel.

HEMODIALYSIS ACCESS

When venous access by central line placement or vascular access device is not possible, usually because of poor venous access, hemodialysis access may be accomplished through upper arm cephalic vein transposition, direct arteriovenous anastomosis, or direct anastomosis of a vein to an artery. In many instances imaging must be performed to visualize the vessels and, in other cases, identify an occlusion and perform the appropriate procedures, including thrombectomy.

STOP AND PRACTICE

Determine the appropriate breakdown and code(s) for the following procedures.

	Anatomic Site	Procedure and Technique	Specifics	Code(s)
1. Removal of pacemaker pulse generator	______	______	______	______
2. Removal of old pacemaker pulse generator	______	______	______	______
Insertion of new pacemaker pulse generator	______	______	______	______
3. Revision of pacemaker skin pocket	______	______	______	______
4. CABG, venous grafting, three vessels	______	______	______	______
5. CABG, arteriovenous grafting, two vessels	______	______	______	______
6. Aortic peripheral atherectomy, open	______	______	______	______
7. Thromboendarterectomy, subclavian thoracic incision	______	______	______	______
8. Balloon angioplasty, percutaneous, iliac vessel	______	______	______	______
9. Blood transfusion	______	______	______	______
10. Venipuncture, age 7	______	______	______	______

STOP AND PRACTICE

Take the following operative reports and assign CPT codes appropriately. Make sure you continue to use the technique of breaking down the information needed to code. Use the guidelines listed above for each subcategory of the cardiovascular system. You may wish to add the "bullets" discussed for each section to your CPT book so those guidelines will be readily available as you search for the appropriate code(s).

1. Operative report

OPERATIVE REPORT

Patient information:

Patient name:
DOB:
MR#:

Date:
Surgeon:
Anesthetist:

Preoperative diagnosis:

Metastatic colon cancer

Postoperative diagnosis:

Metastatic colon cancer

Procedure(s) performed:

1. Placement of a right internal jugular single chamber.
2. Infuse-A-Port placed onto the right anterior chest wall.

Anesthesia:

Assistant surgeon:

Description of procedure:

The patient is a very pleasant 65-year-old male who recently presented to my office with a history of colon cancer and is undergoing chemotherapy. He has very poor peripheral IV access and he presents for the above procedure.
OPERATIVE PROCEDURE:
The patient was taken to the operating room and placed in a supine position on the operating table. After adequate IV sedation was achieved, the patient's right neck and upper chest were prepped and draped in standard surgical fashion. Using 1% lidocaine, I carefully anesthetized an area over the anterior border, sternocleidomastoid muscle, as well as onto the anterior chest wall. Using a Seldinger technique, a guidewire was placed into the right internal jugular vein to the superior vena cava. This was verified using intraoperative fluoroscopy. I then made a pocket under the right anterior chest wall using the 15-blade and electric Bovie cautery, and created it so that the Infuse-A-Port would fit comfortably into the pocket. Then using the dilator introducer system, these were placed over the guidewire into the internal jugular vein. The guidewire and dilator were then removed, and the catheter itself was threaded into the superior vena cava. Again its position was verified using intraoperative fluoroscopy. I then used the tunneling device and tunneled the catheter onto the anterior chest wall, hooked it up to the Infuse-A-Port, placed the Infuse-A-Port into the pocket. I ensured that the Infuse-A-Port worked properly using heparinized saline, both aspirating and then flushing. I then closed the pocket using a 3-0 Vicryl suture and the skin was closed with subcuticular 4-0 Monocryl. The neck incision was also closed with subcuticular 4-0 Monocryl. Benzoin and Steri-strips were placed over the incision.
The patient tolerated the procedure very well and returned to the recovery room in good condition.

GODFREY REGIONAL HOSPITAL
123 Main Street • Aldon, FL 77714 • (407) 555-1234

Step 1: Identify chapter or section of CPT: Surgery
Step 2: Identify anatomic system: ______
Step 3: Identify anatomic site: ______
Step 4: Identify procedure/technique: ______
Step 5: Identify additional specifics: ______
Step 6: Assign CPT code(s): ______
Step 7: Place code(s) in appropriate order: ______
Step 8: Assign modifier code(s) as appropriate: ______

2. Operative report

OPERATIVE REPORT

Patient information:

Patient name:
DOB:
MR#:

Date:
Surgeon:
Anesthetist:

Preoperative diagnosis:

End-stage renal disease, nonmaturation of left arm AV-fistula
CLINICAL HISTORY: The patient is status post left arm AV fistula. She has nonmaturation. Fistulogram shows one moderate size tributary just proximal anastomosis. She presents for elective ligation.

Postoperative diagnosis:

Same

Procedure(s) performed:

Ligation of AV-fistula tributaries

Anesthesia:

Assistant surgeon:

Description of procedure:

DESCRIPTION OF THE PROCEDURE:
The patient had three tributaries marked by ultrasound. One was close to the anastomosis; the other two were more proximal at the arm. We prepped and draped her left arm, anesthetized skin and subcu tissue with local. We dissected down and found the proximal tributary, ligated it, and stapled it. The fistula was still patent after we ligated the tributary. We could not find the more proximal tributary despite dissecting out the fistula for 2 cm. Rather than risk injuring the fistula, I did not proceed with attempts at finding a tributary. We did not attempt to locate the most proximal tributary either. We irrigated the two opened incisions and closed the skin with interrupted 4-0 Biosyn and placed sterile dressing.
The patient is to follow up in one month.

GODFREY REGIONAL HOSPITAL
123 Main Street • Aldon, FL 77714 • (407) 555-1234

Step 1: Identify chapter or section of CPT:	Surgery	Step 5: Identify additional specifics:	_______
Step 2: Identify anatomic system:	_______	Step 6: Assign CPT code(s):	_______
Step 3: Identify anatomic site:	_______	Step 7: Place code(s) in appropriate order:	_______
Step 4: Identify procedure/technique:	_______	Step 8: Assign modifier code(s) as appropriate:	_______

3. Operative report

OPERATIVE REPORT

Patient information:

Patient name:
DOB:
MR#:

Date:
Surgeon:
Anesthetist:

Preoperative diagnosis:

Diatek cath

Postoperative diagnosis:

Procedure(s) performed:

Left Diatek catheter insertion
HISTORY: Malfunction of catheter

Anesthesia:

Assistant surgeon:

Description of procedure:

TECHNIQUE:
The examination was done through the existing tract of the left-sided catheter. A stiff guidewire was initially inserted through the catheter, but the catheter could not be withdrawn. A 0.035 angled Glidewire was inserted through the catheter, and again the indwelling catheter could not be withdrawn. Multiple attempts to release the catheter were unsuccessful. The skin between the exit incision and the internal jugular vein was entered and the catheter removed in its mid-portion and cut. The wire was then inserted through this area for better manipulation. After numerous attempts, the catheter was withdrawn over the wire. The Diatek catheter was then inserted over the wire to the appropriate position. The patient received 1 gram of Ancef intravenously at the start of the procedure, and the old and new tracks of the catheters were flushed with a solution of 1 gram of Ancef and 1 liter of normal saline. The position of the catheter was checked at the termination of the procedure by fluoroscopy. Less than one hour of fluoroscopy time was used for the procedure.
IMPRESSION: Insertion of left-sided Diatek tunneled catheter under fluoroscopic guidance.

GODFREY REGIONAL HOSPITAL
123 Main Street • Aldon, FL 77714 • (407) 555-1234

Step 1: Identify chapter or section of CPT: Surgery
Step 2: Identify anatomic system: ________
Step 3: Identify anatomic site: ________
Step 4: Identify procedure/technique: ________
Step 5: Identify additional specifics: ________
Step 6: Assign CPT code(s): ________
Step 7: Place code(s) in appropriate order: ________
Step 8: Assign modifier code(s) as appropriate: ________

4. Operative report

OPERATIVE REPORT

Patient information:

Patient name:
DOB:
MR#:

Date:
Surgeon:
Anesthetist:

Preoperative diagnosis:

Left leg and thigh, symptomatic varicose veins

Postoperative diagnosis:

Same

Procedure(s) performed:

Varicose vein stripping and ligation of left leg and thigh—primarily lesser, but partial greater saphenous systems

Anesthesia:

Assistant surgeon:

Description of procedure:

The patient was placed in the sitting position for the spinal and then placed supine and in slight Trendelenburg, sterilely prepped and draped. The veins had been marked in the preoperative area. Each marked vein was approached in the following fashion: The skin was incised transversely with a number 11 blade. The vein was teased out. If there were perforator veins or terminal veins, these were ligated with 3-0 Vicryl; otherwise, they were sequentially dissected towards the next mark and then a counter incision was made to connect the dissections. In the lower leg, the veins were small and friable. In the upper thigh, the veins were quite sizable and thick. In this fashion veins were resected from the leg both anteriorly and posteriorly, as well as a significant system on the lateral aspect and on to the thigh initially, laterally, at the knee and extending medially on the more proximal thigh. Every mark had an identified vein that was resected. Skin was closed with 4-0 nylon in interrupted vertical mattress fashion. These were then dressed with Telfa, gauze, Kerlix, and Ace wrap.
She tolerated the procedure well.

GODFREY REGIONAL HOSPITAL
123 Main Street • Aldon, FL 77714 • (407) 555-1234

Step 1: Identify chapter or section of CPT: Surgery
Step 2: Identify anatomic system: ________
Step 3: Identify anatomic site: ________
Step 4: Identify procedure/technique: ________
Step 5: Identify additional specifics: ________
Step 6: Assign CPT code(s): ________
Step 7: Place code(s) in appropriate order: ________
Step 8: Assign modifier code(s) as appropriate: ________

5. Operative report

OPERATIVE REPORT

Patient information:

Patient name:
DOB:
MR#:

Date:
Surgeon:
Anesthetist:

Preoperative diagnosis:

End-stage renal disease; infected Ash catheter
CLINICAL HISTORY: The patient is a 68-year-old white male who was undergoing dialysis. His Ash catheter became infected and required removal. He now presents for a Quinton catheter in his femoral vein.

Postoperative diagnosis:

End-stage renal disease; infected Ash catheter

Procedure(s) performed:

Left femoral Quinton catheter placement

Anesthesia:

Assistant surgeon:

Description of procedure:

The patient was brought to Ambulatory Care, placed in the supine position; right groin was prepped and draped in sterile fashion. We attempted to gain access to right femoral vein, but instead placed the needle into the femoral artery. We were using ultrasound, but the artery and vein were very close together. Patient had some edema from the prior catheter. We held pressure and aborted the procedure after one arterial stick. We then shaved and prepped the left groin and attempted to place the catheter in the left groin. Again, we incurred an arterial puncture. Patient developed a small hematoma. We aborted the left femoral approach. We then attempted the right IJ vein. We were able to gain access but could not thread the guidewire due to a thrombus in the vein. We aborted this procedure, then re-evaluated. The swelling in the left groin had diminished. We again did the ultrasound of the groin and we were able to see the vein with the ultrasound. We prepped and draped and were able to percutaneously enter the left femoral vein without puncturing the artery. We placed the guidewire dilator over the guidewire and then placed the catheter over the guidewire. We sutured it in place and flushed it. It flushed easily.
Plan is to get vancomycin again today, 1 gram. He had only gotten it one time, even though I ordered it with every dialysis; I told the dialysis tech that he needs it with every dialysis. I talked with his primary care physician and our long-term plan is to place a left forearm graft. I will look into the availability for immediate-use graft. If one is not available, we will use the Gore-Tex and wait two weeks to start accessing it.
The patient was transferred to the recovery room in good condition.

GODFREY REGIONAL HOSPITAL
123 Main Street • Aldon, FL 77714 • (407) 555-1234

Step 1: Identify chapter or section of CPT: Surgery
Step 2: Identify anatomic system: ______
Step 3: Identify anatomic site: ______
Step 4: Identify procedure/technique: ______
Step 5: Identify additional specifics: ______
Step 6: Assign CPT code(s): ______
Step 7: Place code(s) in appropriate order: ______
Step 8: Assign modifier code(s) as appropriate: ______

Hemic and Lymphatic Systems (38100-38999)

HEMIC AND LYMPHATIC SYSTEMS SERVICES

Spleen	38100-38200
General	38204-38242
Lymph nodes and lymphatic channels	38300-38999

A limited number of procedures are included in the hemic and lymphatic system. Perhaps the most common is biopsy and/or excision of lymph nodes. CPT makes no distinction when lymph nodes are biopsied versus excised; therefore the same CPT selection would be appropriate. CPT also does not permit separately reporting the biopsy or excision of multiple lymph nodes from the same location or to the same extent. For instance, if multiple lymph node biopsies are performed by open technique on deep cervical nodes, code 38510 would be assigned only once.

Also note that a number of procedures listed elsewhere in CPT already have included the excision of lymph nodes, such as code 19306, mastectomy, radical, including pectoral muscle and axillary and internal mammary lymph nodes. Therefore additional assignment of codes from the hemic and lymphatic section would not be reportable.

A number of codes for bone marrow or stem cell services are also included in the hemic and lymphatic systems. Codes for harvesting, preparing, thawing, aspiration, and other transplantation-related services are included in this section.

Mediastinum and Diaphragm (39000-39599)

Only two subcategories exist for this section, specifically the mediastinum and diaphragm. Procedures for these two subcategories include surgical techniques of incision, excision, repair, and endoscopy as well as unlisted procedures.

Digestive System (40490-49999)

DIGESTIVE SYSTEM SERVICES

Lips	40490-40799
Vestibule of mouth	40800-40899
Tongue and floor of mouth	41000-41599
Dentoalveolar structures	41800-41899
Palate and uvula	42000-42299
Salivary gland and ducts	42300-42699
Pharynx, adenoids, and tonsils	42700-42999
Esophagus	43020-43499
Stomach	43500-43999
Intestines (except rectum)	44005-44799
Meckel's diverticulum and the mesentery	44800-44899
Appendix	44900-44979
Rectum	45000-45999
Anus	46020-46999
Liver	47000-47399
Biliary tract	47400-47999
Pancreas	48000-48999
Abdomen, peritoneum, and omentum	49000-49999

Key Medical Terms

Ablation
Anastomosis
Cholecysto-
Dilation
Entero-
Esophago-
Esophagogastroduodenoscopy (EGD)
Fistula
Gastro-
Hematemesis
Hepato-
Hernia
Laparo-
Snare
Spleno-
Upper gastrointestinal

Subcategories of the digestive system section include the following:

- Lips
- Vestibule of mouth
- Tongue, floor of mouth
- Dentoalveolar structures
- Palate, uvula
- Salivary glands, ducts
- Pharynx, adenoids, tonsils
- Esophagus
- Stomach (Fig. 14-14)
- Intestines (Fig. 14-15)
- Meckel's diverticulum, mesentery
- Appendix
- Rectum
- Anus
- Liver
- Biliary tract
- Pancreas
- Abdomen, peritoneum, omentum

The subcategories by anatomic section begin with the mouth and end with the anus region (Figs. 14-16, 14-17, and 14-18), including internal organs involved in the digestive process.

GENERAL GUIDELINES AND DEFINITIONS

Some coding guidelines should be applied to endoscopic procedures in the digestive disease section, including the following:

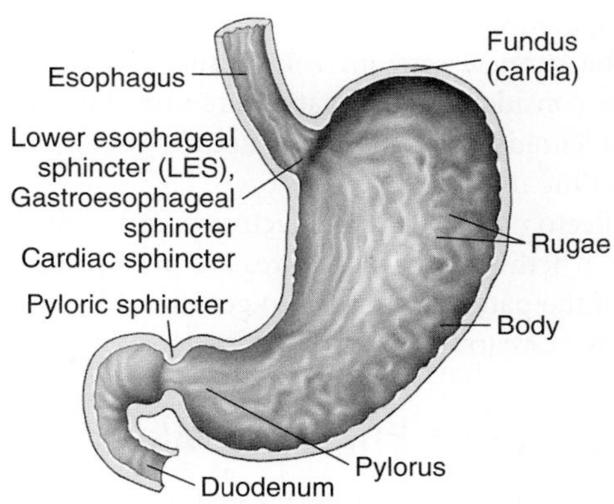

FIGURE 14-14. The stomach.

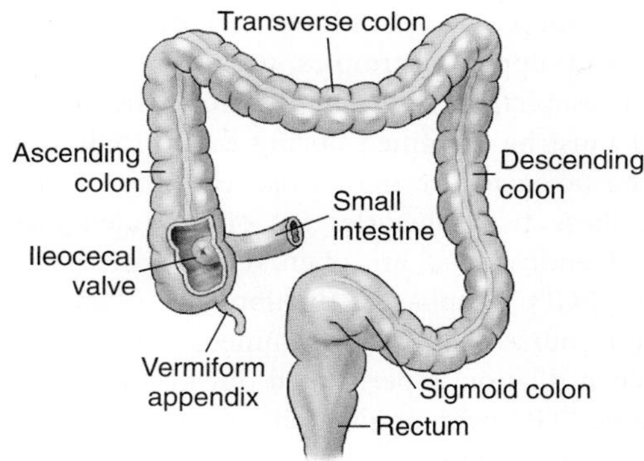

FIGURE 14-15. The large intestine (colon).

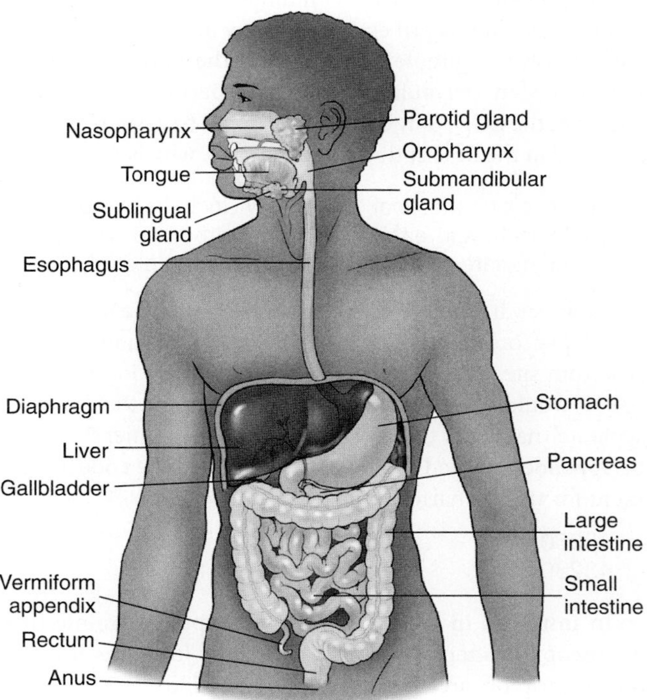

FIGURE 14-16. The gastrointestinal system.

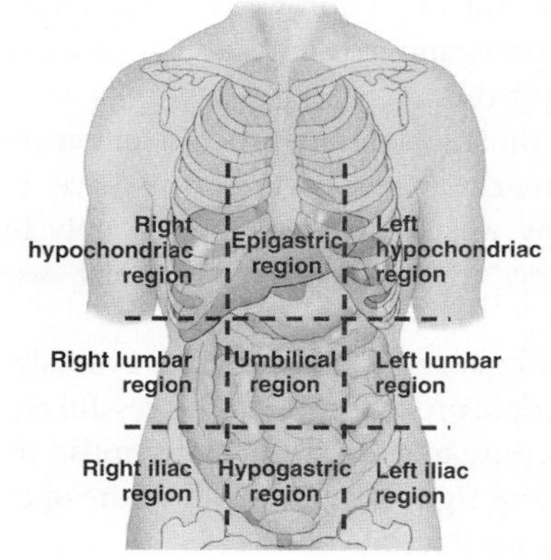

FIGURE 14-17. Abdominopelvic regions.

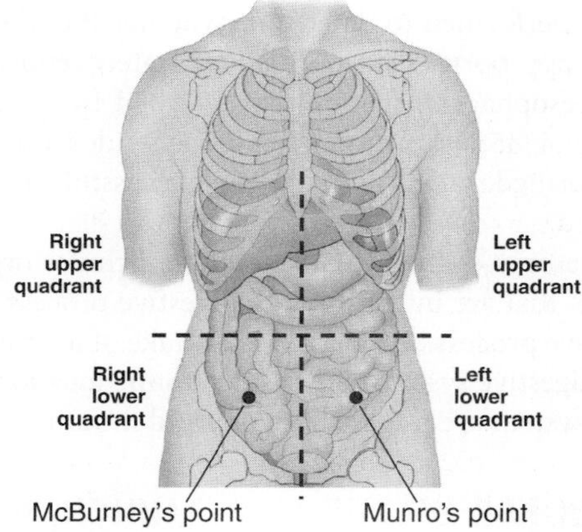

FIGURE 14-18. Abdominopelvic quadrants with Munro's and McBurney's points.

- Codes are assigned based on the technique used, not the number of lesions, tumors, or polyps removed.
- Additional procedures performed on the same anatomic site or sites are assigned modifier 51.
- When multiple anatomic sites are involved, each code for a specific separate site is assigned modifier 59.

As with other global surgical procedures, the approach or vehicle by which a procedure is performed is considered bundled. Therefore when a surgical endoscopy is performed, it includes a diagnostic endoscopy. According to CPT and NCCI guidelines, this would include the following:

- When an endoscopy or enteroscopy is performed as part of another major service, it would not be separately reportable. An example would be when a small intestinal endoscopy is performed during the creation or revision of an enterostomy. In this instance the endoscopy would not be codeable.
- "Scout" endoscopies used to assess anatomic landmarks or extent of disease performed before performing a definitive, surgical procedure.
- Control of bleeding, or hemostasis, which occurs during an endoscopic procedure is considered an integral part of

this service. The exception would be when bleeding is the reason for performing the endoscopic procedure and is the definitive procedure.

- Only the most extensive procedure performed during the encounter may be coded. For instance, if a proctosigmoidoscopy was performed, immediately followed by a colonoscopy, the proctosigmoidoscopy would not be reportable.
- As with other surgical procedures previously discussed, if the endoscopic procedure is not successful and requires an open procedure to successfully accomplish the procedure, only the more significant procedure (the open procedure) would be codeable.
- If a transabdominal colonoscopy or other endoscopic procedure is performed by a colostomy, the endoscopy is not separately reportable. If, however, the endoscopic procedure is performed to determine whether the open procedure is appropriate, it would be separately reportable.
- When esophageal dilation as described by codes 43450 through 43458 is unsuccessful and an endoscopic dilation is performed, only the definitive, successful procedure is reported.

The anatomy of the digestive system includes organs and body parts that are integral to the digestive process. Because the digestive process begins with the intake of food and fluids into the digestive system, the first anatomic locations for the digestive system are the lips, tongue, and mouth.

PROCEDURES OF THE LIPS, MOUTH, PALATE, AND UVULA

Cleft palate is a common birth defect, correctable by a number of different surgical techniques. In some instances a staged technique may be used in which the patient will be returned to the operating room for more than one procedure.

As was seen in the musculoskeletal section, in some instances lacerations or open wounds extend beyond the skin surface. When repairs are performed on the tongue, codes in the range 41250-41252 would be appropriate.

Biopsies of the tongue are categorized by the extent of the biopsy, that is, anterior two thirds versus posterior one third (codes 41100-41105).

A uvulopalatopharyngoplasty is performed to repair the uvula, palate, pharynx, or all of these. This procedure is usually undertaken as the result of obstructive sleep apnea, in which the uvula blocks the airway and causes the patient to momentarily not breathe during sleep. It often results in the patient snoring during sleep and a disruptive sleep pattern.

PROCEDURES OF THE TONSILS AND ADENOIDS

The most common procedure performed on the tonsils and adenoids is the excision of one or both. Depending on the diagnosis, the tonsils may be excised as well as the adenoids during the surgical session. The tonsils, as well as the adenoids, are considered one organ; therefore when both tonsils or both adenoids are excised, it is not necessary or appropriate to add the modifier 50.

Tonsillectomy and adenoidectomy codes are assigned based on whether both procedures are performed as well as the age of the patient—those younger than 12 years or those older than 12 years.

PROCEDURES OF THE ESOPHAGUS

The majority of procedures performed on the esophagus are endoscopic—through the visual examination of the esophagus and other portions of the digestive system—through a scope placed down the esophagus.

Upper endoscopic procedures include esophagoscopies (EGDs) and upper gastrointestinal (GI) endoscopies, in which the esophagus, stomach, and either the duodenum or jejunum must be identified during the procedure. Caution should be taken to use the correct category of procedures because these two categories are often coded incorrectly. Upper GI endoscopies are often referred in the operative report as EGD. Esophageal dilations are often performed during the course of an EGD or immediately after the procedure. When dilation is performed during the course of the endoscopic EGD over a guide wire, code 43248 is assigned. If the scope is removed and dilation is performed subsequent to the endoscopic procedure, codes from the manipulation area are assigned based on the method of dilation.

As previously discussed, multiple services performed through the esophageal endoscope may be separately reportable; however, multiple procedures of the same services are not. For instance, if multiple biopsies are performed during the course of the EGD, only code 43239 would be assigned. This is specified in the description of code 43234, which reads:

> Upper gastrointestinal endoscopy including esophagus, stomach, and either the duodenum and/or jejunum as appropriate; with biopsy, single or multiple 43239

However, if a polyp were excised from the one location by hot biopsy forceps technique (43250) as well as multiple biopsies from sites other than where the polyp was located, code 43239 would also be appropriate. To specify the "distinct, separate" nature of these two procedures, modifier 59 would be appended to the EGD with biopsy code. The code assignment for this scenario would be as follows:

43250
43239-59

In instances in which an EGD or upper gastrointestinal endoscopy is attempted but all anatomic locations listed in the descriptor are not visualized, modifier 52 (reduced services) or modifier 53 (discontinued procedure) would be appropriate.

Endoscopic retrograde cholangiopancreatography (ERCP) requires an endoscope to be advanced into the duodenal papilla to visualize the pancreatic, hepatic, and bile ducts and possibly the gallbladder, depending on the diagnostic presentation. Because the approach for the ERCP is different from that of the EGD, if both are performed it would be appropriate to assign both procedures, with modifier 51 for multiple procedures appended to the secondary, or least significant, procedure. In many instances contrast is injected to visualize all the anatomic structures. The radiologic supervision and interpretation are not included in codes located in the digestive system of the surgery section. These services would be separately reportable by the identity that performs these services.

In addition to the ERCP, when sphincterotomy or insertion of tube or stent is performed it may be assigned code(s) in addition to the primary procedure, with modifier 51 appended. Biliary sludge is often removed during the ERCP, but it does not represent an additional codeable service.

Care should be taken to distinguish procedures accomplished endoscopically (through the visual examination of the site by scope introduced through a body orifice) as opposed to laparoscopically (where the scope is introduced for visualization of an area). Laparoscopic procedures can usually be identified by key terms such as *supraumbilical incision, pseudoperitoneum, trocars, cannula, sheath,* and *Veress needle.*

BARIATRIC SURGERY

A number of surgical procedures to aid in weight loss for the morbidly obese were added to CPT recently. These procedures range from the introduction of an adjustable gastric restrictive device (e.g., Lap Band, Allergan, Inc., Irvine, Calif.) to gastric bypass, in which the stomach is partitioned with a staple line and a short portion of the small intestine is divided and anastomosed to the small upper stomach pouch created.

PROCEDURES OF THE INTESTINES (EXCEPT RECTUM)

Resection of the colon, or colectomy, is often necessary because of a diseased portion of the structure. In some instances only a colectomy (excision of colon or portion of colon) is performed. In other instances the colectomy is performed, and an anastomosis, or surgical connection of the two remaining portions of colon, is performed as well. A colostomy, in some cases temporary and other cases permanent, may also be performed, in which an artificial pouch, or stoma, is created and an abdominal pouch is affixed to empty body waste products. In the case of colonic malignancy the cancerous area is treated, and in the future the anastomosis may be reevaluated and it may or may not be determined that the anastomosis can be reversed, the colon reconnected, and the colostomy "taken down" or eliminated. This may not be the case in some instances, and the amount of time may also vary when this procedure would or could be appropriate.

Note that the colonoscopy procedures are not located in this subsection because the approach for the endoscopy is through the rectum.

PROCEDURES OF THE APPENDIX

An appendectomy performed at the time of another major procedure is considered incidental *(bundled)* and therefore is not coded or billed. Only when the appendectomy is performed for a specific indicated purpose at the time of the other procedure should it be coded and considered for payment. Make certain the medical documentation clearly indicates the medical necessity for the appendectomy.

Appendectomies can be performed open (44950-44960) or laparoscopically (44970-44979), so make certain to review the operative report for the correct approach and definitive procedure.

PROCEDURES OF THE RECTUM

Several types of endoscopic procedures are categorized within the digestive system section, including the following:

- Proctosigmoidoscopy: examination of rectum or sigmoid colon
- Sigmoidoscopy: examination of entire rectum, sigmoid colon, and possibly a portion of descending colon
- Colonoscopy: examination of entire colon, from rectum to cecum, possibly including examination of terminal ileum

All three procedures involve the insertion of the scope through the rectum for purposes of visualizing the anatomic sites identified in the descriptions of the procedures. Care should be taken that the intended procedure is coded. For instance, if a colonoscopy was intended but the surgeon was unable to reach the cecum, it would still be appropriate to code the colonoscopy, but modifier 52 should be appended for reduced services or modifier 53 for discontinued services as appropriate. It would not be appropriate to downcode the service to the extent the procedure was performed.

As mentioned in the discussion regarding esophageal endoscopic procedures, when multiple techniques are used for multiple procedures on distinct anatomic sites, it would be appropriate to code multiple procedure codes within this section. For example:

If a colonoscopy is performed in which polyps, lesions, tumors, or all of these are excised by hot biopsy forceps and additional polyps, lesions, and/or tumors are excised by snare technique, and additional sites are biopsied only, the following codes would be appropriate:

45385 Colonoscopy, flexible, proximal to splenic flexure, with removal of tumor(s), polyp(s), or other lesion(s) by snare technique

45384-51 Colonoscopy, flexible, proximal to splenic flexure, with removal of tumor(s), polyp(s), or other lesion(s) by hot biopsy forceps or bipolar cautery
45380-59 Colonoscopy, flexible, proximal to splenic flexure, with biopsy, single or multiple

Note that the last procedure, 45380, is designated with modifier 59 to indicate that the biopsy site(s) were separate and distinct from the sites where polyp(s), lesion(s), tumor(s), or all three were excised.

PROCEDURES OF THE ANUS

When procedures are performed on the anus, a digital rectal exam is often performed. When performed in conjunction with a surgical procedure, the digital rectal exam is not separately reportable. When performed in conjunction with an evaluation and management service, it should be incorporated in the level of service for that encounter.

Hemorrhoids are a common condition that results from the inflammation of the venous plexus surrounding the anus. They may be inside (internal) the anal canal or outside (external). In addition to designating the hemorrhoids as internal or external, hemorrhoids are also classified in four stages:

- First degree: Do not protrude outside the anal canal
- Second degree: Protrude outside the anal canal; however, retract spontaneously
- Third degree: Protrude outside the anal canal and must be manually reduced
- Fourth degree: Protrude outside the anal canal and cannot be manually reduced; often thrombosed, strangulated, or both

PROCEDURES OF THE LIVER

Liver biopsies can be performed percutaneously, with code 47000 assigned. When performed in conjunction with another surgical procedure, code 47001 would be assigned.

Liver transplants have become more common than they were a few years ago. They involve preparation or harvesting of the donor liver from either a living donor or cadaver, preparation of the graft, and transplantation. All the procedures performed by the provider may be coded. These procedures are complex and time consuming and often involve more than one surgeon; make certain when coding that only those services performed by your surgeon are coded.

BILIARY TRACT

The biliary tract connects the gallbladder to the liver and small intestine. In addition to conditions of the gallbladder, the tract often contains calculi (stones) or tumors. These conditions result in blockage of the tract.

The most common procedure(s) of the biliary tract is a cholecystectomy, or excision of the gallbladder. As with the appendectomy codes, excision of the gallbladder can be performed open, in which case the code would be located under the excision category, or it may be performed laparoscopically. In some instances a cholangiography, or imaging of the biliary duct, may be performed. Codes are located within the excisional and laparoscopic cholecystectomy codes that incorporate the addition of this procedure when performed during the cholecystectomy.

HERNIA REPAIRS

Hernia repairs are divided by the type of hernia (inguinal, femoral, incisional, ventral, epigastric, umbilical). Breakdown for the selection of a hernia repair code is as follows:

- Type of hernia (inguinal, lumbar, femoral, ventral, incisional, umbilical, laparoscopic)
- Initial or recurrent
- Reducible, strangulated, or incarcerated
- Age

STOP AND PRACTICE

Determine the appropriate breakdown and code(s) for the following procedures.

	Anatomic Site	Procedure and Technique	Specifics	Code(s)
1. Exploratory laparotomy	______	______	______	______
2. T & A, age 20	______	______	______	______
3. EGD with polypectomy by snare	______	______	______	______
4. Esophagoscopy with foreign body removal	______	______	______	______
5. Laparoscopic appendectomy	______	______	______	______
6. Initial inguinal hernia repair, age 3	______	______	______	______
7. Cholecystectomy	______	______	______	______
8. EGD with dilation of esophagus	______	______	______	______
9. Colonoscopy, diagnostic with EGD, four biopsies	______	______	______	______
10. Diagnostic anoscopy	______	______	______	______

STOP AND PRACTICE

Take the following operative reports and assign CPT codes appropriately. Make sure you continue to use the technique of breaking down the information needed to code. Use the guidelines listed previously for each subcategory of the digestive system. You may wish to add the "bullets" discussed for each section to your CPT book so those guidelines will be readily available as you search for the appropriate code(s).

1. Operative report

OPERATIVE REPORT

Patient information:

Patient name:
DOB:
MR#:

CONSENT:
Informed consent obtained from the patient after full disclosure of risks and indications to the patient.

Preoperative diagnosis:

Diarrhea. History of colon cancer.

Postoperative diagnosis:

See findings below.

Procedure(s) performed:

Colonoscopy with hot biopsies and cold biopsies

Anesthesia:

Assistant surgeon:

Description of procedure:

After obtaining an informed consent, the patient was brought to the OR and put in the left lateral position. IV line was maintained. IV sedation was given. Vitals were monitored throughout the procedure, which included pulse, pulse oximetry, blood pressure, level of consciousness, and ECG monitoring. Digital rectal examination was done, which showed normal anal tone, no tags, and no hemorrhoids. Scope was introduced and advanced all the way up to the cecum, identified by ileocecal valve and appendicular orifice and entering into the terminal ileum. Patient had lots of stool spread all over, some of this solid, especially in proximal colon. This was washed away repeatedly. Watched colonic mucosa carefully. However, small polyps could have been missed. There was a very small polyp at hepatic flexure, which was biopsied. Terminal ileum appeared normal. Cecum appeared normal. The distal colon area, rectosigmoid, and descending colon appeared a little inflamed. Multiple random biopsies were taken. Biopsy was also taken from the terminal ileum. She had very small to moderate-sized internal hemorrhoids. The rest of the examination revealed normal mucosa. No masses. No AV malformation. No other polyps seen.

FINDINGS:
1. Small polyp in hepatic flexure, hot biopsied and sent for histopathology with good fulguration of the base.
2. Biopsy from the terminal ileum.
3. Erythematous and inflamed-appearing mucosa in the distal colon, especially in the rectal area. Biopsies taken and sent for histopathology from both areas.
4. Poor prep. She had some solid stools spread all over, which were washed away. Mild small to moderate-sized internal hemorrhoids, non-bleeding and non-thrombosed.

PLAN:
Follow up with biopsy results.

Patk Adam MD

GODFREY REGIONAL HOSPITAL
123 Main Street • Aldon, FL 77714 • (407) 555-1234

Step 1: Identify chapter or section of CPT: Surgery
Step 2: Identify anatomic system: ________
Step 3: Identify anatomic site: ________
Step 4: Identify procedure/technique: ________
Step 5: Identify additional specifics: ________
Step 6: Assign CPT code(s): ________
Step 7: Place code(s) in appropriate order: ________
Step 8: Assign modifier code(s) as appropriate: ________

2. Operative report

OPERATIVE REPORT

Patient information:

Patient name:
DOB:
MR#:

Preoperative diagnosis:

Left inguinal pain five years after left inguinal herniorrhaphy

INDICATIONS:
This is a 27-year-old male who has returned to my clinic multiple times complaining of left-sided inguinal pain. He'd had a bilateral inguinal herniorrhaphy five years ago, and then about 2 months or so ago, was lifting something heavy at work and felt what he thought was some tearing and began to have pain in his left groin. Despite rest and nonsteroidal antiinflammatory drugs, he has not been able to resolve this pain. I have examined him multiple times in clinic and can feel no obvious hernia. He is tender in the area. I told him that although his exploration could possibly be negative, I thought that with his persistent pain we could go ahead and explore his left groin.

Postoperative diagnosis:

Same

FINDINGS:
Mesh is intact, negative groin exploration. Of note is that he had a previous McVay with mesh placed over the top. Even with the patient straining and coughing, I couldn't feel any defects or problem with the mesh.

Procedure(s) performed:

Left inguinal exploration

Anesthesia:

Assistant surgeon:

Description of procedure:

The patient was brought to the operating room and placed in a supine position on the operating room table. Anesthesia and some sedation were given. The patient's left groin was prepped and draped in the usual sterile fashion. After the administration of appropriate operative antibiotics, 1% lidocaine mixed with 0.25% Marcaine was used to anesthetize an area in the left groin. An ilioinguinal block was placed. The old incision was re-opened and the dissection was carried sharply down to the external oblique, which was, with some difficulty, dissected free along its anterior extent. The external ring was located and the external oblique opened in line with its fibers, beginning at the external ring. Spermatic cord was isolated, looped, and drawn up. The mesh was palpable beneath. It seemed to be solid; in fact, with patient coughing and straining, there was no defect in the mesh whatsoever. I did feel at both the neo-internal ring of the mesh and at the pubic tubercle as well as all the areas in between. Again, with the patient straining and coughing, there was no palpable hernia defect on direct palpation of his repair mesh. Hemostasis was achieved. The external oblique was closed in a running fashion with 2-0 Vicryl. The skin was closed in a running fashion with 4-0 Monocryl subcuticular stitch. Steri-Strips and a sterile dressing were applied.
The patient was taken to the PACU in good condition.

Patk Olden MD

GODFREY REGIONAL HOSPITAL
123 Main Street • Aldon, FL 77714 • (407) 555-1234

Step 1: Identify chapter or section of CPT:	Surgery	Step 5: Identify additional specifics:	________
Step 2: Identify anatomic system:	________	Step 6: Assign CPT code(s):	________
Step 3: Identify anatomic site:	________	Step 7: Place code(s) in appropriate order:	________
Step 4: Identify procedure/technique:	________	Step 8: Assign modifier code(s) as appropriate:	________

3. Operative report

OPERATIVE REPORT

Patient information:

Patient name:
DOB:
MR#:

CONSENT:
An informed consent was obtained from the patient and his father after explaining the risks, indications, and possible complications. The patient/father gave informed consent.

Preoperative diagnosis:

15-year-old with chronic pyrosis and now losing weight; diarrhea

Postoperative diagnosis:

See findings below.

Procedure(s) performed:

Esophagogastroduodenoscopy

Anesthesia:

Assistant surgeon:

Description of procedure:

After obtaining an informed consent, the patient was brought to the OR, put in the left lateral position. IV line was maintained and IV sedation was given. Vitals were monitored throughout the procedure, which included pulse, pulse oximetry, blood pressure, level of consciousness, and ECG monitoring. Mouth was sprayed with Cetacaine and then mouth block was applied. Esophagogastroduodenoscopy scope was passed in the mouth and easily intubated. Visually guided in the esophagus. The proximal esophagus showed longitudinal ulcer with clean margins at 16 cm. Scope was further advanced. No stricture or masses seen. The distal esophagus appeared normal. Scope was further advanced into the stomach. Rugae appeared normal, which flattened out normally on insufflation. The scope was advanced all the way to pylorus that appeared normal in size and shape. No distortion noticed. Scope was pushed into the duodenal bulb, which appeared normal, and scope was advanced beyond the 3rd part of the duodenum. A couple of biopsies were taken from the small bowel mucosa. Scope was withdrawn all the way back into the antrum. Retroflexion was done. Incisura appeared normal. The scope was dropped down into the fundus and body, both of which appear normal. The scope was straightened out, pulled back all the way up to the GE junction. Excess air was suctioned out. Then re-examined the esophageal ulcer at 16 cm, which extends from 16 to 17 cm, in a longitudinal fashion. One biopsy was taken. However, the patient had difficulty at this time with constant retching. Unable to do any more biopsies. This halted the procedure at this time and the scope was taken out.

FINDINGS:
1. Esophageal ulcer at 16 cm, extending all the way to 17 cm, longitudinal, non-bleeding with clear margins
2. Otherwise normal esophagogastroduodenoscopy with excessive reflux seen on endoscopy

PLAN:
Continue with Prevacid, follow up with biopsy results. Based on the biopsy results, may need another endoscopy after treating with PPI in the next couple of weeks.

Patrick Olsen MD

GODFREY REGIONAL HOSPITAL
123 Main Street • Aldon, FL 77714 • (407) 555-1234

Step 1: Identify chapter or section of CPT: Surgery
Step 2: Identify anatomic system: ________
Step 3: Identify anatomic site: ________
Step 4: Identify procedure/technique: ________
Step 5: Identify additional specifics: ________
Step 6: Assign CPT code(s): ________
Step 7: Place code(s) in appropriate order: ________
Step 8: Assign modifier code(s) as appropriate: ________

4. Operative report

OPERATIVE REPORT

Patient information:

Patient name:
DOB:
MR#:

CONSENT:
Informed consent obtained from the patient after full disclosure of risks and indications to the patient.

Preoperative diagnosis:

Chronic pyrosis. Family history of colon cancer.

Postoperative diagnosis:

See impressions below.

Procedure(s) performed:

Colonoscopy with polypectomies and hot biopsies. Upper endoscopy with biopsy.

Anesthesia:

Assistant surgeon:

Description of procedure:

After obtaining an informed consent, patient was brought to the OR and placed in the left lateral position. Digital rectal examination was done. IV sedation was given. Vitals were monitored throughout the procedure, which included pulse, pulse oximetry, blood pressure, respiratory rate, level of consciousness, ECG monitoring. Colonoscope was introduced in advance all the way up to the cecum, in fact, by ileocecal valve and appendicular orifice. On the way up, had noticed in areas of the sigmoid and the rectum two polyps. Cecum was identified by ileocecal valve and appendicular orifice. Scope was carefully withdrawn. In the descending colon, two small polyps were identified, which were hot-biopsied and totally fulgurated. Good hemostasis and photo documentation obtained. The scope was withdrawn into the sigmoid colon, where there was a large pedunculated polyp. Photo documentation obtained. A small biopsy was taken from the tip of the polyp. Snare was put in. Polyp was snared in toto. Tissue retrieved. Scope was then pulled down into the rectal area. There were two polyps; both were snared. Tissue sent for histopathology. Retroflexion showed large internal hemorrhoids with some tags. No attempt to biopsy them. Scope was taken out. Prep was good. The rest of the examination was within normal limits. Examination was satisfactory. Mouth was sprayed with Cetacaine. IV sedation was given, totaling the dose as described above. With some difficulty, was able to pass scope through the mouth, into esophagus and was advanced all the way into the antrum. He does have a long J-shaped stomach with antrum slightly distorted. However, easily entered into the duodenum. Showed severe duodenitis with lots of edema with at least two pseudo-polyps identified with a central ulceration. Biopsies were taken from the edges of the polyps. Then the scope was withdrawn into the antrum. The antrum looks a little bit deformed. Photo documentation obtained. CLOtest biopsy was taken in the antral area, which showed a few ulcerations as well. Retroflexion revealed two ulcers, healed, on the incisura. Biopsies were taken from one of the ulcers. They were small, non-bleeding. Then the scope was dropped into the body. This showed some atrophic gastritis, but no evidence of any inflammation or any ulcers. Scope was straightened out and pulled up to the GE junction. He has a hiatal hernia approximately 43 cm to 39 cm. Mild distal esophagitis. No evidence of any salmon-colored mucosa seen. In the mid esophagus, he had a bleb appearing like a varix. This was surrounded by a little erythema. Biopsy not attempted, as could be a blood vessel. Scope was further withdrawn. A careful look at the vocal cords appeared normal. Scope was taken out.

FINDINGS: COLONOSCOPY:

1. Two small polyps from the descending colon, both hot-biopsied and sent for histopathology.
2. A large polyp with thick pedicle from sigmoid colon, which was snared in toto and sent for histopathology.
3. Two rectal polyps, one medium sized and one small. Both were snared and sent for histopathology.
4. Large internal hemorrhoids. Small external hemorrhoids.
5. Prep was good. The rest of the examination was essentially normal.

UPPER ENDOSCOPY:

1. Severe duodenitis with edema and ulceration, non-bleeding, well healed with white formation (appears to look like two polyps). Biopsies were taken and sent for histopathology.
2. Antral gastritis with some deformity in the pylorus, CLO test biopsy taken.
3. Ulcers on the incisura are well-healed and non-bleeding. Small in size and two in number; biopsy taken.
4. The rest of the stomach showed atrophic mucosa.
5. Hiatal hernia approximately 3 cm in size, non-inflamed from 41 to 39 cm.
6. Mild distal esophagitis.
7. Varix-like vessel appearing cystic lesion in the mid esophagus with surrounding erythema. Biopsy not taken.

PLAN: COLONOSCOPY:

Follow up with biopsy results. May need colonoscopy in 1 to 2 years for chronic pyrosis, most likely related to his peptic ulcer disease. He has duodenal ulcers. Will re-endoscope to look for duodenal polyps if they persist, even after treatment and on H2 blockers. May need to be snared.

UPPER ENDOSCOPY:

Also will get an esophagogram to delineate further the polyps/varix seen in the upper esophagus. That also needs further endoscopy in the next 4 to 8 weeks.

Patk Adam MD

GODFREY REGIONAL HOSPITAL
123 Main Street • Aldon, FL 77714 • (407) 555-1234

Step 1: Identify chapter or section of CPT: Surgery
Step 2: Identify anatomic system: ________
Step 3: Identify anatomic site: ________
Step 4: Identify procedure/technique: ________
Step 5: Identify additional specifics: ________
Step 6: Assign CPT code(s): ________
Step 7: Place code(s) in appropriate order: ________
Step 8: Assign modifier code(s) as appropriate: ________

5. Operative report

OPERATIVE REPORT

Patient information:

Patient name:
DOB:
MR#:

Preoperative diagnosis:

1) Recurrent tonsillitis. 2) Upper airway obstruction. 3) Hypertrophic tonsils and adenoids.

INDICATION:
4-year-old female with recurrent episodes of tonsillitis. She also has upper airway obstruction manifested by snoring and mouth breathing. Examination reveals hypertrophic tonsils and adenoids.

Postoperative diagnosis:

Same

Procedure(s) performed:

Tonsillectomy and adenoidectomy

Anesthesia:

Assistant surgeon:

Description of procedure:

After consent was obtained, the patient was taken to the operating room and placed on the operating table in supine position. After adequate level of general endotracheal anesthesia was obtained, the patient was turned and draped in appropriate manner for tonsillectomy and adenoidectomy. A McIver mouth gag was then placed to allow visualization of the tonsils. Attention was first focused on the left tonsil. The Allis clamps were placed in the superior pole and tonsils were retracted towards the midline. Then utilizing a needlepoint Bovie, the tonsil was removed in its entirety from superior to inferior direction. Hemostasis was achieved with electrocautery. Similar procedure was then performed on the right tonsil. A cath was then placed through the left nostril to elevate the soft palate. Examination of the nasopharynx showed hypertrophic adenoids. Utilizing suction cautery, the adenoids were removed. Hemostasis was achieved with suction cautery. Tonsillar fossae, as well as the nasopharynx, were then irrigated with saline. Neo-Synephrine spray was then placed in the nasopharynx. Subsequent re-inspection showed no active bleeding. The tension on the mouth gag and the catheter were then released. Re-inspection showed no active bleeding. The mouth gag and catheter were then removed. Prior to removal of mouth gag, 1% Xylocaine with 1:100,000 units of epinephrine was then infiltrated into the retromolar and soft palate areas bilaterally. Patient tolerated the procedure well. There was no break in technique.
The patient was extubated and taken to the post-anesthesia care unit in good condition.

Fluids administered: 1000 cc RL
Estimated blood loss: Less than 10 cc
Pre-operative medications: 4 mg Decadron and 500 mg ampicillin IV

Patk Olan MD

GODFREY REGIONAL HOSPITAL
123 Main Street • Aldon, FL 77714 • (407) 555-1234

Step 1: Identify chapter or section of CPT: Surgery
Step 2: Identify anatomic system: ______
Step 3: Identify anatomic site: ______
Step 4: Identify procedure/technique: ______
Step 5: Identify additional specifics: ______
Step 6: Assign CPT code(s): ______
Step 7: Place code(s) in appropriate order: ______
Step 8: Assign modifier code(s) as appropriate: ______

Urinary System (50010-53899)

URINARY SYSTEM SERVICES

Kidney	50010-50593
Ureter	50600-50980
Bladder	51020-52700
Urethra	53000-53899

Key Medical Terms

Cysto-
Cystourethroscopy
Nephro-
Uretero-
Urethra-
Urinary tract infection (UTI)
Urino-

Subsections of the urinary system section (Fig. 14-19) include the following:

- Kidney (Fig. 14-20)
- Ureter
- Bladder
- Urethra

Cystoscopy, urethroscopy, and cystourethroscopy are included in this section and are broken down by the services performed. According to CPT, when a secondary endoscopic procedure performed at the same anatomic site constitutes more than the usual description for the service, modifier 22 should be appended. Diagnoses for both conditions should be listed, and documentation of the performance of both procedures should be appropriately recorded in the medical record. Many insurance carriers still require that all additional procedures that are not bundled in the primary urologic procedure should be coded and modifier 51 appended to any subsequent services.

Again, the coder must keep in mind the approach of the procedure. A number of procedures performed on the urinary system are performed cystourethroscopically; therefore only that range of codes should be used for these procedures.

Careful consideration should be taken of the subsections of urethroscopic procedures and ureteroscopic procedures performed in order to assign codes appropriately.

Bundling guidelines indicate that when a stent is temporary placed for the purpose of performing a cystourethroscopic procedure, it is considered included in the procedure. However, in instances in which a stent is placed during a cystourethroscopic procedure and left in place after the procedure, that stent placement should be assigned a code.

Insertion of urinary catheters is included in this section as well. However, this is intended only for catheters left in place and not placed for the purpose of collecting a urine specimen. Specific Healthcare Common Procedure Coding System (HCPCS) codes have been established for instances when catheters are placed solely for the purpose of collecting urine specimens.

Additional CPT and NCCI guidelines for urinary procedures are as follows:

- When female or male procedures include placement of a urethral catheter, the catheterization is not separately reportable.
- Bladder irrigation performed to accomplish access or visualize the urinary system is not separately reportable.
- When urethral catheterization or dilation is necessary to accomplish a more extensive or definitive procedure, it is not separately reportable.

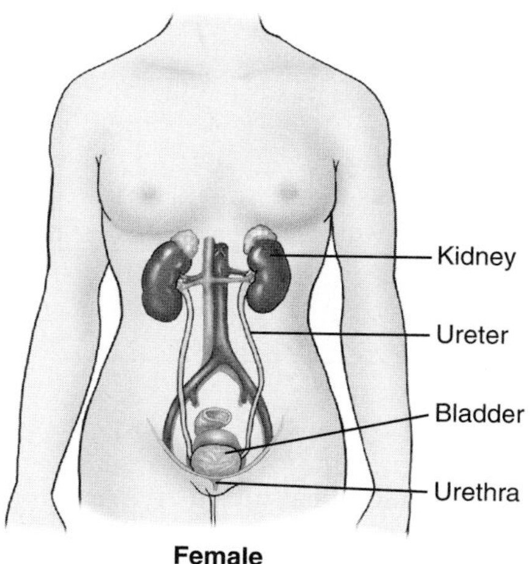

FIGURE 14-19. Female urinary system.

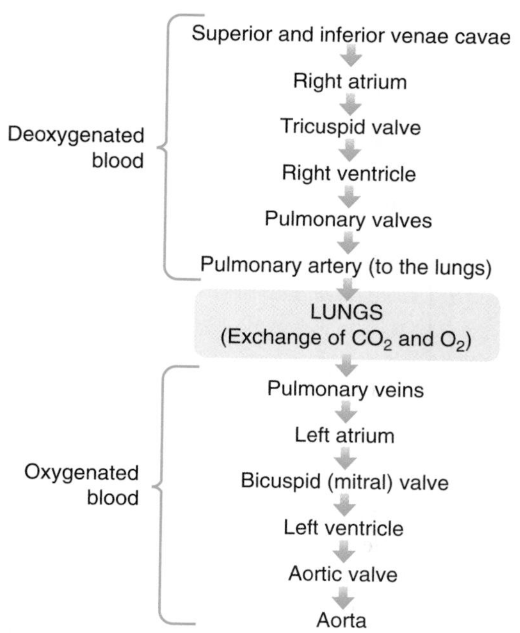

FIGURE 14-20. Cross-section of a kidney.

KIDNEY PROCEDURES

Nephrolithotomy procedures are performed to incise the kidney and, in most cases, remove calculus. In some instances the procedure is performed percutaneously, and various techniques such as lithotripsy, stenting, or extraction by basket are used to remove the calculus.

Kidney transplants are performed when a patient's kidneys stop functioning as the result of disease or renal failure. As with the liver transplantation codes, several surgical procedures are performed to accomplish this task, including harvest of the donor kidney, preparation work, and the transplantation itself.

Nephrectomy may be performed when the kidney is diseased or fails to function. Because most patients have two kidneys, in most instances the removal of one kidney typically leaves one working kidney. Most patients can function with one working kidney, and therefore a kidney transplant would not be necessary. As with a number of other organs located in the abdominal area, the nephrectomy could be performed either laparoscopically or in open surgery.

One of the most common procedures performed in this section is the extracorporeal shock wave lithotripsy. In this procedure shock waves are directed at stones and crushed by radio waves. This is performed with the patient's abdominal area submerged in water or by a cushion filled with water that is placed in the table underneath the patient. The stones are broken in small pieces, making it possible for the stone fragments to pass through the urinary tract.

URETER PROCEDURES

A number of procedures can be performed endoscopically, laparoscopically, or by excision. The operative report must be read carefully to determine the definitive approach for the procedure.

BLADDER PROCEDURES

Urodynamic testing is performed to determine urinary flow and measurement of urinary output. A number of procedures may be performed in an effort to determine whether urinary flow has been obstructed or stress or urge incontinence is responsible for urinary flow problems. When multiple urodynamic procedures are performed, modifier 51 would be appended to all subsequent procedures from this section. Make sure reports specify all procedures performed when coding for these services. Remember, when documentation does not specify whether the procedure was simple or complex, the coder must assume the least significant, which would be the simple procedure.

The introduction of a catheter into the kidney is common in the case of urologic problems. When the catheter is placed nonindwelling or into the urethra and into the bladder for the removal of urine, code 51701 would be assigned. When an indwelling catheter, such as a Foley catheter, is placed, code 51702 or 51703 is assigned based on whether the procedure is simple or complex.

In the case of bladder malignancy, an antineoplastic agent is instilled into the bladder and allowed to stay in the bladder for a prescribed period.

When urinary urge and stress incontinence have been diagnosed, and nonsurgical techniques have failed to resolve or improve the problem, surgical procedures may be performed. The discussion of female genital procedures noted several procedures that may be performed during a vaginal or abdominal hysterectomy. However, when they are performed independently, a laparoscopic technique known as a *sling suspension* is performed. In this procedure, nonabsorbable sutures are placed at the bladder neck and secured to the ipsilateral pectineal ligament. The sutures are then tied in knots, creating a "hammock" or sling suspension of the bladder neck.

A number of endoscopic procedures are performed involving the bladder and other urinary organs as deemed appropriate. These procedures are all located under the heading Endoscopy—Cystoscopy, Urethroscopy, Cystourethroscopy. There are two subheadings within this section: (1) Urethra and Bladder and (2) Ureter and Pelvis. Code selection should be made according to the organ on which the definitive procedure is being performed.

Bladder tumors are often resected, or excised endoscopically. These procedures, referred to as transurethral resection of bladder tumor (TURBT), are coded by the tumor size. NCCI guidelines indicate that regardless of the number of tumors removed, only one unit of service may be coded for these services. For example, if a small tumor is removed as well as a large tumor, despite the fact they are removed from separate areas only one code may be assigned. It would be appropriate to code and bill for only the larger of the tumor resections.

When multiple cystourethroscopic procedures are performed for specific, distinct purposes, it would be appropriate to code for these services, using modifier 51 for subsequent procedures. Keep in mind, however, that any dilation, installation, or catheterization performed to accomplish the definitive procedure or for purposes of visualization or access to the necessary organ of the urinary system is considered bundled and not separately reportable.

Laser vaporization of the prostate, also known as *green light laser,* is performed to eliminate hypertrophic prostate tissue. If transurethral resection of the prostate is also performed, it is not separately reportable.

URETHRAL PROCEDURES

Correction of male urinary incontinence is usually accomplished through a sling procedure performed on the urethra; therefore code 53440 would be appropriate in these instances.

STOP AND PRACTICE

Determine the appropriate breakdown and code(s) for the following procedures.

	Anatomic Site	Procedure and Technique	Specifics	Code(s)
1. Diagnostic cystourethroscopy	______	______	______	______
2. Open drainage of renal abscess	______	______	______	______
3. Injection procedure for cystography	______	______	______	______
4. Needle aspiration of bladder	______	______	______	______
5. Simple cystometrogram	______	______	______	______
Simple uroflowmetry	______	______	______	______
6. Cystourethroscopy with placement of ureteral stent	______	______	______	______
7. Urethral biopsy	______	______	______	______
8. Dilation of urethral stricture with dilator, male	______	______	______	______
9. Laparoscopic radical nephrectomy	______	______	______	______
10. Partial laparoscopic nephrectomy	______	______	______	______

STOP AND PRACTICE

Take the following operative reports and assign CPT codes appropriately. Make sure you continue to use the technique of breaking down the information needed to code. Use the guidelines listed previously for each subcategory of the urinary system. You may wish to add the "bullets" discussed for each section to your CPT book so those guidelines will be readily available as you search for the appropriate code(s).

1. Operative report

OPERATIVE REPORT

Patient information:

Patient name:
DOB:
MR#:

Date:
Surgeon:
Anesthetist:

Preoperative diagnosis:

Bladder neck infection

Postoperative diagnosis:

Same

Procedure(s) performed:

Incision of bladder neck infection

Anesthesia:

General

Assistant surgeon:

Description of procedure:

After the patient was prepped and draped in the lithotomy position, using the resectoscope, the urethra and bladder were inspected. He had about a ten French bladder neck contraction. Guidewire was inserted through the contraction, and then using the Collins knife cutting at the two, ten, seven, and five o'clock positions, the bladder neck was opened. Electrical cautery was used to obtain hemostasis.

Patient tolerated procedure well.

Rachel Perez MD

GODFREY REGIONAL HOSPITAL
123 Main Street • Aldon, FL 77714 • (407) 555-1234

Step 1: Identify chapter or section of CPT: Surgery
Step 2: Identify anatomic system: ________
Step 3: Identify anatomic site: ________
Step 4: Identify procedure/technique: ________
Step 5: Identify additional specifics: ________
Step 6: Assign CPT code(s): ________
Step 7: Place code(s) in appropriate order: ________
Step 8: Assign modifier code(s) as appropriate: ________

2. Operative report

OPERATIVE REPORT

Patient information:

Patient name:
DOB:
MR#:

Date:
Surgeon:
Anesthetist:

Preoperative diagnosis:

1. Right renal colic
2. Mild dilation of the right collecting system, possible right distal ureteral calculus
3. Microscopic hematuria

Postoperative diagnosis:

1. Right renal colic
2. Mild dilation of the right collecting system, possible right distal ureteral calculus
3. Microscopic hematuria
4. Possible spontaneously passed right ureteral calculus

Procedure(s) performed:

1. Cystourethroscopy
2. Right ureteroscopy
3. Right stent insertion

Anesthesia:

General

Assistant surgeon:

Description of procedure:

The patient was placed on the operating table in the lithotomy position after general anesthesia was given. External genitalia were prepped and draped in the usual manner. A #21 panendoscope was inserted transurethrally. Initial inspection of the bladder was not remarkable. Orifices were normal. Right retrograde pyelogram was performed using #8 acorn-tipped catheter, and the study revealed multiple filling defects, which were felt to represent air bubbles but no stones; however, because the patient's symptoms persisted (her microscopic hematuria and the dilation of the collecting system on the right side, which persisted all the way down to the right UVJ), we elected to proceed with right ureteroscopy as follows:

Glidewire was inserted into the right orifice, advanced all the way to the right renal pelvis, following which the distal right ureter was dilated using a Microvasive balloon dilator, size 10 cm in length, 12 French in diameter. After the balloon was removed, a #9 rigid ureteroscope was introduced transurethrally and advanced in the dilated orifice, and ureter was dilated all the way to the right renal pelvis. No stones, tumors, or other abnormalities encountered.

Therefore we felt that the patient's symptoms and abnormal findings on the IVP could have been due to spontaneously passed stone and persistent edema of the right orifice.

Instrument removed. A #24 ureteral stent was inserted over the glidewire and left indwelling between the right renal pelvis and the bladder. The cystoscope was removed.

The patient tolerated the procedure well and was sent to the recovery room in satisfactory condition. She will be discharged home when discharge criteria are met. She will be given Cipro 500 mg bid for a week and she will be advised to continue taking Percocet 10 prn for pain. She will be scheduled for cysto and stent extraction in 5–7 days and further urological management as appropriate.

Rachel Perez MD

GODFREY REGIONAL HOSPITAL
123 Main Street • Aldon, FL 77714 • (407) 555-1234

Step 1: Identify chapter or section of CPT: Surgery
Step 2: Identify anatomic system: ______
Step 3: Identify anatomic site: ______
Step 4: Identify procedure/technique: ______
Step 5: Identify additional specifics: ______
Step 6: Assign CPT code(s): ______
Step 7: Place code(s) in appropriate order: ______
Step 8: Assign modifier code(s) as appropriate: ______

3. Emergency department record

EMERGENCY ROOM RECORD

Name:	Age:	ER physician:
	DOB:	
Allergies/type of reaction:	**Usual medications/dosages:**	
	Flomax, baby aspirin, and saw palmetto	

Triage/presenting complaint: SUBJECTIVE: The patient presents complaining of urinary retention. The patient states that he woke this morning some time ago and was unable to void. States that he had a lot of pressure in the suprapubic area. About 12 years ago, he had a similar problem. They straight-cathed him and he was able to void without problems. After that, the patient has had multiple checks. Nothing ever developed. He has had biopsies done. No cancer noted. He has had an elevated PSA in the past. He did have an episode after some shoulder surgery when he had some urinary retention as well. He had a catheter in for about a week, but after forcing lots of fluids, he was able to come out of that as well. He does have periods where sometimes he can't void, but he just lays down and relaxes and then he is able to void without problems. He increases his fluid intake and this seems to keep things flowing. He is here today to have this checked.

Initial assessment:

Time	T	P	R	BP	Other:				

Medication orders:

Lab work:

X-ray:

Physician's report:

OBJECTIVE:
The patient is a 74-year-old male in no acute distress. He is alert and oriented. Abdomen reveals bowel sounds in all four quadrants. There is definitely some suprapubic pressure and fullness felt there. There is no pain associated with this, just increased pressure. Rectal exam was deferred at this time. Catheter was placed and left indwelling until he drained completely. He had another 500 ml out. Sample was sent to the lab for a urinalysis. Those results are pending. The patient states immediate relief from the catheter, and this will be removed prior to his discharge.

PLAN:
Talked with primary care physician regarding this patient. She felt that as long as he is stating relief, we should be able to send him home, but he should follow up with his regular doctor within the next day or so. If he is unable to void after removal of the catheter, he should recheck with his physician today. Otherwise, he should increase his fluids, keep things flowing, and if there are any further problems, recheck.

Diagnosis:	**Physician sign/date**
IMPRESSION: Urinary retention with past history of enlarged prostate	Nancy Connolly MD
Discharge Transfer Admit Good Satisfactory Other:	

GODFREY REGIONAL HOSPITAL
123 Main Street • Aldon, FL 77714 • (407) 555-1234

Step 1: Identify chapter or section of CPT: Surgery
Step 2: Identify anatomic system: ________
Step 3: Identify anatomic site: ________
Step 4: Identify procedure/technique: ________
Step 5: Identify additional specifics: ________
Step 6: Assign CPT code(s): ________
Step 7: Place code(s) in appropriate order: ________
Step 8: Assign modifier code(s) as appropriate: ________

4. Operative report

OPERATIVE REPORT

Patient information:

Patient name:
DOB:
MR#:

Date:
Surgeon:
Anesthetist:

Preoperative diagnosis:

Recurrent interstitial cystitis with history of gross hematuria

INDICATIONS: This is a 21-year-old female previously referred secondary to recurrent cystitis with associated gross hematuria. Previous antibiotic therapy has included both oral Cipro and Tequin with prior urine culture negative for growth. IVP recently obtained, from which the upper urinary tract was found to be within normal limits with the ureters seen in their entirety and the urinary bladder distended in the absence of intraluminal filling defect. She presents for cystoscopy with hydrodilation of the bladder to complete the lower urinary tract evaluation regarding hematuria, and in addition, to rule out inflammatory bladder disease most consistent with interstitial cystitis. The risks and benefits of the surgical procedure were reviewed preoperatively and include bleeding, infection, urethral injury resulting in stricture formation, bladder perforation, ureteral injury resulting in stricture formation and/or obstruction of the renal unit, postoperative hematuria, and persistent postoperative irritative voiding symptoms and pelvic pain. Full surgical consent was obtained after review of the informed consent document.

Postoperative diagnosis:

Recurrent cystitis with history of gross hematuria; bladder mucosal lesions consistent with inflammatory bladder disease

OPERATIVE FINDINGS: The urethra is within normal limits except for a few inflammatory pseudopolyps present at the anterior bladder neck, which are nonfriable. The bladder neck is open and patent. Careful systematic survey of the bladder demonstrates no evidence of tumor, foreign body, calculus, or mucosal ulceration. Both ureteral orifices are visualized in their normal anatomic positions with clear efflux of urine noted bilaterally. No significant bladder trabeculation is noted with bladder filling or evidence of diverticulum formation. Mucosal changes overlying the trigone consistent with trigonitis present. The bladder was cycled on three consecutive occasions, with final capacity under anesthesia being 650 cc, 800 cc, and 900 cc, respectively. After completion of the second bladder cycle, fine submucosal petechial hemorrhages were present, originating from the left and right lateral bladder walls in addition to posterior bladder wall and bladder dome. Although the degree of erythema was not typical of the usual inflammatory bladder disease, these findings were suggestive of interstitial cystitis where a light terminal hematuria was noted with each completion of bladder cycling.

Procedure(s) performed:

OPERATIVE PROCEDURE: Cystoscopy; hydrodilation of the bladder

Anesthesia:

Assistant surgeon:

Description of procedure:

After informed consent was obtained, the patient was taken to the cystoscopy room, given laryngeal mask anesthesia per protocol, and placed in the lithotomy position. The external genitalia were prepped with Betadine solution and draped in the usual sterile fashion. An umbilical ring was present. The patient did receive one dose of oral antibiotic consisting of Levaquin prior to initiation of the surgical procedure. The 22 French endo sheath and obturator were passed transurethrally to the bladder without difficulty. The obturator was removed and the bladder drained of a scant volume of clear yellow urine in the absence of gross hematuria. Careful systematic survey of the bladder was performed using both the 70-degree and 30-degree lenses, with the findings dictated above. The bladder was then cycled on three consecutive occasions with sterile irrigant, with final bladder capacity under anesthesia being 900 cc. Fine submucosal petechial hemorrhages were noted at completion of the second bladder cycling, most consistent with inflammatory bladder disease suggestive of interstitial cystitis. The bladder was then emptied and the cystoscope slowly retracted to the level of the bladder neck where the entire urethra was visualized using the 12-degree lens. The cystoscope was then removed, as there was no significant postoperative hematuria noted, and the procedure terminated. The patient tolerated the procedure well without complications and was subsequently transferred to the recovery room, extubated, and in stable condition.

Adm Wetz MD

GODFREY REGIONAL HOSPITAL
123 Main Street • Aldon, FL 77714 • (407) 555-1234

Step 1: Identify chapter or section of CPT: Surgery
Step 2: Identify anatomic system: ________
Step 3: Identify anatomic site: ________
Step 4: Identify procedure/technique: ________
Step 5: Identify additional specifics: ________
Step 6: Assign CPT code(s): ________
Step 7: Place code(s) in appropriate order: ________
Step 8: Assign modifier code(s) as appropriate: ________

5. Operative report

OPERATIVE REPORT

Patient information:

Patient name:
DOB:
MR#:

Date:
Surgeon:
Anesthetist:

Preoperative diagnosis:

Bladder symptoms; ureteral colic

Postoperative diagnosis:

Bladder symptoms; ureteral colic

Procedure(s) performed:

Cystoscopy and retrograde stent placement

Anesthesia:

Assistant surgeon:

Description of procedure:

The patient was placed on the operating table in the lithotomy position. She was prepped and draped sterilely. She was sedated with conscious sedation.

Cystoscope was inserted into the bladder. The bladder shows diffuse erythema throughout.

The orifices were in normal placement and configuration. No specific lesions in the bladder. 5 French stent was advanced into the right ureteral orifice. Foley catheter was in place. After removing the Foley, the stent was left in the orifice and tied to the Foley. We are going to do a retrograde film through the stent that was left in place.

Adam Westy MD

GODFREY REGIONAL HOSPITAL
123 Main Street • Aldon, FL 77714 • (407) 555-1234

Step 1: Identify chapter or section of CPT: Surgery
Step 2: Identify anatomic system: ________
Step 3: Identify anatomic site: ________
Step 4: Identify procedure/technique: ________
Step 5: Identify additional specifics: ________
Step 6: Assign CPT code(s): ________
Step 7: Place code(s) in appropriate order: ________
Step 8: Assign modifier code(s) as appropriate: ________

Male Genital System (54000-55899)

MALE GENITAL SYSTEM SERVICES

Penis	54000-54450
Testis	54500-54699
Epididymis	54700-54901
Tunica vaginalis	55000-55060
Scrotum	55100-55180
Vas deferens	55200-55450
Spermatic cord	55500-55559
Seminal vesicles	55600-55680
Prostate	55700-55899

Key Medical Terms

Benign prostatic hyperplasia
Circumcision
Orchido-
Prostate
Vasectomy

Subsections of the male genital system section (Fig. 14-21) include the following:

- Penis
- Testis
- Epididymis
- Tunica vaginalis
- Scrotum
- Vas deferens
- Spermatic cord
- Seminal vesicles
- Prostate

Procedures included in the male genital section include circumcision, vasectomy, and prostate procedures.

Circumcision codes are assigned according to the age of the patient and the technique used. Breakdown for appropriate code selection is as follows:

- Clamp: Device using a regional or ring block
- Surgical excision
- Age (28 days or less, more than 28 days)

The implant of penile prosthesis is included in this section as well. Codes are available for inflatable and noninflatable prosthesis insertion as well as codes for the removal, replacement, or repair of components of the penile prosthesis.

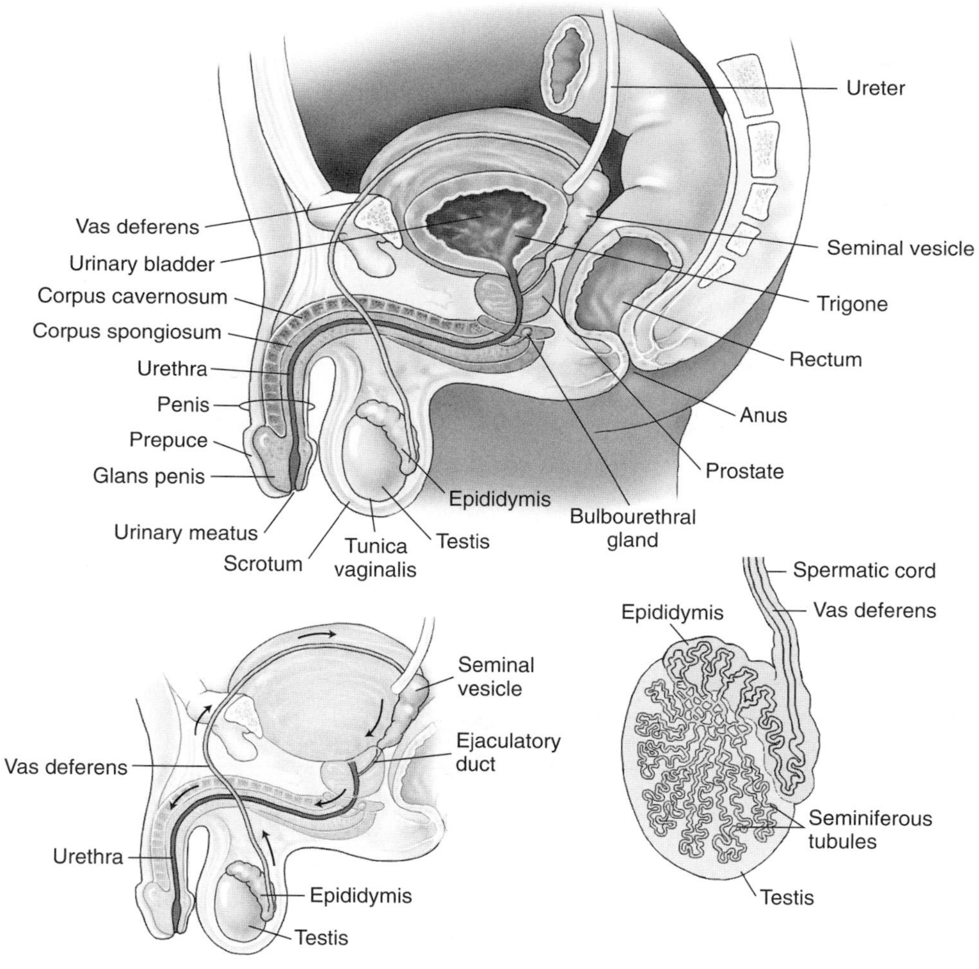

FIGURE 14-21. Male reproductive system with inset of sperm production.

Vasectomies involve the excision or removal of the vas deferens and therefore are listed under that subsection in the male genital system. Note that prostate procedures may be listed in either the male genital system or urinary system based on the specific function of the prostate involved.

Prostate procedures located in the urinary system typically involved the portion of the prostate that is in the vicinity of the bladder neck. The codes for surgical excision of the prostate (prostatectomy) are located in the male genital system section of the CPT and are categorized by the extent of excision: subtotal, total, radical, or retropubic radical. As covered in the discussion of the hematologic and lymphatic system, biopsies or excision of lymph node(s) associated with the prostate gland may already have been included in the prostate procedure; therefore care should be taken in assigning additional lymph node biopsy or excision. An example would be:

Prostatectomy, perineal radical; with lymph node biopsy(s) (limited pelvic lymphadenectomy) 55812

In the this example, it would not be appropriate to assign code(s) from the hematologic or lymphatic system for excision or biopsy of the pelvic lymph nodes in addition to code 55812.

One of the current treatments for prostate cancer involves the placement of radioactive seeds within the prostate for definitive therapy. This involves the placement of devices for guidance or direction of the radiation therapy, CPT code 55876.

Reproductive System Procedures (55920)

Code 55920 is used for the placement of needles or catheters into any organs of the pelvic region or genitalia, except for the prostate (which is assigned code 55876).

Intersex Surgery (55970-55980)

Only two codes exist in this section: one for male-to-female intersex surgery and another for female-to-male surgery. Historically, these are not services covered by third-party carriers.

Female Genital System (56405-58999)

FEMALE GENITAL SYSTEM SERVICES

Vulva, perineum, and introitus	56405-56821
Vagina	57000-57425
Cervix uteri	57452-57800
Corpus uteri	58100-58579
Oviduct/ovary	58600-58770
Ovary	58800-58960
In vitro fertilization	58970-58999

Key Medical Terms

Colpo-
Colpocleisis
Colpourethrocystopexy
Hystero-
Hysteroscopy
Laparoscopy
Marshall-Marchetti-Krantz (MMK)
Meno-
Oophoro-
Salpingo-
Total abdominal hysterectomy
Total abdominal hysterectomy with bilateral salpingo-oophorectomy
Tubal Ligation
Vagino-
Vulvo-

Subsections of the female genital system section (Fig. 14-22) include the following:

- Vulva, perineum, introitus
- Vagina
- Cervix uteri
- Corpus uteri
- Oviduct
- Ovary
- In vitro fertilization

General guidelines for the female genital system are as follows:

- Pelvic examination under anesthesia is included in conjunction with any gynecologic procedure.
- Laparoscopic lysis of adhesions (58660) is not reportable with any surgical laparoscopic procedure.
- Colposcopy is not separately reportable when considered a “scout” procedure to assess the surgical field.

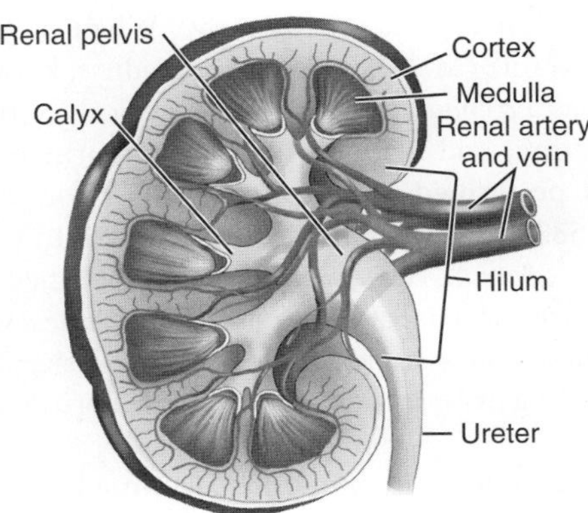

FIGURE 14-22. Cross-section of a kidney.

VULVA, PERINEUM, AND INTROITAL PROCEDURES

Vulvectomy codes are defined as follows:

- Simple: removal of skin and superficial subcutaneous tissue
- Radical: removal of skin and deep subcutaneous tissue
- Partial: removal of less than 80% of vulvar area
- Complete: removal of more than 80% of vulvar area

VAGINAL PROCEDURES

Repair of the vagina is often performed to suture a weakened area of the vaginal wall. This is accomplished through a colporrhaphy. Often the weakened area is the result of a rectocele, enterocele, or urethrocele, which may be repaired as well at the time of the colporrhaphy. In these instances codes from 57230 to 57270 may be used.

When sling procedures are performed on the vagina rather than the bladder, as discussed in the urinary system, codes from the female genital vaginal area are assigned. If the vaginal repair for stress incontinence is performed by open surgery, code 57288 is assigned; code 51992 is assigned when the same procedure is performed laparoscopically.

Colposcopy, the visualization exam of the vagina by scope, would be assigned codes from the endoscopy section (57420-57425).

When loop electrode conization of the cervix is accomplished by colposcopy, code 57461 is assigned. When this same procedure is performed without the use of colposcopy, code 57522 would be assigned.

CORPUS UTERI (UTERUS)

Hysterectomies may be performed vaginally or abdominally based on the patient's condition. Abdominal hysterectomies are assigned codes from the 58150 to 58210 range based on the extent of the procedure. When hysterectomies are performed the excision of the tube(s) or ovary(ies) is included and not assigned codes separately. When a Marshall-Marchetti-Krantz (MMK) or Burch procedure, known in the CPT book as a *colpourethrocystopexy* (surgical fixation of the vagina, urethra, and bladder, typically for urinary incontinency), is performed, assign code 58152 for abdominal approach, 58267 for vaginal, or code 58293 with or without endoscopic control. New codes were established in 2007 when supracervical laparoscopic hysterectomies were performed. These codes are based on the uterus size: 58541-42 for uterus 250 g or less, code 58543-44 for uterus size greater than 250 g.

Appendectomies are commonly performed at the time of hysterectomies. Remember that appendectomies performed with other intraabdominal procedures are considered incidental unless performed for a specified purpose at the time of another surgical procedure.

LAPAROSCOPY AND HYSTEROSCOPY

Procedures may also be performed hysteroscopically, through the uterus with a scope, in which case separate CPT codes from the range 58555 to 58565 should be assigned. Special caution needs to be taken in the assignment of codes in the female genital section because many procedures can be performed laparoscopically, hysteroscopically, vaginally, or abdominally. In some instances a specific procedure may be performed laparoscopically while another is performed hysteroscopically to a different anatomic site during the same encounter.

In other instances surgical repair may be performed in the female genital system, the abdominal cavity, or both. When procedures are performed laparoscopically and extend beyond the tubes and ovaries, laparoscopic codes from the digestive system and abdominal area, code range 49320 to 49329, should be considered. For instance, code 49326 encompasses a surgical laparoscopic omentopexy, which goes beyond the tubes and ovaries.

Tubal ligation may be performed under many circumstances. Codes are located throughout the female genital and maternity care section. This procedure may be performed laparoscopically by clamp or device, by fulguration, at the time of a cesarean section or intraabdominal surgery, or during the period immediately after other delivery during the same hospitalization.

Chromotubation of the oviduct(s) involves the injecting of fluid through the fallopian tubes to determine whether the tubes are obstructed. The procedure is typically performed for the purpose of diagnosing the cause of infertility.

Some of the code ranges for tubal ligation are as follows:

Ligation or transection of fallopian tube(s), abdominal or vaginal approach, unilateral or bilateral	58600
Postpartum, unilateral or bilateral, during same hospitalization (separate procedure)	58605
When done at the time of caesarean delivery or intra-abdominal surgery (not a separate procedure) (list separately in addition to code for primary procedure)	58611
Occlusion of fallopian tube(s) by device (e.g., band, clip, Falope ring) vaginal or suprapubic approach	58615
Laparoscopy, surgical; with fulguration of oviducts (with or without transection)	58670
With occlusion of oviducts by device (e.g., band, clip, falope ring)	58671

Note that the tubal ligation codes indicate ligation or transection of fallopian tube(s); therefore it would not be appropriate to add modifier 50 when both the right and left tubes are ligated or transected.

IN VITRO FERTILIZATION

Codes in this subsection are used when eggs are fertilized outside the body and then reimplanted for fertility purposes.

MATERNITY CARE AND DELIVERY (59000-59899)

Key Medical Terms

Cesarean delivery (C-section)
Gravida
Incomplete abortion
Missed abortion
Para
Vaginal birth after cesarean (VBAC)

The global maternity care package encompasses the antepartum (preoperative care), delivery (surgical care), and postpartum (postoperative) care of the patient. Because this care encompasses a 9-month period, and many patients see another physician or provider during this time, specific CPT codes are assigned for antepartum, postpartum, and delivery care.

GENERAL GUIDELINES AND DEFINITIONS

Antepartum, Delivery, and Postpartum Services

The global obstetric period encompasses the following:

- Antepartum (preoperative): initial and subsequent history, physical examinations, weight, blood pressure, and other recordings
  Routine urinalysis
  Monthly visits (to 28 weeks)
  Biweekly visits (to 36 weeks)
  Weekly visits (to delivery)
- Delivery (operative): admission to hospital
  Uncomplicated labor
  Vaginal delivery (with or without episiotomy; with or without forceps)
  Cesarean delivery
- Postpartum (postoperative): hospital or office visits for normal postpartum care after delivery

All services other than those outlined here may be coded and billed with appropriate codes from correct sections of the CPT. A modifier code probably will be necessary to explain the unusual circumstances (complication) along with medical documentation to establish medical necessity for additional services listed outside the global component.

There is much controversy among third-party carriers regarding what services may be billed in addition to the obstetric package charge. If the practice provides obstetric services regularly, the coder may wish to build these codes into the third-party contract worksheet. For instance, cephalic version (i.e., the manual "turning" of the fetus) obviously involves additional time and surgical risk. Many carriers do not reimburse for this service, with the explanation that this service is commonly provided to obstetric patients.

The coder may wish to refer to the CPT and the coding guidelines established by the obstetric/gynecologic specialty organization(s) to develop a coding method for his or her practice. Keep in mind that the coder must code on the basis of these guidelines, not according to what the individual carrier(s) will accept, recognize, or pay.

High-risk pregnancies, which involve more than the normal number of visits or additional diagnostic or therapeutic services, should be coded with the evaluation and management, surgical, or other CPT codes. A diagnosis should be provided, indicating the reason for the additional services, including the diagnostic code for supervision of high-risk pregnancy.

Multiple deliveries that encompass the entire maternity period (antepartum, delivery, and postpartum) are coded with one code selected from the obstetric package codes based on the delivery type (vaginal, cesarean section [C-section], or successful or unsuccessful vaginal delivery after previous C-section [VBAC]) as well as additional codes for each additional delivery.

Because many maternity patients will not complete their full global period with one physician or group, codes are also available in this section segregated by antepartum visits only, delivery only, and postpartum only. To select the correct code(s) for care provided, the breakdown would be as follows:

- Delivery type
  Vaginal
  C-Section
  VBAC
- Extent work performed
  Whole obstetric package
  Delivery only
  Postpartum only
  Antepartum only

ABORTIONS

Abortions are also listed in the maternity care and delivery section of CPT. Abortion is the spontaneous premature expulsion of the fetus. The codes for treatment are assigned based on whether the abortion is incomplete (products of conception are retained), missed fetus is retained and induced [intentionally terminated pregnancy]), and the method (surgically completed or by dilation and curettage [D&C], injections, or vaginal suppositories).

STOP AND PRACTICE

Determine the appropriate breakdown and code(s) for the following procedures.

	Anatomic Site	Procedure and Technique	Specifics	Code(s)
1. Vaginal delivery only	______	______	______	______
2. Cesarean delivery, antepartum, delivery, postpartum	______	______	______	______
3. Incomplete abortion, completed surgically	______	______	______	______
4. Amniocentesis	______	______	______	______
5. Abdominal hysterectomy with oophorectomy	______	______	______	______
6. Simple vulvectomy	______	______	______	______
7. Transurethral resection of prostate	______	______	______	______
8. Vasectomy	______	______	______	______
9. D&C	______	______	______	______
10. Laparoscopic tubal ligation by fulguration	______	______	______	______

STOP AND PRACTICE

Take the following operative reports and assign CPT codes appropriately. Make sure you continue to utilize our technique of breaking down the information needed to code. Utilize the guidelines listed earlier for each subcategory of the male, female, and maternity systems. You may wish to add the "bullets" we discussed for each section to your CPT book so those guidelines will be readily available as you search for the appropriate code(s).

1. Operative report

OPERATIVE REPORT

Patient information:

Patient name:
DOB:
MR#:

Date:
Surgeon:
Anesthetist:

Preoperative diagnosis:

Postoperative diagnosis:

Procedure(s) performed:

OPERATIVE REPORTS:
This 1-day-old baby is brought into the hospital today for a circumcision. He also is to have his newborn screen blood draw done today. Mom was anxious to go home yesterday and went home in less than 24 hours and was asked to return today. Both mom and father desire to have a circumcision for Jakob. Risks and benefits are discussed, and the parents wish to proceed with the circumcision.

Anesthesia:

Assistant surgeon:

Description of procedure:

The patient was brought to the nursery and placed on the circumcision board. His legs were strapped down. The base of the penis was cleansed with alcohol, and 1% lidocaine without epinephrine was injected at the 10 and 2 o'clock positions. Less than 1 cc of 1% lidocaine was used. Good anesthetic effect. The patient was then prepped and draped in a sterile fashion. Hemostats were placed at the 9 and 3 o'clock positions to help with holding while adhesions were taken down from the glans. Adhesions were taken down, taking great care not to injure the glans. Hemostat was then placed at the dorsum sagittal line down to just distal to the corona. Hemostat was left in place for approximately 1 minute. After removal of the hemostat, an incision was made down to the apex. The foreskin was then retracted and further adhesions were removed. The foreskin was then brought back into place and the Mogen clamp was applied. While trying to bring the foreskin up through the Mogen clamp to the apex of the incision, the skin gave way and tore along the frenulum and along the apex. The Mogen clamp was never completely applied. The Mogen clamp was then removed. Remainder of the foreskin attachment was then cross-clamped with hemostat for approximately 1 minute and then removed with scissors. Trying to maintain esthetics. Good hemostasis in this area. There was, however, oozing of blood along the volar aspect or frenulum part of the penis. Pressure was applied to this area. This was not enough to maintain hemostasis, so silver nitrate sticks were used with good results. The penis was then dressed with Vaseline gauze and patient was placed on observation status to watch for any signs of continued bleeding. Also to watch for urination. Patient was given some Tylenol during the procedure.

During the course of observation, blood began oozing on the dorsal aspect of the penis, and silver nitrate sticks were again used to stop the bleeding. No further bleeding throughout the stay. The patient tolerated diet well. He was given supplement as well as breast feeding while in the hospital. Incident of procedure was discussed with both mom and dad. Patient's pediatrician was contacted by telephone; he felt that all was done appropriately. His colleague was contacted as she was here in the clinic and she was brought to examine the patient. She observed good hemostasis and felt probable good outcome.

The baby was discharged to home approximately at 1:30 p.m. Care of circumcision was discussed with both Mom and Dad. They are strongly urged to come to the clinic with any signs of bleeding or infection. Okay to use Tylenol q4h in the first 24–48 hr. Returnto clinic for recheck on Monday (3 days) and then follow up again at regular scheduled visit on Thursday, one week after delivery.

Upon discussion with Mom after she had taken baby home, he urinated shortly after getting home.

Adm Wetz MD

GODFREY REGIONAL HOSPITAL
123 Main Street • Aldon, FL 77714 • (407) 555-1234

Step 1: Identify chapter or section of CPT: Surgery
Step 2: Identify anatomic system: ________
Step 3: Identify anatomic site: ________
Step 4: Identify procedure/technique: ________
Step 5: Identify additional specifics: ________
Step 6: Assign CPT code(s): ________
Step 7: Place code(s) in appropriate order: ________
Step 8: Assign modifier code(s) as appropriate: ________

2. Operative report

OPERATIVE REPORT

Patient information:

Patient name:
DOB:
MR#:

Date:
Surgeon:
Anesthetist:

Preoperative diagnosis:

Elevated prostatic specific antigen

Postoperative diagnosis:

Elevated prostatic specific antigen, benign prostatic hypertrophy

Procedure(s) performed:

Anesthesia:

Assistant surgeon:

Description of procedure:

The patient was placed on the operating table in the lithotomy position. He was sedated with anesthesia. 10 cc of Xylocaine was injected through the prostate via perineum and 10 cc of Xylocaine jelly was injected per urethra. Cystoscope was inserted. The urethra was unremarkable. The prostate was trilobate and obstructing, quite large through the lumen, and a lot of anterior tissue was projecting into the bladder.

The bladder shows some trabeculation, but no mucosal lesions, no erythema, no stones. The bladder is emptied. Cystoscope is removed.

Finger was inserted into the rectum. His prostate is large. There is a hard, but not rock hard, ridge in the posterolateral prostate towards the apex. The rest of the prostate is just very large and firm. Needle was placed through the perineum, and finger-directed biopsies were taken from all four quadrants of the prostate.

Given the area of abnormality and palpation, he tolerated the procedure without difficulty.

Rachel Perez MD

GODFREY REGIONAL HOSPITAL
123 Main Street • Aldon, FL 77714 • (407) 555-1234

Step 1: Identify chapter or section of CPT: Surgery
Step 2: Identify anatomic system: ________
Step 3: Identify anatomic site: ________
Step 4: Identify procedure/technique: ________
Step 5: Identify additional specifics: ________
Step 6: Assign CPT code(s): ________
Step 7: Place code(s) in appropriate order: ________
Step 8: Assign modifier code(s) as appropriate: ________

3. Operative report

OPERATIVE REPORT

Patient information:

Patient name:
DOB:
MR#:

Date:
Surgeon:
Anesthetist:

Preoperative diagnosis:

Perimenopausal bleeding

Postoperative diagnosis:

Same

Procedure(s) performed:

D&C for control of perimenopausal bleeding. Patient had been seen in the office because of continued bleeding despite trial with hormonal manipulation. The impression was that this was probably related to perimenopausal status. Again, she was requesting to control bleeding and also afford a diagnosis. She was cleared medically by her family doctor who admitted her this morning for the same.

Anesthesia:

Assistant surgeon:

Description of procedure:

On admission an IV line was started. She was then brought to surgery. Procedure was to be done with local IV-monitored anesthesia. She was sedated IV-wise and then placed in the lithotomy position following perineal/vaginal prep. Operation was started. Weighted speculum was inserted into the posterior vagina. The anterior cervix was secured with tenaculum and weighted Hegar's dilators were utilized to size 10, and then a sharp curet was passed in, curetting generous amounts of endometrial tissue until nothing else could be felt except the firm, gritty sensation of myometrium. Operation was terminated at this point.

Patient was then taken from surgery to the recovery room in a satisfactory condition. She will be discharged today and will follow up with her primary care physician for continued care.

Adam Westgate MD

GODFREY REGIONAL HOSPITAL
123 Main Street • Aldon, FL 77714 • (407) 555-1234

Step 1: Identify chapter or section of CPT:	Surgery	Step 5: Identify additional specifics:	______
Step 2: Identify anatomic system:	______	Step 6: Assign CPT code(s):	______
Step 3: Identify anatomic site:	______	Step 7: Place code(s) in appropriate order:	______
Step 4: Identify procedure/technique:	______	Step 8: Assign modifier code(s) as appropriate:	______

4. Operative report

OPERATIVE REPORT

Patient information:

Patient name:
DOB:
MR#:

Date:
Surgeon:
Anesthetist:

Preoperative diagnosis:

1. Pelvic pain
2. Right ovarian cyst

Postoperative diagnosis:

1. Stage III endometriosis
2. Pelvic adhesions

Procedure(s) performed:

1. Exam under anesthesia
2. Laparoscopy
3. Lysis of adhesions

Anesthesia:

Assistant surgeon:

Description of procedure:

The patient was taken to the operating room and placed under adequate general anesthesia. She was then examined under anesthesia because prior ultrasound showed a 5 × 8 cm mass; however, on pelvic examination, the cystic lesion on the right side did not feel as big as what was seen on ultrasound. Therefore, repeat ultrasound was done under anesthesia. There was a 3-cm cyst noted on the right ovary. At that point, decision was made to perform a laparoscopy. Consent for the laparoscopy was obtained from the patient's husband.

The patient was placed in the lithotomy position and prepped and draped in the usual fashion. Foley catheter was placed in the bladder. Hulka tenaculum was then placed in the uterus for manipulation.

A small 5-mm infraumbilical incision was made, through which a Veress needle was passed without difficulty. After adequate insufflation with carbon dioxide gas, a 5-mm trocar was passed without difficulty. The laparoscope was passed through this and an intra-abdominal adhesion was noted. A suprapubic incision was made, 5 mm, in the midline, through which a 5-mm trocar was passed under direct visualization. The pelvis was inspected and the findings were as follows.

First, there were adhesions between the lower sigmoid colon and the posterior wall of the uterus with involved endometrial-type blebs. There were also deep black endometriotic implants along both uterosacral ligaments. Deeper in the cul-de-sac were red endometriotic implants. The right ovary was adhered to the right side of the uterine wall, and this was taken down bluntly. The cyst in the ovary opened up, and brown fluid could be seen coming from the cyst, which would be consistent with an endometrioma. It was opened completely and irrigated. The right adnexa was completely dissected off the uterus by blunt dissection. The lower sigmoid, upper rectal area was also dissected off the posterior wall of the uterus by blunt dissection. The sigmoid colon on the left, however, was adhered to a point just below the left ovary. This made it difficult to see the left ovary completely. However, the laparoscope was passed through the suprapubic cannula, and this allowed us to see the distal part of the tube. Both fimbriae appeared to be normal. There were some brown implants of endometriosis on the left ovary. The pelvis was extensively irrigated. At this point, there was no bleeding from the adhesiolysis.

A decision was made that the patient would benefit from a four- to six-month course of Lupron Depot to allow time for the pelvis to heal and some of the endometriosis to regress. At that point, a second-look laparoscopy will be performed with a laser to treat any residual endometriosis. Therefore, at this point, the procedure was terminated. The suprapubic cannula was removed under direct visualization without subsequent bleeding. CO_2 gas was released through the umbilical cannula, which was then removed. Both incisions were closed with Dermabond. Hulka tenaculum was removed from the cervix without subsequent bleeding. Needle and sponge counts were reported as correct by the circulating nurse.

General anesthesia was reversed and the patient was sent to the recovery room in stable condition.

Rachel Perez MD

GODFREY REGIONAL HOSPITAL
123 Main Street • Aldon, FL 77714 • (407) 555-1234

Step 1: Identify chapter or section of CPT: Surgery
Step 2: Identify anatomic system: ________
Step 3: Identify anatomic site: ________
Step 4: Identify procedure/technique: ________
Step 5: Identify additional specifics: ________
Step 6: Assign CPT code(s): ________
Step 7: Place code(s) in appropriate order: ________
Step 8: Assign modifier code(s) as appropriate: ________

5. Operative report

OPERATIVE REPORT

Patient information:

Patient name:
DOB:
MR#:

Date:
Surgeon:
Anesthetist:

Preoperative diagnosis:

Incomplete abortion at eight weeks' gestation, twin gestation noted

Postoperative diagnosis:

Same

Procedure(s) performed:

Suction D&C under ultrasound guidance

Anesthesia:

Assistant surgeon:

Description of procedure:

The patient was prepped and draped in the usual fashion for suction D&C. Under adequate general anesthesia, and with ultrasound guidance, the cervix was dilated and a #10 suction cannula was introduced. The anterior, posterior, and lateral walls of the endometrial cavity were curetted, yielding a moderate amount of products of conception. No endometrial defects were encountered. A medium-sized sharp curette was then introduced. The anterior, posterior, and lateral walls of the endometrial cavity were gently curetted, yielding a scant amount of additional tissue. Again, no endometrial defects were encountered. No injury to the uterus was noted. A Foley catheter was used to fill the bladder for proper visualization during the procedure. IV oxytocin was infused as well as Methergine 0.2 mg IM, and after the procedure, two 100 mg tablets of Cytotec were placed intrarectally.

The patient tolerated the procedure well, left the operating room in good condition, breathing spontaneously, vital signs stable. All sponge, instrument, and needle counts were correct at the end of the procedure.

Rachel Perez MD

GODFREY REGIONAL HOSPITAL
123 Main Street • Aldon, FL 77714 • (407) 555-1234

Step 1: Identify chapter or section of CPT: Surgery
Step 2: Identify anatomic system: ________
Step 3: Identify anatomic site: ________
Step 4: Identify procedure/technique: ________
Step 5: Identify additional specifics: ________
Step 6: Assign CPT code(s): ________
Step 7: Place code(s) in appropriate order: ________
Step 8: Assign modifier code(s) as appropriate: ________

Endocrine System (60000-60699)

ENDOCRINE SYSTEM SERVICES

Thyroid gland	60000-60300
Parathyroid, thymus, adrenal glands, pancreas, and carotid body	60500-60699

Subsections of the endocrine system section include:

- Thyroid gland
- Parathyroid, thymus, adrenal glands, carotid body

Nervous System (61000-64999)

NERVOUS SYSTEM SERVICES

Skull, meninges, and brain	61000-62258
Spine and spinal cord	62263-63746
Extracranial nerves, peripheral nerves, and autonomic nervous system	64400-64999

Key Medical Terms

Anesthesia
Cerebrospinal fluid
Cranio-
Encephalo-
Laminectomy
Lamino-
Laminotomy
Myelo-
Neuro-
Neurolytic substance

Subsections of the nervous system section include:

- Skull, meninges, brain (Figs. 14-23 and 14-24)
- Spine, spinal cord (Fig. 14-25)
- Extracranial nerves, peripheral nerves, autonomic nerves

Procedures included in this section are categorized as follows:

- Arthrodesis: surgical fixation of joint by fusion of joint surfaces
- Corpectomy: removal of entire vertebral body or vertebral body resection
- Diskectomy: excision of intervertebral disk
- Laminectomy: incision of posterior arch of vertebra
- Laminotomy: division of lamina of vertebra

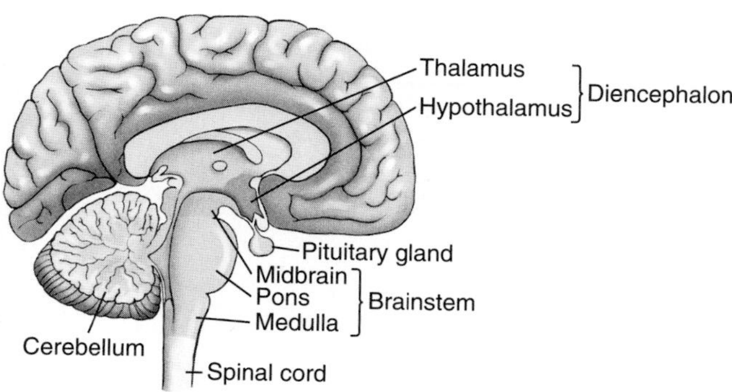

FIGURE 14-23. The brain.

SKULL, MENINGES, AND BRAIN

Surgical procedures performed on the skull, meninges, and brain often involve taps, punctures, drainage, or other procedures necessary to alleviate pressure on the brain. CPT guidelines specify that when these "temporary" procedures are necessary to alleviate pressure before the definitive procedure, they are not separately reportable. When these procedures are performed as part of a staged procedure, they may be coded with modifier 58 to designate they were planned as staged procedures.

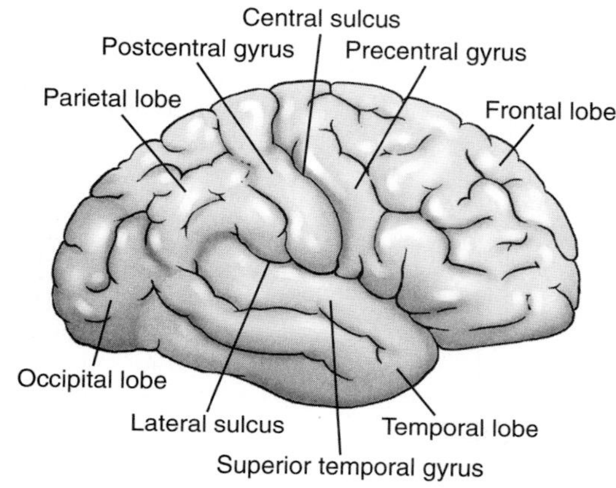

FIGURE 14-24. The cerebrum.

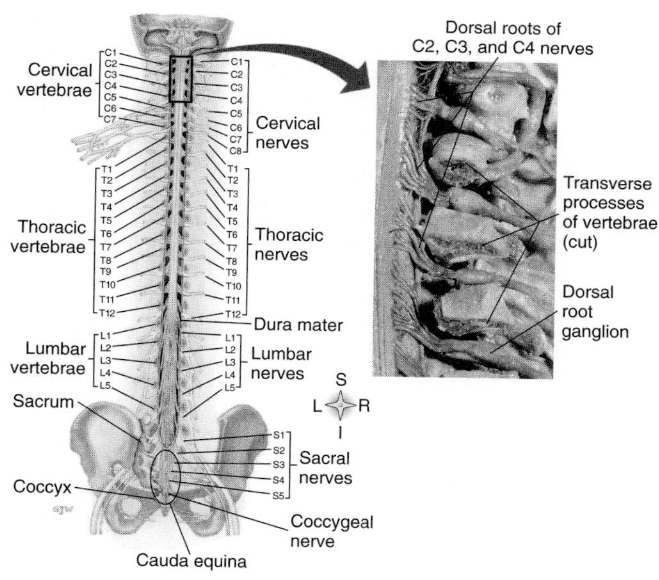

FIGURE 14-25. The spinal cord.

Other CPT and NCCI guidelines for the skull, meninges, and brain are as follows:

- Craniectomies and craniotomies when performed as "scout" procedures or for exploration purposes are not reportable when a definitive procedure is performed.
- Spinal taps, or lumbar punctures, include any anesthetic necessary to perform the procedure.
- When a cerebrospinal fluid leak occurs during a spinal procedure, repair of the leak is not separately reportable. Procedures of the skull base include the following:
  - Approach: procedure necessary to expose the lesion
  - Definitive: repair, biopsy, resection, excision of lesions, and primary closure
  - Repair or reconstruction: extensive grafting or repair required

As discussed when assigning codes for pacemakers and defibrillators, this is the second area in CPT where guidelines allow assignment of codes for all procedures performed on the skull base. Therefore if the surgeon performs both the approach and definitive procedure, it would be appropriate to assign the appropriate code(s) for both procedures. Because these procedures are usually quite lengthy, it is not unusual for each portion of the procedure to be performed by a different surgeon.

NERVOUS SYSTEM SHUNTS

Cerebrospinal fluid shunts are placed for the proper drainage of fluid from the brain. When obstructions or congenital abnormalities do not allow appropriate drainage and circulation of cerebrospinal fluid, a shunt is placed.

SPINE AND SPINAL CORD PROCEDURES

The insertion of spinal catheters for pain management is also included in the nervous system surgical section. This procedure involves the placement of a permanent catheter for back pain management.

Other pain management codes are included in this section for epidural, lumbar, cervical, and thoracic injections not performed through an indwelling catheter. These are found in the injection, drainage, and aspiration subsection of the spine and spinal cord section. When neurolytic substances intended to destroy or numb are injected, codes from the range 62280 to 62282 are used. When diagnostic or therapeutic substances—such as anesthetics, antispasmodics, opioids, steroids, or other therapeutic substances—are injected, codes from the 62310 to 62319 range are assigned. Codes are also based on the specific part of the spine the injections are performed on: cervical, lumbar, or thoracic. Remember that the operative report will typically designate these locations by the abbreviations C (cervical), L (lumbar), and T (thoracic), followed by the segment. For example, the first cervical vertebra would be designated as C1. The first vertebral interspace (the space between the vertebrae) would be designated as C1-C2. The vertebrae are divided as follows:

Cervical vertebrae (seven)	C1-C7
Thoracic vertebrae (12)	T1-T12
Lumbar vertebrae (5)	L1-L5
Sacral vertebrae (5)	S1-S5
Coccygeal vertebrae (4)	
Coccyx/tailbone	

Procedures of the spine and spinal cord include laminectomy (surgical excision of lamina) and laminotomy (incision of lamina). Although other sections of CPT have codes that bundle multiple procedures or approaches, the same is not true for some spinal surgery. Because of the delicate nature of surgery, the approach, definitive, and repair or reconstructive procedure are typically all billable under CPT guidelines. The coder should note any exclusions; however, in this section, multiple procedures are codeable or billable for these intricate and complex procedures.

Procedures for carpal tunnel syndrome are included in the nervous system. When the procedure is performed surgically, code 64721 is assigned. However, when the procedure is performed arthroscopically, code 29848 is assigned. Notes to that effect are included in both the musculoskeletal section and the nervous system section of CPT.

EXTRACRANIAL NERVES, PERIPHERAL NERVES, AND AUTONOMIC NERVOUS SYSTEM PROCEDURES

Procedures performed on the nerves are divided by the procedure performed (nerve block, transection, suturing, repair, excision) as well as the specific nerve type or nerve involved.

When repair of the median nerve at the carpal tunnel is performed open, code 64721 would be assigned. Keep in mind when this procedure is performed arthroscopically, code 29848 is assigned instead. Note that CPT has notated this "cross walk" information following both codes as a guide to correct coding.

Eye and Ocular Adnexa (65091-68899)

EYE AND OCULAR ADNEXA SERVICES

Eyeball	65091-65290
Anterior segment	65400-66999
Posterior segment	67005-67299
Ocular adnexa	67311-67999
Conjunctiva	68020-68899

Key Medical Terms

Blepharo-
Cataract
Conjunctivo-

Enucleation
Extraocular muscles intact (EOMI)
Extracapsular
Intracapsular
Kerato-
OD (right eye)
OS (left eye)
OU (both eyes)
Phacoemulsification
Pupils equal, round, and reactive to light and accommodation (PERRLA)
Sclero
Strabismus

Subsections of the eye and ocular adnexa sections include the following:

- Eyeball (Fig. 14-26)
- Anterior segment
- Posterior segment
- Ocular adnexa
- Conjunctiva

Ophthalmologic examinations and refractions are NOT included in the eye and ocular adnexa section because they are not considered surgical. They are located in the medicine section of CPT, which is discussed in Chapter 17.

To properly code procedures that involve the eye, the coder must be familiar with the anatomic landmarks of the eye. Take a look at Figure 14-26 along with the introductory words for the eye and ocular adnexa in the previous lists. If a more detailed review is necessary, keep in mind that the Professional Edition of CPT includes anatomic illustrations for visualization and reference.

Of note, blepharoplasty, when involving only the eyelid, is typically assigned codes from the integumentary section. When the procedure involves more than the eyelid, codes from the eye and ocular adnexa section would be appropriate.

Some general CPT and NCCI guidelines that relate to coding the eye and ocular adnexa are as follows:

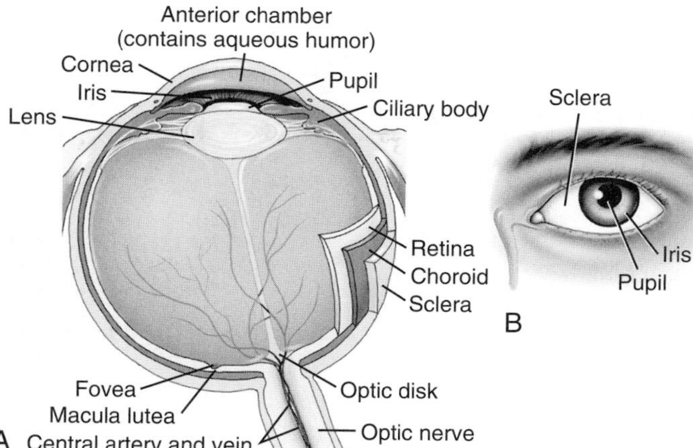

FIGURE 14-26. A, The eyeball viewed from above. **B,** The anterior view of the eyeball.

- When a subconjunctival injection is performed as part of a more extensive procedure, the injection is not separately reportable.
- Iridectomy, trabeculectomy, and anterior vitrectomy performed in conjunction with a cataract removal are considered an integral part of the cataract extraction, except when performed for a different diagnosis and separate purpose.
- The various approaches for removing a cataract are mutually exclusively when performed on the same eye. In other words, only one definitive procedure may be assigned for cataract extraction for the same eye.
- Incision, drainage, and excision of conjunctiva codes are included in all conjunctivoplasties.
- Canthoplasty is included in repair procedures, including blepharoplasties.

ANTERIOR SEGMENT PROCEDURES

Procedures performed on the cornea would be located in the anterior segment subsection of the eye. Radial keratotomy is performed by making incisions into the cornea that result in improved vision. Code 64771 is assigned to this procedure.

CATARACT EXTRACTION PROCEDURES

When assigning codes for cataract extraction, the coder must determine whether the extraction was extracapsular or intracapsular and whether the intraocular lens prosthesis was placed at the time of the cataract extraction or later. Remember that when the procedure is not specific, it would be assumed that the procedure was performed extracapsular (outside the capsule), which would be the least significant. When additional techniques or procedures are necessary to complete the cataract extraction, code 66982 would be assigned. These additional techniques may include procedures such as the insertion of an iris expansion device or suture support to ensure the intraocular lens prosthesis stays in place.

If complications occur during the procedure, the surgeon may elect to extract the cataract only and implant the intraocular lens at a future time. In this case, codes for the cataract extraction should not include the intraocular lens implant. At a later date the surgeon may elect to implant the intraocular lens. At that time, code 66985 would be assigned. Keep in mind that the procedures for cataract extraction would typically require the designation of RT or LT for right or left eye. Remember that the medical designation of OD, OS, or OU indicates the right eye (OD), left eye (OS), or both eyes (OU).

OCULAR ADNEXA PROCEDURES

Strabismus procedures involve the straightening or stretching of vertical or horizontal muscles or both to correct what typically is referred to as "crossed eyes" or "lazy eye." The coder must determine whether the muscles involved are horizontal or vertical as well as the number of muscles corrected.

CONJUNCTIVA PROCEDURES

Procedures relating to the lacrimal duct, or tear duct, are included in this section. When the tear duct is obstructed, repair, probing, or closure of a lacrimal fistula may be necessary.

Auditory System (69000-69990)

AUDITORY SYSTEM SERVICES

External ear	69000-69399
Middle ear	69400-69799
Inner ear	69801-69990

Key Medical Terms

AD (right ear)
AS (left ear)
AU (both ears)
Cerumen
Cochlear
Head, eyes, ears, nose, and throat (HEENT)
Labyrintho-
Myringo-
Oto-
Pressure-equalization (PE) tube
Stapes
Tympano-
Ventilating tube

Subsections of the auditory system section include the following:

- External ear (Fig. 14-27)
- Middle ear
- Inner ear
- Temporal bone, middle fossa approach

Hearing and other diagnostic auditory evaluations are not included in the auditory section of the surgery section but rather in the medicine section of CPT.

The auditory system is divided into the three parts of the ear: external, middle, and inner.

EXTERNAL EAR PROCEDURES

Removal of impacted cerumen is included in the common procedures performed on the external ear. CPT guidelines indicate this procedure should be assigned only when the procedure note is clear that the cerumen is "impacted." When assigned, the procedure is coded only once whether performed on one or both ears; therefore the anatomic modifiers RT, LT, and 50 would not be appropriate.

Removal of foreign bodies from the ear is also a common procedure, especially in children. This may be performed without general anesthesia (69200) or may require general anesthesia (69205) because of the nature of the foreign body or the child's age.

MIDDLE EAR PROCEDURES

The most commonly performed procedure from this section is the insertion of ventilating tubes into the ear (typically performed on children). Codes are assigned based on whether a myringotomy only (incision) is performed or whether a new opening is created (for placement of a tube). A tympanostomy, or new opening, would include the incision required to insert the ventilating tube and create the new opening. Codes are also assigned based on whether general or local

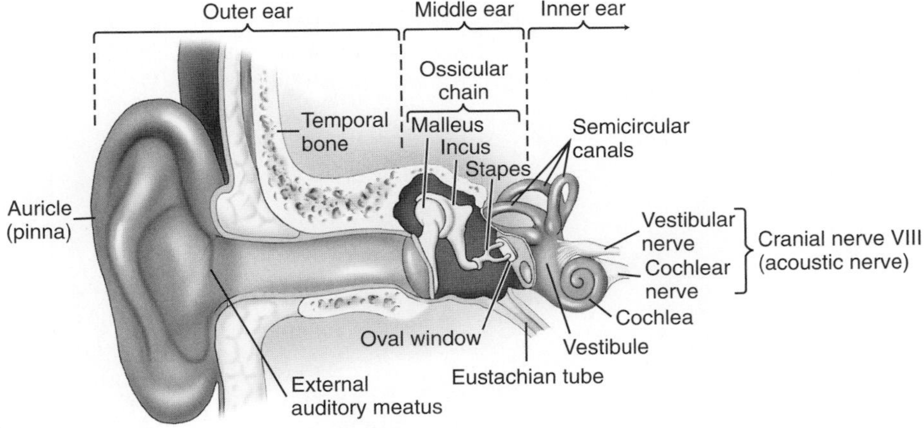

FIGURE 14-27. The ear.

anesthesia is used as well as the patient's age. Because this procedure may be performed on either the left ear (AS), right ear (AD), or both ears (AU) the anatomic modifiers RT, LT, or 50 would be appropriate with these codes.

The inner ear includes the labyrinth and the cochlea, a cone-shaped cavity forming one of the divisions of the inner ear. The most common procedure in the past decade from this section may be cochlear device implantation (code 69930) in persons whose natural cochlea is deformed, not present, or damaged, causing hearing loss. Implantation of this device usually restores hearing to an otherwise deaf individual.

STOP AND PRACTICE

Determine the appropriate breakdown and code(s) for the following procedures.

	Anatomic Site	Procedure and Technique	Specifics	Code(s)
1. Extracapsular cataract extraction with intraocular lens	______	______	______	______
2. Strabismus surgery, two horizontal muscles, right eye	______	______	______	______
3. Creation of subarachnoid/subdural-peritoneal shunt	______	______	______	______
4. Elevation of simple skull fracture	______	______	______	______
5. Nerve block, by anesthetic, facial nerve	______	______	______	______
6. Implantation of neurostimulator electrodes, percutaneous	______	______	______	______
7. Suture three digital nerves of hand	______	______	______	______
8. Repair of carpal tunnel nerve	______	______	______	______
9. Tympanostomy with tube placement bilateral with general anesthesia	______	______	______	______
10. Removal of cerumen	______	______	______	______

STOP AND PRACTICE

Take the following operative reports and assign CPT codes appropriately. Make sure you continue to utilize our technique of breaking down the information needed to code. Utilize the guidelines listed earlier for each subcategory of the nervous, eye, and ear systems. You may wish to add the "bullets" we discussed for each section to your CPT book so those guidelines will be readily available as you search for the appropriate code(s).

1. Operative report

OPERATIVE REPORT

Patient information:

Patient name:
DOB:
MR#:

Date:
Surgeon:
Anesthetist:

Preoperative diagnosis:

Postoperative diagnosis:

Procedure(s) performed:

Spinal cord stimulator trial; intraoperative spinal cord stimulator screening

Anesthesia:

Assistant surgeon:

Description of procedure:

After an IV was started, the patient was taken to the operating room and placed prone on the operating table. A couple of pillows were placed under the abdomen to straighten out the spinal flexion. The lumbar area was prepped and draped in the usual sterile fashion using DuraPrep, and under direct fluoroscopy the T10 to L2 spinous processes were identified and marked. The skin overlying the L1-2 interspace was infiltrated with 5–6 cc of a mixture of 1% lidocaine and 0.5% bupivacaine.

A small stab wound was made in the L1-2 interspace just above the spinous process. A 15-gauge Tuohy needle was inserted under direct fluoroscopy control through the stab wound and guided into the L1-2 interspace. Under direct fluoroscopy control, the needle was then advanced further until the epidural space was identified using the loss-of-resistance technique. After negative aspiration for blood or CSF was confirmed, a guidewire was inserted through the Tuohy needle and advanced up into the epidural space without any problems. The system was then inserted through the Tuohy needle, and under direct fluoroscopy control, was gradually advanced up into the epidural space in the midline. The final positioning of the tip of the lead was noted to be at the mid body of the T10 vertebra.

The stylet inside the quad lead was removed and a shorter lead connector was inserted into the lead system. This connector was then attached to the screening cable and locked into place. The patient was allowed to wake up at this time in preparation for the intraoperative screening. Various combinations were tried intraoperatively, and the final settings of the screener were noted before the lead was disconnected from the screening cable. The Tuohy needle was then withdrawn into the subcutaneous tissue very carefully, and the positioning of the lead was confirmed after the needle was withdrawn. The lead was basically noted to be intact after the needle was withdrawn and removed. The lead was then fixed in place using Steri-Strips, and an extension lead was connected to the quad lead system. Sterile dressing was applied over the lead system, and the patient was transported to the recovery area where she was observed for a few minutes before being discharged home.

POSTOPERATIVE SCREENING:
In the recovery area the patient was educated in detail about the use of the screener and the final settings were as follows: Lead 0 was negative, lead 1 was positive, 2 was off, and 3 was off. Pulse width was 390, rate was at 40, and aptitude was 4.1. The patient was shown how to use the machine and was discharged home on Keflex 500 mg po q8h for seven days and was told to come back for follow-up in one week, at which time we will consider further options, depending on her response to this modality of treatment. Until such time the patient will continue her OxyContin and baclofen and will also continue her physical therapy exercises. At the time of discharge, the patient reported excellent pain relief as far as her burning neuropathic pain is concerned; however, she continued to have some dull aching, spasmodic pain in the hip joint and in the muscles of the leg.

The patient reported good coverage in both her lower extremities with a slight predominance on the left side.

Rachel Perez MD

GODFREY REGIONAL HOSPITAL
123 Main Street • Aldon, FL 77714 • (407) 555-1234

Step 1: Identify chapter or section of CPT:	Surgery	Step 5: Identify additional specifics:	_______
Step 2: Identify anatomic system:	_______	Step 6: Assign CPT code(s):	_______
Step 3: Identify anatomic site:	_______	Step 7: Place code(s) in appropriate order:	_______
Step 4: Identify procedure/technique:	_______	Step 8: Assign modifier code(s) as appropriate:	_______

2. Operative report

OPERATIVE REPORT

Patient information:

Patient name:
DOB:
MR#:

Date:
Surgeon:
Anesthetist:

Preoperative diagnosis:

Cervical radiculopathy; dystrophy, right upper extremity; headaches

Postoperative diagnosis:

Cervical radiculopathy; dystrophy, right upper extremity; headaches

Procedure(s) performed:

Cervical epidural steroid injections under fluoroscopy and sedation, trigger point injection to right paravertebral neck and suprascapular region on the right side

Anesthesia:

Assistant surgeon:

Description of procedure:

The patient was taken to the operating room. IV fluids given, 200 cc lactated Ringer's preoperatively as prehydration. Monitors placed. IV with sedation given.

Surgical scrub to lower neck under fluoroscopic guidance. C7-C8 intervertebral space was identified. The skin was infiltrated with 1% lidocaine 2 cc. Epidural needle #17 Tuohy, loss-of-resistance technique; loss of resistance positive. Needle position confirmed by fluoroscopy, and 2 cc of 0.25% bupivacaine injected as a test dose. Test dose was negative. No CSF, no heme on aspiration. Then 5 cc of normal saline preservative-free with 40 mg of Depo-Medrol was injected though the epidural space and the needle was removed. Two trigger points were done on the right side, one at the right paravertebral neck and the second at the right suprascapular region. Each trigger point was injected with 2.5 cc of 0.25% bupivacaine and 20 mg of Depo-Medrol to each side.

OPERATIVE REPORT: The patient tolerated the procedure well. Vital signs are stable. The patient was taken to PACU.

POSTOPERATIVE PLAN: Discharge home, ice packs to lower back, follow-up in the office in seven days.

COMPLICATIONS: Nil

Adam Westgate MD

GODFREY REGIONAL HOSPITAL
123 Main Street • Aldon, FL 77714 • (407) 555-1234

Step 1: Identify chapter or section of CPT: Surgery
Step 2: Identify anatomic system: ________
Step 3: Identify anatomic site: ________
Step 4: Identify procedure/technique: ________
Step 5: Identify additional specifics: ________
Step 6: Assign CPT code(s): ________
Step 7: Place code(s) in appropriate order: ________
Step 8: Assign modifier code(s) as appropriate: ________

3. Operative report

OPERATIVE REPORT

Patient information:

Patient name:
DOB:
MR#:

Date:
Surgeon:
Anesthetist:

Preoperative diagnosis:

Carpal tunnel syndrome, left wrist

Postoperative diagnosis:

Carpal tunnel syndrome, left wrist

Procedure(s) performed:

Left carpal tunnel release

Anesthesia:

Assistant surgeon:

Description of procedure:

SURGICAL TECHNIQUE: The patient was brought to the operating room and placed in the supine position. After adequate block, the arm was prepped with DuraPrep and sterilely draped in the usual manner. We made a small incision directly over the carpal ligament and deep and via careful scissors dissection to the ligament itself. The ligament was then sharply incised. Once we accessed tunnel, the ligament was released under direct visualization, both proximally and distally at its entire length. The nerve was initially quite pale and then turned purple. We made sure the nerve was free and we irrigated the wound and closed the skin with 4-0 nylon. The patient tolerated the procedure well and was placed in a splint and taken to the recovery room in good condition.

Adam Westy MD

GODFREY REGIONAL HOSPITAL
123 Main Street • Aldon, FL 77714 • (407) 555-1234

Step 1: Identify chapter or section of CPT: Surgery
Step 2: Identify anatomic system: ________
Step 3: Identify anatomic site: ________
Step 4: Identify procedure/technique: ________
Step 5: Identify additional specifics: ________
Step 6: Assign CPT code(s): ________
Step 7: Place code(s) in appropriate order: ________
Step 8: Assign modifier code(s) as appropriate: ________

4. Operative report

OPERATIVE REPORT

Patient information:

Patient name:
DOB:
MR#:

Date:
Surgeon:
Anesthetist:

Preoperative diagnosis:

Cataract, right eye

Postoperative diagnosis:

Cataract, right eye

Procedure(s) performed:

Phacoemulsification of the lens of the right eye, with posterior chamber intraocular lens implant

Anesthesia:

Topical

Assistant surgeon:

Description of procedure:

The patient was brought to the anesthesia waiting area and administered a drop of tetracaine in the eye. The patient was then taken into the operating room and placed in the supine position. Two drops of viscous lidocaine were placed in the conjunctival cul-de-sac of the eye. The patient was administered a mild sedative intravenously. The patient was then prepared and draped in the usual sterile fashion.

A 15-degree blade was used to make a stab incision at approximately two o'clock to the left of the temporal meridian. One-half cc of unpreserved 1% lidocaine was then irrigated into the anterior chamber. The anterior chamber was filled with Vitrax. A 2.65-mm keratome was advanced through the temporal limbus into the anterior chamber. A stab capsulotomy was then made with a 25-gauge bent-tip cystotome. Forceps were used to complete the circular capsulorrhexis.

The nucleus of the lens was hydrodissected with balanced salt solution. Phacoemulsification of the nucleus of the lens was carried out using a phaco chop method in 1 minute and 17 seconds with an EPT of 33 seconds. The residual cortex was aspirated from the cul-de-sac. The posterior capsule was polished. The capsular bag was filled with BioLon. An Allergen model AR 40, 20 diopter posterior chamber lens was then introduced into the capsular bag. The residual BioLon was removed from the eye.

The wound was hydrated wih balanced salt solution. The wound was stable without leakage. Drops of Ocuflox, Pred Forte, and Timoptic 0.5% were placed in the eye. The patient was taken to the recovery area in a stable condition.

ADDENDUM: Because of preexisting extreme density of the nucleus, BSS 1 was employed. Following the emulsification of half of the nucleus, additional Vitrax was placed into the anterior chamber. The cornea was clear at the end of the case.

Linda Patrick MD

GODFREY REGIONAL HOSPITAL
123 Main Street • Aldon, FL 77714 • (407) 555-1234

Step 1: Identify chapter or section of CPT: Surgery
Step 2: Identify anatomic system: ________
Step 3: Identify anatomic site: ________
Step 4: Identify procedure/technique: ________
Step 5: Identify additional specifics: ________
Step 6: Assign CPT code(s): ________
Step 7: Place code(s) in appropriate order: ________
Step 8: Assign modifier code(s) as appropriate: ________

5. Operative report

OPERATIVE REPORT

Patient information:

Patient name:
DOB:
MR#:

Preoperative diagnosis:

29-year-old female with history of recurrent episodes of otitis media. She now has a chronic right otitis media with effusion and mild right conductive hearing loss. Patient presents now for right PE tube per discussion.
1) Recurrent right otitis media with effusion.
2) Right mild conductive hearing loss.
3) Sclerotic right tympanic membrane.

Postoperative diagnosis:

Same

Procedure(s) performed:

Right myringotomy with tympanostomy tube placement

Anesthesia:

Assistant surgeon:

Description of procedure:

After consent was obtained, the patient was taken to the operating room and placed on the operating table in the supine position. After an adequate level of IV sedation was obtained, the patient was draped in the appropriate manner for right PE tube. Utilizing the ear speculum and ear microscope, the external canal was cleared of cerumen. The tympanic membrane was very sclerotic in the posterior aspect. As such, a myringotomy incision was placed in the anterior quadrant. Serous effusion was suctioned. A Bobbin tympanostomy tube was then placed without difficulty. Cortisporin otic suspension and cotton ball were then placed. The patient tolerated the procedure well; there was no break in technique. The patient was awakened and taken to the recovery room in good condition.

James Elliott MD

GODFREY REGIONAL HOSPITAL
123 Main Street • Aldon, FL 77714 • (407) 555-1234

Step 1: Identify chapter or section of CPT: Surgery
Step 2: Identify anatomic system: ________
Step 3: Identify anatomic site: ________
Step 4: Identify procedure/technique: ________
Step 5: Identify additional specifics: ________
Step 6: Assign CPT code(s): ________
Step 7: Place code(s) in appropriate order: ________
Step 8: Assign modifier code(s) as appropriate: ________

Chapter in Review

Certification Review

- Laceration repairs are classified as simple, intermediate, or complex.
- Lesions may be removed by excision, destruction, or shaving.
- The antepartum period of maternity care correlates with the preoperative period for other surgical services.
- The postpartum period of maternity care correlates with the postoperative period for other surgical services.
- Fracture repairs are classified as open or closed procedures, and they do not necessarily correlate with the injury description of open or closed.
- The proper use of modifier codes for surgery services often determines whether services typically included in the global component should be considered for payment.
- When a diagnostic approach is undertaken followed by a definitive surgery procedure, the diagnostic approach is considered incidental or bundled in the major surgery procedure.
- The codes for application of casts are included in the surgery section. The initial cast is considered part of the global component when it is applied at the time of the surgical procedure and by the same physician. Additional casts, or those placed by someone other than the surgeon, may be coded separately.

Student Assignments

- Study Chapter 14.
- Review the Learning Objectives for Chapter 14.
- Complete the Stop and Practice exercises for Chapter 14.
- Review the Certification Review for Chapter 14.
- Complete the Chapter Review exercise, assigning the appropriate CPT codes and modifiers.
- Complete the practice exercises on the companion Evolve site for reinforcement of the concepts contained in Chapter 14.
- Complete Workbook exercises for Chapter 14 as assigned by your instructor.

Chapter Review Exercise

Review the surgical components and assign the appropriate CPT codes and modifiers. If directed by your instructor, assign ICD-9-CM code(s) as well.

1. Left breast mass
   Preoperative diagnosis: Rule out breast carcinoma
   Postoperative diagnosis: Same

A 55-year-old female presented with a left breast mass, which was recommended for left breast biopsy. The options, risks, alternative treatments, and exact nature of the procedure were described in detail to the patient, and she seemed to understand.

Patient was taken to the operating room; under general anesthesia, left breast was prepped and draped in a sterile fashion. Left infraareolar incision was made and mass was dissected free of surrounding tissue. Hemostasis was obtained and wound was closed with interrupted 0-Vicryl, 4-0 Vicryl subcutaneous to the skin. Patient tolerated the procedure well and was taken to the recovery room in stable condition.

Adam Westgate, MD

CPT Procedure Code(s): ________ ________

ICD-9-CM Code(s): ________ ________

2. Cholecystectomy
   Preoperative diagnosis: Cholecystitis, cholelithiasis
   Postoperative diagnosis: Same
   Operation: Cholecystectomy with operative cholangiogram

A 31-year-old white female presented with midepigastric and right upper quadrant pain increasing in intensity. Evaluation revealed multiple gallstones, and surgery was recommended. The options, risks, alternative treatments, and exact nature of the procedure were described in detail, and the patient seemed to understand well.

Patient was taken to the operating room; under adequate general anesthesia, the abdomen was prepped and draped in a sterile fashion. The stomach and bladder were drained and supraumbilical incision was made. The Veress needle was used for institution of the pneumoperitoneum. A 10-mm port was placed, as well as the usual upper paramedian 10-mm port and lateral 5-mm ports. Gallbladder was retracted up to its bed using blunt dissection and cautery. The cystic duct was identified, and an intraoperative cholangiogram was read as normal. The cystic duct and cystic artery were ligated and divided. The gallbladder was dissected free of surrounding tissue with cautery and was removed through the upper paramedian port. The right upper quadrant was then irrigated. After hemostasis was ensured, wounds were closed with 2-0 Vicryl and 4-0 Vicryl subcuticular. Skin incisions were then infiltrated with Marcaine, at which time the patient was taken to the recovery room in stable condition.

Adam Westgate, MD

CPT Procedure Code(s): 47563
ICD-9-CM Code(s): 574.10

3. Right breast mass

Preoperative diagnosis: Right breast mass

Postoperative diagnosis: Same

Operation: Right subcutaneous mastectomy

This is a 70-year-old male who presented with enlarging right breast mass, unresponsive to conservative treatment. He was recommended for mastectomy. The options, risks, alternative treatments, and exact nature of the procedure were described in detail to the patient, and he seemed to understand adequately.

The patient was taken to the operating room, where, under general anesthesia, the right breast was prepped and draped in a sterile fashion. An inferior incision was made, the large mass was dissected free of surrounding tissue, and all breast tissue was removed down to the pectoralis muscle. Clinically, it appeared to be benign. There was a fair amount of dead space after the resection; a Penrose drain was placed in the depths of the wound, brought out through the inferior wound, and sutured in place with 2-0 silk. The wound was then closed in layers with interrupted 2-0 Vicryl and 4-0 Vicryl subcuticular on the skin. Sterile pressure dressing was applied. Patient was taken to the recovery room in stable condition, with drain in place and functioning well.

Rachel Perez, MD

CPT Procedure Code(s): 19304-RT
ICD-9-CM Code(s): 611.72

4. Cataract, right eye

Patient is a 75-year-old gentleman with a visually significant cataract of the right eye. He was seen preoperatively by his family physician and cleared for local anesthetic. Patient was brought into the outpatient surgical suite and underwent uncomplicated phacoemulsification and posterior lens implant of the right eye under local standby using topical anesthetic. He was taken to the recovery room in good condition.

Linda Patrick, MD

CPT Procedure Code(s): 66984-RT
ICD-9-CM Code(s):

5. Hiatal hernia

Preoperative diagnosis: Dysphagia

Postoperative diagnosis: Hiatal hernia with reflux and distal esophageal stricture

Operation: Upper GI endoscopy with biopsy

Esophageal dilatation

This is an 81-year-old male who presented with increasing dysphagia and trouble swallowing. He was recommended for endoscopy after the options, risks, alternative treatments, and exact nature of the procedure were described in detail, and the patient seemed to understand. Patient was taken to the endoscopy suite under adequate topical anesthesia. The Olympus endoscope was inserted without difficulty. The proximal and midesophagus were normal. The distal esophagus showed a circumferential stricture, which was biopsied. There was also a hiatal hernia. Upon entering the stomach, mild inflammation was noted and the antrum was biopsied for *Helicobacter.* The pyloric channel and duodenum were clean. J-maneuver revealed no fundic abnormalities. The endoscope was withdrawn. The patient tolerated the procedure well. He was then dilated to a 42-French Maloney dilator.

Rachel Perez, MD

CPT Procedure Code(s): 43220
43239 = biopsy
ICD-9-CM Code(s):

Practical Application

Take the following operative reports, extract the key words, assign the appropriate CPT code(s) and ICD-9-CM code(s), put them in order, and add the appropriate modifier(s). After assigning the appropriate code(s) for each procedure, access the Evolve site and view the available surgical procedures to put the operative report and codes into perspective.

1. Operative report

OPERATIVE REPORT

Patient information:

Patient name:
DOB:
MR#:

Date:
Surgeon:
Anesthetist:

Preoperative diagnosis:

Extensive basal cell carcinoma in the left retroauricular area

Postoperative diagnosis:

Same

Procedure(s) performed:

OPERATION:
1. Wide excision basal cell carcinoma of the left auricular area
2. Harvesting skin graft of the left thigh and then skin graft application to the area of excisional therapy left auricular area

The patient had been seen in referral from his family doctor. He had local extensive basal cell carcinoma. Because of its size, 4 × 5 cm, it was clear that primary repair could not be accomplished, so I advised that possible skin graft would be necessary. I advised them to go home and talk it over, and if they wished to go through with the procedure, I would be delighted to do that. So, after they talked it over, the wife called me and they gave their consent to proceed. The procedure was done under local.

Anesthesia:

Assistant surgeon:

Description of procedure:

He was brought to surgery. The area in the left retroauricular area was shaved. The area in question, lesion with ulcerations, etc., was marked out. Then, starting on the left thigh, the appropriate area was chosen, cleaned with Betadine, and draped. 2% Xylocaine was then infiltrated, and appropriate split-thickness skin graft of appropriate thickness was harvested using the disposable Dynatome. This was saved in ice, wrapped in a sponge soaked in ice. Then the lesion behind the left ear was now addressed. This was infiltrated again with 2% Xylocaine. Once anesthesia took, the lesion was excised completely and submitted to Pathology for clearance. No marginal involvement was identified. Hemostasis was achieved. Then the graft harvested previously was now fashioned by nicking it in several places to allow for adequate drainage, and then sutured to the skin margins. In the lowermost aspect the graft was inadequate, so the wound defect was closed for now with 2-0 nylon with total closure of the wound with the graft. Operation terminated. Appropriate dressings were applied to the donor site on the left thigh as well as the op site in the left retroauricular area.

Patient was discharged to follow up on Friday just to check the status of the wound. Nursing was then advised to make sure patient doesn't pull off the dressings, or we are back to square one.

Stanley Krosett, MD

GODFREY REGIONAL HOSPITAL
123 Main Street • Aldon, FL 77714 • (407) 555-1234

CPT codes

____

____

ICD-9-CM code(s):

____

____

2. Operative report

OPERATIVE REPORT

Patient information:

Patient name:
DOB:
MR#:

Date:
Surgeon:
Anesthetist:

Preoperative diagnosis:

Chondromalacia patella, lateral patellar tilt and lateral retinacular tightness

Postoperative diagnosis:

Same

Procedure(s) performed:

Right knee arthroscopy and chondroplasty of patella; right knee arthroscopy lateral release

Anesthesia:

Assistant surgeon:

Description of procedure:

After suitable general anesthesia had been achieved, the patient's right knee was prepped and draped in the usual manner. Prior to prepping, a thigh tourniquet was applied, and after draping, inflated to 300 mm of mercury. Inflow cannula was inserted to the suprapatellar pouch on the medial side. The arthroscope was inserted through an anterior lateral portal. The medial compartment was examined first. There was noted to be intact stable medial meniscus and intact articular surfaces. Examination of the notch revealed intact and stable ACL and PCL. Examination of the lateral compartment revealed intact articular surfaces and intact and stable lateral meniscus. Examination of the patellofemoral joint revealed localized chondromalacia at the lateral aspect of the inferior pole of the patella. This was smoothed with a shaver and further smoothing was done using an Oratec probe. The patient was noted to have a small medial synovial plica and this was trimmed with the shaver as well. Using an arthroscopic cautery, arthroscopic lateral release was done from the superior pole of the patella to the joint line. Following this, the knee joint was thoroughly irrigated and the arthroscope removed. Patellar tracking was then reassessed and the patella lateral retinaculum tightness had been corrected. Knee joint was thoroughly irrigated again and no bleeding was noted. Dressing was applied. Tourniquet was released. Following tourniquet release, good circulation was noted to return to the foot.

The patient tolerated the procedure well and returned to the recovery room in stable condition.

GODFREY REGIONAL HOSPITAL
123 Main Street • Aldon, FL 77714 • (407) 555-1234

CPT codes

____

____

ICD-9-CM code(s):

____

____

3. Operative report

OPERATIVE REPORT

Patient information:

Patient name:
DOB:
MR#:

Date:
Surgeon:
Anesthetist:

Preoperative diagnosis:

1. Right lateral epicondylitis
2. Possible loose body, right elbow

INDICATIONS FOR PROCEDURE: A 56-year-old gentleman with a history of bilateral radial head fractures, nondisplaced treated non-operatively, and persistent pain in his right elbow. Resulting symptoms of lateral epicondylitis had been treated with physical therapy, injections, splinting, and anti-inflammatory medications. He continues to have discomfort. After discussion of the options, risks, and benefits of surgery including bleeding, infection, nerve damage, continued pain and discomfort, all questions were answered and consents were signed. The patient was taken to the operating room.

Postoperative diagnosis:

Right lateral epicondylitis

Procedure(s) performed:

Right lateral tennis elbow release with elbow arthrotomy and exploration

Anesthesia:

Assistant surgeon:

Description of procedure:

COMPLICATIONS: None

The patient was taken to the operating room and placed supine on the operating room table. General anesthesia was obtained. The right arm was prepped and draped in the usual sterile fashion. A standard lateral incision was made directly over the lateral epicondyle. Subcutaneous tissue was dissected down to the deep fascia. The deep fascia was identified and the interval between the ECU and extensor carpi radialis longus was identified and split. As this was separated, we identified the extensor carpi radialis brevis. It was subsequently released from its origin onto the lateral humeral epicondyle, and there was significant scar tissue beneath this. This was subsequently rongeured off, and we inspected the radial capitello joint, found no evidence of any loose bodies with good smooth articular cartilage. We then closed the capsule up with 3-0 Ticron. It was then irrigated out copiously. The tourniquet was let down. Hemostasis was obtained with electrocautery. The superficial extensors were then sutured together with 2-0 Vicryl, the subcutaneous tissue with 2-0 Vicryl, and the skin was sutured with 4-0 nylon in a running fashion.

The patient tolerated the procedure well, was extubated in the operating room, transferred from the operating table to his bed, and taken to the postanesthesia recovery room in stable condition.

GODFREY REGIONAL HOSPITAL
123 Main Street • Aldon, FL 77714 • (407) 555-1234

CPT codes

ICD-9-CM code(s):

4. Operative report

OPERATIVE REPORT

Patient information:

Patient name:
DOB:
MR#:

Date:
Surgeon:
Anesthetist:

Preoperative diagnosis:

Left carpal tunnel

Postoperative diagnosis:

Left carpal tunnel

Procedure(s) performed:

Laparoscopic carpal tunnel release

Anesthesia:

Monitored anesthesia care, local

Assistant surgeon:

Description of procedure:

The patient was taken to the operating room. The left upper extremity was prepped and draped in the usual sterile fashion. The arm was elevated and the tourniquet inflated to 250 mm Hg. The portals were marked out per routine and anesthetized with local infiltration of 1% lidocaine.

The proximal portal was opened with a 15-blade. Blunt spreading exposed the retinaculum, which was opened, allowing instrumentation to be placed in the canal and brought out distally through the distal portal that was opened with a 15-blade. A scope was placed within the cannula and the undersurface of the retinaculum was cleared, confirmed, and sectioned with good spreading of the retinaculum.

Instrumentation was removed. The portal was closed with Steri-strips. Compressive Ace was applied. Pressure was held and the tourniquet was dropped.

The patient was removed from the operating room in satisfactory condition.

GODFREY REGIONAL HOSPITAL
123 Main Street • Aldon, FL 77714 • (407) 555-1234

CPT codes

____

____

ICD-9-CM code(s):

____

____

5. Operative report

OPERATIVE REPORT

Patient information:

Patient name:
DOB:
MR#:

Date:
Surgeon:
Anesthetist:

Preoperative diagnosis:

Symptomatic hardware of the right knee

Postoperative diagnosis:

Symptomatic hardware of the right knee and ganglion cyst

Procedure(s) performed:

Excision of symptomatic hardware and ganglion cyst

Anesthesia:

Assistant surgeon:

Description of procedure:

The patient was taken to the operating room, and after IV sedation was administered, her right lower extremity was prepped and draped in sterile fashion. A mixture of 1% lidocaine and 1⁄2% Marcaine without epinephrine was used for local anesthesia. Approximately a 3-cm skin incision was made, with sharp dissection and blunt dissection down to bone being performed. A ganglion cyst was encountered. It was not a discrete cyst, but the fluid in it was definitely that of a ganglion cyst. This was opened up and cauterized as needed.

The hardware was identified and the screws removed. The bone had grown over the edges of the washer and some bone resection was required to get the washer out. Once this washer had been retrieved, the wound was irrigated out copiously and the screw hole was curetted. Copious amounts of antibiotic irrigation were used. The wound was closed in layers with Vicryl for the subcutaneous tissue, and Biosyn and Steri-strips were applied to the skin.

Sterile dressing was applied. The patient was taken to the recovery room in good condition.

GODFREY REGIONAL HOSPITAL
123 Main Street • Aldon, FL 77714 • (407) 555-1234

CPT codes

____

____

ICD-9-CM code(s):

____

____

6. Operative report

OPERATIVE REPORT

Patient information:

Patient name:
DOB:
MR#:

Date:
Surgeon:
Anesthetist:

Preoperative diagnosis:

Chronic right maxillary/ethmoid sinusitis

CLINICAL NOTE:
The patient is a 27-year-old white female with chronic right cheek tenderness and pain that has not responded to conservative medical treatment. Preoperative CT scan showed opacification of the maxillary sinus with obstruction of the osteomeatal complex. The remaining sinuses were clear.

Postoperative diagnosis:

Mucocele of the right maxillary sinus with obstruction of the osteomeatal complex

Procedure(s) performed:

1. Endoscopic right anterior ethmoidectomy
2. Right meatal antrostomy with removal of right maxillary sinus mucocele

Anesthesia:

General

Assistant surgeon:

Description of procedure:

The patient was brought in to the operating room and placed on the operating room table in a supine position. General endotracheal anesthesia was performed. The right nose was vasoconstricted with topical Afrin and injected with 3 cc of 1% lidocaine with 1:100,000 parts epinephrine to the right middle turbinate and lateral nasal wall mucosa adjacent. After the face was prepped and draped, a TV monitor was used for visualization attached to a zero-degree sinus endoscope. The mucosa around the hiatus, semiluminaris, and the middle meatus was removed with straight biting forceps. Using a Bolger probe, the antrum of the right maxillary sinus was entered. Using a power microdebrider and Blakesley forceps, anterior ethmoidectomy and 1-cm maxillary antrostomy were performed. Using 30- and 70-degree sinus endoscopes, the right maxillary sinus was examined, and there was no evidence of fungus or mucopurulent debris present. It appeared that there was a large right mucous retention cyst completely filling the right maxillary sinus that was removed upon entering the right maxillary sinus. Large curved suction was placed into the sinus and was irrigated copiously with normal saline and suctioned dry. MeroGel was placed into the right anterior ethmoid sinus cavity, followed with a slim Kennedy nasal tampon into the right middle meatal region. The posterior nasal cavity and oropharynx were suctioned dry, and there was adequate hemostasis present.

The patient was awakened from general anesthesia, extubated, and brought to the recovery room in stable condition, having tolerated the procedure well.

ESTIMATED BLOOD LOSS: Less than 10 cc

Maurice Doater, MD

GODFREY REGIONAL HOSPITAL
123 Main Street • Aldon, FL 77714 • (407) 555-1234

CPT codes

____

____

ICD-9-CM code(s):

____

____

7. Emergency department record

EMERGENCY ROOM RECORD

Name:	Age:	ER physician:
	DOB:	Robert Rais

Allergies/type of reaction:	Usual medications/dosages:

Triage/presenting complaint: CC: Nosebleed on anticoagulants

Patient complains that immediately prior to arrival, she experienced a nosebleed, unable to stop.

Initial assessment:

ROS: Negative for chest pain, dyspnea, negative excessive bruising, fever, nausea, dizziness, syncope, vomiting
PMH/SH: Negative

Time	T	P	R	BP	Other:				

Medication orders:

Lab work:

X-ray:

Physician's report:

EXAM:
Vital signs are noted, patient appears well nourished, in mild distress

HEENT: Nose, dried blood right anterior nasal mucosa. Fresh clots right anterior nasal mucosa.
Pharynx: Unremarkable.
Chest: No visible signs of trauma
CV: All distal pulses are 2+
MS: Normal ROM, no swelling or deformities
Neuro: Alert, oriented to person, time, and place

TREATMENT:
Clots were cleared from nasal passages and oozing of flow continued. Both nares were treated with cauterization and the bleeding appeared to be well controlled at that time.

Diagnosis:	Physician sign/date
Anterior epistaxis	Robert Rais MD
Discharge Transfer Admit Good Satisfactory Other:	

GODFREY REGIONAL HOSPITAL
123 Main Street • Aldon, FL 77714 • (407) 555-1234

CPT codes

____

____

ICD-9-CM code(s):

____

____

8. Operative report

OPERATIVE REPORT

Patient information:

Patient name:
DOB:
MR#:

Date:
Surgeon:
Anesthetist:

Preoperative diagnosis:

Diatek cath

Postoperative diagnosis:

Procedure(s) performed:

Left Diatek catheter insertion

HISTORY: Malfunction of catheter

Anesthesia:

Assistant surgeon:

Description of procedure:

TECHNIQUE:
The examination was done through the existing tract of the left-sided catheter. A stiff guidewire was initially inserted through the catheter, but the catheter could not be withdrawn. A 0.035 angled Glidewire was inserted through the catheter, and again the indwelling catheter could not be withdrawn. Multiple attempts to release the catheter were unsuccessful. The skin between the exit incision and the internal jugular vein was entered and the catheter removed in its mid-portion and cut. The wire was then inserted through this area for better manipulation. After numerous attempts, the catheter was withdrawn over the wire. The Diatek catheter was then inserted over the wire to the appropriate position. The patient received 1 gram of Ancef intravenously at the start of the procedure, and the old and new tracks of the catheters were flushed with a solution of 1 gram of Ancef and 1 liter of normal saline. The position of the catheter was checked at the termination of the procedure by fluoroscopy. Less than one hour of fluoroscopy time was used for the procedure.

IMPRESSION: Insertion of left-sided Diatek tunneled catheter under fluoroscopic guidance.

GODFREY REGIONAL HOSPITAL
123 Main Street • Aldon, FL 77714 • (407) 555-1234

CPT codes

____

____

ICD-9-CM code(s):

____

____

9. Operative report

OPERATIVE REPORT

Patient information:

Patient name:
DOB:
MR#:

Preoperative diagnosis:

Esophageal food bolus

INDICATION:
This 77-year-old male came to the emergency room several hours after eating steak and felt it get stuck in his esophagus. He has had this problem before and refuses to undergo dilatation because he thinks he will need it frequently after that.

Postoperative diagnosis:

Same

Procedure(s) performed:

EGD with removal of food bolus

Anesthesia:

Assistant surgeon:

Description of procedure:

The patient was taken to the operating room and put into the left lateral decubitus position on the operating room table. After the induction of anesthesia, the flexible fiberoptic scope was passed through the oropharynx and into the esophagus without difficulty. The scope was advanced through the esophagus. There was a large amount of what appeared to be meat in the esophagus. Upon reaching the lower portion of the esophagus, it was packed full, and we were unable to clearly identify a direction in which to push the food bolus through and it would not push through easily. Therefore the pelican forceps were used to remove large amounts of the meat so that the distal end of the esophagus and GE junction could be identified, and the remainder was pushed through. The patient tolerated the procedure well. The scope was removed. No apparent esophageal carcinoma was noted.

The patient was transferred to recovery in stable condition.

Patrick Olson MD

GODFREY REGIONAL HOSPITAL
123 Main Street • Aldon, FL 77714 • (407) 555-1234

CPT codes

ICD-9-CM code(s):

10. Operative report

OPERATIVE REPORT

Patient information:

Patient name:
DOB:
MR#:

CONSENT:
Signed and on chart

Preoperative diagnosis:

INDICATION:
Anemia, history of heme-positive stools, history of polyps

Postoperative diagnosis:

Colonic AVMs, polyps, diverticulosis coli, external hemorrhoids

Procedure(s) performed:

Colonoscopy with polypectomy and electrocoagulation with arteriovenous malformation

Anesthesia:

Assistant surgeon:

Description of procedure:

Prior to the procedure, the patient was consented. He was then taken to the endoscopy suite, placed in the left lateral decubitus position, and adequately sedated.

Next, digital rectal exam was performed revealing no mass, external hemorrhoids, good tone, and enlarged prostate.

Next, the Olympus CP-160L colonoscope was introduced into the patient's rectum and passed throughout the colon into the cecum. Free intubation of ileocecal valve and terminal ileum was not achieved. In the cecum, there were a couple of AVMs. These were treated with 7 French BICAP probe, 20 watt setting. Successful obliteration of AVMs. There was another one in the ascending colon that was also electrocoagulated. There were a few scattered diverticula noted in the right colon and ascending colon. There was a 5-mm polyp removed by hot snare polypectomy and placed in jar B. In the transverse colon, there were a few scattered diverticula, but no polyps, no AVMs. In the descending and sigmoid colon, there were scattered diverticula, but no polyps, no AVMs. The endoscope was brought back into the rectum. There were a couple of 2-mm polyps removed by fulguration polypectomy. On retroflexed view, he did not have enlarged internal hemorrhoids. The endoscope was straightened, reintroduced around the colon into the cecum. The patient was placed in the supine position. The endoscope was gradually withdrawn. The colon was deflated. No additional lesions were noted. The endoscope was then removed.

The patient tolerated the procedure well.

MEDICATIONS UTILIZED:
Versed 10 mg IV in increments; Demerol 130 mg IV in increments

IMPRESSION:
1. Colon polyps
2. AVMs
3. Diverticulosis coli
4. External hemorrhoids

PLAN:
At this time is to check biopsy results. Continue on iron supplements as previously mentioned. If he develops recurrent iron deficiency, we will need to place him on IV iron, as he has had previous antrectomy.

Patrick Adams MD

GODFREY REGIONAL HOSPITAL
123 Main Street • Aldon, FL 77714 • (407) 555-1234

CPT codes

ICD-9-CM code(s):

11. Operative report

OPERATIVE REPORT

Patient information:

Patient name:
DOB:
MR#:

CONSENT:
Informed consent was obtained from the patient after full disclosure of risks and indications to the patient.

Preoperative diagnosis:

History of polyps in the past

Postoperative diagnosis:

See assessment below.

Procedure(s) performed:

Colonoscopy with biopsies

Anesthesia:

Assistant surgeon:

Description of procedure:

After obtaining informed consent, the patient was brought to the OR and put in the left lateral position. IV line was maintained. IV sedation was given and vitals were monitored throughout the procedure that included pulse, pulse oximetry, blood pressure, and level of consciousness. Digital rectal examination was done, which revealed normal anal tone. No masses palpable. The scope was introduced and advanced all the way up to the cecum, identified by ileocecal valve and appendical orifice. The scope was withdrawn, watching all of the colonic mucosa. There were several pockets of liquid stools at various stages. Most of them were washed and cleaned away as much as possible, and a closer examination of the mucosa was performed. No AV malformation noticed, no masses, no polyps. Up until the sigmoid region there were two polyps adjacent to each other, one a little larger than the other, both of them less than 5 mm, which were hot-biopsied and sent for histopathology. In the rectum, retroflexion was done, which showed moderate-sized abdominal hemorrhoids non-bleeding, non-thrombosed, and the scope was straightened out and pulled out.

The patient tolerated the procedure well. Prep was fair. There were a few pockets of liquid stool that may have obscured the vision. Small polyps may have been missed. No gross abnormality was seen.

ASSESSMENT:
Two sigmoid polyps hot-biopsied, small in size, approximately less than 5 cm in size, sent for histopathology. Moderate-sized internal hemorrhoids. Otherwise normal exam.

PLAN:
Follow up with biopsy results.

Patk Olam MD

GODFREY REGIONAL HOSPITAL
123 Main Street • Aldon, FL 77714 • (407) 555-1234

CPT codes

____

____

ICD-9-CM code(s):

____

____

12. Operative report

OPERATIVE REPORT

Patient information:

Patient name:
DOB:
MR#:

Preoperative diagnosis:

Umbilical hernia

Postoperative diagnosis:

Umbilical hernia

Procedure(s) performed:

Repair of umbilical hernia

Anesthesia:

Assistant surgeon:

Description of procedure:

Under spinal anesthesia, the patient was prepped and draped in the usual sterile manner. 0.5% Marcaine with epinephrine was injected along the incisional lines. An elliptical incision was made around the umbilicus. The incision was carried through subcutaneous tissue, basically all the way to the fascia level. The hernia sac was opened and excised along with the umbilicus. Limited exploration was done. The peritoneum was closed with #0 Vicryl sutures. The fascia was dissected above and below. The fascia was closed in imbricating fashion, pushing the lower edge under the upper part of the fascia. Mattress sutures were taken from above, a distance away from the edge, and the edge was then incorporated. Then on the way back, we took the suture from the edge to a distance away from the upper part of the fascia. This was tightened and tied so the lower edge would go underneath the upper part of the fascia. Eight of these interrupted sutures were made and they were tightened and tied.

The upper edge was then sutured to the fascia below with a running suture of #1 Vicryl. There was good hemostasis. The subcutaneous tissue was closed with two layers of 2-0 Vicryl and skin was closed with 4-0 Dexon subcuticular sutures.

The patient tolerated the procedure well and left the operating room in good condition.

INDICATIONS AND/OR FINDINGS:
This patient had a large umbilical hernia. The defect measured 3 cm.

Patrick Adams MD

GODFREY REGIONAL HOSPITAL
123 Main Street • Aldon, FL 77714 • (407) 555-1234

CPT codes

ICD-9-CM code(s):

13. Operative report

OPERATIVE REPORT

Patient information:

Patient name:
DOB:
MR#:

Date:
Surgeon:
Anesthetist:

Preoperative diagnosis:

Infertility

Postoperative diagnosis:

1. Infertility
2. Tubo-ovarian adhesions

FINDINGS: Filmy adhesions of the ovary and tube down to the pelvic sidewall bilaterally. The left fallopian tube was completely clubbed and no fimbria were visualized. The right fallopian tube was visualized and slightly clubbed; however, fimbria were visualized slightly. The bowel, liver, and gallbladder appeared normal.

Procedure(s) performed:

1. Diagnostic laparoscopy
2. Lysis of adhesions
3. Fimbriectomy

Anesthesia:

Assistant surgeon:

Description of procedure:

The patient was taken to the operating room in the supine position. After general endotracheal anesthesia was induced, she was prepped and draped in a sterile fashion. A vertical incision was made in the umbilicus and taken down bluntly to the fascia. The abdomen was extended with the operator's hand and a Veress needle was inserted and directed toward the pelvis. Hanging drop test was performed. Pneumoperitoneum was created with 2½ liters of CO_2 gas, with pressure being maintained below 12 mm of mercury. Once pneumoperitoneum was created, the Veress needle was removed. 12-mm trocar was inserted directly toward the pelvis. Visualization of the abdomen and pelvis revealed the above-noted findings, and photographs were taken. There was no evidence of trauma due to entry.

An accessory trocar was placed in the left lower quadrant lateral to the inferior epigastric vessels. It was placed under direct visualization. Sharp and blunt dissection was used to free up the adhesions of the ovaries to the sidewall. It was also used to free up the adhesions of the right fallopian tube distally to expose more of the fimbria. The areas were hemostatic. Once this was performed, the ovaries were wrapped in Interceed. The pneumoperitoneum was then allowed to escape. Trocar was removed. Fascial incision to the umbilicus was closed with a figure-of-eight stitch of 0 Vicryl. The skin was closed with subcuticular stitch of 3-0 Vicryl. The accessory trocar site was closed with a single stitch of 3-0 nylon.

The patient tolerated the procedure well and went to the recovery room in stable condition. All needle, sponge, and instrument counts were correct.

ESTIMATED BLOOD LOSS: Minimal

COMPLICATIONS: None

SPECIMENS: None

Alan Wexty, MD

GODFREY REGIONAL HOSPITAL
123 Main Street • Aldon, FL 77714 • (407) 555-1234

CPT codes

____

____

ICD-9-CM code(s):

____

____

14. Operative report

OPERATIVE REPORT

Patient information:

Patient name:
DOB:
MR#:

Date:
Surgeon:
Anesthetist:

Preoperative diagnosis:

Urinary retention

Postoperative diagnosis:

Urinary retention

Procedure(s) performed:

Cystoscopy and percutaneous placement of suprapubic catheter

Anesthesia:

Assistant surgeon:

Description of procedure:

The patient was placed on the operating table in the lithotomy position. His perineum was prepped and draped sterilely. 10 cc of Xylocaine jelly was injected per urethra. The scope was inserted. His urethra is unremarkable. Prostate is very large with trilobated hypertrophy and a big median bar that you have to go up and over.

The bladder shows a lot of catheter cystitis and a lot of trabeculation, just diffusely inflamed. The bladder was filled under vision with the cystoscope. I then approached him two fingerbreadths suprapubically infiltrated with Xylocaine through the skin and fascia until I accessed the bladder and could aspirate bladder. I looked in the bladder and I could see the needle coming in the dome of the bladder. I then made a stab incision, and using the Amplatz dilator, dilated to 28 French, leaving the sheath, and placed a 24 French Foley catheter. This was sewn in place. The cystoscope was removed.

He tolerated the procedure without difficulty.

Rachel Perez MD

GODFREY REGIONAL HOSPITAL
123 Main Street • Aldon, FL 77714 • (407) 555-1234

CPT codes

____

____

ICD-9-CM code(s):

____

____

15. Operative report

OPERATIVE REPORT

Patient information:

Patient name:
DOB:
MR#:

Date:
Surgeon:
Anesthetist:

Preoperative diagnosis:

Postmenopausal bleeding, cervical polyp

Postoperative diagnosis:

Postmenopausal bleeding, cervical polyp

Procedure(s) performed:

Evaluation under anesthesia, removal of cervical polyp, dilation and curettage

Anesthesia:

General endotracheal

Assistant surgeon:

Description of procedure:

Patient was taken to the operating room. After adequate level of general endotracheal anesthesia, the patient was placed in a modified lithotomy position. Patient was draped and prepped in usual sterile fashion. Evaluation under anesthesia revealed a normal uterus. No adnexal masses. Weighted vaginal speculum was placed in the vagina. Cervix was grasped with single-tooth tenaculum. There was a small polyp or redundant cervix, which was removed. Cervix had been dilated to a #21 French Bratt dilator, and an endometrial curettage revealed scant tissue. The single-tooth tenaculum was removed, as was the weighted vaginal speculum.

The patient tolerated the procedure well and was sent to recovery room in satisfactory condition.

ESTIMATED BLOOD LOSS: 10 cc

PATHOLOGY: Endocervical polyp, endometrial curetting

GODFREY REGIONAL HOSPITAL
123 Main Street • Aldon, FL 77714 • (407) 555-1234

CPT codes

____

____

ICD-9-CM code(s):

____

____

16. Operative report

PAIN MANAGEMENT REPORT

Patient information:

Patient name:
DOB:
MR#:

Date:
Surgeon:
Anesthetist:

Preoperative diagnosis:

Postoperative diagnosis:

Procedure(s) performed:

Trigger point injections

Anesthesia:

Assistant surgeon:

Description of procedure:

Mary Smythe is a 58-year-old lady who has myofascial pain syndrome. She was doing better after the last set of trigger point injections; however, she went to a funeral out of town, and from riding that distance, she states that her back pain had increased.

PROCEDURE:
Risks, benefits, and options discussed. Written consent was obtained. Vital signs stable, afebrile. The patient is placed in the sitting position. Palpation of the longissimus muscle and also the multifidus muscle reveals eight total trigger points. These trigger points were marked, skin prepped with alcohol, aseptic technique. 26-gauge needle and Marcaine 0.25% 1 cc was injected into each trigger point. The patient tolerated the procedure well and left the clinic in stable condition.

ASSESSMENT AND PLAN:
Myofascial pain syndrome in the lower lumbar and upper sacral areas. The patient received trigger point injections as above. The patient will return to clinic in one week for repeat trigger point injections. Will consider MRI of the lumbar spine if series of trigger point injections does not improve her low back. The patient is to continue physical therapy.

Thank you for letting us participate in this patient's care.

Rachel Perez MD

GODFREY REGIONAL HOSPITAL
123 Main Street • Aldon, FL 77714 • (407) 555-1234

CPT codes

____

____

ICD-9-CM code(s):

____

____

17. Operative report

PAIN MANAGEMENT REPORT

Patient information:

Patient name:
DOB:
MR#:

Date:
Surgeon:
Anesthetist:

Preoperative diagnosis:

Postoperative diagnosis:

Procedure(s) performed:

Bilateral injections of steroids into the wrists

Anesthesia:

Assistant surgeon:

Description of procedure:

A 24-year-old lady has bilateral wrist pain with occasional radiation of the pain into the arms and elbows. She was involved in a motor vehicle accident. The patient states that she continues to have bilateral wrist pain and it has not improved. I talked to her about possibly injecting some steroids between the articular processes in her wrists bilaterally. The risks, benefits, and options were discussed. She understood and accepted.

After oral and written consent, sterile prep with Betadine and alcohol, a 22-gauge needle was used to inject 0.125% bupivacaine plain along with Kenalog, approximately 6 mg per cc. The patient's wrists were injected on the dorsal side. She received an injection near the articular fossa of the ulna and the pisiform bone; 1 cc was injected in a fanlike manner in that area. Then another 1 cc was injected between the lunate and the radius in a fanlike manner and this was again done at the radius and the scaphoid bone. This was done on both wrists.

The patient tolerated the procedure well. She stated relief prior to leaving the clinic. Patient will return to the clinic in 1 to 2 weeks for possible repeat injection.

ASSESSMENT/PLAN:
Patient was involved in a motor vehicle accident in January of this year. Most of her aches and pains have been getting gradually better except for her wrists bilaterally. She did not have wrist pain before the accident. She has wrist pain after the accident. Patient was unable to be seen by orthopedic service due to her current lawsuit situation. Patient received injection of steroids at the wrists to decrease possible inflammation in the dorsal wrist area of bone and ligaments. Patient will return to the clinic in 1 to 2 weeks for possible repeat injection. Thank you for letting us participate in the patient's care.

Adm Wntz MD

GODFREY REGIONAL HOSPITAL
123 Main Street • Aldon, FL 77714 • (407) 555-1234

CPT codes

____

____

ICD-9-CM code(s):

____

____

18. Operative report

OPERATIVE REPORT

Patient information:

Patient name:
DOB:
MR#:

Date:
Surgeon:
Anesthetist:

Preoperative diagnosis:

Carpal tunnel syndromes, thenar paresis, right

Postoperative diagnosis:

Carpal tunnel syndromes, thenar paresis, right

Procedure(s) performed:

Carpal tunnel release, with median external neurolysis and release motor branch (right)

Anesthesia:

Assistant surgeon:

Description of procedure:

OPERATION:
After informed consent and complete discussion of the alternatives, potentials, and complications, and no guarantees implied or given, the patient was taken to the operating room. After an adequate level of regional and intravenous anesthesia had been obtained, the patient's upper extremity was surgically scrubbed with Betadine soap and prepped with Betadine solution. Draping occurred in the usual sterile fashion. Following Esmarch exsanguination, the forearm tourniquet was elevated to 150 mm Hg above systolic pressure.

A thenar incision was utilized. Dissection was carried down through the subcutaneous fat and fascia under 3½ power loupe magnification.The superficial nerves were kept out of harm's way throughout the procedure.

The palmar fascia was divided longitudinally and the transverse carpal ligament was then carefully identified. A hemostat was placed under the ligament, and under direct visualization, the ulnar border of the transverse carpal ligament was released. Care was taken to release the most proximal border of the transverse carpal ligament by tunneling proximally with elevation of the proximal skin and speculum retractor until a complete release of the proximal carpal ligament and distal forearm fascia had been performed. Following this, a digit could be placed in the carpal tunnel, demonstrating complete release.

Next, the external neurolysis was performed with freeing of the scarred fascicles. Marked hourglass constriction and scarring were noted locally in the median nerve and motor branch. The sensory and motor branches were carefully dissected and released of the constricting tissue. The motor branch was identified and followed into the thickened abductor pollicis brevis fascia, and the constricting fascia was released.

Next, the thickened synovial layer between the medial nerve and tendons was released. The small finger could be placed in the carpal tunnel, demonstrating that the ligament was completely released over the median nerve, using the nasal speculum to directly view the ligament. Irrigation was carried out with triple antibiotic solution. Marcaine, 0.5%, and Decadron were instilled. The skin was re-approximated with subcuticular 3-0 Vicryl for the palmar fascia and interrupted 4-0 Prolene. Steri-Strips were applied. A bulky sterile hand dressing with volar and radial splint supports was applied with the thumb held in the protected position with adduction and opposition.

Following release of the tourniquet, good capillary fill was noted in the fingers. The patient tolerated the operative procedure and anesthesia satisfactorily. No breaks in sterile technique occurred. No complications occurred. The patient did receive cephalosporin antibiotics thirty minutes prior to the procedure prophylactically. The patient was taken to the recovery room with stable vital signs in satisfactory condition.

The patient was instructed preoperatively on the need for physiotherapy to maximize healing during the rehabilitation period.

Adam Westgate MD

GODFREY REGIONAL HOSPITAL
123 Main Street • Aldon, FL 77714 • (407) 555-1234

CPT codes

ICD-9-CM code(s):

19. Operative report

OPERATIVE REPORT

Patient information:

Patient name:
DOB:
MR#:

Date:
Surgeon:
Anesthetist:

Preoperative diagnosis:

Ectropion, left lower lid

Postoperative diagnosis:

Same

Procedure(s) performed:

Wedge resection, left lower lid
COMPLICATIONS:
None

Anesthesia:

Local, with standby

Assistant surgeon:

Description of procedure:

NARRATIVE DESCRIPTION:
The patient was brought to the operating room directly from outpatient status. He was placed on the operating table and made secure and comfortable. Anesthesia administered medication that produced profound sedation. While sedated, he was given a local injection in the left lower lid of 2% Xylocaine with epinephrine. Prepping and draping were carried out in the usual manner. The globe was anesthetized with tetracaine so that the patient would not be uncomfortable when we touched the eye. Stevens scissors was used to resect a large-base triangular wedge between the medial and the lateral thirds of the lower lid close to the end of the tarsal plate. Hemostasis was obtained with cautery. The defect was then closed with interrupted 6-0 Vicryl. Two sutures were put through the tarsal plate and securely tied, giving good apposition. A third suture was placed through the grey line, reestablishing the lid margins, and three sutures were placed to close the skin. The wound was medicated with Maxitrol ointment. The eye was left open and without a patch. The patient was awake and alert and appeared to tolerate the procedure well.

There was no evidence of any surgical or anesthetic complications, and he left the operating room awake, alert, and in good condition.

Linda Patrick MD

GODFREY REGIONAL HOSPITAL
123 Main Street • Aldon, FL 77714 • (407) 555-1234

CPT codes

____

____

ICD-9-CM code(s):

____

____

20. Operative report

OPERATIVE REPORT

Patient information:

Patient name:
DOB:
MR#:

Preoperative diagnosis:

8-year-old brought in to the emergency room by father after child accidentally put foreign body in left ear. Denies any hearing problem. No drainage apparent from the ear.

ALLERGIES: none

Postoperative diagnosis:

Procedure(s) performed:

Anesthesia:

Assistant surgeon:

Description of procedure:

Alert, oriented × 3. Temp 98.1, pulse 100, respiratory rate 20. Does not appear to be in any distress.

Ear exam revealed left ear canal with a small plastic object. Right ear within normal limits.

FB in left ear with auditory canal which was removed after washing and using Alligator forceps. Under direct visual guidance, object was grasped and taken out in one piece. Reexam reveals no ulcers, slight erythema around the area where the item was sitting. Rest of the exam is unremarkable.

Patient was discharged in the care of the father in stable condition.

Nancy Connolly MD

GODFREY REGIONAL HOSPITAL
123 Main Street • Aldon, FL 77714 • (407) 555-1234

CPT codes

____

____

ICD-9-CM code(s):

____

____

15

Radiology Services

LEARNING OBJECTIVES

After completing this chapter, the student will be able to:

- Understand the documentation for radiology services.
- Grasp the proper usage of modifiers for radiology services.
- Understand the appropriate application of technical and professional components.
- Identify the different types of radiologic services.
- Understand coding complexities for radiologic services.
- Apply the radiology coding concepts to practical coding scenarios.

KEY TERMS

Computed Tomography (CT)
Magnetic Resonance Imaging (MRI)
Mammography
Professional Component
Technical Component

Radiology Documentation and Coding Guidelines

RADIOLOGY SERVICES

Initial documentation for radiologic services is provided the radiology request form, the clinical history, and information regarding the patient's clinical history. Unless the information contained in the request form is documented as reviewed, it must be incorporated in the actual radiology report to be used for coding purposes. Although the charge document or encounter form is often used for billing purposes, care should be taken to substantiate all services. This includes the correct number of views and location (Figs. 15-1 and 15-2), administration of contrast, and other services, all of which must be recorded in the medical chart or medical documentation. Subsections of the radiology chapter are as follows:

Diagnostic radiology (diagnostic imaging)	70010-76499
Diagnostic ultrasound	76506-76999
Radiological guidance	77001-77032
Breast, mammography	77051-77059
Bone/joint studies	77071-77084
Radiation oncology	77280-77799
Nuclear medicine	78000-79999

A written interpretive report is imperative for billing. The report should include the following:

- Symptoms
- Physical findings or clinical indication
- Procedure performed
- Final impression or diagnosis
- Number of views
- Contrast(s)

Without the radiologic report, billing for the interpretation is not appropriate. In some instances more than one physician will actually interpret the report, sometimes referred to as an *overread*. Overreads occur when the ordering physician initially reads the radiology report because of time restraints or the need to initiate treatment. Sometimes the facility where the services are performed requires the x-ray films be reviewed by a radiologist, so both the ordering physician and the radiologist may interpret the films. In these instances Medicare and many other insurance carriers indicate that the physician who performs the interpretation independently without the need for additional interpretation or advice may code and bill for that service.

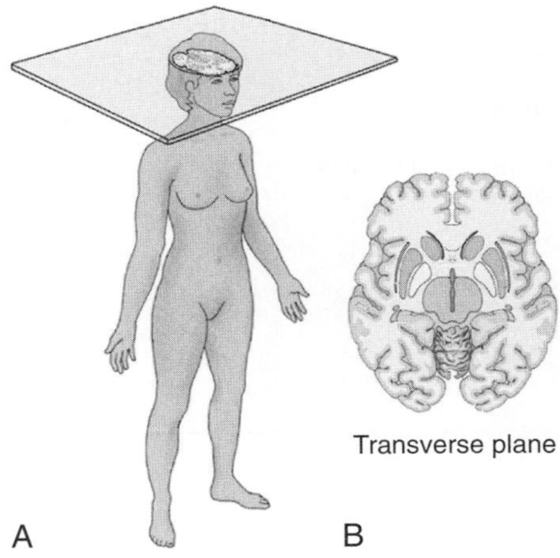

FIGURE 15-1. A, Transverse plane. **B,** Transverse section of the brain.

In Table 10-1, look at the radiology column in at the steps and components needed for coding according to Current Procedural Terminology (CPT).

CPT CODING STEPS: RADIOLOGY EXAMPLES

Step 1: Identify Chapter

Type of service	X-rays MRI/CT Ultrasounds Nuclear medicine
Range of codes	70010-79999

Step 2: Determine Type or Location

Type of service	Diagnostic Ultrasound

Step 3: Determine Specific Type

Anatomic part	Chest Lower extremity

Step 4: Determine Specific Procedure Information

Views/contrast	Two views with contrast

Step 5: Determine Extent/Specifics

Additional guidelines

Review the radiology report on the next page and identify key words in determining the radiologic service performed.

Review the chart component listing and extract the key words needed to assign CPT code(s) for these services.

CPT CODING STEPS

Type/Service	Radiology Examples	Chart Information
Step 1: Identify Chapter		
	X-rays radiology MRI/CT Ultrasounds Nuclear medicine	
Range of codes	70010-79999	70010-79999
Step 2: Determine Type/Location		
	X-ray Diagnostic Ultrasound	
Step 3: Determine Specific Type		
Anatomic part	Leg/knee Chest Lower extremity	

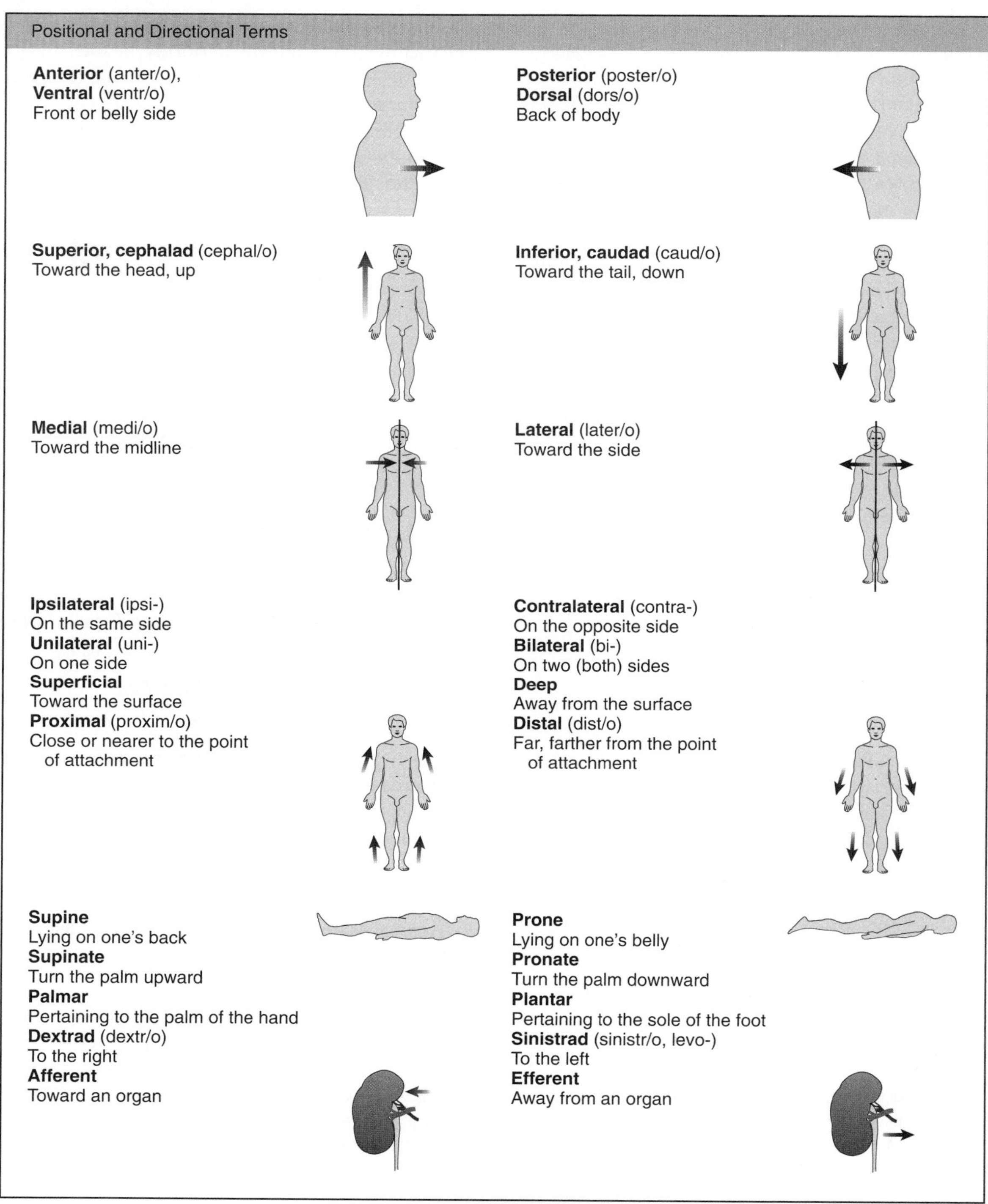

FIGURE 15-2. Positional and directional terms.

Type/Service	Radiology Examples	Chart Information
Step 4: Determine Specific Procedure Information		
	Views/contrast	Standing anteroposterior Both knees
	Two views with contrast	
Step 5: Determine Extent/Specifics		
	Additional guidelines	

In summary, the breakdown process for this procedure would be as follows:

Radiology code	70000-79999
Diagnostic x-ray section	70000-76499
Lower extremity	73500-73725
Knee	73560-73580
Anteroposterior standing view(s)	73565

These categories make locating the appropriate code(s) simple.

Medical Necessity of Radiologic Services

Providers of radiology and other ancillary services are subject to requirements by third-party carriers for diagnostic codes that justify ancillary services performed. Because many radiology services are ordered and performed to rule out certain diagnoses, and rule-out diagnoses cannot be used for physician coding, the coder is often forced to submit signs, symptoms, and ill-defined conditions as the medical necessity for services performed.

The basis for required documentation of medical necessity for ancillary services stems from years of reimbursement by third-party carriers for services that may not have been medically necessary for a given condition. The coder must view this scenario from the carrier's perspective to appreciate the significance. For example,

> Consider a room full of 30 students, all of whom arrive at the physician's office with "chest pain." All these patients must be examined and, in some cases, baseline studies, such as an electrocardiogram (ECG), must be done. As the result of abnormal or questionable ECG results, a few of these "patients" need additional testing, such as an exercise stress test. If the stress test detects an abnormality, an even smaller number of these individuals may need a thallium stress test. By requiring documented medical necessity for each level of service, the third-party carrier has authorized reimbursement of the thallium stress test in only a few individuals, thereby representing a substantial savings to the carrier.

Take a look at this example in dollars and cents:

30 students need ECGs ($60.00)	$1800.00
Five students with abnormal ECGs require a stress test ($200.00)	$1000.00
Two students with abnormal stress tests require thallium stress tests ($1500.00)	$3000.00
Total cost:	$5800.00
Compared with:	
30 students receive thallium stress tests ($1500.00)	$45,000.00

The third-party carrier wants to make certain that all ancillary services are medically necessary and that costs for these services are controlled.

Radiology Coding Guidelines

GENERAL GUIDELINES

One of the distinctions of radiology services is that many of the procedures performed are provided by two individuals: the technician, who completes the **technical component**, and the physician or radiologist, who provides supervision and written interpretation of the results, thus fulfilling the **professional component**. The combination of technical and professional components constitutes the global component, as described in Chapter 13.

Of the procedures with both technical and professional components, many may have only one component performed, so procedures in the radiology section may already be separated into these components. In those instances it is not necessary to include a modifier indicating that only the professional component has been performed. For example, code 72275, epidurography, radiologic supervision and interpretation is assigned only for the professional portion of this procedure; therefore appending modifier 26 to this procedure is not appropriate or necessary. The coder should take note that not all procedures in the radiology section have been divided as outlined here.

When only the radiologic interpretation or professional services are performed and the code has not been already separated by definition, modifier 26 would be appended to that service. An example would be code 71010, radiologic exam, chest, single view, frontal. If the entire procedure, both the technical and professional portions, is performed, code 71010 would be appropriate. If only the professional portion is performed, modifier 26 should be appended, and it would appear as 71010-26.

NATIONAL CORRECT CODING INITIATIVE GUIDELINES

In addition to the guidelines outlined by CPT, additional guidelines by the National Correct Coding Initiative (NCCI) specify what procedures may be coded or what services are considered bundled:

- When radiographic images must be repeated because of substandard quality, only one unit of service for that code may be reported.
- When limited comparative radiographic studies are performed, such as postreduction, postcatheter, postintubation, CPT codes for comprehensive radiographic services should be reported by appending modifier 52.
- When services are provided both with and without contrast, they should be assigned codes that include both, not coded with both "with" codes and "without" codes.
- When diagnostic angiography, such as venography or arteriography, is performed in conjunction with intravascular interventional procedures, it should be reported by appending modifier 59.
- Injection of radiopharmaceuticals is included as part of the nuclear medicine study.
- Xeroradiography, such as CPT code 76150, is not separately reportable with any mammographic studies.
- Guidance for placement of radiation fields by CT scan or ultrasound for the same anatomic fields is not separately reportable.
- Code 76970, ultrasound study follow-up, cannot be reported with echocardiography or ultrasound guidance procedures performed during the same encounter.
- Bone studies involve a series of radiologic films; therefore coding for individual radiographs is not appropriate.
- CPT codes 70540 to 70543 are used for MRI imaging of the orbit, face, neck, or all of these. Only one code in this series may be reported regardless of whether one or all of these areas are evaluated during an imaging session.
- An MRI of the brain and MRI of the orbit are separately reportable only when they are medically necessary. An incidental finding during the MRI of the brain does not constitute a medically necessary reason for additional studies.

MODIFIERS

The following modifier codes are appropriate for use with codes in the radiology section of CPT:

Modifier 22	Unusual procedural services
Modifier 26	Professional component only
Modifier 32	Mandated services
Modifier 50	Bilateral procedures
Modifier 51	Multiple procedures
Modifier 52	Reduced services
Modifier 53	Discontinued procedures
Modifier 58	Related or staged procedure by same physician during global surgical period
Modifier 59	Distinct procedure services
Modifier 62	Two surgeons
Modifier 66	Surgical team
Modifier 76	Repeat procedure by same physician
Modifier 77	Repeat procedure by another physician
Modifier 78	Return to operating room for related procedure during global or postoperative period
Modifier 79	Unrelated procedure or service by same physician during global or postoperative period
Modifier 80	Assistant surgeon
Modifier 90	Outside or reference laboratory services
Modifier 99	Multiple modifiers

Descriptions of these modifiers have previously been provided. Refer to the descriptions in the modifier section, the CPT Modifier Reference Tool 9-4, the complete outline of modifier codes in Chapter 9, and the Modifier Appendix located in the CPT code book.

When bilateral services are performed, they should be coded with the modifier 50, bilateral procedures. If the carrier recognizes modifier codes from the Healthcare Common Procedure Coding System (HCPCS), use RT (right) and LT (left). HCPCS modifiers are discussed later.

When additional views not listed in CPT are necessary, the appropriate CPT code should be used with modifier 22. A documented explanation should be included regarding additional views and the medical necessity for such.

When fewer views than those listed in CPT are performed, the appropriate CPT code should be used with modifier 52. The number of views performed should be recorded in the medical documentation.

Second readings or interpretations of radiography are not reimbursable by most third-party carriers.

SUPERVISION AND INTERPRETATION CODES

Supervision and interpretation (S & I) codes are used to code the personal supervision of the radiologic procedure and the interpretation. To bill for the supervision and interpretation, the physician must be present during the procedure. The interpretation itself may be performed at a later time. When the supervision (S) portion of an S & I code is performed by one entity and the (I) portion is performed by another, both providers should bill the S & I code with modifier 52 appended to indicate they have not performed all the services assigned to that code.

INTERPRETATION OF RADIOLOGIC AND DIAGNOSTIC SERVICES

In general, third-party carriers pay for only one interpretation of diagnostic services, including radiologic services. Only in the case of questionable findings would an interpretation of images perhaps be paid more than once. Any provider may code or bill for the interpretation of diagnostic results when the interpretation is made without the assistance of another provider or physician. For instance, if the emergency department (ED) physician requests or is required to seek the assistance of the radiologist in interpretation of an x-ray film, the emergency department physician may not code for that service.

When third-party carriers receive two claims for the interpretive services, they typically pay for the first claim received. If a second claim is received, the carrier will have to determine which physician's interpretation contributed to the diagnosis and treatment of that patient and pay accordingly. Another consideration would be whether the radiologist's interpretation was conveyed to the treating physician in time to contribute to the diagnosis and treatment of the patient.

CODING FOR CONTRASTS

When radiologic services are performed that involve the use of contrast, only contrasts that are administered other than rectally or orally will be considered. A number of codes, especially for CT and MRI scans, cover the performance of scans with, without, or with and without contrast. In the case of "with and without" contrast, the area is scanned initially without any contrast. The radiologic report should indicate that contrast was administered after images without contrast were taken to establish the legitimate use of the "with and without" contrast code.

RADIOPHARMACEUTICALS

When radiopharmaceuticals (drugs for radiologic imaging services over and above those incidental to the imaging) are used, coding for the provision of these supplies is appropriate. An appropriate HCPCS code such as A4641 should be assigned for these services.

Steps in Coding Radiology Services

We have already taken a look earlier in this chapter at the basic steps in breaking down the coding of radiology services. They were as follows:

Step 1 Identify appropriate CPT chapter: Radiology
Step 2 Identify the appropriate subsection in the radiology section
Step 3 Determine the anatomic part
Step 4 Locate the appropriate code(s)
Step 5 Determine extent of the procedure (number of views; limited or complete; with, without, or with and without contrast)
Step 6 Assign appropriate procedure code or modifier code(s)

Following is a more detailed look at each of these steps in the process of identifying the appropriate code(s).

Step 1: Identify Appropriate CPT Chapter: Radiology

The radiology section of CPT encompasses services where radiant energy is used to visualize affected areas and, in some cases, provide therapeutic treatment with radiation.

Step 2: Identify the Appropriate Subsection in the Radiology Section

The radiology section of CPT encompasses procedures typically performed in the radiology facility of a provider's office or in an outpatient or hospital setting. These codes may be used by any physician or facility in any setting, however, as long as the definitions are met.

Radiology services include diagnostic services such as the common chest x-ray as well as diagnostic ultrasound, radiation oncology, and nuclear medicine. The radiology section of CPT is divided into the following areas:

- Diagnostic radiology: encompasses the radiologic imaging performed with typical x-ray equipment. This includes such services as skeletal x-rays, MRI, and CT or CAT (computerized axial tomography) scans.
- Diagnostic ultrasound: involves sound waves producing an image. A-mode, M-mode, B-scan, or real-time scans are used for ultrasonic imaging.
- Radiation oncology: involves the services of teletherapy and brachytherapy in the provision of therapeutic radiation treatments. These treatments are typically used to treat neoplasms, most often those already diagnosed as malignant.
- Nuclear medicine: includes radiographic imaging with the injection or infusion of radioelements for the purpose of visualizing the organ or system.

STOP AND PRACTICE

Identify under which subsection within the radiology area the following procedures would be located.

Subsection

1. Chest x-ray ____________
2. Pelvic ultrasound ____________
3. Fluoroscopic guidance central venous catheter placement ____________
4. Screening mammogram ____________
5. CT head without contrast ____________
6. Kidney, ureters, bladder (KUB) ____________
7. Radiation treatment delivery ____________
8. Bone density study ____________
9. Bone imaging ____________
10. Foot x-ray ____________

Step 3: Determine the Anatomic Part

As much as possible, the codes in each subsection are arranged in anatomic order. For example, in the diagnostic radiology section, codes for the head and neck are first, followed by shoulder and upper extremities, and progressing down the anatomic structure of the body. Of course, there are some anatomic areas, such as veins and arteries, that would be difficult to place in order because they are located throughout the body.

STOP AND PRACTICE

Place the following diagnostic x-ray images in the order one would expect to find them in the diagnostic radiology section of CPT. (*1V* Stands for one view, *2V* stands for two views, and *3V* stands for three views.)

1. X-ray, elbow, 2V __________
2. X-ray, radius, 2V __________
3. X-ray, knee, 3V __________
4. X-ray, spine, cervical, 2V __________
5. X-ray, clavicle, 2V __________
6. X-ray, tibia, 3V __________
7. X-ray, chest, 1V __________
8. X-ray, hip, 2V __________
9. X-ray, wrist, 2V __________
10. X-ray, forearm, 2V __________

Step 4: Locate the Appropriate Code(s)

Once the anatomic part has been identified, locate the appropriate range of codes for the specific part. For example, in question 1 in the previous Stop and Practice exercise, X-ray, elbow, the following would apply:

Step 1 Determine chapter of CPT: Radiology
Step 2 Determine subsection: Diagnostic radiology
Step 3 Determine anatomic part: Elbow
Step 4 Locate appropriate codes: 73070-73085

STOP AND PRACTICE

Use the questions from the previous Stop and Practice exercise and identify the appropriate range of codes. All the services listed in this exercise are located in the diagnostic radiology section of CPT; therefore it is only necessary to determine the specific anatomic part (step 3 of the process) and the appropriate code(s) to consider (step 4).

	Anatomic Part	Appropriate Code(s)
1. X-ray, elbow, 2V	Elbow	73070-73085
2. X-ray, radius, 2V	________	________
3. X-ray, knee, 3V	________	________
4. X-ray, spine, cervical, 2V	________	________
5. X-ray, clavicle, 2V	________	________
6. X-ray, tibia, 3V	________	________
7. X-ray, chest, 1V	________	________
8. X-ray, hip, 2V	________	________
9. X-ray, wrist, 2V	________	________
10. X-ray, forearm, 2V	________	________

Step 5: Determine the Extent of the Procedure (Number of Views, Limited or Complete, With or Without or With and Without Contrast)

Once you have determined the appropriate range of codes, review the radiologic report to determine the number of views that were taken of the anatomic site. In the case of CT scans and MRIs, codes for without contrast, with and without contrast, followed by with contrast may be assigned. Keep in mind the NCCI guideline that indicates it would not be appropriate to assign a code for without contrast and a code for with contrast when a combination code, without contrast followed by with contrast, exists.

STOP AND PRACTICE

Review again the questions started in the previous exercises and assign the appropriate code for the services as indicated.

	Step 4: Appropriate Code(s)	Step 5: Code Assignment
1. X-ray, elbow, 2V	73070-73085	73070
2. X-ray, radius, 2V	________	________
3. X-ray, knee, 3V	________	________
4. X-ray, spine, cervical, 2V	________	________
5. X-ray, clavicle, 2V	________	________
6. X-ray, tibia, 3V	________	________
7. X-ray, chest, 1V	________	________
8. X-ray, hip, 2V	________	________
9. X-ray, wrist, 2V	________	________
10. X-ray, forearm, 2V	________	________

Step 6: Assign Procedure Code(s) and Modifier Code(s)

After identifying the appropriate CPT code(s) for services, determine whether modifier code(s) would be appropriate. For instance, in question 1, where code 73070 was determined to be appropriate, it would also be appropriate to assign an anatomic modifier of LT. Therefore the most appropriate answer for the service would be 73070-LT.

STOP AND PRACTICE

Assign the appropriate codes and modifiers to the following questions.

	Step 4: Appropriate Code(s)	Step 5: Code Assignment	Step 6: Modifier(s)
1. X-ray, elbow, 2V, Left	73070-73085	73070	LT
2. X-ray, radius, 2V, left	________	________	________
3. X-ray, knee, 3V, right	________	________	________
4. X-ray, spine, cervical, 2V	________	________	________
5. X-ray, clavicle, 2V, left	________	________	________
6. X-ray, tibia, 3V, right	________	________	________
7. X-ray, chest, 1V	________	________	________
8. X-ray, hip, 2V, left	________	________	________
9. X-ray, wrist, 2V, left	________	________	________
10. X-ray, forearm, 2V, right	________	________	________

Coding of Specific Radiologic Categories

Once the student understands the basic processes of assigning radiology codes, it is important to further understand additional coding guidelines for the specific subsections in the radiologic section.

DIAGNOSTIC RADIOLOGY (70010-76499)

Diagnostic Radiology Services

Head and neck	70010-70559
Chest	71010-71555
Spine and pelvis	72010-72295
Upper extremities	73000-73225
Lower extremities	73500-73725
Abdomen	74000-74190
Gastrointestinal tract	74210-74363
Urinary tract	74400-74485
Gynecologic and obstetric	74710-74775
Heart	75557-75564
Vascular procedures	75600-75996
Other procedures	76000-76499

Procedures in the diagnostic radiology subsection are divided by anatomic site and by the number of views. Diagnostic radiology includes plain x-ray films, CT scans, MRI, magnetic resonance angiography (MRA), and angiography. Anatomic sites begin with the head, chest, and upper extremities and progress to the lower extremities, as in other sections of CPT.

A brief review of the imaging procedures is appropriate at this time. Plain x-ray films are the most common radiologic studies performed. These procedures involve images obtained by x-ray technology and typically are used for evaluating fractures of bones or joints and other anatomic abnormalities. CT scans involve the use of specialized computerized equipment and software to produce three-dimensional images. This technology is typically used for evaluating internal structures of the body and produces images in slices to allow for highly detailed analysis.

MRI produces images that contrast the various parts and abnormalities that may exist in the body area or system being imaged. MRA uses this same technique but adds the injection of dye into vessels to better visualize the size and condition of the vessels. CT and MRI scans may also involve the injection of contrast to best visualize the areas of concern.

Radiologic services may be performed with contrast, without contrast, or with and without contrast. Oral contrast given before or during a study does not constitute "with contrast" and should be assigned a "without contrast" code unless other nonoral contrast is also given.

Care should be taken to make certain the appropriate code is assigned for the radiologic service that may or may not involve contrast. Following is an example of coding for a CT scan of the chest to visualize the many code choices available:

CODE	DESCRIPTION
71250	CT, thorax, without contrast material
71260	CT, thorax, with contrast
71270	CT, thorax, without contrast, followed by contrast
71275	CT, angiography, chest, with contrast material, including noncontrast images, if performed, and image postprocessing
71550	MRI, chest, without contrast
71551	MRI, chest, with contrast
71552	MRI, chest, without contrast, followed by contrast
71555	MRA, chest, with or without contrast material

Remember that when images are performed both with and without contrast, only the "without contrast, followed by contrast" code should be assigned. It would not be appropriate and would be considered unbundling to assign the code for without contrast as well as the code for with contrast in lieu of the combination code for this service.

It is also important that the interpretation clearly indicates that images are performed without contrast, followed by the administration of contrast, and additional images after the contrast is administered are taken.

Interventional radiologists are physicians who perform radiologic studies under interventional guidance, which usually involves the administration of contrast into the vessels. Many of these studies are performed to determine abnormalities of the vessels, such as congenital defects, obstructions, or aneurysms.

STOP AND PRACTICE

Try these diagnostic radiologic exercises.

Example: Chest x-ray, 2V

Step 1: Chapter: Radiology
Step 2: Radiology subsection: Diagnostic
Step 3: Anatomic part: Chest
Step 4: Appropriate code(s): 71010-71035
Step 5: Extent of procedure (number views, limited, complete): 2 V
Step 6: Procedure code(s) and modifier code(s): 71020

1. CT brain without contrast
   Step 1: Chapter: Radiology
   Step 2: Radiology subsection: ____________
   Step 3: Anatomic part: ____________
   Step 4: Appropriate code(s): ____________
   Step 5: Extent of procedure (number views, limited, complete): ____________
   Step 6: Procedure code(s) and modifier code(s): ____________
2. Upper gastrointestinal study
   Step 1: Chapter: Radiology
   Step 2: Radiology subsection: ____________
   Step 3: Anatomic part: ____________
   Step 4: Appropriate code(s): ____________
   Step 5: Extent of procedure (number views, limited, complete): ____________
   Step 6: Procedure code(s) and modifier code(s): ____________
3. Knee, left, 3V
   Step 1: Chapter: Radiology
   Step 2: Radiology subsection: ____________
   Step 3: Anatomic part: ____________
   Step 4: Appropriate code(s): ____________
   Step 5: Extent of procedure (number views, limited, complete): ____________
   Step 6: Procedure code(s) and modifier code(s): ____________
4. MRI, knee, right
   Step 1: Chapter: Radiology
   Step 2: Radiology subsection: ____________
   Step 3: Anatomic part: ____________
   Step 4: Appropriate code(s): ____________
   Step 5: Extent of procedure (number views, limited, complete): ____________
   Step 6: Procedure code(s) and modifier code(s): ____________
5. CT abdomen with and without contrast
   Step 1: Chapter: Radiology
   Step 2: Radiology subsection: ____________
   Step 3: Anatomic part: ____________
   Step 4: Appropriate code(s): ____________
   Step 5: Extent of procedure (number views, limited, complete): ____________
   Step 6: Procedure code(s) and modifier code(s): ____________
6. C Spine, 2V
   Step 1: Chapter: Radiology
   Step 2: Radiology subsection: ____________
   Step 3: Anatomic part: ____________
   Step 4: Appropriate code(s): ____________
   Step 5: Extent of procedure (number views, limited, complete): ____________
   Step 6: Procedure code(s) and modifier code(s): ____________
7. Tibia/fibula, 2V, left
   Step 1: Chapter: Radiology
   Step 2: Radiology subsection: ____________
   Step 3: Anatomic part: ____________
   Step 4: Appropriate code(s): ____________
   Step 5: Extent of procedure (number views, limited, complete): ____________
   Step 6: Procedure code(s) and modifier code(s): ____________
8. Lt foot, 2V/ Lt ankle, 2V
   Step 1: Chapter: Radiology
   Step 2: Radiology subsection: ____________
   Step 3: Anatomic part: ____________
   Step 4: Appropriate code(s): ____________
   Step 5: Extent of procedure (number views, limited, complete): ____________
   Step 6: Procedure code(s) and modifier code(s): ____________
9. Venography, bilateral extremity, S & I
   Step 1: Chapter: Radiology
   Step 2: Radiology subsection: ____________
   Step 3: Anatomic part: ____________
   Step 4: Appropriate code(s): ____________
   Step 5: Extent of procedure (number views, limited, complete): ____________
   Step 6: Procedure code(s) and modifier code(s): ____________
10. Radiologic examination, surgical specimen
    Step 1: Chapter: Radiology
    Step 2: Radiology subsection: ____________
    Step 3: Anatomic part: ____________
    Step 4: Appropriate code(s): ____________
    Step 5: Extent of procedure (number views, limited, complete): ____________
    Step 6: Procedure code(s) and modifier code(s): ____________

STOP AND PRACTICE

Now that you are familiar with the appropriate coding guidelines for diagnostic radiology, try some of the following radiological reports by assigning the CPT code(s).

1. Radiology report

RADIOLOGY REPORT

MR#:
DOB:
Dr.

Clinical summary:

CLINICAL DIAGNOSIS:
Atypical headaches

PART TO BE EXAMINED:
CT head with and without contrast

Abdomen:

Conclusion:

HEAD CT:

INDICATIONS:
Atypical headaches

REPORT:
CT of the head performed without and with IV contrast. Demonstrates no evidence of intracranial hemorrhage, mass effect, or midline shift. There are no enhancing cerebral masses.

IMPRESSION:
Negative head CT

Ddt/mm

D:
T:

Lisa Valhas, M.D. Date

GODFREY REGIONAL HOSPITAL
123 Main Street • Aldon, FL 77714 • (407) 555-1234

CPT code(s)

____
____

2. Radiology report

RADIOLOGY REPORT

MR#:
DOB:
Dr.

Clinical summary:

DIAGNOSIS:
Constipation

PART TO BE EXAMINED:
Barium enema

Abdomen:

Conclusion:

BARIUM ENEMA:
Negative colon and terminal ileum

Ddt/mm

D:
T:

Lisa Valhas, M.D. Date

GODFREY REGIONAL HOSPITAL
123 Main Street • Aldon, FL 77714 • (407) 555-1234

CPT code(s)

____

____

3. Radiology report

RADIOLOGY REPORT

MR#:
DOB:
Dr.

Clinical summary:

DIAGNOSIS:
Abdominal/pelvic pain

PART TO BE EXAMINED:
Abdomen/pelvis

Abdomen:

Conclusion:

TRANSABDOMINAL PELVIC ULTRASOUND:
Transabdominal pelvic ultrasound was performed by the ultrasound technologist. Thirty static images are submitted for review. Without the benefit of endovaginal scanning of the pelvis, this exam is incomplete. The uterus was of normal size. Uterus is grossly negative for mass. The endometrium is not well visualized on any of the images. On one static image, the endometrial thickness is measured at approximately 5 mm. In the postmenopausal patient, this is at the upper limits of normal. If the patient is having vaginal bleeding, this finding should be further evaluated with follow-up ultrasound. Neither ovary is definitively identified. The visualized portions of both adnexa are very grossly negative for mass or fluid collections. If pelvis mass is a consideration, I would recommend an endovaginal ultrasound examination of the pelvis or a CT scan.

Ddt/mm

D:
T:

Lisa Valhas, M.D. Date

GODFREY REGIONAL HOSPITAL
123 Main Street • Aldon, FL 77714 • (407) 555-1234

CPT code(s)

____

____

4. Radiology report

RADIOLOGY REPORT

MR#:
DOB:
Dr.

Clinical summary:

DIAGNOSIS:
Weight loss

PART TO BE EXAMINED:
CXR

Abdomen:

Conclusion:

PA AND LATERAL CHEST:
Normal heart size and pulmonary vascularity. A small amount of pleural fluid or pleural thickening has developed bilaterally since the previous exam of three years ago. There is also mild bibasilar atelectasis. The remainder of the exam is unchanged. There are old bilateral rib fractures. Mildly tortuous thoracic aorta.

Ddt/mm

D:
T:

Lisa Valhas, M.D. Date

GODFREY MEDICAL ASSOCIATES
1532 Third Avenue, Suite 120 • Aldon, FL 77713 • (407) 555-4000

CPT code(s)

____

____

5. Radiology report

RADIOLOGY REPORT

MR#:
DOB:
Dr.

Clinical summary:

Abdomen:

Conclusion:

LUMBAR SPINE MRI:
T1 and T2 sagittal and selected axial images
The sagittal images demonstrate anterior spondylolisthesis of L5, displaced forward by approximately 9 mm relative to the sacrum and 4–5 mm relative to L4. There is evidence of bilateral spondylolysis at L5. The findings cause deformity of the spinal canal at LS-S1 with increase in AP diameter. Degenerative disk disease with narrowing at L5-S1 interspace. Moderate posterior bulging of the disks at L1, L2, and L3 interspaces associated with degenerative changes in the facet joints. This results in spinal stenosis, moderately severe at L2-L3 and moderate at L1-L2 and L3-L4. Moderate degenerative changes in the interspaces anteriorly. Anterior wedging of the body of T12 with mild to moderate bulging of the disk at this level.

SUMMARY:
Significant spondylolisthesis of L5 with forward subluxation. Moderately severe spinal stenosis at L1-L2 and L3-L4. There is high-signal material associated with the right kidney on the T2 images. Suggest obtaining an ultrasound exam to evaluate further.

Ddt/mm

D:
T:

Lisa Valhas, M.D. Date

GODFREY REGIONAL HOSPITAL
123 Main Street • Aldon, FL 77714 • (407) 555-1234

CPT code(s)

____

____

DIAGNOSTIC ULTRASOUND (76506-76645)

Diagnostic Ultrasound Services

Head and neck	76506-76645
Abdomen and retroperitoneum	76700-76776
Spinal canal	76800
Pelvis	76801-76857
Genitalia	76870-76873
Extremities	76880-76886
Ultrasonic guidance procedures	76930-76965
Other procedures	76970-76999

Diagnostic ultrasound involves the use of high-frequency sound waves to provide images of anatomic structures. This imagery is then used to determine the cause of specific disease or illness. Four types of ultrasounds are outlined in the CPT coding manual:

- Real-time scan: one-dimensional display that outlines the structure. A-Mode: *amplitude* of sound waves. Ultrasound imaging relies on high-frequency sound waves that reflect off anatomic structures and return like an echo. The return time is calculated and an image created on the screen from the distances and intensities of the echoes (*A* is for *amplitude*).
- M-Mode: one-dimensional display of movement of anatomic structures (*M* is for *motion*).
- B-Scan: two-dimensional display of tissues and organs (*B* is for *brightness*).
- Real-time scan: two-dimensional display that shows the structure and motion of tissues and organs.

Most codes in the diagnostic ultrasound section include codes for limited and complete. Limited codes are typically assigned when a specific organ or body part is imaged. For example, a kidney ultrasound would be coded as limited because the images were of only one organ in the area. Complete codes are justified when all structures or organs in the specific area are imaged.

STOP AND PRACTICE

Try the following ultrasonic radiologic exercises.

1. Breast ultrasound, right
   Step 1: Chapter: Radiology
   Step 2: Radiology subsection: ________________
   Step 3: Anatomic part: ________________
   Step 4: Appropriate code(s): ________________
   Step 5: Extent of procedure (number views, limited, complete): ________________
   Step 6: Procedure code(s) and modifier code(s):
   ____
2. Gallbladder ultrasound
   Step 1: Chapter: Radiology
   Step 2: Radiology subsection: ________________
   Step 3: Anatomic part: ________________
   Step 4: Appropriate code(s): ________________
   Step 5: Extent of procedure (number views, limited, complete): ________________
   Step 6: Procedure code(s) and modifier code(s):
   ____
3. Transplanted kidney ultrasound
   Step 1: Chapter: Radiology
   Step 2: Radiology subsection: ________________
   Step 3: Anatomic part: ________________
   Step 4: Appropriate code(s): ________________
   Step 5: Extent of procedure (number views, limited, complete): ________________
   Step 6: Procedure code(s) and modifier code(s):
   ____
4. Obstetric ultrasound, sizes and dates
   Step 1: Chapter: Radiology
   Step 2: Radiology subsection: ________________
   Step 3: Anatomic part: ________________
   Step 4: Appropriate code(s): ________________
   Step 5: Extent of procedure (number views, limited, complete): ________________
   Step 6: Procedure code(s) and modifier code(s):
   ____
5. Intraoperative ultrasound guidance
   Step 1: Chapter: Radiology
   Step 2: Radiology subsection: ________________
   Step 3: Anatomic part: ________________
   Step 4: Appropriate code(s): ________________
   Step 5: Extent of procedure (number views, limited, complete): ________________
   Step 6: Procedure code(s) and modifier code(s):
   ____
6. Ultrasound scrotum
   Step 1: Chapter: Radiology
   Step 2: Radiology subsection: ________________
   Step 3: Anatomic part: ________________
   Step 4: Appropriate code(s): ________________
   Step 5: Extent of procedure (number views, limited, complete): ________________
   Step 6: Procedure code(s) and modifier code(s):
   ____

STOP AND PRACTICE—cont'd

7. Transvaginal ultrasound
   Step 1: Chapter: Radiology
   Step 2: Radiology subsection: ____________________
   Step 3: Anatomic part: ____________________
   Step 4: Appropriate code(s): ____________________
   Step 5: Extent of procedure (number views, limited, complete): ____________________
   Step 6: Procedure code(s) and modifier code(s): ____________________
8. Ultrasound guidance pericardiocentesis S & I
   Step 1: Chapter: Radiology
   Step 2: Radiology subsection: ____________________
   Step 3: Anatomic part: ____________________
   Step 4: Appropriate code(s): ____________________
   Step 5: Extent of procedure (number views, limited, complete): ____________________
   Step 6: Procedure code(s) and modifier code(s): ____________________
9. Transvaginal obstetric ultrasound
   Step 1: Chapter: Radiology
   Step 2: Radiology subsection: ____________________
   Step 3: Anatomic part: ____________________
   Step 4: Appropriate code(s): ____________________
   Step 5: Extent of procedure (number views, limited, complete): ____________________
   Step 6: Procedure code(s) and modifier code(s): ____________________
10. Limited retroperitoneal ultrasound
   Step 1: Chapter: Radiology
   Step 2: Radiology subsection: ____________________
   Step 3: Anatomic part: ____________________
   Step 4: Appropriate code(s): ____________________
   Step 5: Extent of procedure (number views, limited, complete): ____________________
   Step 6: Procedure code(s) and modifier code(s): ____________________

STOP AND PRACTICE

Now try assigning the appropriate CPT codes to the following real-life radiologic studies.

1. Radiology report

RADIOLOGY REPORT

MR#:
DOB:
Dr.

Clinical summary:

ABDOMINAL ULTRASOUND

INDICATION:
Nausea and abdominal pain

Abdomen:

Conclusion:

REPORT:
Abdominal ultrasound demonstrates normal echogenicity of the liver with no focal masses. No evidence of intra- or extrahepatic bile duct dilation. The gallbladder is normal. The pancreatic head appears normal. The body and tail of the pancreas are not well seen due to overlying bowel gas. Proximal aorta appears normal. The distal aorta is poorly visualized due to bowel gas. Both kidneys are negative for hydronephrosis. The right kidney measures 10.5 cm and the left 9.4 cm pole to pole. Normal spleen.

Ddt/mm

D:
T:

Lisa Valhas, M.D. Date

GODFREY REGIONAL HOSPITAL
123 Main Street • Aldon, FL 77714 • (407) 555-1234

CPT code(s)

____

____

2. Radiology report

RADIOLOGY REPORT

MR#:
DOB:
Dr.

Clinical summary:

OB ULTRASOUND

INDICATION:
Size and dates, history of hypertension

Abdomen:

Conclusion:

REPORT:
Single intrauterine viable pregnancy with the fetus in the cephalic position. The placenta is located anteriorly in the upper uterine segment. Normal amount of amniotic fluid. Fetal cardiac motion observed by the technologist with rate of approximately 137 beats per minute. Fetal anatomy appears normal on the images provided. The estimated ultrasound due date is 4/15/xx. Please see obstetrical worksheet for measurements.

Ddt/mm

D:
T:

Lisa Valhas, M.D. Date

GODFREY REGIONAL HOSPITAL
123 Main Street • Aldon, FL 77714 • (407) 555-1234

CPT code(s)

____

____

3. Radiology report

RADIOLOGY REPORT

MR#:
DOB:
Dr.

Clinical summary:

Abdomen:

Conclusion:

PELVIC ULTRASOUND:
Retroverted uterus is slightly enlarged in a generalized manner, measuring 9.0 cm in length and 7 cm in its AP and width. Thickness of the endometrium 1.0 cm. There is a light nonhomogenicity to the parenchymal pattern within the uterus, but subtle 4.7-cm × 3.6-cm area of slightly increased echogenicity anteriorly in the lower body area of the uterus, which could represent a uterine fibroid. Both ovaries are top normal in size, with the right ovary measuring 4.3 cm in its greatest dimension, and it contains a 1.8-cm cyst. Left ovary measures 4.1 cm and contains two cysts, measuring 1.6 cm and 1.7 cm in their greatest dimensions. No free fluid in the pelvis.

Ddt/mm

D:
T:

Lisa Valhas, M.D. Date

GODFREY REGIONAL HOSPITAL
123 Main Street • Aldon, FL 77714 • (407) 555-1234

CPT code(s)

____

____

4. Radiology report

RADIOLOGY REPORT

MR#:
DOB:
Dr.

Clinical summary:

US BILAT LOWER EXT ARTERIAL

REASON FOR EXAM:
Claudication, calf pain

Abdomen:

Conclusion:

FINDINGS:
Right common femoral artery, proximal, mid, and distal superficial femoral arteries, popliteal artery, and posterior tibial artery show triphasic wave signals. Dorsalis pedis shows the same. Left common femoral artery, proximal, mid, and distal superficial femoral arteries, popliteal artery, posterior tib, and dorsalis pedis show triphasic signal also. ABI at the right ankle is 1.19; at the right dorsalis pedis, 1.04. On the left, 1.17 and 1.19 respectively. These are normal ratios. Velocities on the right show a mild gradient in proximal superficial femoral artery to the mid superficial femoral artery on the right only. The mid superficial femoral artery to the distal superficial femoral artery shows a small gradient.

The color Doppler images are not showing any high-grade stenosis.

IMPRESSION:
No evidence of any arterial stenosis. Normal triphasic signals and ABIs throughout both lower extremities.

Ddt/mm

D:
T:

Lisa Valhas, M.D. Date

GODFREY REGIONAL HOSPITAL
123 Main Street • Aldon, FL 77714 • (407) 555-1234

CPT code(s)

____

____

5. Radiology report

RADIOLOGY REPORT

MR#:
DOB:
Dr.

Clinical summary:

CLINICAL INFORMATION:
History of CVA

Abdomen:

Conclusion:

DUPLEX CAROTID ULTRASOUND:
Examination of the left carotid demonstrated extensive plaque formation in the bulb extending into the origin of the left internal carotid. Doppler frequency spectrum analysis demonstrated velocities of up to 344 cm per second within the left internal carotid. Systolic ratio is 6.7, indicating greater than 60% diameter stenosis. There is normal flow in the left vertebral artery.

Examination of the right carotid demonstrated moderate amount of plaque in the bulb extending into the origins of the internal and external carotids. Doppler frequency spectrum analysis, however, demonstrated no hemodynamically significant stenosis. There is normal flow in the right vertebral artery.

CONCLUSION:
Greater than 60% diameter stenosis of the left internal carotid

Ddt/mm

D:
T:

Lisa Valhas, M.D. Date

GODFREY REGIONAL HOSPITAL
123 Main Street • Aldon, FL 77714 • (407) 555-1234

CPT code(s)

____

____

FLUOROSCOPIC GUIDANCE (77001-77032)

Fluoroscopic Guidance Services

Fluoroscopic guidance	77001-77003
Computed tomography guidance	77011-77014
Magnetic resonance guidance	77021-77022
Other radiologic guidance	77031-77032

BREAST MAMMOGRAPHY (77051-77059)

Many states have laws that require insurance carriers to cover screening mammograms for all insured clients. The guidelines are usually modeled after federal guidelines that cover all Medicare patients or after the American Cancer Society screening guidelines.

Screening mammograms are furnished to a patient who has no signs or symptoms of breast disease or personal or family history of breast disease. These services are typically covered for the purpose of early detection of breast cancer. A diagnostic code, such as V76.12, screening mammogram, would be appropriate. Because CPT code 77057 indicates bilateral screening, the use of modifier 50 would not be appropriate.

Diagnostic mammograms are performed in the presence of signs or symptoms or a personal or family history of breast disease in male or female patients. There are two codes for diagnostic mammograms, unilateral (77055) and bilateral (77056), so it is not necessary to append modifier 50 to these codes.

BONE AND JOINT STUDIES (77071-77084)

Studies that involve multiple images of the bones and joints are assigned from this section. The most common procedure from this section would be the dual-energy x-ray absorptiometry (DEXA) scan, a bone scan performed to determine osteopenia or osteoporosis.

STOP AND PRACTICE

Try the following radiology exercises.

1. CT guidance, needle placement
   - Step 1: Chapter: Radiology
   - Step 2: Radiology subsection: ________________
   - Step 3: Anatomic part: ________________
   - Step 4: Appropriate code(s): ________________
   - Step 5: Extent of procedure (number views, limited, complete): ________________
   - Step 6: Procedure code(s) and modifier code(s): ________________
2. MRI guidance, needle placement
   - Step 1: Chapter: Radiology
   - Step 2: Radiology subsection: ________________
   - Step 3: Anatomic part: ________________
   - Step 4: Appropriate code(s): ________________
   - Step 5: Extent of procedure (number views, limited, complete): ________________
   - Step 6: Procedure code(s) and modifier code(s): ________________
3. Fluoroscopic guidance, needle placement
   - Step 1: Chapter: Radiology
   - Step 2: Radiology subsection: ________________
   - Step 3: Anatomic part: ________________
   - Step 4: Appropriate code(s): ________________
   - Step 5: Extent of procedure (number views, limited, complete): ________________
   - Step 6: Procedure code(s) and modifier code(s): ________________
4. Screening mammogram, bilateral
   - Step 1: Chapter: Radiology
   - Step 2: Radiology subsection: ________________
   - Step 3: Anatomic part: ________________
   - Step 4: Appropriate code(s): ________________
   - Step 5: Extent of procedure (number views, limited, complete): ________________
   - Step 6: Procedure code(s) and modifier code(s): ________________
5. Diagnostic mammogram, right
   - Step 1: Chapter: Radiology
   - Step 2: Radiology subsection: ________________
   - Step 3: Anatomic part: ________________
   - Step 4: Appropriate code(s): ________________
   - Step 5: Extent of procedure (number views, limited, complete): ________________
   - Step 6: Procedure code(s) and modifier code(s): ________________
6. Diagnostic mammogram
   - Step 1: Chapter: Radiology
   - Step 2: Radiology subsection: ________________
   - Step 3: Anatomic part: ________________
   - Step 4: Appropriate code(s): ________________
   - Step 5: Extent of procedure (number views, limited, complete): ________________
   - Step 6: Procedure code(s) and modifier code(s): ________________

STOP AND PRACTICE—cont'd

7. MRI right breast
   Step 1: Chapter: Radiology
   Step 2: Radiology subsection: ____________________
   Step 3: Anatomic part: ____________________
   Step 4: Appropriate code(s): ____________________
   Step 5: Extent of procedure (number views, limited, complete): ____________________
   Step 6: Procedure code(s) and modifier code(s): ____________________

8. Bone age studies
   Step 1: Chapter: Radiology
   Step 2: Radiology subsection: ____________________
   Step 3: Anatomic part: ____________________
   Step 4: Appropriate code(s): ____________________
   Step 5: Extent of procedure (number views, limited, complete): ____________________
   Step 6: Procedure code(s) and modifier code(s): ____________________

9. DEXA scan, axial skeleton
   Step 1: Chapter: Radiology
   Step 2: Radiology subsection: ____________________
   Step 3: Anatomic part: ____________________
   Step 4: Appropriate code(s): ____________________
   Step 5: Extent of procedure (number views, limited, complete): ____________________
   Step 6: Procedure code(s) and modifier code(s): ____________________

10. Joint survey, two joints, one view
    Step 1: Chapter: Radiology
    Step 2: Radiology subsection: ____________________
    Step 3: Anatomic part: ____________________
    Step 4: Appropriate code(s): ____________________
    Step 5: Extent of procedure (number views, limited, complete): ____________________
    Step 6: Procedure code(s) and modifier code(s): ____________________

STOP AND PRACTICE

Now that we have completed our review of the ultrasonic guidance and mammography codes, try the following practical real-life radiology reports. Assign CPT code(s) and modifiers as appropriate for the following.

1. Radiology report

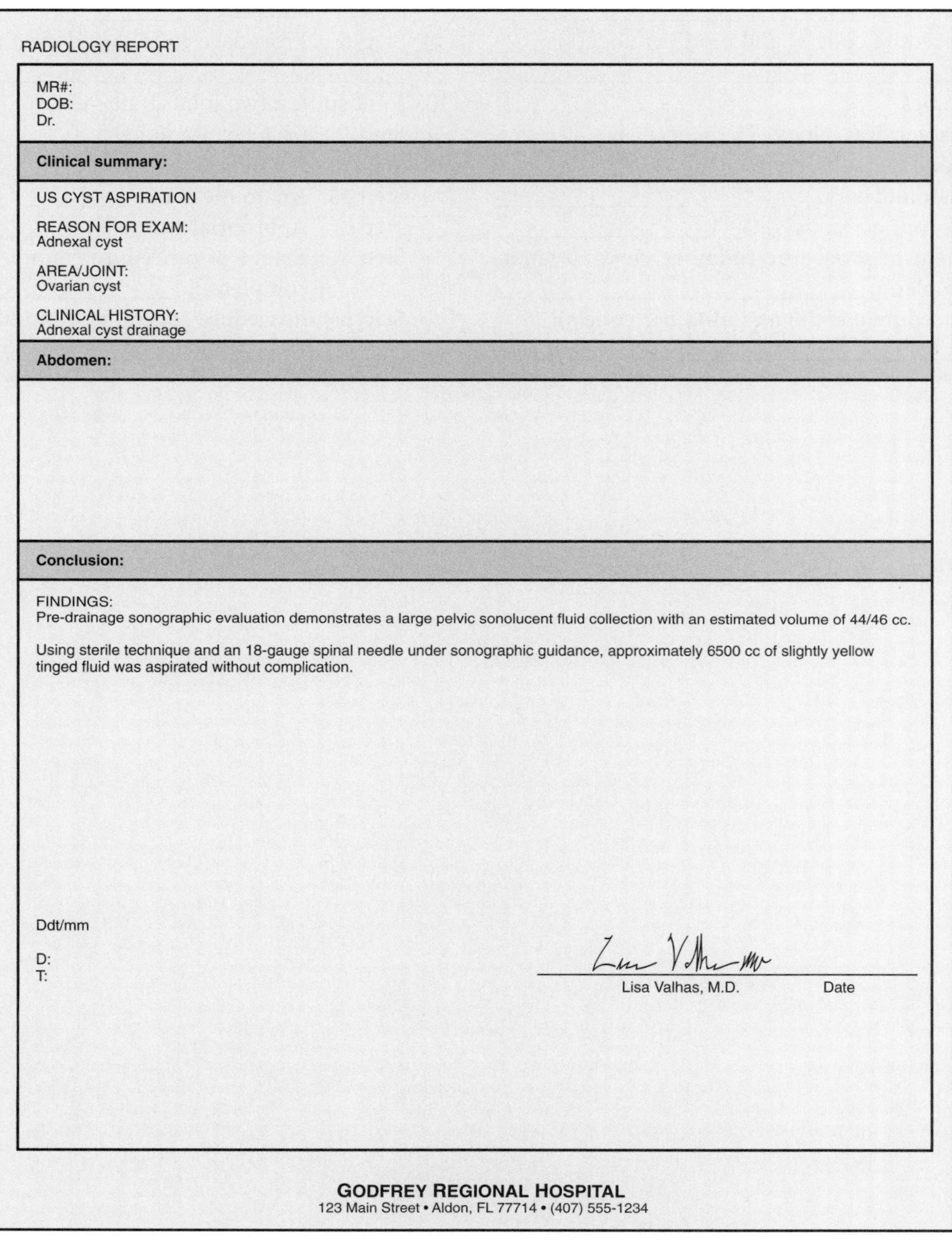

RADIOLOGY REPORT

MR#:
DOB:
Dr.

Clinical summary:

US CYST ASPIRATION

REASON FOR EXAM:
Adnexal cyst

AREA/JOINT:
Ovarian cyst

CLINICAL HISTORY:
Adnexal cyst drainage

Abdomen:

Conclusion:

FINDINGS:
Pre-drainage sonographic evaluation demonstrates a large pelvic sonolucent fluid collection with an estimated volume of 44/46 cc.

Using sterile technique and an 18-gauge spinal needle under sonographic guidance, approximately 6500 cc of slightly yellow tinged fluid was aspirated without complication.

Ddt/mm

D:
T:

Lisa Valhas, M.D. Date

GODFREY REGIONAL HOSPITAL
123 Main Street • Aldon, FL 77714 • (407) 555-1234

CPT code(s)

____

____

2. Radiology report

RADIOLOGY REPORT

MR#:
DOB:
Dr.

Clinical summary:

CLINICAL INFORMATION:
Follow-up to a mammogram

Abdomen:

Conclusion:

Magnification views were obtained to evaluate a questioned area of spiculation on the upper, inner quadrant of the left breast described on the prior exam. On magnification views, this resolves into overlapping parenchyma. There are no radiographic signs of breast carcinoma.

CONCLUSION:
No radiographic signs of breast carcinoma

Ddt/mm

D:
T:

Lisa Valhas, M.D. Date

GODFREY REGIONAL HOSPITAL
123 Main Street • Aldon, FL 77714 • (407) 555-1234

CPT code(s)

____

____

3. Radiology report

RADIOLOGY REPORT

MR#:
DOB:
Dr.

Clinical summary:

CLINICAL INFORMATION:
Chest nodule

Abdomen:

Conclusion:

CT OF THE CHEST:
There is a prior chest radiograph obtained four years ago. The patient's recent chest radiograph, obtained at a Godfrey Regional Hospital, has not been delivered for review.
Axial scans were obtained through the chest at 10-mm intervals. Subsequently, 2-mm scans were obtained though a 10-mm nodule in the left upper lobe. Subsequently, the patient was given 150 ccs of Isovue intravenously, and axial scans were obtained through the chest at 7-mm intervals. Following this, 2-mm scans were obtained through the nodular density in the left upper lobe.
The slightly ovoid lobule in the left upper lobe measures 10 mm in diameter. It has a Hounsfield density of 27 on the pre-enhanced images and approximately 28 on the post-enhanced images. This indicates that it is not enhancing.
Since the nodule was apparently identifiable on a chest radiograph, it must contain sufficient calcification to be identifiable at this small size. Hounsfield measurements are probably artifactually low due to partial volume affect. For this reason, the finding is most consistent with small granuloma. Review of an old chest radiograph obtained here two years ago shows a marginal density overlying the left 7th rib in about this location, so it has probably been present since that time.
When the old chest radiograph arrives, we will compare it with the current study.
No additional pulmonary abnormality is identified. The major bronchi are normal. The hilar mediastinal structures are normal.
Scans into the upper abdomen show numerous calculi in the gallbladder. The adrenals are normal.

1. Small non-enhancing nodule left upper lobe (see discussion above)
2. The old radiographs will be reviewed when they arrive.
3. Cholelithiasis

Ddt/mm

D:
T:

Lisa Valhas, M.D. Date

GODFREY REGIONAL HOSPITAL
123 Main Street • Aldon, FL 77714 • (407) 555-1234

CPT code(s)

____

____

4. Radiology report

RADIOLOGY REPORT

MR#:
DOB:
Dr.

Clinical summary:

Abdomen:

EXCRETORY UROGRAPHY:
The plain film of the abdomen demonstrates a considerable amount of stool throughout the colon, although the patient reports having received a colon prep last night.

Intravenous injection of 100 ccs of Isovue produced no adverse reaction. There is a prominent symmetrical nephrogram demonstrating normal, smoothly marginated kidneys. This is best seen on the nephrotomography.

Contrast appears in the collecting structures at two minutes bilaterally.

Conclusion:

1. Normal excretory urography
2. Minimal bladder trabeculation

Ddt/mm

D:
T:

Lisa Valhas, M.D. Date

GODFREY REGIONAL HOSPITAL
123 Main Street • Aldon, FL 77714 • (407) 555-1234

CPT code(s)

____

____

5. Radiology report

RADIOLOGY REPORT

MR#:
DOB:
Dr.

Clinical summary:

CLINICAL INFORMATION:
Right breast density

Abdomen:

Conclusion:

ADD VIEWS OF A RIGHT MAMMOGRAM:
CC and MLO magnification spot films of a nodular density in the lower outer quadrant of the right breast were obtained.

The density has somewhat lobular margins with some minimal breaking at one point. No unusual calcification is seen.

CONCLUSION:
Stable nodule in the right breast

ULTRASONOGRAPHY OF THE RIGHT BREAST: Right breast ultrasonography shows a 6-mm diameter hypodense nodule in the right breast at the 8 o'clock position. It does not contain any internal echoes. It does not, however, show significant enhancement through transmission. It probably corresponds to the nodule seen on mammography. One could attempt to aspirate this with ultrasound guidance to see if it is a cyst, but if it is not cystic or cannot be accurately aspirated, then excision would be recommended, as it has increased in size since the previous mammogram.

CONCLUSION: Ultrasonography shows a hypodense lesion in the right breast at the 8 o'clock position (see discussion above)

FDA CATEGORY:
4—Suspicious abnormality

Ddt/mm

D:
T:

Lisa Valhas, M.D. Date

GODFREY REGIONAL HOSPITAL
123 Main Street • Aldon, FL 77714 • (407) 555-1234

CPT code(s)

____

____

RADIATION ONCOLOGY (77261-77799)

Radiation Oncology Services

Clinical treatment planning	
External and internal sources	77261-77299
Medical radiation physics, dosimetry, treatment devices, and special services	77300-77370
Stereotactic radiation treatment delivery	77371-77373
Other procedures	77399
Radiation treatment delivery	77401-77421
Neutron beam treatment delivery	77422-77423
Radiation treatment management	77427-77499
Proton beam treatment delivery	77520-77525
Hyperthermia	77600-77615
Clinical intracavitary hyperthermia	77620
Clinical brachytherapy	77750-77799

The radiation oncology section of CPT contains services performed by or under the supervision of the radiation oncologist. This physician typically provides services to patients who have already received a diagnosis of a tumor or malignant neoplasm (other diagnoses are sometimes treated). The patient who receives treatment from the radiation oncologist usually has been diagnosed at the time of the initial treatment. Patients may continue to visit the oncologist for further diagnoses, treatments, and evaluation. The radiation oncology subsection is divided into the following groups.

Clinical Treatment Planning

Treatment planning includes test interpretation, tumor localization, and volume determination, or amount of radiation to be delivered. Time and dosage determination, treatment modality, number and size of treatment ports, appropriate treatment devices, and other procedures necessary to a treatment plan are also included.

Codes are assigned as simple, intermediate, or complex as follows:

Simple	Single port or simple parallel opposed ports with simple or no blockingSingle treatment area
Intermediate	Three or more converging ports Two separate treatment areas Multiple blocks of special time-dose constraints
Complex	Complex blocking Custom shielding blocks Tangential ports Special wedges or compensators Three or more treatment areas Rotational or special beam considerations Combination of therapeutic modalities

Therapeutic Radiology Simulation

This category has codes that cover the use of a simulator to determine the various treatment portal outlines and orientation to be used in the course of radiation therapy. A simulator, which is incapable of delivering radiation therapy, can generate radiation in the diagnostic x-ray range. It permits the orientation of a radiation beam that simulates the beam(s) proposed for therapy, while at the same time providing radiologic visualization of the area. Therapeutic radiology simulation requires the involvement of the physician, the technician, and all equipment necessary to provide this service. Therapeutic radiologic simulation is also categorized as simple, intermediate, or complex. Definitions for these categories are the same as previously listed. In addition, three-dimensional computer-generated reconstruction of tumor volume and surrounding critical normal tissue structures from direct CT scans, MRI data, or both may be assigned CPT code 77295.

Radiation Physics

The radiation physics subcategory comprises the decisions made by the physician about the type of treatment indicated, including appropriate doses, dose calculations, and the development of treatment devices.

Radiation Treatment Management

The codes in this section are used to bill for weekly management of the delivery of radiation therapy. Weekly management is defined in CPT as five treatments equaling 1 week of treatment, regardless of breaks between treatment days. It is not necessary that the radiation oncologist personally examine the patient for each fraction, only that an evaluation of the patient's data be performed. Multiple fractions furnished on the same date may be counted as long as there has been a distinct break in therapy sessions and the fractions consist of services that under normal circumstances would have been performed on different days.

Clinical Brachytherapy

Placement of radioactive material into or around a tumor site is coded in the clinical brachytherapy subsection. Placement may be defined as simple, intermediate, or complex, as defined by the CPT radiology guidelines.

STOP AND PRACTICE

Try the following radiology exercises.

1. Proton treatment delivery, simple
   Step 1: Chapter: Radiology
   Step 2: Radiology subsection: ____________
   Step 3: Anatomic part: ____________
   Step 4: Appropriate code(s): ____________
   Step 5: Extent of procedure (number views, limited, complete): ____________
   Step 6: Procedure code(s) and modifier code(s): ____________
2. Radiation dosimetry calculation
   Step 1: Chapter: Radiology
   Step 2: Radiology subsection: ____________
   Step 3: Anatomic part: ____________
   Step 4: Appropriate code(s): ____________
   Step 5: Extent of procedure (number views, limited, complete): ____________
   Step 6: Procedure code(s) and modifier code(s): ____________
3. Therapeutic radiation treatment planning, single treatment area
   Step 1: Chapter: Radiology
   Step 2: Radiology subsection: ____________
   Step 3: Anatomic part: ____________
   Step 4: Appropriate code(s): ____________
   Step 5: Extent of procedure (number views, limited, complete): ____________
   Step 6: Procedure code(s) and modifier code(s): ____________
4. Radiation treatment, single area, 5 MeV
   Step 1: Chapter: Radiology
   Step 2: Radiology subsection: ____________
   Step 3: Anatomic part: ____________
   Step 4: Appropriate code(s): ____________
   Step 5: Extent of procedure (number views, limited, complete): ____________
   Step 6: Procedure code(s) and modifier code(s): ____________
5. Therapeutic radiation treatment planning, two treatment areas
   Step 1: Chapter: Radiology
   Step 2: Radiology subsection: ____________
   Step 3: Anatomic part: ____________
   Step 4: Appropriate code(s): ____________
   Step 5: Extent of procedure (number views, limited, complete): ____________
   Step 6: Procedure code(s) and modifier code(s): ____________
6. Therapeutic radiation simulation-aided field setting, one area
   Step 1 Chapter: Radiology
   Step 2: Radiology subsection: ____________
   Step 3: Anatomic part: ____________
   Step 4: Appropriate code(s): ____________
   Step 5: Extent of procedure (number views, limited, complete): ____________
   Step 6: Procedure code(s) and modifier code(s): ____________
7. Intracavitary radiation source application
   Step 1: Chapter: Radiology
   Step 2: Radiology subsection: ____________
   Step 3: Anatomic part: ____________
   Step 4: Appropriate code(s): ____________
   Step 5: Extent of procedure (number views, limited, complete): ____________
   Step 6: Procedure code(s) and modifier code(s): ____________
8. Proton treatment delivery complex
   Step 1: Chapter: Radiology
   Step 2: Radiology subsection: ____________
   Step 3: Anatomic part: ____________
   Step 4: Appropriate code(s): ____________
   Step 5: Extent of procedure (number views, limited, complete): ____________
   Step 6: Procedure code(s) and modifier code(s): ____________
9. Surface application of radiation source
   Step 1: Chapter: Radiology
   Step 2: Radiology subsection: ____________
   Step 3: Anatomic part: ____________
   Step 4: Appropriate code(s): ____________
   Step 5: Extent of procedure (number views, limited, complete): ____________
   Step 6: Procedure code(s) and modifier code(s): ____________
10. Radiation treatment, two treatment areas, 20 MeV
    Step 1: Chapter: Radiology
    Step 2: Radiology subsection: ____________
    Step 3: Anatomic part: ____________
    Step 4: Appropriate code(s): ____________
    Step 5: Extent of procedure (number views, limited, complete): ____________
    Step 6: Procedure code(s) and modifier code(s): ____________

NUCLEAR MEDICINE

Nuclear Medicine Services

Diagnostic	78000-78999
Therapeutic	79005-79999

The specialty of radiologic nuclear medicine comprises the placement and monitoring of radioactive nuclides within the body. This section is subsectioned according to anatomic site. As with all of CPT, if the documentation does not substantiate multiple determinations, uptakes, or views, the coder must select a single uptake or view. Feedback should be provided to the physician regarding the possibility of documenting and coding additional items when appropriate to obtain additional reimbursement. The provision of the radiopharmaceutical should also be coded and billed with the appropriate supply or HCPCS code(s).

Positron emission tomography (PET) scans are also located in the nuclear medicine section of the radiology chapter of CPT. These codes are found in the nuclear medicine section by anatomic location.

STOP AND PRACTICE

Try the following radiology exercises.

1. Thyroid uptake
   Step 1: Chapter: Radiology
   Step 2: Radiology subsection: ________________
   Step 3: Anatomic part: ________________
   Step 4: Appropriate code(s): ________________
   Step 5: Extent of procedure (number views, limited, complete): ________________
   Step 6: Procedure code(s) and modifier code(s): ________________
2. Myocardial perfusion with ejection fraction
   Step 1: Chapter: Radiology
   Step 2: Radiology subsection: ________________
   Step 3: Anatomic part: ________________
   Step 4: Appropriate code(s): ________________
   Step 5: Extent of procedure (number views, limited, complete): ________________
   Step 6: Procedure code(s) and modifier code(s): ________________
3. Whole-body bone imaging
   Step 1: Chapter: Radiology
   Step 2: Radiology subsection: ________________
   Step 3: Anatomic part: ________________
   Step 4: Appropriate code(s): ________________
   Step 5: Extent of procedure (number views, limited, complete): ________________
   Step 6: Procedure code(s) and modifier code(s): ________________
4. Liver and spleen imaging
   Step 1: Chapter: Radiology
   Step 2: Radiology subsection: ________________
   Step 3: Anatomic part: ________________
   Step 4: Appropriate code(s): ________________
   Step 5: Extent of procedure (number views, limited, complete): ________________
   Step 6: Procedure code(s) and modifier code(s): ________________
5. Thyroid imaging only
   Step 1: Chapter: Radiology
   Step 2: Radiology subsection: ________________
   Step 3: Anatomic part: ________________
   Step 4: Appropriate code(s): ________________
   Step 5: Extent of procedure (number views, limited, complete): ________________
   Step 6: Procedure code(s) and modifier code(s): ________________
6. Bone marrow imaging, limited
   Step 1: Chapter: Radiology
   Step 2: Radiology subsection: ________________
   Step 3: Anatomic part: ________________
   Step 4: Appropriate code(s): ________________
   Step 5: Extent of procedure (number views, limited, complete): ________________
   Step 6: Procedure code(s) and modifier code(s): ________________
7. Esophageal motility
   Step 1: Chapter: Radiology
   Step 2: Radiology subsection: ________________
   Step 3: Anatomic part: ________________
   Step 4: Appropriate code(s): ________________
   Step 5: Extent of procedure (number views, limited, complete): ________________
   Step 6: Procedure code(s) and modifier code(s): ________________
8. Single-photon emission CT (SPECT) liver imaging
   Step 1: Chapter: Radiology
   Step 2: Radiology subsection: ________________
   Step 3: Anatomic part: ________________
   Step 4: Appropriate code(s): ________________
   Step 5: Extent of procedure (number views, limited, complete): ________________
   Step 6: Procedure code(s) and modifier code(s): ________________

STOP AND PRACTICE—cont'd

9. Brain imaging, four views
   Step 1: Chapter: Radiology
   Step 2: Radiology subsection: ____________________
   Step 3: Anatomic part: ____________________
   Step 4: Appropriate code(s): ____________________
   Step 5: Extent of procedure (number views, limited, complete): ____________________
   Step 6: Procedure code(s) and modifier code(s): ____________________

10. Cerebrospinal fluid flow imaging, ventriculography
    Step 1: Chapter: Radiology
    Step 2: Radiology subsection: ____________________
    Step 3: Anatomic part: ____________________
    Step 4: Appropriate code(s): ____________________
    Step 5: Extent of procedure (number views, limited, complete): ____________________
    Step 6: Procedure code(s) and modifier code(s): ____________________

STOP AND PRACTICE

Assign CPT code(s) and modifiers as appropriate for the following.

1. Radiology report

RADIOLOGY REPORT

MR#:
DOB:
Dr.

Clinical summary:

Abdomen:

Conclusion:

RADIONUCLIDE RENOGRAM:
10.2 millicuries of technetium 99m DTPA used.

On the perfusion scan over 60 seconds, the perfusion curve for each kidney is relatively flattened, with the curve for the right kidney reduced in amplitude compared with the left. The aortic bolus curve is normal in configuration; these findings are not specific, but could be seen with bilateral renal artery stenosis or nephrosclerosis. Suggest further evaluation with duplex ultrasound if not already done.

Considering the function study performed over 45 minutes, the renogram curve on the left is relatively flattened. The curves do decrease in amplitude over time, and percent contribution on the right is 44, and percent contribution on the left is 56. It may be helpful to repeat the study using Lasix if indicated clinically.

Ddt/mm

D:
T:

Lisa Valhas, M.D. Date

GODFREY REGIONAL HOSPITAL
123 Main Street • Aldon, FL 77714 • (407) 555-1234

CPT code(s)

____

____

2. Radiology report

RADIOLOGY REPORT

MR#:
DOB:
Dr.

Clinical summary:

DIAGNOSIS:
Cyst on liver

PART TO BE EXAMINED:
CT abdomen

Abdomen:

Conclusion:

CT ABDOMEN:
Exam performed both with and without IV contrast. Oral contrast also given. Lung bases are clear. There is no pleural fluid. Liver of normal size. There is a 3 1/2 × 3 centimeter benign cyst inferior on medial aspect of the right lobe of liver. Several other additional small benign cysts measuring up to 0.9 centimeters are elsewhere on the right and left lobes of liver. Recent ultrasound exam of the liver demonstrates a 1.3-centimeter focal area of increased echogenicity in left lobe of liver, but this is not visualized with certainty on the CT exam. Might obtain follow-up ultrasound exam in three months or so to make sure there is no interval change. Gallbladder is normal with no biliary ductal dilatation. Spleen and pancreas are normal. Kidneys are normal except for several small benign cysts in the left kidney. Abdominal aorta normal size. No ascites or adenopathy. No abnormality involved in the bowel.

Ddt/mm

D:
T:

Lisa Valhas, M.D. Date

GODFREY REGIONAL HOSPITAL
123 Main Street • Aldon, FL 77714 • (407) 555-1234

CPT code(s)

____

____

3. Radiology report

RADIOLOGY REPORT

MR#:
DOB:
Dr.

Clinical summary:

DIAGNOSIS:
Menopausal, hypothyroid, breast CA

PART TO BE EXAMINED:
Bone density

Abdomen:

Conclusion:

DEXA BONE DENSITY:
T values obtained for the lumbar spine range from 11.1 to 20.0. At the hip, the values range from 20.2 to 20.6. No evidence of osteoporosis.

The standards for the T-scores are as follows:
Osteopenia: 21 to 22.5 S.D.
Osteoporosis: below 22.5 S.D.
Established osteoporosis: below 22.5 S.D. plus fracture

Ddt/mm

D:
T:

Lisa Valhas, M.D. Date

GODFREY REGIONAL HOSPITAL
123 Main Street • Aldon, FL 77714 • (407) 555-1234

CPT code(s)

____

____

4. Radiology report

RADIOLOGY REPORT

MR#:
DOB:
Dr.

Clinical summary:

DIAGNOSIS:
Increased kyphosis (thoracic)

PART TO BE EXAMINED:
Bone density

Abdomen:

Conclusion:

DEXA BONE DENSITY:
T values obtained for the lumbar spine range from 24.2 to 25.5, consistent with osteoporosis. At the hip, the values are from 22.0 to 22.8.

The standards for the T-scores are as follows:
Osteopenia: 21 to 22.5 S.D.
Osteoporosis: below 22.5 S.D.
Established osteoporosis: below 22.5 S.D. plus fracture

Ddt/mm

D:
T:

Lisa Valhas, M.D. Date

GODFREY REGIONAL HOSPITAL
123 Main Street • Aldon, FL 77714 • (407) 555-1234

CPT code(s)

____

____

5. Radiology report

RADIOLOGY REPORT

MR#:
DOB:
Dr.

Clinical summary:

DIAGNOSIS:
Chronic parotitis

PART TO BE EXAMINED:
R sialogram

Abdomen:

Conclusion:

PAROTID SIALOGRAM:
After the exam was explained to the patient, it was carried out under sterile conditions. The tip of the sialogram catheter was positioned within the opening to the right parotid duct, and 2 ccs of Renografin 60 was gently injected under fluoroscopic visualization. The main right parotid duct is of normal size and without filling defect. The intraglandular branches are normal to slightly decreased in size. Would question possible displacement of the intraglandular branching ducts and might further evaluate with CT or MRI scan of the right parotid gland.

Ddt/mm

D:
T:

Lisa Valhas, M.D. Date

GODFREY REGIONAL HOSPITAL
123 Main Street • Aldon, FL 77714 • (407) 555-1234

CPT code(s)

Chapter in Review

Certification Review

- All radiologic services are considered global and have two components: technical and professional.
- Diagnostic radiology encompasses the radiologic imaging performed with traditional x-ray equipment.
- Diagnostic ultrasound involves the use of ultrasound for imaging.
- Nuclear medicine involves use by injection or infusion of radioelements to allow visualization of a specified area.
- Modifier 50 or HCPCS modifiers RT and LT (depending on carrier guidelines) should be used for radiologic services when services are performed bilaterally.
- Radiologic services must include a diagnostic statement to the highest level of specificity to justify the medical necessity of performing the requested tests.

Student Assignments

- Study Chapter 15.
- Review the Learning Objectives for Chapter 15.
- Review the Certification Review for Chapter 15.
- Complete the Chapter Review exercise to reinforce concepts learned in the chapter.
- Complete the practice exercises on the companion Evolve site for reinforcement of radiology concepts.
- Complete the Practical Application exercises for real-life scenarios.
- Complete the Workbook exercises, as assigned by your instructor, or individually for additional practice.

Chapter Review Exercise

Assign codes for the following scenarios. Because the ICD-9-CM requires noting the medical necessity for radiologic services, assign both the ICD-9-CM and CPT code(s) for these services. Unless otherwise specified, both technical and professional components of these radiologic services have been provided.

1. A patient visits the family physician with the complaint of cough and symptoms suggestive of upper respiratory infection. The family physician sends the patient to the radiology department and requests posteroanterior and lateral chest x-rays to rule out pneumonia.

   CPT code: 71020 ICD-9-CM code: ______

2. A patient arrives in the radiology department with physician orders for x-rays of the forearm, posteroanterior and lateral, for shaft fracture of the left radius.

   CPT code: ______ ICD-9-CM code: ______

3. A patient is brought to the radiology section for a two-view x-ray of the right wrist with the diagnosis of wrist fracture.

   CPT code: ______ ICD-9-CM code: ______

4. A patient is brought to the radiology section for multiple x-rays after an automobile accident. The patient complains of ankle pain along with pain in the clavicular area. X-rays of the right ankle and clavicle are ordered to rule out fracture.

   CPT code: ______ ICD-9-CM code: ______

5. A patient arrives in the radiology department with physician order to perform vaginal core irradiation, special treatment.

   CPT code: ______ ICD-9-CM code: ______

6. A radiologist performs an A-scan ultrasound to determine intraocular lens power in preparation for a cataract extraction with lens implantation.

   CPT code: ______ ICD-9-CM code: ______

7. A patient with breast cancer who will begin radiation therapy arrives in the radiation oncology department for application of an intracavitary radioactive source.

   CPT code: ______ ICD-9-CM code: ______

8. A patient with a cerebral brain tumor arrives for stereotactic radiation treatment management.

   CPT code: ______ ICD-9-CM code: ______

9. A limited abdominal real-time echography with image documentation and interpretation is performed for an abdominal mass.

   CPT code: 76705 ICD-9-CM code: ______

10. Radiology provides ultrasonic guidance for the performance of a needle biopsy for a breast mass.

    CPT code: ______ ICD-9-CM code: ______

11. A pelvic ultrasound is performed for determination of fetal age because of small size for dates.

    CPT code: ______ ICD-9-CM code: ______

12. A patient arrives in the radiology department for bone imaging of the right leg for diagnosis of osteomyelitis.

CPT code: _______ ICD-9-CM code: _______

13. Patient arrives for mammogram as a result of a suspected right breast mass.

CPT code: _______ ICD-9-CM code: _______

14. Ultrasound of the kidney is performed to determine size and location of kidney mass.

CPT code: _______ ICD-9-CM code: _______

15. Patient arrives for CT of the abdomen due to right upper quadrant pain. After several initial images are taken, contrast is introduced and additional images are obtained.

CPT code: _______ ICD-9-CM code: _______

16. Patient presents with a history of arthritis of the right wrist for bilateral wrist x-rays. Two views of the right and left wrist are performed that confirm arthritis in both joints.

CPT code: _______ ICD-9-CM code: _______

17. Patient presents with a month-long history of low back pain for a four-view radiologic exam of the lumbosacral spine. Diagnosis is ankylosing spondylitis of L4-L6.

CPT code: _______ ICD-9-CM code: _______

18. Patient with history of chronic obstructive pulmonary disease (COPD) presents with chronic cough and fever. Chest PA is performed to determine whether reoccurrence of pneumonia has occurred. No pneumonia is found, exacerbation of COPD is confirmed.

CPT code: _______ ICD-9-CM code: _______

19. Radiologist performs the preoperative placement of a radiologic marker for the performance of breast lesion excision by surgeon later the same day.

CPT code: 77032 ICD-9-CM code: _______

20. Pregnant female presents for a repeat transabdominal ultrasound to reevaluate fetal size and possible abnormality.

CPT code: _______ ICD-9-CM code: _______

Practical Application

Assign the appropriate CPT code(s), modifier(s), and ICD-9-CM code(s) to the following radiology reports.

1. Radiology report

RADIOLOGY REPORT

MR#:
DOB:
Dr.

Clinical summary:

DIAGNOSIS:
Abdominal pain, nausea

PART TO BE EXAMINED:
UGI

Abdomen:

Conclusion:

UPPER GI:
There is mild esophageal dismotility, with loss of the primary peristalsis, followed by multiple non-propulsive tertiary contractions in the distal esophagus. The esophageal mucosa appears normal. Small sliding-type esophageal hiatal hernia. No evidence of esophagitis at this time. The stomach is negative. There are mild to moderately thickened folds in the duodenal bulb, consistent with duodenitis. No ulcer demonstrated.

Ddt/mm

D:
T:

Lisa Valhas, M.D. Date

GODFREY REGIONAL HOSPITAL
123 Main Street • Aldon, FL 77714 • (407) 555-1234

CPT code(s) ____________________

ICD-9-CM codes ____________________

2. Radiology report

RADIOLOGY REPORT

MR#:
DOB:
Dr.

Clinical summary:

Abdomen:

Conclusion:

OB ULTRASOUND EXAMINATION:
The technologist performed the exam and hard-copy images were reviewed.

Single intrauterine pregnancy with fetus in the breech position. The placenta is located anteriorly and to the right. The lower margin of the placenta covers or partially covers the internal cervical os and this is considered to represent a "partial placenta previa."

Fetal cardiac motion observed by the technologist. Fetal anatomy is within normal limits on the images provided. Average ultrasound age estimated to be 21 weeks and 9 days.

The technologist estimates amniotic fluid index at 17.2 cm, which is in the 90th percentile for known gestational age.

Refer to the obstetrical worksheet for other measurements.

Ddt/mm

D:
T:

Lisa Valhas, M.D. Date

GODFREY REGIONAL HOSPITAL
123 Main Street • Aldon, FL 77714 • (407) 555-1234

CPT code(s)

____

____

ICD-9-CM codes

____

____

3. Radiology report

RADIOLOGY REPORT

MR#:
DOB:
Dr.

Clinical summary:

PROCEDURE:
Abdominal and pelvic CT

Abdomen:

Oral and IV contrast material used. Nonenhanced sections made of the liver.

Since 7/21/xx, the ion density mass described in the upper left abdomen has been resected. The patient has a history of gastric sarcoma. There are surgical staples at the greater curvature of the stomach. The bowel is not dilated. The bolus of contrast material is relatively weak, but the liver appears uniform in density. 2-cm low-density mass in posterior left kidney, probably a cyst. Small cortical cyst, right kidney. Atheromatous changes, abdominal aorta. No evidence of retroperitoneal adenopathy.

PELVIC CT:
Oral and IV contrast material used. Moderate enlargement of the prostate gland. No other evidence of a pathologic pelvic mass.

Conclusion:

Ddt/mm

D:
T:

Lisa Valhas, M.D. Date

GODFREY REGIONAL HOSPITAL
123 Main Street • Aldon, FL 77714 • (407) 555-1234

CPT code(s)

____

____

ICD-9-CM codes

____

____

4. Radiology report

RADIOLOGY REPORT

MR#:
DOB:
Dr.

Clinical summary:

Abdomen:

Conclusion:

RIGHT KNEE MRI:
Selected sagittal, axial, and coronal images obtained without additional contrast. Most of the medial meniscus is absent. Lateral meniscus intact. The anterior cruciate ligament is not visualized clearly but it is most likely intact. Posterior cruciate ligament intact. Collateral ligaments intact. Moderately degenerative changes, medial compartment of the knee with moderate narrowing of the joint space and with at least a moderate amount of loss of articulating cartilage. A small to moderate sized nonspecific joint effusion.

IMPRESSION:
Extensive degenerative tear involving the medial meniscus. Moderate degenerative changes, medial compartment of the right knee.

Ddt/mm

D:
T:

Lisa Valhas, M.D. Date

GODFREY REGIONAL HOSPITAL
123 Main Street • Aldon, FL 77714 • (407) 555-1234

CPT code(s) ______________________

ICD-9-CM codes ______________________

5. Radiology report

RADIOLOGY REPORT

MR#:
DOB:
Dr.

Clinical summary:

UPPER GI WITH AIR CONTRAST

REASON FOR EXAM:
Abdominal pain, nausea daily off and on

Abdomen:

Conclusion:

Patient ingested gas crystals, then barium. Multiple spot and overhead images were obtained of the upper GI tract.

Stomach is normal in shape, size, and contour. There is mild irregularity of the duodenal wall folds, small lucent filling defects in the base of the duodenum. Duodenal sweep is remarkable for the second part showing a little spiculation of the folds; the third part of the sweep, the fourth, and the jejunum appear normal. GE reflux is demonstrated into the lower esophagus. Neither hernia nor stricture.

IMPRESSION:
Films suggest mild duodenitis affecting the bulb and the second part of the sweep, GE reflux into the lower esophagus.

Ddt/mm

D:
T:

Lisa Valhas, M.D. Date

GODFREY REGIONAL HOSPITAL
123 Main Street • Aldon, FL 77714 • (407) 555-1234

CPT code(s) ______

ICD-9-CM codes ______

6. Radiology report

RADIOLOGY REPORT

MR#:
DOB:
Dr.

Clinical summary:

CT ABDOMEN WITH CONTRAST

CT PELVIS WITH CONTRAST

REASON FOR EXAM:
LLQ pain

Abdomen:

Conclusion:

CT (spiral, 8-mm collimation) through the abdomen and pelvis with oral and IV contrast, 150 ml of Omnipaque 300.

The study is abnormal because there is a thickened abnormal loop of bowel in the left lower quadrant of the abdomen. The bowel wall is clearly thickened, with small air lucencies around it, and there is blurred definition with pericolonic hazy soft tissue attenuating inflammatory changes. There is about a 4-cm fluid attenuating density in the left parametrial level near the fundus; this could represent fluid-filled focus of colon, early formation of abscess (no air in it), ovarian cyst; it's probably part of the inflammatory colonic process. There is no free fluid.

Punctate 5–7 mm nodule in the right lung base, probably a granuloma but it should be followed up with CT scan.

The liver has a uniform attenuation; small contracted gallbladder; the spleen is normal. Pancreas, kidneys, stomach are normal. Small and large bowel are as described. There are tiny studs of lymph nodes in the periaortic retroperitoneum, but they are not pathologically enlarged; they may be a response to this inflammatory process in the abdomen. There is no clear approachable area of abscess formation. The uterus is unremarkable, as are the urinary bladder and the inguinal region.

IMPRESSION:
Abnormal left lower quadrant inflammatory process, at least a 10-cm segment of inflamed thickened colon; differential includes diverticulitis, colitis, possible early abscess formation (not approachable by CT). GYN etiology for inflammation can also cause a similar presentation.

Ddt/mm

D:
T:

Lisa Valhas, M.D. Date

GODFREY REGIONAL HOSPITAL
123 Main Street • Aldon, FL 77714 • (407) 555-1234

CPT code(s)

____

____

ICD-9-CM codes

____

____

7. Radiology report

RADIOLOGY REPORT

MR#:
DOB:
Dr.

Clinical summary:

ABD FLAT/UPRIGHT

REASON FOR EXAM:
Abdominal pain

CLINICAL HISTORY:
Abdominal pain

Abdomen:

Conclusion:

FINDINGS:
There is a 4-cm round bony deformity in left lateral iliac crest; correlate for intervention here versus exostoses or primary bone process. Bowel pattern is negative; lung bases are clear. No pathologic calcifications; punctate pelvic phleboliths on the left.

IMPRESSION:
Punctate pelvic phleboliths on the left just below the level of the ischial spine. Deformity in left lateral iliac crest; exostoses/bone process versus postbiopsy site.

Ddt/mm

D:
T:

Lisa Valhas, M.D. Date

GODFREY MEDICAL ASSOCIATES
1532 Third Avenue, Suite 120 • Aldon, FL 77713 • (407) 555-4000

CPT code(s)

ICD-9-CM codes

8. Radiology report

RADIOLOGY REPORT

MR#:
DOB:
Dr.

Clinical summary:

CLINICAL INFORMATION:
Bruise over third finger

Abdomen:

Conclusion:

RIGHT HAND, THREE VIEWS:
There is no fracture or dislocation. Degenerative changes are seen at the first metacarpal phalangeal joint with joint space narrowing and marginal osteophyte formation and subchondral sclerosis. Mild degenerative change is seen at the interphalangeal joints throughout.

CONCLUSION:
Degenerative changes; no fracture is identified

Ddt/mm

D:
T:

Lisa Valhas, M.D. Date

GODFREY MEDICAL ASSOCIATES
1532 Third Avenue, Suite 120 • Aldon, FL 77713 • (407) 555-4000

CPT code(s) ______________________ ______________________

ICD-9-CM codes ______________________ ______________________

9. Radiology report

RADIOLOGY REPORT

MR#:
DOB:
Dr.

Clinical summary:

CLINICAL INFORMATION:
Wrist pain

Abdomen:

Conclusion:

LEFT WRIST:
Three views of the left wrist were obtained. No acute fracture is identified. There is considerable degenerative change of the right carpal joint with joint space narrowing and subchondral sclerosis. Degenerative changes are seen at the articulation between the greater multiangular and the navicular bones. On the lateral view a dorsal osteophyte rises from the mid carpus, probably arising from the lunate. Moderate soft tissue swelling is seen dorsally and ventrally. There are a few small calcific densities in the soft tissue ventrally. I cannot determine whether these are vascular or soft tissue, or even small avulsions. At this age I would suspect they are vascular.

CONCLUSION:
Degenerative changes, no definite fractures

Ddt/mm

D:
T:

Lisa Valhas, M.D. Date

GODFREY MEDICAL ASSOCIATES
1532 Third Avenue, Suite 120 • Aldon, FL 77713 • (407) 555-4000

CPT code(s)

____

____

ICD-9-CM codes

____

____

10. Radiology report

RADIOLOGY REPORT

MR#:
DOB:
Dr.

Clinical summary:

CLINICAL INFORMATION:
SOB

Abdomen:

Conclusion:

CHEST PA AND LATERAL:
Comparison is made with the study of six years ago.

The heart size and the vasculature are normal. There is no infiltrate or effusion. Senescent changes are seen throughout the chest.

CONCLUSION:
No active disease in the chest

Ddt/mm

D:
T:

Lisa Valhas, M.D. Date

GODFREY MEDICAL ASSOCIATES
1532 Third Avenue, Suite 120 • Aldon, FL 77713 • (407) 555-4000

CPT code(s)

ICD-9-CM codes

16

Pathology Services

LEARNING OBJECTIVES

After completing this chapter, the student will be able to:

- Understand the documentation used for pathology services.
- Identify types of pathology services and explain proper application of coding rules for each category of services.
- Comprehend the various modifier codes used for coding pathology services and use them in actual coding scenarios.
- Understand and use the basic steps for coding pathology services.
- Apply pathology coding concepts to practical coding scenarios.

KEY TERMS

Anatomic Pathology

Automated

Clinical Laboratory Improvements Amendments (CLIA)

Dipstick

Disease-Oriented Panels

Evocative/Suppression Testing

Manual

Surgical Pathology

Urinalysis

Pathology Documentation and Coding Guidelines

PATHOLOGY SERVICE CODES

Documentation for pathology services is provided in both the pathology request form and the actual laboratory report. Typically, the pathology laboratory or pathologist does not examine the patient and relies on information provided on the pathology order form for suspected conditions, signs, or symptoms. Pathology services typically require the use of data and statistical analysis for the determination of a diagnosis. As is the case with radiology services, for both professional and technical components of the global service to be coded and billed, documentation must contain both the technical performance and the professional interpretation. The interpretation may be documented on the actual laboratory slip (Fig. 16-1) or dictated as part of the medical record documentation (Fig. 16-2). Subsections of the pathology chapter are as follows:

Organ or disease-oriented panels	80047-80076
Drug testing	80100-80103
Therapeutic drug assays	80150-80299
Evocative/suppression testing	80400-80440
Consultations (clinical pathology)	80500-80504
Urinalysis	81000-81099
Chemistry	82000-84999
Hematology and coagulation	85002-85999
Immunology	86000-86804
Tissue typing	86805-86849
Transfusion medicine	86850-86999
Microbiology	87001-87999
Anatomic pathology	88000-88099
Cytopathology	88104-88199
Cytogenetic studies	88230-88299
Surgical pathology	88300-88399
Transcutaneous procedures	88720-88741
Other procedures	89049-89240
Reproductive medicine procedures	89250-89356

Review the components needed for determining the laboratory service performed. Look at the key elements in Figure 10-1, specifically pathology services.

CPT CODING STEPS: PATHOLOGY EXAMPLES

Step 1: Identify Chapter

Study of Body Substances	
Range of codes	80048-89399

Step 2: Determine Type/Location

Type of service	Chemistry Hematology

Step 3: Determine Specific Type

Specific test	Hemoglobin Hematocrit

Step 4: Determine Specific Procedure Information

Automated or manual	Automated Manual

Step 5: Determine Extent/Additional Specifics

Additional guidelines

Step 6: Assign CPT Codes Appropriately

Overview

The pathology section of Current Procedural Terminology (CPT) is composed of services performed on specimens collected by the physician or facility. The physician's office or facility may charge for the collection or preparation of the specimen based on CPT guidelines.

In general, pathology specimens are prepared and/or screened by laboratory personnel under the direction and supervision of the pathologist directing the laboratory. Certain tests require review of the specimens or tests by the pathologist. Patient contact for services performed in the pathology section are limited; however, because the pathologist is a physician, codes from the evaluation and management section may be assigned by the pathologist when a patient encounter is performed and history, exam, and medical decision making are performed and documented.

GENERAL CODING AND BILLING GUIDELINES

Automated and Manual

Pathology services may be performed by different methods, namely, automated, manual, and dipstick. Dipstick use is specific to urinalysis and involves dipping a chemically treated urine strip into the specimen and analyzing visual changes. Automated analysis involves the introduction of a urine specimen into a urine analysis system that provides a printout of the findings from multiple analyses for review by the physician. Manually analyzed specimens are subjected to several diagnostic protocols, each one separate, usually by a pathologist or a lab technician under the supervision of the pathologist.

When laboratory services are performed and the methods unspecified, the coder must use the least significant code. All **automated** services, with the exception of **urinalysis**, will be considered least significant because reduced provider involvement and analysis are required compared with **manual** services. With urine specimens, the **dipstick** method is considered the least significant.

CLIA Requirements

In 1988 the **Clinical Laboratory Improvements Amendments (CLIA)** were enacted to ensure that laboratories consistently provide accurate procedures and services. Each laboratory is assigned a CLIA certificate number or certificate

Patient name: ____________ Room #: ____________
Age: ______ Sex: ______ Accession #: ____________
Collected: ____________ Received: ____________
Reported: ____________ Req. #/Med. Rec. #: ____________
Requesting Phys: ____________ Pt. ID #: ____________

Test name	Results		Reference range	TL
	Out of range	In range		

Testing location (see reverse side)

GODFREY CLINICAL LABORATORIES
465 Dogwood Court • Aldon, FL 77712 • (407) 555-9876

FIGURE 16-1. Laboratory slip.

SURGICAL PATHOLOGY REPORT

Name:______________________________Hosp. No.:__________________Path. No.:__________________
Date:______________Room:________Age:______Sex:______Surgeon: ______________________________M.D.
Operation:____
Material submitted:____
Pre-op diagnosis:____
Post-op diagnosis:____
Previous material:____________________Pertinent history: _____________________________________

Diagnosis:

Gross description:

Specimen consist of an elongated fragment of membranous and fatty tissue measuring approximately 17 cms in length x 3 cms at the widest part x 2 mms in average thickness. One surface is smooth and glistening and the opposite surface shows areas of hemorrhage. Representative sections are submitted.

Micro description:

Section consists of fragments of fatty tissue traversed by dense bands of connective tissue with congested capillaries. One of the fragments appears to have a lining of mesothelial cells.

Maria Callingmo M.D.
Pathologist

GODFREY CLINICAL LABORATORIES
465 Dogwood Court • Aldon, FL 77712 • (407) 555-9876

FIGURE 16-2. Pathology report.

of waiver number, which must be listed on the CMS-1500 claim form in Box 23. The facility's CLIA certification specifies what laboratory services may or may not be performed at the facility or physician's office. The Healthcare Common Procedure Coding System (HCPCS) modifier QW is appended to laboratory services performed in the physician's office to signify the services are CLIA-waived services.

Specimen Collection and Drawing Fee

Specific procedure codes have been established for the collection of specimens. These codes are located in the surgery and medicine sections of CPT and are typically used only when the specimen is prepared to send to an outside laboratory for processing.

Specimen handling codes (99000-99002) are assigned to specimens that must be collected, prepared, and labeled. Appropriate forms must be prepared for the specimen to be forwarded to another facility for processing.

Specimen drawing fees (36400-36425) are used for venipuncture to obtain specimens. These codes are assigned based on the patient's age and how the specimen is obtained (e.g., percutaneous, cutdown). When carriers require the use of HCPCS codes, G0001, in lieu of CPT code 36415, is used for the routine venipuncture for collection of specimen(s). Code P9615 is used for catheterization for collection of specimen(s).

CORRECT CODING INITIATIVE GUIDELINES

Most of the National Correct Coding Initiative (NCCI) guidelines address services that are bundled in panel or group codes in the pathology section. Guidelines indicate that when multiple services are performed that can be assigned one pathology code, it is inappropriate to unbundle these services and assign more than one pathology code.

An excellent example would be the services located in the organ- and disease-oriented panels. Although each of the services contained in one of these codes may be performed independently, and in those instances would be assigned an individual code, when all services included in one of the panel codes are performed at the same time the appropriate panel code should be assigned.

In addition, the following services are not additionally reportable for the pathology section:

- Multiple tests performed to identify the same analyte, marker, or infectious agent
- Duplicate testing
- Only one code reported for all flow cytometry performed on the same specimen
- Total thyroxine with or without thyroid hormone binding ratio when free thyroxine is reported

In instances in which a test is ordered and additionally related tests are necessary to provide or verify the result, those tests would be considered part of the ordered test. However, in instances in which an initial positive result necessitates additional testing that is NOT performed to complete the ordered test, those services would be separately reportable.

For example, both an automated hemogram (85027) and a manual differential white blood cell (WBC) count (85007) may be coded. However, the provider cannot report an automated hemogram with an automated differential WBC (85025) with a manual differential WBC count (85007) because this would represent some duplication of services.

TYPES OF PATHOLOGY SERVICES

The pathology section of CPT is divided into the following subsections:

- Organ- or **disease-oriented panels**
- Drug testing
- Therapeutic drug assays
- **Evocative/suppression testing**
- Consultations (clinical pathology)
- Urinalysis
- Chemistry
- Hematology and coagulation
- Immunology
- Transfusion medicine
- Microbiology
- **Anatomic pathology**
- **Surgical pathology**

As with the radiology section of CPT, diagnostic coding that identifies the medical necessity for pathology services is necessary as well. One of the most common reasons that laboratory services are not paid or are paid incorrectly by third-party carriers is that diagnosis codes do not match the pathology service. For example, if pathology service codes are for a urine specimen, a diagnosis code for blood analysis, such as anemia, would not be appropriate.

Steps in Coding Pathology Services

The steps involved in determining the appropriate pathology code or codes for services performed require the following breakdown of information:

- Step 1: Identifies that the services were performed on body substances from a specimen submitted for examination and diagnosis.
- Step 2: Identifies the subsection within the laboratory section and typically details the type of services performed. Subsections are listed earlier, under types of pathology services. A discussion of each of these subsections is presented later in this chapter.
- Step 3: Identifies the specific test within the subsection identified for the specific service. In many instances, procedures within a subsection are listed in alphabetical order, making the location of these services simpler. However, abbreviations for a number of these tests are often used, so familiarity with laboratory tests becomes important.

- Step 4: Identifies the method used for performing the specific test. In some instances the test may be specified as automated or manual. In other instances it may be qualitative versus quantitative. Different methods are typically coded and billed with different CPT codes.
- Step 5: Identifies any additional information regarding the services being performed.
- Step 6: Assign CPT codes appropriately.

This narrowing down process is important, especially in CPT sections such as pathology, because of the volume of services and the number of subsections contained in this section.

Also, keep in mind one of the basic rules of coding: *If it is not documented, it did not happen.* When the method used for testing is not specified, the least significant method will be assigned.

Review of Pathology Subsections

ORGAN- OR DISEASE-ORIENTED PANELS (80047-80076)

Panel tests should not be reported separately when performed on the same day. Twelve panels of tests are commonly performed for definitive testing: basic metabolic, electrolyte, comprehensive metabolic, general health, obstetric, hepatic function, hepatitis, lipids, arthritis, TORCH antibody, thyroid, and thyroid with thyroid-stimulating hormone (TSH). Refer to the current CPT manual for a list of the included procedures. Note that all tests included in a specific panel must be performed before panel codes can be assigned. If even one of these tests is not medically necessary or not performed, each test must be ordered and billed independently.

DRUG TESTING (80100-80103)

Initial testing procedures from this section, codes 80100 and 80101, are usually confirmed with an additional technique by using code 80102. Testing is categorized by the classification of drugs, such as barbiturates and amphetamines. Testing from this section identifies only the presence or absence of drugs, not the specific drug or amount.

Code 80100 is considered a qualitative screen for multiple drug classes. In other words, the test indicates only whether drugs are present in the specimen. Code 80101 is a qualitative test as well, known as an *immunoassay,* in which only one drug class is tested at a time.

THERAPEUTIC DRUG ASSAYS (80150-80299)

Tests in this section are performed quantitatively; they identify the presence of the drug(s) as well as the exact amount or quantity present. These codes are used when the drug identified is to be measured or quantitated. These tests are usually ordered to determine whether the patient is receiving a therapeutic level of a prescribed medication. Drugs listed in CPT are by generic categories; therefore the coder may find it helpful to use a drug book or the *Physicians' Desk Reference* (PDR) to identify the classification for the specific drug.

Examples of the types of medications tested in this section include the following:

- Antiarrhythmics
- Antibiotics
- Anticonvulsants
- Antidepressants
- Sedatives
- Tranquilizers

STOP AND PRACTICE

Assign the appropriate CPT code(s) for the following services from the organ- and disease-oriented panel, drug testing, and drug assay sections.

1. Comprehensive metabolic panel
   Step 1: Chapter: Pathology ____________
   Step 2: Subsection: ____________
   Step 3: Specific service: ____________
   Step 4: Specific technique: ____________
   Step 5: Additional information: ____________
   Step 6: CPT codes: ____________
2. Opiate drug testing, qualitative, single drug class method
   Step 1: Chapter: Pathology ____________
   Step 2: Subsection: ____________
   Step 3: Specific service: ____________
   Step 4: Specific technique: ____________
   Step 5: Additional information: ____________
   Step 6: CPT codes: ____________
3. Digoxin drug assay
   Step 1: Chapter: Pathology ____________
   Step 2: Subsection: ____________
   Step 3: Specific service: ____________
   Step 4: Specific technique: ____________
   Step 5: Additional information: ____________
   Step 6: CPT codes: ____________
4. Lithium drug assay
   Step 1: Chapter: Pathology ____________
   Step 2: Subsection: ____________

STOP AND PRACTICE—cont'd

Step 3: Specific service: ____________
Step 4: Specific technique: ____________
Step 5: Additional information: ____________
Step 6: CPT codes: ____________

5. Drug confirmation testing
Step 1: Chapter: Pathology ____________
Step 2: Subsection: ____________
Step 3: Specific service: ____________
Step 4: Specific technique: ____________
Step 5: Additional information: ____________
Step 6: CPT code(s): ____________

6. Carbon dioxide
Chloride
Potassium
Sodium
Step 1: Chapter: Pathology ____________
Step 2: Subsection: ____________
Step 3: Specific service: ____________
Step 4: Specific technique: ____________
Step 5: Additional information: ____________
Step 6: CPT code(s): ____________

7. Renal function panel
Step 1: Chapter: Pathology ____________
Step 2: Subsection: ____________
Step 3: Specific service: ____________
Step 4: Specific technique: ____________
Step 5: Additional information: ____________
Step 6: CPT code(s): ____________

8. Carbon dioxide
Potassium
Step 1: Chapter: Pathology ____________
Step 2: Subsection: ____________
Step 3: Specific service: ____________
Step 4: Specific technique: ____________
Step 5: Additional information: ____________
Step 6: CPT code(s): ____________

9. Lidocaine drug assay
Step 1: Chapter: Pathology ____________
Step 2: Subsection: ____________
Step 3: Specific service: ____________
Step 4: Specific technique: ____________
Step 5: Additional information: ____________
Step 6: CPT code(s): ____________

10. Cholesterol, serum, total lipoprotein, direct measurement, high-density cholesterol triglycerides
Step 1: Chapter: Pathology ____________
Step 2: Subsection: ____________
Step 3: Specific service: ____________
Step 4: Specific technique: ____________
Step 5: Additional information: ____________
Step 6: CPT code(s): ____________

EVOCATIVE/SUPPRESSION TESTING (80400-80440)

These codes are used for procedures that measure the effects of administered drugs. CPT guidelines may specify the method used with specific instructions. They are arranged in alphabetical order by name, and many of the services contained in this section include multiple administrations of identical tests. For example, the glucagon tolerance panel (code 80422) includes three glucose tests (code 82947) and three insulin studies (code 83525). The service for all six tests would be coded and billed as 80422, with days or units of one.

CONSULTATION (CLINICAL PATHOLOGY) (80500-80504)

Codes 80500 and 80502 are for use by the pathologist only. These codes apply to the opinion rendered by request from a pathologist concerning a pathologic specimen (pathology consultation). In instances in which the consultation is limited to an expert opinion only with the review of the patient's records, code 80500 would be appropriate. When patient records are reviewed as part of the consultant's response to the requesting party, code 80502 would be appropriate.

Evaluation and management consultation codes may also be used when the consultation or requested opinion concerning the patient's condition requires that the pathologist consider history, examination, and medical decision making.

Codes 88321 to 88334 are also consultation codes used by the pathologist for opinions on slides only, which are discussed later in this chapter.

URINALYSIS (81000-81099)

This section includes codes for several methods of urinalysis. When not specified in documentation, the most basic level of service is implied. In the case of pathology, the most basic service is an automated test rather than a manual one. Automated tests require less medical decision making and are less complex for the pathologist. In the urinalysis section, dipstick urinalysis is considered the least significant, followed by automated urinalysis.

STOP AND PRACTICE

Using the steps covered thus far in this chapter, capture the appropriate information for the following pathology services.

1. Adrenocorticotropic hormone (ACTH) stimulation panel for adrenal insufficiency
   Step 1: Chapter: Pathology ______
   Step 2: Subsection: ______
   Step 3: Specific service: ______
   Step 4: Specific technique: ______
   Step 5: Additional information: ______
   Step 6: CPT code(s): ______
2. Dipstick urinalysis
   Step 1: Chapter: Pathology ______
   Step 2: Subsection: ______
   Step 3: Specific service: ______
   Step 4: Specific technique: ______
   Step 5: Additional information: ______
   Step 6: CPT code(s): ______
3. Automated urinalysis
   Step 1: Chapter: Pathology ______
   Step 2: Subsection: ______
   Step 3: Specific service: ______
   Step 4: Specific technique: ______
   Step 5: Additional information: ______
   Step 6: CPT code(s): ______
4. Limited clinical consultation
   Step 1: Chapter: Pathology ______
   Step 2: Subsection: ______
   Step 3: Specific service: ______
   Step 4: Specific technique: ______
   Step 5: Additional information: ______
   Step 6: CPT code(s): ______
5. Urine pregnancy test
   Step 1: Chapter: Pathology ______
   Step 2: Subsection: ______
   Step 3: Specific service: ______
   Step 4: Specific technique: ______
   Step 5: Additional information: ______
   Step 6: CPT code(s): ______
6. Glucagon tolerance panel
   Step 1: Chapter: Pathology ______
   Step 2: Subsection: ______
   Step 3: Specific service: ______
   Step 4: Specific technique: ______
   Step 5: Additional information: ______
   Step 6: CPT code(s): ______
7. Growth hormone stimulation panel
   Step 1: Chapter: Pathology ______
   Step 2: Subsection: ______
   Step 3: Specific service: ______
   Step 4: Specific technique: ______
   Step 5: Additional information: ______
   Step 6: CPT code(s): ______
8. Qualitative urinalysis
   Step 1: Chapter: Pathology ______
   Step 2: Subsection: ______
   Step 3: Specific service: ______
   Step 4: Specific technique: ______
   Step 5: Additional information: ______
   Step 6: CPT code(s): ______
9. Insulin tolerance panel (for ACTH insufficiency)
   Step 1: Chapter: Pathology ______
   Step 2: Subsection: ______
   Step 3: Specific service: ______
   Step 4: Specific technique: ______
   Step 5: Additional information: ______
   Step 6: CPT code(s): ______
10. Microscopic qualitative urinalysis
    Step 1: Chapter: Pathology ______
    Step 2: Subsection: ______
    Step 3: Specific service: ______
    Step 4: Specific technique: ______
    Step 5: Additional information: ______
    Step 6: CPT code(s): ______

CHEMISTRY (82000-84999)

Performance of blood chemistry analysis is included in this section. Multiple codes may be available for testing of one agent, such as glucose. Codes are arranged in alphabetical order and can encompass multiple procedures. Tests are considered quantitative unless otherwise specified by the procedure definition.

HEMATOLOGY (85002-85999)

This section encompasses hematology and coagulation studies, including blood counts. Keep in mind that services are provided only as specified. If the method for a test is not specified, the least complicated method will be assumed. In this case, automated is less significant than manual.

IMMUNOLOGY (86000-86804)

This section identifies codes used for antibody studies and for blood bank services. Conditions of the immune system caused by the action of identified antibodies are also included.

TISSUE TYPING (86805-86849)

Services from the tissue typing section are performed for identifying antigens (e.g., human leukocyte antigen [HLA]) present on tissue (bone marrow, kidney) for the purpose of transplantation, transfusion, or assessment of the risk of genetically related diseases such as ankylosing spondylosis (HLA B-27).

STOP AND PRACTICE

Using the steps covered thus far in this chapter, capture the appropriate information for the following pathology services from the subsections just covered.

1. Albumin, serum
   Step 1: Chapter: Pathology ____________
   Step 2: Subsection: ____________
   Step 3: Specific service: ____________
   Step 4: Specific technique: ____________
   Step 5: Additional information: ____________
   Step 6: CPT code(s): ____________
2. Total bilirubin
   Step 1: Chapter: Pathology ____________
   Step 2: Subsection: ____________
   Step 3: Specific service: ____________
   Step 4: Specific technique: ____________
   Step 5: Additional information: ____________
   Step 6: CPT code(s): ____________
3. Bleeding time
   Step 1: Chapter: Pathology ____________
   Step 2: Subsection: ____________
   Step 3: Specific service: ____________
   Step 4: Specific technique: ____________
   Step 5: Additional information: ____________
   Step 6: CPT code(s): ____________
4. Automated complete blood count (CBC)
   Step 1: Chapter: Pathology ____________
   Step 2: Subsection: ____________
   Step 3: Specific service: ____________
   Step 4: Specific technique: ____________
   Step 5: Additional information: ____________
   Step 6: CPT code(s): ____________
5. Antibody, *Bordetella*
   Step 1: Chapter: Pathology ____________
   Step 2: Subsection: ____________
   Step 3: Specific service: ____________
   Step 4: Specific technique: ____________
   Step 5: Additional information: ____________
   Step 6: CPT code(s): ____________
6. Skin test, *Candida*
   Step 1: Chapter: Pathology ____________
   Step 2: Subsection: ____________
   Step 3: Specific service: ____________
   Step 4: Specific technique: ____________
   Step 5: Additional information: ____________
   Step 6: CPT code(s): ____________
7. Infectious antigen detection,
   Step 1: Chapter: Pathology ____________
   Step 2: Subsection: ____________
   Step 3: Specific service: ____________
   Step 4: Specific technique: ____________
   Step 5: Additional information: ____________
   Step 6: CPT code(s): ____________
8. Fungi culture, yeast
   Step 1: Chapter: Pathology ____________
   Step 2: Subsection: ____________
   Step 3: Specific service: ____________
   Step 4: Specific technique: ____________
   Step 5: Additional information: ____________
   Step 6: CPT code(s): ____________
9. Culture, bacterial, blood
   Step 1: Chapter: Pathology ____________
   Step 2: Subsection: ____________
   Step 3: Specific service: ____________
   Step 4: Specific technique: ____________
   Step 5: Additional information: ____________
   Step 6: CPT code(s): ____________
10. Pinworm exam
   Step 1: Chapter: Pathology ____________
   Step 2: Subsection: ____________
   Step 3: Specific service: ____________
   Step 4: Specific technique: ____________
   Step 5: Additional information: ____________
   Step 6: CPT code(s): ____________

TRANSFUSION MEDICINE (86850-86999)

Most blood bank procedures are located in this section.

MICROBIOLOGY (87001-87999)

This section includes bacteriology, virology, and parasitology assays. These codes include culture, organism identification, and sensitivity studies. When it is medically necessary to perform the same test on multiple specimens or sites, modifier 59 should be appended to the subsequent codes.

ANATOMIC PATHOLOGY (88000-88099)

This section includes postmortem examinations, including autopsies, and cytopathologic and cytogenetic studies. Codes from 88141 to 88175 are used to report cervical and vaginal tests. Codes from 88150 to 88154 should be used for Pap smears that are examined with a method other than the Bethesda method. Codes from 88164 to 88167 should be used for Pap smears with the Bethesda method. For specimens collected in fluid, commonly known as Thin-Prep, codes from 88142 to 88143 should be assigned.

SURGICAL PATHOLOGY (88300-88399)

Surgical pathology involves gross and microscopic specimens sent to pathology for examination and evaluation. Each specimen is identified by the anatomic location from which it came, type of pathologic examination requested, and tissue type. When multiple tissues are received together as a single specimen or are not individually identified, they may not be charged separately.

Services are divided into the following six levels:

Level I	Specimens that normally do not need microscopic evaluation
Level II	Tissue removed, no probability of malignancy
Level III	Tissue with low probability of malignancy
Level IV	Tissue with a higher probability for malignancy or other possible disease
Level V	Complex pathology evaluations
Level VI	Examination of neoplastic tissue or complex specimens

STOP AND PRACTICE

Using the steps covered thus far in this chapter, capture the appropriate information for the following pathology services from the subsections just covered.

1. Blood typing, ABO
   Step 1: Chapter: Pathology ____________
   Step 2: Subsection: ____________
   Step 3: Specific service: ____________
   Step 4: Specific technique: ____________
   Step 5: Additional information: ____________
   Step 6: CPT code(s): ____________
2. Blood typing, Rh
   Step 1: Chapter: Pathology ____________
   Step 2: Subsection: ____________
   Step 3: Specific service: ____________
   Step 4: Specific technique: ____________
   Step 5: Additional information: ____________
   Step 6: CPT code(s): ____________
3. Cytopathology, cervical
   Step 1: Chapter: Pathology ____________
   Step 2: Subsection: ____________
   Step 3: Specific service: ____________
   Step 4: Specific technique: ____________
   Step 5: Additional information: ____________
   Step 6: CPT code(s): ____________
4. Surgical pathology, appendix
   Step 1: Chapter: Pathology ____________
   Step 2: Subsection: ____________
   Step 3: Specific service: ____________
   Step 4: Specific technique: ____________
   Step 5: Additional information: ____________
   Step 6: CPT code(s): ____________
5. Surgical pathology, induced abortion
   Step 1: Chapter: Pathology ____________
   Step 2: Subsection: ____________
   Step 3: Specific service: ____________
   Step 4: Specific technique: ____________
   Step 5: Additional information: ____________
   Step 6: CPT code(s): ____________
6. Surgical pathology, spontaneous abortion
   Step 1: Chapter: Pathology ____________
   Step 2: Subsection: ____________
   Step 3: Specific service: ____________
   Step 4: Specific technique: ____________
   Step 5: Additional information: ____________
   Step 6: CPT code(s): ____________
7. Surgical pathology, mastectomy, regional lymph nodes
   Step 1: Chapter: Pathology ____________
   Step 2: Subsection: ____________
   Step 3: Specific service: ____________
   Step 4: Specific technique: ____________
   Step 5: Additional information: ____________
   Step 6: CPT code(s): ____________
8. Postmortem examination, gross only
   Step 1: Chapter: Pathology ____________
   Step 2: Subsection: ____________
   Step 3: Specific service: ____________
   Step 4: Specific technique: ____________
   Step 5: Additional information: ____________
   Step 6: CPT code(s): ____________
9. Irradiation of blood product, two units
   Step 1: Chapter: Pathology ____________
   Step 2: Subsection: ____________
   Step 3: Specific service: ____________
   Step 4: Specific technique: ____________
   Step 5: Additional information: ____________
   Step 6: CPT code(s): ____________
10. Leukocyte transfusion
   Step 1: Chapter: Pathology ____________
   Step 2: Subsection: ____________
   Step 3: Specific service: ____________
   Step 4: Specific technique: ____________
   Step 5: Additional information: ____________
   Step 6: CPT code(s): ____________

TRANSCUTANEOUS IN VIVO PROCEDURES (88400-88741)

When bilirubin and hemoglobins are assessed transcutaneously on a viable fetus, codes from this subsection are used rather than codes from the chemistry or hematology sections.

REPRODUCTIVE MEDICINE PROCEDURES (89250-89356)

Codes in this subsection include those for studies related to the reproductive process, such as semen and sperm analysis; preservation, storage, and thawing of embryos; and other procedures necessary for reproduction and fertilization techniques.

Pathology Modifiers

After identifying services (steps 1 and 2), determining method (step 3), gathering all specific information for a service (steps 3, 4, and 5), and assigning appropriate CPT code(s) (step 6), the coder's last step (step 8) of the pathology coding process involves assigning modifier codes when appropriate. (Step 7 may be eliminated for pathology services because the order of services does not affect reimbursement hierarchy.)

Many of the modifier codes for use in the pathology section have already been discussed. They are only mentioned again for purposes of inclusion in the pathology section of this textbook.

GENERAL MODIFIERS

Modifier 22	Unusual procedural services
Modifier 26	Professional component only
Modifier 32	Mandated services
Modifier 52	Reduced services
Modifier 53	Discontinued procedures
Modifier 59	Distinct procedural services

SPECIFIC PATHOLOGY SECTION MODIFIERS

Modifier 90: Reference (Outside) Laboratory

This modifier is unique to the pathology section, although it is used minimally in some other sections of CPT as well. When services are performed by an outside laboratory, but the physician's office is billing the patient's third-party insurer for these services, modifier 90 should be appended. This enables the third-party insurer to recognize which provider rendered the services and which provider is authorized to bill for these services. If the laboratory also attempts to bill for these services, the third-party insurer can ascertain that the billing arrangement was for the physician's office to bill the insurer and the laboratory to bill the physician's office.

Centers for Medicare and Medicaid Services Alert: Note that Medicare does not allow an arrangement such as this. Medicare guidelines specify that only the party providing the services may bill for those services. This applies to all services, not just pathology services, provided to Medicare recipients.

Also of note, laboratory services (all codes within the 80000 series) are reimbursed at 100% of the Medicare allowance. Make certain the practice receives the appropriate reimbursement for these services and ensure that patients are not charged 20% coinsurance.

Modifier 91: Repeat Pathology Services

This is a relatively new modifier code specifically designed for pathology services. This modifier should be appended to pathology services only when repeat services are medically necessary. The modifier should not be used for repeat services because inadequate or insufficient specimens were previously submitted. It should be used only when the repeat pathology services are represented by the identical CPT code.

Chapter in Review

Certification Review

- Pathology services are billed as automated (least significant) when not specified as automated or manual.
- The most commonly performed pathologic services for specific diagnostic testing are grouped in the organ- and disease-oriented panels.
- The organ- and disease-oriented panels may be used only when all components are ordered. In the event that any of the services contained with the organ panel is not requested, the coder must only code each individual test performed.
- Drug testing determines whether drugs are present in the patient's system.
- Drug assays determine quantity and specific drug(s) that are present.
- Surgical pathology specimens are assigned six levels of service based on the complexity of the specimen, not necessarily the size.
- When surgical pathology specimens are not received or identified separately, they may not be charged separately.
- Two specific modifiers are used in the pathology sections, namely, modifier 90, reference (outside)

laboratory, and modifier 91, repeat pathology services.

- Medicare guidelines specify that only the provider of pathology services may bill for those services. Arrangements with pathology laboratories for physician coding or billing of laboratory-performed testing are prohibited by federal Medicare guidelines.

Student Assignments

- Study Chapter 16.
- Review the Learning Objectives for Chapter 16.
- Review the Certification Review for Chapter 16.
- Complete the Chapter Review exercise to reinforce concepts learned in the chapter.
- Complete the practice exercises on the companion Evolve site for reinforcement of pathology coding concepts.
- Complete the Practical Application exercises for real-life coding scenarios.
- Complete the Workbook exercises as assigned by your instructor, or individually for additional practice.

Chapter Review Exercise

Code the following. In some instances "no code" or "insufficient information" may be appropriate. When information is not sufficient, document the additional information required to assign an appropriate code(s).

1. Specimen received for sodium, glucose, and chloride profile
   CPT code(s): 84295, 82947, 82435
2. Automated hemogram and platelet count with complete WBC count
   CPT code(s): 85027
3. Antinuclear antibody titer
   CPT code(s): 86039
4. ABO and RH blood typing
   CPT code(s): 86900, 86901
5. Prostate specimen from a transurethral resection of the prostate
   CPT code(s): 88305
6. Thyroid disease panel
   CPT code(s): not enough info.
7. Test for presence of barbiturates, opiates, amphetamines, qualitative method
   CPT code(s): 80100 x 3
8. Metabolic panel
   CPT code(s): not enough info.
9. Surgical pathology, appendix (not incidental)
   CPT code(s): 88304
10. Bacterial culture, urine
    CPT code(s): 87086
11. PSA (prostate specific antigen)
    CPT code(s): 84152
12. Therapeutic assay, digoxin
    CPT code(s): 80162
13. Carbon dioxide, chloride, potassium, sodium (PANEL)
    CPT code(s): 80051
14. Potassium level
    CPT code(s): 84132
15. Glucose
    CPT code(s): 82947
16. Bilirubin, total
    CPT code(s): 82247
17. Surgical pathology, malignant neoplasm with partial mastectomy
    CPT code(s): 88307
18. Surgical pathology, oophorectomy
    CPT code(s): 88305
19. Chemical analysis, arsenic
    CPT code(s): 82175
20. Hemoglobin
    CPT code(s): 85018

Practical Application

Assign the appropriate CPT code(s), modifier(s), and ICD-9-CM code(s) for the following pathology reports.

1. Surgical pathology report

SURGICAL PATHOLOGY REPORT

Name: ______ Hosp. No.: ______ Path. No.: ______
Date: ______ Room: ______ Age: ______ Sex: ______ Surgeon: ______ M.D.
Operation: ______
Material submitted: Nasal Polyps
Pre-op diagnosis: ______
Post-op diagnosis: ______
Previous material: ______ Pertinent history: Sinonasal Polyposis and Pansinusitis

Diagnosis:

Nasal cavity, excision. Mild to moderate chronic sinusitis, and inflammatory nasal polyps.

Gross description:

Submitted in formalin, labeled with patient's name and "nasal polyps" are multiple fragments of tan polypoid mucosal tissue measuring approximately 1 × 1 × 0.5 cm in aggregate. Submitted in toto.

Micro description:

Slide shows multiple sections of upper respiratory mucosa and submucosa with delicate trabecular bone. Some of the fragments appear polypoid and edematous. The submucosal bowel fragments demonstrate mild to focally moderate infiltrates of small lymphocytes, plasma cells and scattered neutrophils and eosinophils.

Maria Callingwood M.D.
Pathologist

GODFREY CLINICAL LABORATORIES
465 Dogwood Court • Aldon, FL 77712 • (407) 555-9876

CPT code: ______ ICD-9-CM code: ______

2. Surgical pathology report

SURGICAL PATHOLOGY REPORT

Name: ______ Hosp. No.: ______ Path. No.: ______
Date: ______ Room: ______ Age: ______ Sex: ______ Surgeon: ______ M.D.
Operation: ______
Material submitted: Cervical Lymph Nodes
Pre-op diagnosis: ______
Post-op diagnosis: ______
Previous material: ______ Pertinent history: Recently detected several left adenopathy, R/O Malignancy

Diagnosis:

Changes consistent with lymphoid reactive hyperplasia

Gross description:

Specimen received in two parts.

The first part received in saline on crushed ice and identified "lt cervical lymph node" is a beige fragment of soft tissue which measures 2.0 × 0.5 × 1.5 cm.

The cut surface is tan-brown and focally hemorrhagic. The specimen is divided and placed in RPMI solution for cell marker study.

The second part of the specimen received in formalin and identified "lt cervical lymph node" is 1.5 × 0.5 × 0.5 cm. The cut surface is tan-brown and smooth.

The specimen is entirely submitted in two cassettes.

Micro description:

Maria Callingno M.D.
Pathologist

GODFREY CLINICAL LABORATORIES
465 Dogwood Court • Aldon, FL 77712 • (407) 555-9876

CPT code: ______ ICD-9-CM code: ______

3. Surgical pathology report

SURGICAL PATHOLOGY REPORT

Name: ______ Hosp. No.: ______ Path. No.: ______
Date: ______ Room: ______ Age: ______ Sex: ______ Surgeon: ______ M.D.
Operation: ______
Material submitted: Lung, Surgical Biopsy, Liver Needle, Surgical Biopsy
Pre-op diagnosis: ______
Post-op diagnosis: ______
Previous material: ______ Pertinent history: Lung Mass, ? Liver Mets

Diagnosis:

A. Biopsy, lung
Poorly differentiated malignancy, consistent with small cell carcinoma
B. Needle, biopsy, liver
Poorly differentiated malignancy, consistent with small cell carcinoma

Gross description:

A. Specimen is labeled as lung biopsy. Specimen consists of three tan-brown tissue fragments each measuring less than 1 mm in greatest dimension.
B. Specimen is labeled as liver biopsy. Specimen consists of four tan-brown tissue fragments each measuring less than 1 mm each.

Micro description:

Slides reviewed

Maria Callignon M.D.
Pathologist

GODFREY CLINICAL LABORATORIES
465 Dogwood Court • Aldon, FL 77712 • (407) 555-9876

CPT code: ______ ICD-9-CM code: ______

4. Hematology tests

Test Names	Result	Normal Range
Protime	10.6	10.5-13.0 seconds
International normalized ratio	0.8 L	2.0-3.0 ratio
Partial thromboplastin time	30.9	22.0-35.0 seconds

CPT code: ______ ICD-9-CM code: ______

5. Autopsy report

Microscopic Examination

Heart: Sections of the heart show thin epicardium. Marked hypertrophy of myocardial fibers. Nuclei quite large, irregular in shape and size.

Lungs: Multiple sections of lung show large distended alveolar spaces filled in some areas with fibrinous exudates and numbers of neutrophils. Alveolar walls are thickened and edematous. Vessels are congested, moderate numbers of neutrophils. Some of the bronchi are quite dilated. Cross-section of a small artery shows the lumen filled with a thrombus. Focal areas of fibrosis of the lung are also noted.

Liver: Multiple small fatty vacuoles are noted in the cytoplasm of the hepatocytes, particularly in the peripheral zones.

Pancreas: Shows normal lobular pattern.

Diagnosis:

Hypertrophic cardiomyopathy
Edema and congestion of lungs
Hypostatic bronchopneumonia, bilateral
Small infarct of lung
Fatty changes of liver

CPT code: ______ ICD-9-CM code: ______

17

Medicine Services

LEARNING OBJECTIVES

After completing this chapter, the student will be able to:

- Understand the proper documentation for medicine services.
- Understand the proper coding guidelines for each subsection of the medicine section of CPT.
- Identify the services encompassed in the medicine section of CPT.
- Comprehend the proper use of modifier codes for services provided in the medicine section of CPT.
- Understand how to code medicine section services in conjunction with other services provided in CPT by using previously acquired bundling versus separate guidelines.
- Apply medicine coding concepts to practical coding scenarios.

KEY TERMS

Chiropractic

Infusion

Injection

Intramuscularly (IM)

Intravenously (IV)

Osteopathic

Otorhinolaryngologic

Rehydration

Documentation

Because the services in the medicine section of CPT are varied, the documentation guidelines vary greatly as well. All services contained in the medicine section are considered diagnostic or therapeutic in nature; thus a physician request or order form is required, thereby beginning the documentation process. As with other ancillary services such as radiology and pathology, only documentation that is verified as reviewed may be used to determine diagnosis and procedural coding information. Many of the services contained in the medicine section include not only the request, but also the imaging services performed as well as a written or dictated report. In the absence of a written or dictated report, written documentation contained on the actual imaging can serve as documentation as long as the interpreting physician indicates the written review, date, and signature (see Chapter 2).

MEDICINE SERVICE CODES

Immune globulins	90281-90399
Immunization or vaccination administration	90465-90474
Vaccines or toxoids	90476-90749
Rehydration	90760-90761
Infusions	90760-90779
Therapeutic or diagnostic injections	90765-90779
Psychiatry	90801-90899
Biofeedback	90901-90911
Dialysis	90918-90999
Gastroenterology	91000-91299
Ophthalmology	92002-92499
Special otorhinolaryngologic services	92502-92700
Cardiovascular medicine	93000-93662
Noninvasive vascular diagnostic studies	93668-93893
Pulmonary medicine	94002-94799
Allergy and clinical immunology	95004-95199
Neurology or neuromuscular procedures	95805-96020
Central nervous system assessments	96101-96125
Health and behavior assessment or intervention	96150-96155
Chemotherapy administration	96401-96549
Photodynamic therapy	96567-96571
Special dermatologic services	96900-96999
Physical medicine and rehabilitation	97001-97799
Medical nutrition therapy	97802-97804
Acupuncture	97810-97814
Osteopathic manipulative treatment	98925-98929
Chiropractic manipulative treatment	98940-98943
Education and training for patient self-management	98960-98962
Non–face-to-face nonphysician services	98966-98968
Special supplies and services	99000-99091
Sedation with or without analgesia	99143-99150
Other services	99170-99199
Home health services	99500-99602

Because many of the services are also based on the number of units, such as extremities or hours, documentation must include information to code for the specific unit of service specified in the descriptor. Keep in mind that services must coincide verbatim with the CPT procedure code to justify assignment of that specific code. For example, if code 94681, oxygen uptake, expired gas analysis, including CO_2 output and percentage oxygen extracted, is to be assigned, the patient must have undergone a protocol that includes all the components specified by the descriptors.

Following is a breakdown of information needed to correctly assign CPT code(s) for medicine services.

CPT Coding Steps: Medicine Examples

Step 1

Identify chapter	Diagnostic Therapeutic
Range of codes	90281-99199 99500-99600

Step 2

Determine type/location	Specialty type Allergy Pulmonary

Step 3

Specific type	Specific test Pulmonary function test

Step 4

Specific procedure information	Tests

Step 5

Extent/additional specifics	Additional guidelines

A multitude of reports are used for these services because of their great variation. This section is unique in that it encompasses a variety of services rather than simply evaluation and management or surgical services. The formats in which the information is presented vary greatly. Figures 17-1, 17-2, and 17-3 show forms of documentation. As with radiologic and pathology services, for the coding or billing entity to be coded or billed for the global service, the coding or billing provider must document both the technical and interpretive reports.

Coding Guidelines

The medicine section of CPT encompasses a variety of services. Several guidelines apply specifically to each subsection of the medicine section. These are discussed later in this chapter. It is important to differentiate the services found in the medicine section of CPT from those found in the surgery section because they are often confused. Remember from the surgery section discussion of CPT (see Chapter 13) that services in the surgery section are defined as invasive,

Place top of report No. 3 here

PULMONARY FUNCTION REPORT

Name: ______
ID #: ______
Age: ______ Ht: ______ Wt: ______
Reason for test: ______
Smoker? ______
Dyspnea: ______
Lung surgery: ______
Frequent cough: ______
Pain breathing? ______
Heart disease? ______
Wheeze/asthma? ______
Abnormal X-ray? ______

Test	PRED	ACTL	%PRED
FVC	4.76		81%
FEV1	3.77		88%
FEV1/FVC	81%		107%
FEF 25%–75%	4.64		124%
MMET (sec.)	0.68		49%
FEF max	9.14		127%
FEF 25%	8.43		126%
FEF 50%	6.26		118%
FEF 75%	3.17		56%
ET (sec.)	—		—
Maximal FVC	4.76		81%
Maximal FEV1	3.77		88%
MVV (L/min.)	154.7		100%

BTPS factor: ______ Last cal: ______
Primary normals source: Knudson.

Base: ______
T ______

Operator: ______

Physician: ______

GODFREY CLINICAL LABORATORIES
465 Dogwood Court • Aldon, FL 77712 • (407) 555-9876

FIGURE 17-1. Pulmonary report.

ELECTROMYOGRAPHY LABORATORY REPORT

Nerve conduction studies

Name: ______________________
Clinic number: ____________ Age: ____
Birthdate: ________ Date: __________
Referring physician: ______________

NR = No response
M = Motor
S = Sensory
Mx = Mixed
• = no increment after 10 sec. exercise
† = no decrement to 2/sec x3
X = Forearm median to ulnar crossover

Nerve stimulated	(Recording site)	**Amplitude** (Sensory = uV; Meter = mV) Distal			Proximal		**Distal/peak latency** (mSec)			**Conduction velocity** (M/sec)			**F-wave latency** (mSec)		
		Right	Left	Normal	Rt	Lt	Rt	Lt	Normal	Rt	Lt	Normal	Rt	Lt	Normal
Lower right															
Sural (S) Pt.B	ankle						NH								
Peroneal (M) knee	EDB	3.0					14.8			45					
Peroneal (M) ankle	EDB	3.0					4.8								
Posterior tibia (M) knee	AH	1.0					14.8			41					
Posterior tibia (M) ankle	AH	1.5					4.2								
H-reflex							NR	NR							
Med (s) wrist	1st	9.0					3.6								
Med (m) elbow	thenar	2.8					9.6			58					
Med (m) wrist	thenar	2.8					4.4								
Ulnar (s) wrist	5th	1440					2.8								

Needle examination:

Summary:

Impression:

__________________, M.D.

GODFREY CLINICAL LABORATORIES
465 Dogwood Court • Aldon, FL 77712 • (407) 555-9876

FIGURE 17-2. Electromyography.

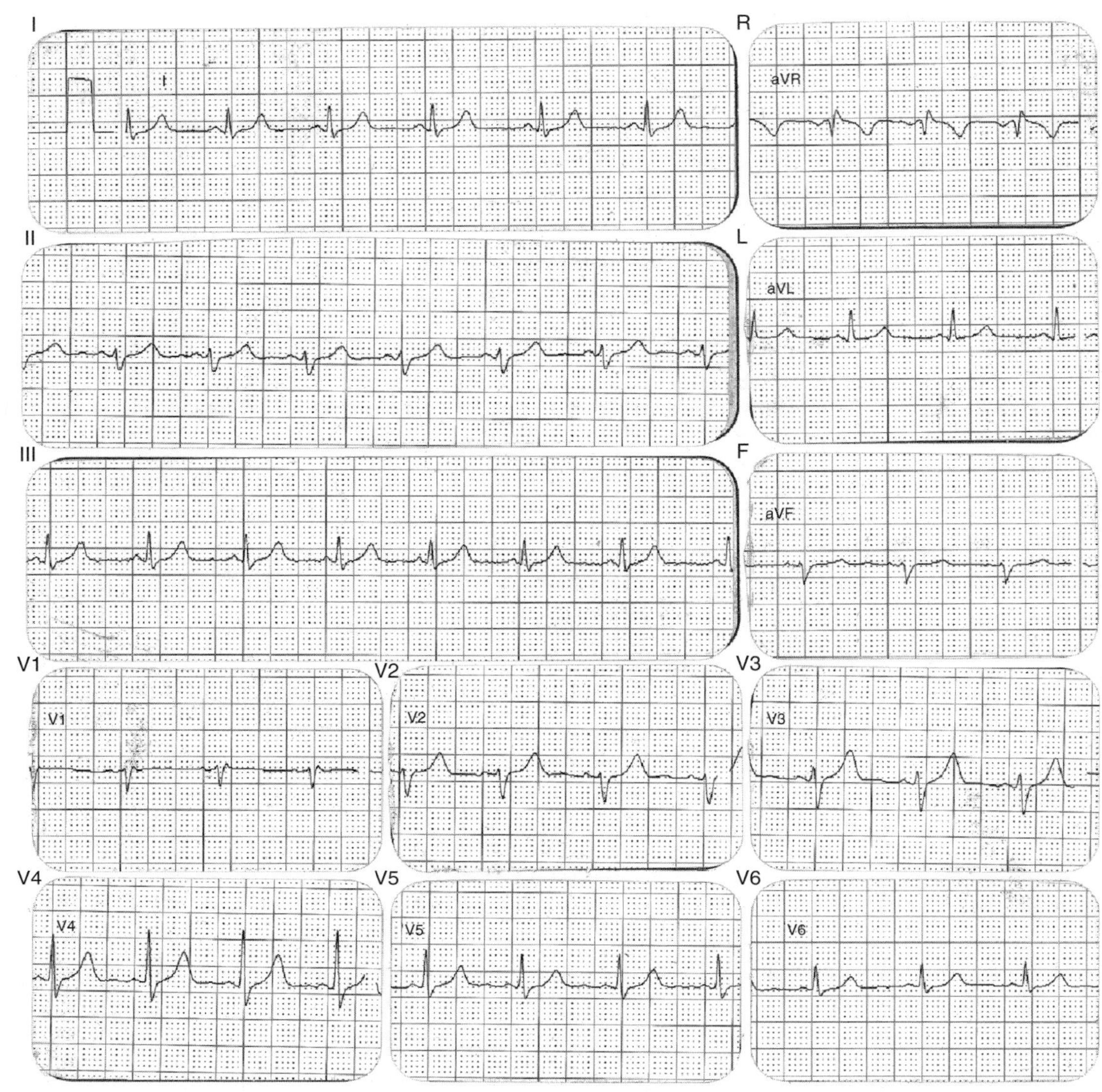

CLIN. DIAG.: Chest Pain

ECG DESCRIPTION: Stat 12 Lead

INTERPRETATION:

PATIENT: Jane Doe

DIG ( ) QUIN. ( ) AGE 29 SEX F B.P. 120/80

ECG REQUEST BY Dr. Hope U. Arewell

ATR. RATE 90 VENTR. RATE 90

INTERVALS: P-R .12 QRS .08 QTc

AXIS: Left Axis shift

RHYTHM: Normal Sinus Rhythm

INTERPRETED BY: H. Arewell MD

DATE:

FIGURE 17-3. Electrocardiography.

definitive, or restorative. Services contained in the medicine section, in contrast, are typically diagnostic, therapeutic, or both. Most of the services contained in this section will not necessarily resolve a condition but rather diagnose or treat the problem.

MODIFIERS

Because the explanation regarding modifiers for the medicine section have been presented in other sections of this book, they are listed here only for convenience.

Modifier 22	Unusual procedural services
Modifier 26	Professional component only
Modifier 32	Mandated services
Modifier 50	Bilateral procedures
Modifier 51	Multiple procedures
Modifier 52	Reduced services
Modifier 53	Discontinued procedures
Modifier 58	Related or staged procedure by same doctor during global surgical period
Modifier 59	Distinct procedure services
Modifier 62	Two surgeons
Modifier 66	Surgical team
Modifier 76	Repeat procedure by same physician
Modifier 77	Repeat procedure by another physician
Modifier 78	Return to OR for related procedure during global or postoperative period
Modifier 79	Unrelated procedure or service by same doctor during global or postoperative period
Modifier 80	Assistant surgeon
Modifier 90	Outside or reference laboratory services
Modifier 99	Multiple modifiers

Refer to Chapter 9 for a complete summary of codes, their definitions, and their proper use.

CORRECT CODING INITIATIVE GUIDELINES

There are a number of National Correct Coding Initiative (NCCI) guidelines pertinent to medicine services. Because the services vary greatly from one subsection to another, specific guidelines will be provided with each subsection.

STEPS IN CODING FROM THE MEDICINE SECTION

Step 1: Determine the specific subsection for medicine services.
Step 2: Identify the procedure performed.
Step 3 Determine extent of procedure performed.
Step 4: Select appropriate code(s).
Step 5: Assign modifier code(s) when appropriate.

Coding of Specific Medicine Subsections

IMMUNE GLOBULINS (CODES 90281-90399)

These codes identify the immune globulin product only. For administration of these products, the coder must select the appropriate injection code from codes 96365 through 96375. Immune globulins are proteins produced in lymph tissue that function as antibodies in the immune response.

Codes from the immune globulin subsection are assigned for the product only and are categorized by the type of immune globulin, method of administration, and the type of dose, such as full dose or mini-dose.

IMMUNIZATION OR VACCINATION ADMINISTRATION (CODES 90465-90474)

These codes include the administration of the vaccine only, not the vaccine material for **injection**. Codes from range 90476 to 90749 should be assigned as well as the appropriate administration code(s). Codes from this subsection are divided according to the route of administration, such as oral, intranasal, injection, or percutaneous. Codes are further categorized by the age of the patient as well as whether the administration is for a single vaccine or toxoid or a multiple-combination vaccine or toxoid. An example of a multiple-combination vaccine would be the measles, mumps, and rubella (MMR) vaccine, which is administered prophylactically.

VACCINES OR TOXOIDS (CODES 90476-90749)

The codes in this section are intended for the provision of vaccine or toxoid supplies only. If the vaccine or toxoid is provided and administered, make certain to bill the appropriate administration code (90465-90474), as well as the proper vaccine or toxoid code. Note that many codes in this section are age specific, so make certain that information on patient age is considered when the code is selected.

Many of the services defined in this section are preventive in nature, so some insurance carriers will not reimburse for these services. Medicare, however, does cover the pneumococcal pneumonia vaccination and the hepatitis B vaccine in specific instances.

PSYCHIATRY (CODES 90801-90899)

Because many services performed by psychiatric staff may not meet the requirements for evaluation and management (E & M) services, these services are encompassed in the psychiatric subsection of the medicine section.

A word of caution when coding and billing for services provided from the psychiatric section: many insurance carriers will not pay for services provided by other than a licensed physician or credentialed provider. Make certain to incorporate this information in the third-party contract worksheet to ensure only authorized providers render these services.

Many codes listed in the psychiatry medicine section specify where the services are provided, and some may be physician specific. Make certain the services are provided only by authorized providers and that the claim correctly reflects this information.

Psychiatric therapeutic services are categorized as insight oriented, behavior modifying, or interactive and are divided according to location. Interactive therapy is typically provided to children or individuals who have difficulty communicating for other reasons. Insight-oriented or behavior-modifying psychotherapy involves the use of supportive interaction and discussion to provide therapeutic change.

Time is an integral component to assigning the correct code for psychotherapy. Codes are assigned based on 20- to 30-minute, 45- to 50-minute, or 75- to 80-minute increments. Obviously the psychiatric provider must make certain this time element is documented to code these services correctly.

In instances when psychotherapy is provided in conjunction with an E & M service, combination codes such as 90805, individual psychotherapy, insight oriented, behavior modifying and/or supporting, in an office or outpatient facility, approximately 20 to 30 minutes face-to-face with the patient; with medical evaluation and management services, would be appropriate.

The following steps are used to determine the correct psychiatry codes:

Step 1: Determine whether the service should be coded from the E & M section or from the psychiatry/medicine section.

Step 2: Determine procedure performed.

Services are divided by the following:

- Office or other outpatient
- Inpatient, partial hospital, or residential care

Step 3: Determine extent or type of service

- Insight oriented or behavior modifying
- Development of behavior modification and of insight and supportive therapy necessary to provide therapeutic change
- Interactive
- Use of play equipment, physical devices, or other means of nonverbal communication to effect therapeutic change

Step 4: Determine appropriate code(s) based on time

- Keep in mind the "rounding" rule: half or more of a time unit must be provided before a specific code can be used. This means that all psychiatric medicine codes involving time MUST include its proper documentation.

In addition to the insight-oriented and interactive psychotherapy codes, other psychotherapy codes are included in the psychiatry/medicine section; these encompass group and family therapy and psychiatric services such as electroconvulsive therapy.

BIOFEEDBACK (CODES 90901-90911)

Biofeedback training is encompassed in these codes; a code is included for each modality as well as specific codes for perianal, anorectal, or urethral sphincter training. Biofeedback includes the process of giving the patient information to gain control of physiologic processes such as blood pressure control, pain control, or urinary incontinence control.

DIALYSIS (CODES 90935-90999)

Dialysis is not considered a surgical procedure. Dialysis codes are found in the medicine section. Because services for dialysis patients are typically provided on a scheduled basis in the course of a month, many of the units for these codes include months.

Patients with end-stage renal disease (ESRD) require regular dialysis and management. The breakdown for codes that cover these services is as follows:

- Age of the patient (codes are specific to patient age)
- Length of time services were performed (codes available for full or partial month)
- The type of services (ESRD or hemodialysis)

Training and hemoperfusion codes are also included in the dialysis section. Remember that services performed that meet criteria for codeable services should be coded and billed whether or not a given carrier provides reimbursement.

Codes 90967 to 90970, referred to as *end-stage renal disease services,* are intended to encompass renal services necessary for the patient with ESRD during a specified period. Codes 90951 to 90966 are intended to be used when an entire calendar month of services is performed, whereas codes 90967 to 90970 are intended to be used when less than a full month of services is performed. Note this code range is specified as "per day"; therefore for each date of service these ESRD services are provided an additional unit of service should be assigned. For example:

ESRD services, 80 year old, 02/02/10-02/05/10

These services were provided for 4 days only; therefore codes from the 90967 to 90970 range should be assigned. Four units of services were provided, so the services would be coded as follows:

90970 Days/units: 4

Dialysis services are categorized by hemodialysis, or the routing of blood and waste products outside the body, and peritoneal dialysis, which uses the peritoneal cavity. In the case of Medicare patients receiving dialysis services, note that applicable HCPCS codes should be assigned for these services. Codes G0308 to G0319 are used for hemodialysis and G0320 to G0327 for peritoneal dialysis for Medicare-eligible patients.

STOP AND PRACTICE

Using guidelines for vaccine, immunization, infusion and injection, psychiatry, biofeedback, and dialysis services, determining the correct code(s) for the following:

1. Supportive psychotherapy, 25 minutes, office
   Step 1 Subsection medicine services: ____________
   Step 2 Procedure performed: ____________
   Step 3 Extent of procedure performed: ____________
   Step 4 Appropriate code(s): ____________
   Step 5 Assign modifier code(s) when appropriate: ____________
2. ESRD services, 02/01-02/24, 21-year-old male
   Step 1 Subsection medicine services: ____________
   Step 2 Procedure performed: ____________
   Step 3 Extent of procedure performed: ____________
   Step 4 Appropriate code(s): ____________
   Step 5 Assign modifier code(s) when appropriate: ____________
3. Administration and provision of tetanus/diphtheria toxoid, absorbed
   Step 1 Subsection medicine services: ____________
   Step 2 Procedure performed: ____________
   Step 3 Extent of procedure performed: ____________
   Step 4 Appropriate code(s): ____________
   Step 5 Assign modifier code(s) when appropriate: ____________
4. Anthrax toxoid administration and provision, SQ
   Step 1 Subsection medicine services: ____________
   Step 2 Procedure performed: ____________
   Step 3 Extent of procedure performed: ____________
   Step 4 Appropriate code(s): ____________
   Step 5 Assign modifier code(s) when appropriate: ____________
5. IV hydration, 1 hour 45 minutes
   Step 1 Subsection medicine services: ____________
   Step 2 Procedure performed: ____________
   Step 3 Extent of procedure performed: ____________
   Step 4 Appropriate code(s): ____________
   Step 5 Assign modifier code(s) when appropriate: ____________
6. Administration of IV Pepcid, 1 hr 10 minutes
   Step 1 Subsection medicine services: ____________
   Step 2 Procedure performed: ____________
   Step 3 Extent of procedure performed: ____________
   Step 4 Appropriate code(s): ____________
   Step 5 Assign modifier code(s) when appropriate: ____________
7. Administration of IM antibiotics
   Step 1 Subsection medicine services: ____________
   Step 2 Procedure performed: ____________
   Step 3 Extent of procedure performed: ____________
   Step 4 Appropriate code(s): ____________
   Step 5 Assign modifier code(s) when appropriate: ____________
8. Inpatient supportive psychotherapy, 20 minutes
   Step 1 Subsection medicine services: ____________
   Step 2 Procedure performed: ____________
   Step 3 Extent of procedure performed: ____________
   Step 4 Appropriate code(s): ____________
   Step 5 Assign modifier code(s) when appropriate: ____________
9. Family psychotherapy with patient present
   Step 1 Subsection medicine services: ____________
   Step 2 Procedure performed: ____________
   Step 3 Extent of procedure performed: ____________
   Step 4 Appropriate code(s): ____________
   Step 5 Assign modifier code(s) when appropriate: ____________
10. Administration of IV Heparin, 10:00 AM to 1:15 PM
    Step 1 Subsection medicine services: ____________
    Step 2 Procedure performed: ____________
    Step 3 Extent of procedure performed: ____________
    Step 4 Appropriate code(s): ____________
    Step 5 Assign modifier code(s) when appropriate: ____________

GASTROENTEROLOGY (CODES 91000-91299)

Some gastroenterologic (GI) procedures are included in the medicine section rather than the surgical section because many are noninvasive. Keep in mind that guidelines for the medicine section should be followed for these services, but GI surgical procedures follow surgery guidelines for coding and billing. Placement of tubes (intestinal bleeding tubes, esophageal intubation) and GI studies are included in this section. Also, providers who are not GI physicians commonly use the gastric intubation code 91105.

A relatively new procedure referred to as *capsule endoscopy* is also located in the gastroenterology section. This procedure involves endoscopy of the GI system through the use of a capsule placed in the GI tract for imaging. The capsule captures imaging for a period and then is expelled through the natural digestive process over time.

OPHTHALMOLOGY (CODES 92002-92499)

As with psychiatry, a number of services provided by ophthalmologists do not meet the E & M guidelines for physician services. Again, services provided in the medicine section of CPT are considered diagnostic or therapeutic rather than invasive, restorative, or definitive in nature. The breakdown is as follows:

- New patient or established patient status

  Keep in mind the new patient rules previously discussed. If the patient has already been seen by the physician or a member of his or her group within the last 3 years, that patient is considered an established patient.
- Level of service provided

  Intermediate—includes history, general medical observation, external ocular and adnexal examination, and other diagnostic procedures.

  Comprehensive—includes a general evaluation of the **complete** visual system. These services constitute a single service, but they may be provided over more than one visit. These services include the following:
  - History
  - General medical observation
  - External or ophthalmoscopic examination
  - Gross visual fields
  - Basic sensorimotor examination

  Special—includes special evaluation of part of the visual system.

In addition, the following special ophthalmologic services are included in this section:

- Refractive state determination
- Contact lens fitting
- Visual field examination
- Tonometry
- Tonography
- Ophthalmoscopy

The ophthalmology section differentiates between contact lens services provided for the patient with impaired vision, such as myopia, and those performed for the patient with aphakia. Make certain that the correct code is selected on the basis of the medical data and that these data are included in the medical record. In many instances third-party carriers do not reimburse for contact lens services other than for the diagnosis of aphakia, so when this diagnosis is appropriate it is important that it be included for proper reimbursement.

The codes for the fitting of eyeglasses are similarly divided into nonaphakia and aphakia diagnoses, as are the supply codes listed in this section.

SPECIAL OTORHINOLARYNGOLOGIC SERVICES (CODES 92502-92700)

Only ear-nose-throat (ENT) services not typically included in a comprehensive E & M visit are listed in this section. Again, note that these services are typically diagnostic or therapeutic in nature. These include the following:

- Treatment of speech disorders
- Vestibular function tests
- Audiologic function tests (include such tests as hearing tests, hearing aid checks or testing, and other hearing-specific diagnostic testing)

A number of codes in the otorhonolaryngologic section are specific to the provider-type. NCCI guidelines indicate the following regarding providers of services for these ENT services:

- Codes 92507, 92508, and 92525 are intended for use by speech-language pathologists.
- Codes 97110, 97112, 097150, 97530, and 97532 are typically performed by occupational or physical therapists.

With the increasing use of cochlear implants for the correction of hearing defects, additional codes have been added for the diagnostic analysis of these implants (92601, 92603) and subsequent reprogramming (92602, 92604).

CARDIOVASCULAR MEDICINE (CODES 92950-93799)

The practice of cardiology is typically divided into at least the following three subspecialties:

1. Noninvasive cardiology
2. Cardiovascular surgery
3. Electrophysiology

Procedures typically performed by the cardiovascular surgeon have already been discussed in the cardiac subsection of the surgery section. Procedures that are noninvasive appear in the medicine section of CPT.

For this section, the coder may disregard the rule that includes approach for a procedure within the procedure code. When cardiac catheterization is provided in conjunction with other cardiac services listed in this section, such as balloon angioplasty, both services may be billed. Note that procedures in this section are somewhat progressive in nature. Many of the more involved cardiac procedures are inclusive of services listed elsewhere. For example, atherectomy includes performance with or without balloon angioplasty.

A problem encountered in coding these noninvasive procedures is that some procedures (e.g., placement of stents, balloon angioplasty, atherectomy) are coded and billed by each vessel treated. For purposes of coding these services, CPT and the American College of Cardiology recognize only three main vessels and the corresponding modifiers:

LC	Left circumflex coronary artery
LD	Left anterior descending coronary artery
RC	Right coronary artery

Branch vessels from these three arteries are included in the services. For example, when two stents are placed in the same vessel (e.g., right coronary), only one code (92980) should be selected. The three vessels are identified by modifiers LC, LD, and RC to denote the specific vessel. These modifier codes represent HCPCS national level II modifier codes and are not recognized by all third-party carriers. Should the practice perform these services, the coder must incorporate into the submission of claims the codes for which third-party carriers want these modifiers to be included.

As with many specialized services, there is a progression of both service level and associated medical necessity for these services. The scenario in Chapter 14 in which a few students rather than the whole group received thallium stress tests is an example. This is especially true in the cardiology section. Medicare and many other third-party carriers have specific diagnostic codes considered medically necessary for low-level services, such as electrocardiograms (ECGs); higher level services require a more specific comprehensive diagnostic statement before reimbursement will be considered.

Cardiac catheterization is the medical diagnostic procedure that involves introduction, positioning, and repositioning of the catheter in addition to the recording of measurements. When angiography is performed in conjunction with a cardiac catheterization, each angiography code may be billed in addition to the cardiac catheterization. Angiography requires dye injection. Codes for the injection, the angiography, and heart catheterization are therefore appropriate. Modifier 51 is not necessary for these services because it is assumed multiple codes or services are provided during one session. According to NCCI guidelines, when withdrawing the catheter during a cardiac catheterization, providers may inject a small amount of dye to examine the renal arteries and/or iliac arteries. If these services are medically necessary, they may be reported with HCPCS codes G0275 or G0278. Code 75722 and 75724 should not be assigned for the renal arteries unless the renal artery is catheterized and a complete renal angiogram is performed and interpreted. Any ECG tracings performed during the course of the cardiac catheterization are not separately reportable as well as any fluoroscopy codes.

Figure 17-4 outlines the components in assigning codes for the performance of a cardiac catheterization and associated services.

Electrophysiologic procedures are also included in the noninvasive cardiology subchapter of the medicine section. Note that the procedures in this section are noninvasive, and the implantation or removal of pacemakers and stimulators is included in the cardiac surgery section. Analysis of pacemaker function is included in the "other vascular studies" section of the cardiology subsection.

A number of other services are included in the cardiovascular subsection of the Medicine section of CPT. Some of these services may be performed by a number of physicians, not just cardiologists. For example, ECGs are performed in many physician offices as well as in the hospital. In some instance codes are provided for the global services (including both the technical and professional components), such as 93000, as well as codes for the same service for only the professional component (code 93010) and a code for only the technical component (code 93005). It would be inappropriate to code both 93005 and 93010 for the global ECG (technical and professional components) rather than code or bill 93000.

Cardiopulmonary resuscitation (CPR) is also included in the cardiovascular subsection. When CPR is performed independently without other physician evaluation services, code 92950 would be assigned. If critical care or other time-driven evaluation and management services are performed during the same encounter, the time required for CPT is not included in the critical care time.

Routine cardiac rhythm monitoring should not be assigned codes 93040 to 03042 because these codes were intended for diagnostic rhythm ECG testing only.

NONINVASIVE VASCULAR DIAGNOSTIC STUDIES (CODES 93875-93990)

Noninvasive vascular diagnostic studies are divided into the following groups:

- Cerebrovascular arterial studies
- Extremity arterial studies
- Extremity venous studies
- Visceral and penile vascular studies
- Extremity arteriovenous studies

STOP AND PRACTICE

Using the guidelines for gastroenterology, ophthalmology, otorhinolaryngology, cardiovascular and vascular studies, determine the correct code(s) for the following:

1. Gastric intubation
   Step 1 Subsection medicine services: ____________
   Step 2 Procedure performed: ____________
   Step 3 Extent of procedure performed: ____________
   Step 4 Appropriate code(s): ____________
   Step 5 Assign modifier code(s) when appropriate: ____________

2. Fitting of bifocal lenses (spectacles)
   Step 1 Subsection medicine services: ____________
   Step 2 Procedure performed: ____________
   Step 3 Extent of procedure performed: ____________
   Step 4 Appropriate code(s): ____________
   Step 5 Assign modifier code(s) when appropriate: ____________

3. Auditory evoked potential
   Step 1 Subsection medicine services: ____________
   Step 2 Procedure performed: ____________

STOP AND PRACTICE—cont'd

Step 3 Extent of procedure performed: ___________
Step 4 Appropriate code(s): ___________
Step 5 Assign modifier code(s) when appropriate: ___________

4. Gastric motility study
   Step 1 Subsection medicine services: ___________
   Step 2 Procedure performed: ___________
   Step 3 Extent of procedure performed: ___________
   Step 4 Appropriate code(s): ___________
   Step 5 Assign modifier code(s) when appropriate: ___________
5. ECG, interpretation and report only
   Step 1 Subsection medicine services: ___________
   Step 2 Procedure performed: ___________
   Step 3 Extent of procedure performed: ___________
   Step 4 Appropriate code(s): ___________
   Step 5 Assign modifier code(s) when appropriate: ___________
6. Left heart catheterization
   Right coronary injection/angiography
   Left ventricle injection/angiography
   Step 1 Subsection medicine services: ___________
   Step 2 Procedure performed: ___________
   Step 3 Extent of procedure performed: ___________
   Step 4 Appropriate code(s): ___________
   Step 5 Assign modifier code(s) when appropriate: ___________
7. Left heart catheterization
   Right coronary injection/angiography
   Left ventricle injection/angiography
   2 Stents, coronary vessel
   1 Balloon angioplasty, coronary vessel
   Step 1 Subsection medicine services: ___________
   Step 2 Procedure performed: ___________
   Step 3 Extent of procedure performed: ___________
   Step 4 Appropriate code(s): ___________
   Step 5 Assign modifier code(s) when appropriate: ___________
8. Cardiovascular stress test, technical, tracing only
   Step 1 Subsection medicine services: ___________
   Step 2 Procedure performed: ___________
   Step 3 Extent of procedure performed: ___________
   Step 4 Appropriate code(s): ___________
   Step 5 Assign modifier code(s) when appropriate: ___________
9. Visual fields exam, limited
   Step 1 Subsection medicine services: ___________
   Step 2 Procedure performed: ___________
   Step 3 Extent of procedure performed: ___________
   Step 4 Appropriate code(s): ___________
   Step 5 Assign modifier code(s) when appropriate: ___________
10. Diagnostic analysis, cochlear implant, 12-year-old child
   Step 1 Subsection medicine services: ___________
   Step 2 Procedure performed: ___________
   Step 3 Extent of procedure performed: ___________
   Step 4 Appropriate code(s): ___________
   Step 5 Assign modifier code(s) when appropriate: ___________

PULMONARY MEDICINE (CODES 94002-94799)

The pulmonary medicine services listed in this section are diagnostic procedures and interpretations only. When E & M services are provided in addition to these services, they may be reported with the appropriate E & M code(s).

The coder must ensure that these services are performed by the billing provider. In some instances these services may be performed in an inpatient hospital setting; in this case the services are provided by hospital staff and are only interpreted by the medical provider. When this occurs a code specific only to interpretation and reading should be used, or the appropriate code should have modifier 26 appended.

One of the most common services from this section is a nebulizer treatment, used primarily for treating asthma. The treatment involves the use of a device known as a *nebulizer* that produces a spray that, when inhaled, treats the symptoms of asthma.

Also in this section is spirometry, which is a measurement of air capacity. Also known as a *pulmonary function test* (PFT), the test may be performed by itself, as in code 94010, or before and after bronchodilators are administered to determine the effect of the bronchodilators on the patient's condition. In this case 94060 would be assigned for both before and after bronchodilator PFT.

ALLERGY AND CLINICAL IMMUNOLOGY (CODES 95004-95199)

Allergy testing encompasses procedures performed percutaneously by scratch, puncture, or prick to determine allergy sensitivities. Allergy testing may also be performed intracutaneously or with patch application.

CARDIAC CATHETERIZATION CODING

1 **Access site**

Venous/right	Codes 93501/93530
Arterial/left	Codes 93510–93524
Combined left/right	Codes 93526–93533
Catheterization performed subsequent day for therapeutic services (PTCA, stent, atherectomy where left heart cath not performed)	Code 93508

2 **Injection/imaging codes**

	Injection	Imaging
Arterial conduit	93539	93556
Aortocoronary venous bypass	93540	93556
Pulmonary	93541	93566
Selective right ventricular/atrial	93542	93555
Left ventricular/atrial	93543	93555
Aorta	93544	93556
Selective coronary	93545	93556

Coding guidelines:
Duplicate imaging codes should be deleted. Modifier 51 need not be assigned.

3 **Therapeutic procedures (when applicable)**

	1st vessel	Each addtl. vessel
PTCA (balloon angioplasty)	92982	92984
Intracoronary stent(s)	92980	92981
Atherectomy	92995	92996

Coding guidelines:
Definitive procedure only may be coded per vessel
Vessel modifiers:

LC	Left circumflex
LD	Left anterior descending
RC	Right coronary

FIGURE 17-4. Cardiac catheterization coding.

The allergen immunotherapy procedure includes professional services for the administration of allergy immunotherapy but does not include provision of the allergenic extract. Codes 95120 through 95170 include the provision of the extract as well as administration of the allergy immunotherapy. E & M codes can be billed in addition to allergen immunotherapy codes only if other E & M services are performed.

Keep in mind that the medical documentation for these services should include a verbal or written order for all allergenic extracts as well as documentation by the billing provider of allergen immunotherapy either provided or supervised by the billing provider.

Many patients with allergies present to their physicians for the sole purpose of receiving allergy immunotherapy. In many instances these patients arrive with their vials of allergenic extract, or the extract may be stored at the physician's office. In these instances only the codes for administration of that extract should be charged.

E & M codes may also be assigned for patient encounters in which a provider evaluates and manages the patient by performing a history, examination, and medical decision making during the course of the encounter. When patients present solely for the purpose of allergy immunotherapy and no history, examination, or medical decision making is performed, it would not be appropriate to assign an E & M code.

NEUROLOGY AND NEUROMUSCULAR PROCEDURES (CODES 95805-96020)

Services in this section include electroencephalogram (EEG), electromyelogram (EMG), evoked potential, and sleep services. These may be billed in addition to any E & M services provided over and above the neurologic procedures.

Routine EEG is coded according to the technique used and time. For instance, 95812 and 94813 are based on time (41 to 60 minutes and more than 1 hour, respectively), whereas codes 95816 to 95827 are based on the state of awareness (awake, drowsy, asleep, coma, all night).

EMG is assigned codes according to the number of extremities the studies are performed on, such as 95860, needle EMG, one extremity.

CENTRAL NERVOUS SYSTEM ASSESSMENTS (CODES 96101-96125)

These services, which are typically provided for testing cognitive functions, include assessment of aphasia and speech and neurobehavioral, neuropsychological, and psychological evaluation. This testing typically involves either psychological testing (96101-96103) or developmental testing (96110-96111). Other methods may also be used, including neurobehavior or neuropsychological examination or testing.

HYDRATION, THERAPEUTIC, PROPHYLACTIC, AND DIAGNOSTIC INJECTIONS AND INFUSIONS (CODES 96360-96549)

Codes from this subsection are selected according to the technique by which the medication is administered. Coding guidelines require that only one "initial" code be assigned per encounter. For instance, if an initial therapeutic infusion code is assigned and hydration is also performed, the subsequent hydration code would be required to be used. The initial code should be chosen not by which infusion or injection is performed first, but by the code that best describes the primary reason for the encounter.

When infusion codes are assigned, the following services are included and should not be coded separately:

- Any use of local anesthetic
- Intravenous start
- Access to indwelling intravenous line, such as a port or catheter
- Flushing the catheter or port at the conclusion of the infusion
- Standard tubing, syringes, and supplies necessary to perform the infusion

NCCI Guidelines

- When fluid administration is for the sole purpose of maintaining patency of access, the infusion of that substance is not separately reportable. This is often referred to in medical documentation as TKO ("to keep open") or KVO ("keep vein open").
- When fluids are administered between units of blood or blood products transfusion to maintain the line, they are not separately reportable.
- Code 99211 is not separately reportable unless a separately reportable evaluation and management service at the time of another procedure is performed.
- When services are performed in the facility setting, the infusion codes are not intended for physician use; however, they may be assigned when appropriate in the office or clinic setting.
- Flushing of a line before, during, or after administration of fluids or medications is not separately reportable.
- Drug administration services related to a surgical procedure are not separately reportable by the physician performing the procedure.

Rehydration

Codes were added to cover infusion of fluids for rehydration purposes. These codes require the initial service (code 96360) to encompass 31 minutes or more of infusion for the purpose of rehydration. This is usually accomplished with prepackaged fluids, which include fluids and sometimes the addition of potassium. Normal saline or lactated Ringer's solution are examples of fluids given for rehydration. When medications are added to the fluids, only the infusion of medications (listed under therapeutic or diagnostic injections or infusions) are coded. Additional infusion of fluids is assigned the code 96361 for each additional hour (minimum of 31 minutes per unit is required).

THERAPEUTIC OR DIAGNOSTIC INFUSIONS (EXCLUDING CHEMOTHERAPY)

These codes are intended for use in prolonged intravenous **infusion**. Code 96365 should be used when the time of infusion does not exceed 1 hour. More than 15 minutes must be documented before this service can be coded and billed. Additional 1-hour increments may be billed with code 96366. For each additional hour an infusion requiring more than half an hour (>31 minutes) must have been performed and documented. Note that when CPT codes contain the term "each," those services should NOT be billed as multiple or repeat procedures, but rather with the appropriate code and in multiple units of service in the units column of the claim form.

NCCI guidelines indicate that hydration, infusion, and chemotherapy infusion and injection codes are reportable by physicians for services performed in the physician's office. However, when performed in the hospital outpatient, inpatient, or emergency department, these services are not separately reportable by the physician. However, the facility may code or bill for these services because they are typically provided by facility personnel.

THERAPEUTIC OR DIAGNOSTIC INJECTIONS

When injections are performed subcutaneously, **intramuscularly (IM)**, intraarterially, or **intravenously (IV)**, codes from this section should be used. Make certain when coding for injection services that the name, strength, dosage, and route of medication are specified.

It is important to distinguish between an IV infusion, in which the medication is placed in a bag and infused or dripped through an IV line at a specified rate over a prolonged period, and an IV injection, sometimes referred to as *an intravenous push,* which is usually injected directly into the IV line for a quicker response to the medication. IV push or IV injections are often given for pain medications or cardiac drugs in the event of a cardiac arrest. In these circumstances fast-acting medications are essential to resolve the patient's problem, and a prolonged infusion may not be performed quickly enough.

Figure 17-5 contains the code ranges necessary for injection services. Note that a minimum of two codes are necessary in most cases (one for the provision of the drugs and one for the administration).

If chemotherapy is provided at the same encounter as the physician E & M service, both may be billed if two separate services have been provided.

Chemotherapy administration includes only the administration of the chemotherapeutic agent. The chemotherapeutic agents or drugs must be listed separately, usually with an appropriate HCPCS code (see Chapter 18).

Chemotherapy services may be provided by several routes, such as the following:

- Subcutaneous
- Intramuscular
- Intravenous
- Infusion
- Intraarterial
- Directly into the pleural cavity

Codes are also available in this section to bill for the refilling and maintenance of portable or implanted chemotherapy pumps.

Several chemotherapy administration codes are listed by the hour and, as in the diagnostic injection or infusion section, the rounding-up rule applies. Units of service are used rather than a modifier code for multiple services.

Time is important to correct coding, so documentation should include the amount of time spent performing these services. See Figure 17-5 for the ranges for coding and billing chemotherapy administration and drugs. As is the case with IV injection codes, current CPT guidelines allow only one initial infusion service per calendar date. For instance, if a patient receives chemotherapy infusion as well as another medication infusion, only the chemotherapy may be coded with an initial chemotherapy code. The medication infusion will be assigned a subsequent infusion code, as would any chemotherapy or medication IV injection during the encounter.

Also keep in mind that the chemotherapy administration codes are intended to be used for the administration of antineoplastic substances only; therefore when antiemetics are administered in conjunction with chemotherapy, these medications would be assigned codes from the medication infusion or injection codes regarding the chemotherapy administration.

According to NCCI guidelines, the flushing or irrigation of an implanted vascular access port or device before or after the administration of chemotherapeutic or nonchemotherapeutic drugs is not separately reportable.

SPECIAL DERMATOLOGIC SERVICES (CODES 96567-96999)

Actinotherapy and photochemotherapy services are included in this section. For the most part the services of the dermatologist are included in the E & M section or the integumentary subsection of the surgery section. Photodynamic therapy is the injection of an agent into the patient's body. When the substance has dissipated from the normal cells, a laser is used to destroy the remaining malignant cells.

ADMINISTRATION/PROVISION OF DRUGS/VACCINES

	Immune globulins	Vaccine/ toxoids	Medications	Chemotherapy
ADMINISTRATION	90765–90779	90465–90474	90765–90779	96400–96542
PROVISION OF MEDICINE/AGENT	90281–90399	90476–90749	99070 or HCPCS as required by specific carrier	96545 or HCPCS as required by specific carrier

FIGURE 17-5. Administration and provision of drugs, medicines, or vaccines.

PHYSICAL MEDICINE AND REHABILITATION (CODES 97001-97546)

Physical therapy is provided through the following two mechanisms:

1. *Modalities:* Any physical agent applied that produces therapeutic changes in tissue. Agents include light, mechanical, electric energy, and thermal applications. They may be delivered by two methods:
   - Supervised—Does not require the direct supervision of the provider
   - Constant attendance—Requires one-on-one contact with the provider
2. *Therapeutic procedures:* Methods that attempt to improve functionality through the application of clinical skills. The provider is required to have one-on-one contact for the services performed in this section. Procedures such as massage, gait training, and manual therapy are included in this subsection.

Many of the codes in this section are time driven (15-minute increments). Third-party (insurance) guidelines stipulate that half of that time unit must be used to code and bill for a unit of service.

ACTIVE WOUND CARE MANAGEMENT (CODES 97597-97606)

Codes from this section are used for the removal of devitalized or dead tissue to promote healing. These codes are intended for treatment of chronic, nonhealing wounds that require selective or nonselective debridement. *Selective* debridement refers to treating a specific portion of the wound, whereas *nonselective* refers to treating the entire wound and not concentrating on a particular region or area. Note that the codes from this section are designated according to square centimeters of the wound, which would be determined by the measurement of the length multiplied by the width of the wound.

OSTEOPATHIC MANIPULATIVE TREATMENT (CODES 98925-98929)

This section involves procedures performed by the physician who provides manual treatment to reduce, alleviate, or eliminate impairment. Codes from this section are assigned by the number of body regions involved, including the following:

98925	One to two body regions
98926	Three to four body regions
98927	Five to six body regions
98928	Seven to eight body regions
98929	Nine to 10 body regions

Body regions are defined as head, cervical, thoracic, lumbar, sacral, pelvic, lower extremities, upper extremities, rib cage, abdomen, and visceral regions.

CHIROPRACTIC MANIPULATIVE TREATMENT (CODES 98940-98943)

Chiropractic treatment involves procedures designed to improve joint and neurophysiologic function. These codes are assigned by the number of spinal regions, including the following:

- Cervical
- Thoracic
- Lumbar
- Sacral
- Pelvic

Five extraspinal regions are also identified as the following:

- Upper extremities
- Lower extremities
- Rib cage
- Head
- Abdomen

A premanipulation assessment of the patient is included in this section and may be coded in addition to an E & M service if the patient's condition requires significantly separately identifiable services above the usual work associated with the premanipulation assessment.

EDUCATION AND TRAINING FOR PATIENT SELF-MANAGEMENT (CODES 98960-98962)

When education or training is provided for the patient to self-manage his or her medical problem, codes from this section are used based on the number of patients.

NON–FACE-TO-FACE NONPHYSICIAN SERVICES (CODES 98966-98969)

Additional services were added to CPT in 2008 to cover the advancement of medical technology. Codes 98966 to 98968 are intended to be assigned in instances in which assessment and management of the patient are performed by telephone by a nonphysician health care professional. These codes are time based; therefore documentation of time is necessary to assign the appropriate code.

In addition, online medical evaluations are assigned code 98969 when the medical evaluation is made by electronic communication rather than face-to-face by a nonphysician health care professional.

SPECIAL SUPPLIES AND SERVICES (CODES 99000-99091)

This category represents the miscellaneous portion of the medicine section and codes that do not fit in any other category in CPT. Many services listed in this section are coded and billed. Many insurance carriers do not reimburse for these services, which include items such as educational supplies, physician educational services, and office services provided outside normal hours or the normal confines of the office. Some of these codes are delineated in the following sections.

Specimen Handling (99000)

This code should be used when a specimen must be prepared for transfer from the provider's office to a laboratory for testing. This code is discussed in the pathology section of this text (Chapter 16).

Postoperative Follow-up Care (99024)

Normal postoperative care that is an integral part of the global surgical procedure is billed with code 99024. There is usually no charge or fee associated with this code. It serves as a placeholder for counting services provided. It also statistically tracks the average number of follow-up postoperative visits needed for specific surgical cases.

This code would NOT be used for other-than-normal postoperative follow-up care. Those services would be billed with the appropriate E & M service code and the appropriate modifier code(s). This is discussed in Chapter 13 of this text (in the surgery section of CPT).

Miscellaneous Supplies and Materials (99070)

This code should NOT be used for items normally used by the physician supplying the normal E & M service. An invoice delineating the cost of the item is often requested. Make certain when using this code for medications that the name, strength, and dosage of each medication are documented on the claim.

When the provision of drugs or biologicals is coded with 99070, it is necessary to include the name of the drug, strength, dosage, and route of administration on the second line of the CMS-1500 claim form. The use of this code is shown in Figure 17-4.

SEDATION WITH OR WITHOUT ANALGESIA (CONSCIOUS SEDATION) (CODES 99143-99150)

This medical procedure, which induces a medically controlled state of reduced consciousness, may be performed IV or IM or through inhalation, oral, rectal, or intranasal routes.

OTHER SERVICES (CODES 99170-99199)

This category includes services such as administration of ipecac (99175), use of hyperbaric oxygen therapy or hypothermia, assembly and operation of oxygenator or heat exchanger, and phlebotomy when performed for therapeutic purposes.

HOME HEALTH SERVICES (CODES 99500-99602)

This category, added in 2002, incorporates codes for services and visits provided by home health providers. A physician's office would not use these codes.

STOP AND PRACTICE

Using guidelines for pulmonary, allergy, neurology, central nervous system, chemotherapy, dermatologic, physical medicine, active wound management, osteopathic and chiropractic, non–face-to-face, and special services, determine the correct code(s) for the following:

1. IV push, Antineoplastic (chemotherapy)
   Step 1 Subsection medicine services: ___________
   Step 2 Procedure performed: ___________
   Step 3 Extent of procedure performed: ___________
   Step 4 Appropriate code(s): ___________
   Step 5 Assign modifier code(s) when appropriate: ___________
2. Gait training, 27 minutes
   Step 1 Subsection medicine services: ___________
   Step 2 Procedure performed: ___________
   Step 3 Extent of procedure performed: ___________
   Step 4 Appropriate code(s): ___________
   Step 5 Assign modifier code(s) when appropriate: ___________
3. Specimen handling, from physician's office to laboratory
   Step 1 Subsection medicine services: ___________
   Step 2 Procedure performed: ___________
   Step 3 Extent of procedure performed: ___________
   Step 4 Appropriate code(s): ___________
   Step 5 Assign modifier code(s) when appropriate: ___________
4. Pulmonary function test
   Step 1 Subsection medicine services: ___________
   Step 2 Procedure performed: ___________
   Step 3 Extent of procedure performed: ___________
   Step 4 Appropriate code(s): ___________
   Step 5 Assign modifier code(s) when appropriate: ___________

STOP AND PRACTICE—cont'd

5. Neurostimulator analysis with reprogramming
   - Step 1 Subsection medicine services: ____________
   - Step 2 Procedure performed: ____________
   - Step 3 Extent of procedure performed: ____________
   - Step 4 Appropriate code(s): ____________
   - Step 5 Assign modifier code(s) when appropriate: ____________
6. Electric stimulation, constant attendance, 30 minutes
   - Step 1 Subsection medicine services: ____________
   - Step 2 Procedure performed: ____________
   - Step 3 Extent of procedure performed: ____________
   - Step 4 Appropriate code(s): ____________
   - Step 5 Assign modifier code(s) when appropriate: ____________
7. PFT with and without bronchodilator
   - Step 1 Subsection medicine services: ____________
   - Step 2 Procedure performed: ____________
   - Step 3 Extent of procedure performed: ____________
   - Step 4 Appropriate code(s): ____________
   - Step 5 Assign modifier code(s) when appropriate: ____________
8. Laser treatment psoriasis, 350 cm
   - Step 1 Subsection medicine services: ____________
   - Step 2 Procedure performed: ____________
   - Step 3 Extent of procedure performed: ____________
   - Step 4 Appropriate code(s): ____________
   - Step 5 Assign modifier code(s) when appropriate: ____________
9. Physical therapy evaluation
   - Step 1 Subsection medicine services: ____________
   - Step 2 Procedure performed: ____________
   - Step 3 Extent of procedure performed: ____________
   - Step 4 Appropriate code(s): ____________
   - Step 5 Assign modifier code(s) when appropriate: ____________
10. Pressurized nebulizer treatment
    - Step 1 Subsection Medicine services: ____________
    - Step 2 Procedure performed: ____________
    - Step 3 Extent of procedure performed: ____________
    - Step 4 Appropriate code(s): ____________
    - Step 5 Assign modifier code(s) when appropriate: ____________

Chapter in Review

Certification Review

- Services listed in the medicine section may be coded and billed by any provider who meets the description of services outlined.
- The codes for immunization or vaccine administration are to be used for administration only. Supply of the vaccine material is coded 90476 through 90749.
- When code descriptions contain the word "each," the code is used for each unit of service provided. For example, when 8 hours of a particular service are provided and the code specifies "each" hour, the service should be coded with the correct CPT code once only, with the days or units of services designated as eight.
- Services outlined in the psychiatry section indicate that some specific services must be provided by physicians only.
- Many of the psychiatry codes are divided into two categories: interactive and insight oriented.
- Several codes in the dialysis subsection are billed on a monthly basis.
- Gastroenterology services in the medicine section should follow guidelines from the medicine section, but gastroenterology services from the surgical section should follow surgical guidelines.
- Cardiovascular services recognize three main vessels for purposes of coding or billing: left circumflex, left anterior descending, and right coronary artery.
- In coding for allergy services, an E & M service may NOT be billed unless documentation supports a separately identifiable E & M service.
- The supply of drugs is coded or billed using 99070 from CPT unless the specific carrier dictates the use of HCPCS codes for medication supplies.
- Specimen handling codes are to be used only when a specimen must be prepared for transfer from a facility to the laboratory for testing purposes.
- The postoperative follow-up care code 99024 designates services that are an integral component

of the global surgery procedure. As such, they typically hold no dollar value but serve as a tracking mechanism for the number of postoperative follow-up visits needed for specific cases.

- When other-than-normal uncomplicated follow-up care is performed, the use of 99024 is NOT appropriate. Use the appropriate E & M code.

Student Assignments

- Study Chapter 17.
- Review the Learning Objectives for Chapter 17.
- Review the Certification Review for Chapter 17.
- Complete the Chapter Review exercise to reinforce concepts learned in the chapter.
- Complete the practice exercises on the companion Evolve site for reinforcement of medicine coding concepts.
- Complete the Workbook exercises as assigned by your instructor, or individually for additional practice.

Chapter Review Exercise

Complete the following coding exercises using the medicine section of CPT.

1. Cardiac catheterization, left with stent placement to the left circumflex coronary artery
   CPT code(s): 93510, 92980-LC
2. ECG, interpretation and report only
   CPT code(s): 93010
3. Cardiac echocardiograph with cardiac color flow Doppler imaging
   CPT code(s): 93306
4. MMR vaccine
   CPT code(s): 90707
5. Chemotherapy, infusion, IV, 2 hours
   CPT code(s): 96413, 96416
6. Dermatologic ultraviolet light treatment
   CPT code(s): ____________
7. ESRD, dialysis, per month, less than age 2 years
   CPT code(s): ____________
8. Prescription and fitting of contact lenses
   CPT code(s): ____________
9. Laryngeal function studies
   CPT code(s): ____________
10. Cardiopulmonary resuscitation
    CPT code(s): ____________
11. Percutaneous transluminal coronary angioplasty left circumflex, right coronary
    CPT code(s): ____________
12. Spirometry
    CPT code(s): ____________
13. Postoperative follow-up visit
    CPT code(s): ____________
14. Intraoperative neurophysiology testing, 1 hour
    CPT code(s): ____________
15. Patch allergy test(s), 15 tests
    CPT code(s): ____________
16. Doppler study of intracranial arteries, limited, transcranial
    CPT code(s): ____________
17. Bronchospasm evaluation
    CPT code(s): ____________
18. Cardiovascular stress test, complete
    CPT code(s): ____________
19. Allergy immunotherapy, administration only
    CPT code(s): 95115
20. Comprehensive ophthalmologic examination, new patient
    CPT code(s): ____________

Practical Application

Assign CPT code(s) and appropriate modifier(s) and list code(s) in the correct order for the following scenarios.

1. Office visit

OFFICE NOTE

Chief complaint: Coughing up blood

Date: ________________

Vital signs: BP______ P______ R______

History:

SUBJECTIVE: 73-year-old who presents with episodes of coughing up blood in the morning. Patient has a history of nasopharygeal carcinoma. Patient states that he has had similar episodes where he was diagnosed with pulmonary congestion.

Chest X-Ray shows some degree of cardiomegaly, no pleural effusion. No pulmonary congestion.

Labs are normal.

Exam:

Alert and oriented times three. Does not appear to be in acute distress. HEENT: PERRLA, EOMI, Throat clear. Chest: Clear, few basal crackles. Abdomen: Soft, non-tender, Extremities: No edema, no cyanosis

Diagnosis/assessment:

Hemoptysis, apparently no evidence of current bleeding at this time. Advised to return to the office immediately if develops any dizziness, increased tiredness or black, tarry stool or hematemesis.

Maurice Doater, MD

Patient name: ________________

Date of service: ________________

GODFREY MEDICAL ASSOCIATES

1532 Third Avenue, Suite 120 • Aldon, FL 77713 • (407) 555-4000

CPT code(s): ________________

2. Office visit

OFFICE NOTE

Chief complaint: ______________________

Date: ______________

Vital signs: BP______ P______ R______

History:

62-year-old with longstanding asthma/COPD, complaining of shortness of breath.

Exam:

On exam, she is afebrile. Temp 97, Pulse 92, respirations 20. She is alert, oriented and is in no obvious distress and only mildly dyspneic at rest. Pupils equal, round, reactive. Conjunctiva noninjected. TMs nondistended. Nasopharynx noncongested. Lung sounds revealed diffuse, coarse, expiratory wheezes throughout both lungs. Heart sounds are distant and regular without murmur. Abdomen is soft, nontender. Extremities are without cyanosis. There is no edema. She was given Albuterol nebulizer without any improvement. An additional Albuterol nebulizer was given and her dyspnea Improved but she continued to have coarse wheezes. She was also given Solu-Medrol 125 mg IM. Chest x-ray shows a questionable early right lower lobe infiltrate.

Diagnosis/assessment:

IMPRESSION:
Early acute right lower lobe pneumonia
Exacerbation of COPD/asthma

Jay Corman MD

Patient name: ______________________

Date of service: ______________

GODFREY MEDICAL ASSOCIATES
1532 Third Avenue, Suite 120 • Aldon, FL 77713 • (407) 555-4000

CPT code(s): ______________________

3. Emergency department record

EMERGENCY ROOM RECORD

Name:	Age:	ER physician:
	DOB:	
Allergies/type of reaction:	**Usual medications/dosages:**	

Triage/presenting complaint:

This is an 84-year-old female who suddenly became unresponsive. Upon arrival of EMS personnel, she was shocked and was able to be revived. The best rhythm they could maintain was a pulseless electrical activity.

Initial assessment:

Time	T	P	R	BP	Other:					

Medication orders:

Lab work:

X-ray:

Physician's report:

Upon arrival, CPR was continued. One (1) additional mg of epinephrine was given IV push and this generated some electrical activity but no pulse. Because of the extremely poor prognosis, and the fact that the patient has incurable cancer, we opted to cease CPR and the patient was pronounced at 10:15 AM.

Diagnosis:	Physician sign/date
	Robert Rai MD
Discharge Transfer Admit Good Satisfactory Other:	

GODFREY REGIONAL HOSPITAL
123 Main Street • Aldon, FL 77714 • (407) 555-1234

CPT code(s): ______________________

4. Office visit

OFFICE NOTE

Chief complaint: ____________________

Date: ____________________

Vital signs: BP______ P______ R______

History:

This is an established 79-year-old with COPD, CAD and hypertension. He was recently placed on Levaquin and Prednisone. He completed his doses in the last couple days, and now reports increased shortness of breath. He has a dry nonproductive cough, no fever, chills, or sore throat. No peripheral edema, no angina or other symptoms.

Exam:

On exam, temp 98.9, on oxygen chronically. Throat is negative. He has no JVD and no adenopathy. Lungs, some bilateral expiratory wheezing and a few rales in the right base. Heart sounds mildly irregular. No murmurs. Abdomen negative, no peripheral edema.

Diagnosis/assessment:

Impression: LRI with exacerbation of COPD

He already has a nebulizer. We can give him Solu-Medrol, 100 mg IV, and Kenalog, 60 mg IM. He was prescribed Levaquin 500 mg as directed.

William Obert MD

Patient name: ____________________

Date of service: ____________________

GODFREY MEDICAL ASSOCIATES
1532 Third Avenue, Suite 120 • Aldon, FL 77713 • (407) 555-4000

CPT code(s): ____________________

5. Emergency department record

EMERGENCY ROOM RECORD

Name:	Age:	ER physician:
	DOB:	

Allergies/type of reaction:	Usual medications/dosages:

Triage/presenting complaint:

70-year-old who apparently fell backwards, hitting the crown of her head. She has a 2.5 cm laceration of the occiput. She has not received a tetanus shot for over 10 years.

Initial assessment:

Time	T	P	R	BP	Other:				

Medication orders:

Lab work:

X-ray:

Physician's report:

Temperature, 98, pulse, 90, repirations 20. The site is cleaned and anesthetized. Three (3) Ethilon interrupted sutures are utilized to bring the wound together. The edges appear well approximated. The patient is also given a tD Immunization to update her immunization status.

2.5 cm scalp laceration

Patient should follow up in 7 days for suture removal or sooner if signs of infection.

Diagnosis:	Physician sign/date
	Nancy Connelly MD
Discharge Transfer Admit Good Satisfactory Other:	

GODFREY REGIONAL HOSPITAL
123 Main Street • Aldon, FL 77714 • (407) 555-1234

CPT code(s): ______________________

6. Office visit

OFFICE NOTE

Chief complaint: ______________________________

Date: ______________

Vital signs: BP______ P______ R______

History:

77-year-old male presents with history of intermittent shortness of breath at rest. States the shortness of breath seems to increase when he takes a deep breath. Denies any chest pain, chest pressure.

Exam:

Temperature, 97.8, pulse 77, respirations 24. EOMI PERRL. Throat clear, neck supple with no apparent JVD. Some crackles noted on the right side of the chest greater than the left. Abdomen is soft and nontender. 2+ lower extremity edema on the right side. Left side has a prosthesis. Lab work is normal, chest x-ray shows some slight increase in fluid on the right side. ECG shows normal sinus rhythm.

Diagnosis/assessment:

Given 20 mg IM of Lasix in the office with instructions to start taking additional 10 mg po Lasix daily and return on Friday to be rechecked.

Stacy Kratt, MD

Patient name: ______________________________

Date of service: ______________

GODFREY MEDICAL ASSOCIATES
1532 Third Avenue, Suite 120 • Aldon, FL 77713 • (407) 555-4000

CPT code(s): ______________________

7. Office visit

OFFICE NOTE

Chief complaint: ______

Date: ______

Vital signs: BP______ P______ R______

History:

Patient presents with complaints of chest pain. States he has had a CABG done three years ago. He has been doing fairly well until about two months ago. He started having some twinges of chest pain which has gradually worsened over the last 2 months. Upon arrival, his pain resolved with just lying down and putting on some O_2.

Exam:

Chest clear, heart regular rate and rhythm without murmurs. ECG showed some nonspecific ST-T wave changes. Chest X-Ray appears to be clear.

Diagnosis/assessment:

Chest pain, appears to be stable worsening angina.

Instructed to stop Norvasc, start on Metoprolol, 250 mg bid. Recommended follow-up in two weeks.

Patient name: ______

Date of service: ______

GODFREY MEDICAL ASSOCIATES

1532 Third Avenue, Suite 120 • Aldon, FL 77713 • (407) 555-4000

CPT code(s): ______

8. Emergency department record

EMERGENCY ROOM RECORD

Name:	Age:	ER physician:
	DOB:	
Allergies/type of reaction:	**Usual medications/dosages:**	

Triage/presenting complaint: 45-year-old male transported by ambulance to ER after being involved In MVA. He seems to have lost control either because of falling asleep or because of alcohol, which I could smell in the ER. He crossed the median, and headed towards another van that he hit head-on. He had to be extricated from his vehicle.

On arrival, he was in moderate distress from pain, complaining of severe pain to his left lower extremity, which was completely deformed. His left foot was rotated 90 degrees to the outside. The patient does not remember the accident or any details.

He denies headache, blurred or double vision, neck pain, chest pain or shortness of breath. Denies abdominal pain. Most of his pain is in his left lower extremity. Past medical history is significant for IDDM, asthma and Hep C.

Initial assessment:

Time	T	P	R	BP	Other:					

Medication orders:

Lab work:

X-ray:

Physician's report: PHYSICAL EXAM: On physical exam, he was awake, alert, and oriented. He was in moderate distress from pain, especially when being moved. HEENT: head normocephalic, atraumatic. Some abrasions to the upper part of his forehead. His cranial nerves appear intact. There was no bleeding from his ears or nostrils. Chest was symmetrical, there was no deformity, no tenderness. Lungs clear to auscultation. Heart, regular, rate and rhythm. Patient had a very tender left hip. He had a deformed left thigh. He had a deformed left leg with a long laceration almost 12 cm in length involving skin, subcutaneous tissue and muscle. Patient has his left foot externally rotated. Both feet were warm and pink. He had positive dorsalis pedis pulses and good capillary filling of his toes. He had a swollen right hand, mostly on the dorsal aspect. Good radial pulses bilaterally and good range of motion of shoulders, elbows and wrist joints.

ER COURSE:

An IV line was established and the patient was placed on saline wide open, X-rays were performed of the right wrist, right hand, left hip, chest, c-spine, left lower leg. Urinalysis, CBC CMP were performed.

X-rays revealed comminuted intertrochanteric fracture and left distal comminuted transverse fracture of the femur. Also possibility of distal phalanx of right thumb.

Diagnosis:

ASSESSMENT: Status post MVA with comminuted fx left intertrochanteric femur, left distal femur, frank hematuria.

Patient was given 4 mc IV morphine push before transfer to neighboring facility.

Physician sign/date

Robert Rai MD

Discharge **Transfer** **Admit** **Good** **Satisfactory** **Other:**

GODFREY REGIONAL HOSPITAL
123 Main Street • Aldon, FL 77714 • (407) 555-1234

CPT code(s): ______________________________

9. Operative report

OPERATIVE REPORT

Patient information:

Patient name:
DOB:
MR#:

Date:
Surgeon:
Anesthetist:

Preoperative diagnosis:

Postoperative diagnosis:

Procedure(s) performed:

Anesthesia:

Assistant surgeon:

Description of procedure:

Access was via the left femoral vein

Imaging was obtained of the pulmonary, coronary and left and right ventricles

Obstruction was noted in the right coronary vessels ×3 and the left circumflex ×4

PTCA (Angioplasty) was performed × 3 in the Right Coronary Vessel, two of which required the placement of an intracoronary stent. The left circumflex received four (4) angioplasties only.

GODFREY REGIONAL HOSPITAL
123 Main Street • Aldon, FL 77714 • (407) 555-1234

CPT code(s): ______________________

10. Operative report

OPERATIVE REPORT

Patient information:

Patient name:
DOB:
MR#:

Date:
Surgeon:
Anesthetist:

Preoperative diagnosis:

Postoperative diagnosis:

Procedure(s) performed:

Anesthesia:

Assistant surgeon:

Description of procedure:

Access via the left femoral artery

Imaging was obtained of the left and right ventricles, the aorta and coronary arteries. Obstructions were identified in the circumflex, the descending and the coronary vessel appeared clear.

Angioplasties × 3 were performed in the left circumflex, followed by stent placement; however, neither were successful and atherectomy was performed to the three (3) obstructed areas in the left circumflex. Angioplasties × 2 were performed in the left descending, one followed by stent placement.

GODFREY REGIONAL HOSPITAL
123 Main Street • Aldon, FL 77714 • (407) 555-1234

CPT code(s): ______________________

18

HCPCS Level II Codes

LEARNING OBJECTIVES

After completing this chapter, the student will be able to:

- Know when CPT codes versus HCPCS codes should be coded and billed.
- Comprehend and apply the rules for selecting the appropriate HCPCS level II codes.
- Identify the individual sections and subsections of HCPCS level II and the types of services that are included.
- Apply HCPCS coding concepts to practical coding scenarios.

CODING REFERENCE TOOLS

Tool 18-1
HCPCS Code Book Index

Tool 18-2
Rules for Selecting HCPCS Level II National Codes

KEY TERMS

Healthcare Common Procedure Coding System (HCPCS)

Level I HCPCS Codes

Level II HCPCS Codes

In addition to the CPT codes already discussed in Chapters 10 through 17, **Healthcare Common Procedure Coding System** (**HCPCS**) codes may be used for coding medical services. At the beginning of the CPT discussion, the HCPCS system was introduced as being composed of two levels:

Level I	Physicians Current Procedural Terminology (CPT)
Level II	HCPCS National Codes

Chapters 10 through 17 discussed **level I HCPCS codes** found in the current CPT code book. CPT, however, does not contain all the codes needed to report medical services and supplies. As a result, the Centers for Medicare and Medicaid Services (CMS) developed the second level of codes to address items not found in CPT.

Level II HCPCS codes primarily identify products, supplies, and services not included in the level I CPT coding system, such as ambulance, durable medical equipment, prosthetics, orthotics, other supplies, and drugs. These codes are used by most Medicare and Medicaid carriers for reporting these items rather than the codes listed under special supplies in the medicine section of CPT. The HCPCS codes define specific services, often identifying the name of the supply or the drug, its dosage, and its strength. HCPCS codes eliminate the need for CPT codes such as 99070, which require manual listing of additional information and a manual review process by the third-party carrier. As with all services coded and billed to third-party carriers, HCPCS code assignments are driven by the documentation contained in the medical record. In some instances this information will be documented first by oral order of the physician or by medical personnel in the office. In other instances it will be contained on a separate document, such as a medication log. Despite where the documentation originates or who documents the original service order, the physician is still responsible for validation by signature and date so that service can be billed and reimbursed. HCPCS codes are used on a regular basis by durable medical equipment (DME) companies because they code and bill for these types of services on a regular basis.

CMS has mandated the use of HCPCS codes on Medicare claims; many Medicaid carriers require them as well. These codes obviously improve the providers ability to effectively communicate what services have been provided without the need for narrative descriptions and detailed attachments.

Format

The HCPCS national codes are used for reporting medical services and supplies; they use an alpha prefix followed by four numeric characters. Additional modifier codes have been included with HCPCS level II national codes; they appear as 2-digit alpha characters as opposed to the 2-digit numeric characters of CPT. A complete listing of HCPCS modifiers is outlined in the introduction to CPT in Chapters 9 and 10.

There are several types of HCPCS level II codes depending on the purpose for the codes. National permanent HCPCS codes serve the function of a standardized coding system as dictated by CMS in the Health Insurance Portability and Accountability Act (HIPAA) requirement of a standardized coding system. Dental codes are a separate section of HCPCS level II national codes, which include codes established by the American Dental Association (ADA) known as Current Dental Terminology (CDT). Responsibility for changes, additions, and deletions to these codes is maintained by the ADA rather than CMS but are included in HCPCS level II. Miscellaneous codes are codes for which there is no existing national code. These codes allow a provider to bill for services with a standardized code while consideration is being given to the assignment of a national permanent code. Temporary national codes are usually assigned for short periods until the HCPCS workgroup determines whether permanent codes will be added in the current year HCPCS code book. Because the permanent national codes are only updated annually on January 1, temporary codes may be assigned in the interim. Following are types of temporary HCPCS codes:

C codes	Identify items that may qualify for "pass through" payments for hospital outpatient services. These typically include new technology or devices that have not yet been assigned a permanent CPT code or national HCPCS code.
G codes	Codes that usually would be assigned a CPT code for which there is no CPT code assignment to date.
Q codes	Services that typically would not be assigned CPT codes, such as drugs, biologicals, medical equipment, and supplies.
S codes	Assigned for services such as drugs and supplies for which codes are needed for the private insurance sector for policies, programs, or claims processing. These codes are typically not payable by Medicare or other federal government programs.
H codes	Used by state Medicaid agencies to identify mental health services such as alcohol and drug treatment services.

LAYOUT

General

Sections are outlined according to the type of supplies or materials that are being provided. Within each section are subsections defining specific supplies and materials within the section.

CONTENTS

General

Tool 18-1 outlines the contents of the HCPCS code book. As with CPT, the coder should select the appropriate HCPCS code, following a step-by-step process as outlined in Tool 18-2.

Additional information is contained in the appendixes of the level II HCPCS national codes. These appendixes provide information regarding coverage issues, specifically outlining covered and noncovered services and describing service limitations. A general section overview follows below.

Transportation Services, Including Ambulance (A0021-A0999)

This section covers the transportation of patients from their place of residence or where the injury occurs to the hospital. In some instances the transportation of the patient is for nonemergent transport and in other cases it may involve the return of the patient from the treating facility. In addition,

TOOL 18-1

HCPCS CODE BOOK INDEX

A0000-A0999	Transportation Services
A4000-A8999	Medical and Surgical Supplies
A9000-A9999	Administrative, Misc/Investigational Supplies
B4000-B9999	Enteral/Parenteral Therapy
D0000-D9999	Dental Procedures
E0100-E9999	Durable Medical Equipment (DME)
G0000-G9999 (Temporary)	Procedures/Professional Services
J0000-J8999	Drugs Administered by Other than Oral Method
J9000-J9999	Chemotherapy Drugs
K0000-K9999	Assigned by DME Regional Carriers
L0000-L4999	Orthotic Procedures
L5000-L9999	Prosthetic Procedures
M0000-M0302	Medical Services
P0000-P9999	Pathology/Laboratory Services
Q0000-Q9999	Temporary Nationally Assigned
R0000-R5999	Diagnostic Radiology Services
S0009-S9999	Temporary National Codes (Non-Medicare)
V0000-V2999	Vision Services

TOOL 18-2

RULES FOR SELECTING HCPCS LEVEL II NATIONAL CODES

1. Determine where services will be billed from CPT or HCPCS national codes (usually determined by carrier).
2. Consult the index to HCPCS codes to determine the appropriate section of HCPCS codes to consult.
3. Locate the appropriate HCPCS code listed in alphabetical order with the appropriate HCPCS section.
4. Determine the appropriate number of units. Unlike CPT, the rounding rule does not apply. If any portion of the unit(s) of service is met, the code may be used. For example, an injection of tetracycline 150 mg would be coded as "J0120, injection, tetracycline" up to 250 mg. Note the description indicates "up to"; therefore the requirement has been met.
5. When multiple units of service are provided, the days or units entry should be made. For example: "Injection, tetracycline, 600 mg" would be billed as J0120, 3 units.

codes are assigned according to the level of care that needs to be provided to the patient during transport (e.g., basic life support, advance life support).

A 2-digit alpha modifier code is usually required in addition to the HCPCS code for services to indicate the origin of the transport and the destination. The applicable modifiers are as follows:

D	Diagnostic or therapeutic site (other than provider or hospital)
E	Residential, domiciliary, custodial
G	Hospital-based dialysis center
H	Hospital
I	Site of transfer
J	Non-hospital–based facility
N	Skilled nursing facility
P	Physicians office
R	Residence
S	Scene of accident
X	Intermediate stop at physicians office en route to hospital (destination code only)

Therefore one would expect to see a 5-digit HCPCS code followed by a 2-digit modifier indicating the origin (first digit) and the destination (second digit).For example, "ambulance nonemergency transport from home to hospital, basic life support only" would be coded as follows:

A0428-RH	Ambulance service, basic life support, nonemergency transport from residence to hospital

Medical and Surgical Supplies (A4206-A8004)

This section includes supplies and materials that may be used in the performance of a visit or procedure. Keep in mind that codes listed in HCPCS, as is also the case with CPT codes, do not necessarily guarantee that each insurance carrier will consider that service or supply for reimbursement. Also keep in mind that HCPCS and CPT guidelines state that the highest level of specificity should be used when assigning procedure codes for services performed. Therefore HCPCS level II codes should be used in lieu of CPT code 99070 when appropriate.

Several subcategories are included within the medical and surgical supply section as follows:

General	A4206-A4290
Vascular catheters	A4300-A4306
Incontinence appliances and care supplies	A4310-A4316
Urinary catheters	A4320-A4355
External urinary supplies	A4356-A4358
Ostomy supplies	A4361-A4434
Additional miscellaneous supplies	A4450-A4608
Supplies for oxygen/related respiratory	A4611-A4629
Other durable medical equipment	A4630-A4640
Supplies for radiologic procedures	A4641-A4650
End-stage renal disease supplies	A4651-A4932
Additional ostomy supplies	A5051-A5093
Additional incontinence supplies	A5102-A5114
Incontinence/ostomy appliances	A5120-A5200
Diabetic shoes, fitting, modifications	A5500-A5513
Dressing, wound care, burn supplies	A6000-A6550
Respiratory supplies	A7000-A8004
Administrative, miscellaneous and investigational supplies	A9150-A9999

Enteral and Parenteral Therapy (B4034-B9999)

Supplies and materials used in the administration of therapy performed by infusion and other introduction into the system other than oral administration are contained in this section. This includes the supplies needed, such as catheters and tubing, as well as the solutions administered by these routes. Subcategories for this section are as follows:

Enteral formula supplies	B4034-B4262
Parenteral nutrition solution and supplies	B4264-B5200
Enteral and parental pumps	B9000-B9999

Enteral supplies are used in the administration of therapy to the gastrointestinal tract, whereas parenteral supplies are used for therapy through other than the gastrointestinal tract.

Pass-Through Items (C1300-C9728)

The codes in this section are only used by hospital outpatient facilities. In some instances carriers give additional consideration to devices and materials used in the performance of a procedure that are of significant cost to allow for additional reimbursement.

There are no subsections for the pass-through items; however, the needed item can be easily located because the services for this section are in alphabetical order.

Dental Procedures (D0120-D9999)

Codes from this section are copyrighted and maintained by the ADA. In some instances, you may find an HCPCS level II book that does not include the dental codes because a royalty fee must be paid to this organization to reproduce these codes.

Items in this section range from the diagnostic care and treatment of the teeth and gums to prosthetic devices. Many of the services in this section are not covered by the Medicare program. Prosthetic devices, however, are a covered Medicare benefit because they replace a malfunctioning, missing, or inoperable internal body area or organ.

Subcategories for the dental section are as follows:

Diagnostic	D0120-D0999
Preventive	D1110-D1555
Restorative	D2140-D2999
Endodontics	D3110-D3999
Periodontics	D4210-D4999
Prosthodontics (removable)	D5110-D6199
Prosthodontics (fixed)	D6205-D6999
Oral/maxillofacial surgery	D7111-D8999
Adjunctive general services	D9110-D9999
Durable medical equipment	(E0100-E8002)

Durable medical equipment is a term used to describe certain Medicare benefits, including iron lungs, oxygen tents, hospital beds, and wheelchairs used in the patients home.* This term does not include equipment furnished by a supplier who has used it to demonstrate its function or who has not met such minimum training standards as the Secretary may establish regarding the demonstration. Regarding a seat-lift chair, such term includes only the seat-lift mechanism and does not include the chair. This information is defined by Title XVIII of the Social Security Act and pertains to Medicare recipients. Other carriers and insurances may interpret the guidelines for coverage for durable medical equipment differently.

Included in the durable medical equipment section are such items as:

- Cane and crutches
- Walkers
- Commodes
- Decubitus care equipment
- Bath and toilet aids
- Hospital beds
- Oxygen and related equipment
- Humidifiers and nebulizers
- Transcutaneous electrical nerve stimulators
- Infusion pump equipment and supplies
- Wheelchairs and accessories
- Artificial kidney machines

Procedures and Professional Services (G0008-G9140)

A number of services and procedures that have not been included in CPT are contained within this section. In many instances, Medicare has mandated that a specific code be used for a specific service or screening, and again the HCPCS level II code would supersede the use of the appropriate CPT code.

For example, when screening colonoscopies are performed on Medicare beneficiaries, the following codes would be used in lieu of CPT code 45378, screening colonoscopy:

G0105 Colorectal cancer screening; colonoscopy on individual at high risk†

*This may include a power-operated vehicle that may be appropriately used as a wheelchair, but only when the use of such a vehicle is determined to be necessary on the basis of the individuals medical and physical condition. The vehicle must meet prescribed safety requirements. "Home" includes institutions used as a home other than an institution that meets the requirements of subsection (e)(1) of this section or section 1819(a)(1)), whether furnished on a rental basis or purchased. Durable medical equipment also includes blood-testing strips and blood glucose monitors for individuals with diabetes. (*CMS Coders Manual*, part 3, Chapter 11).

†Medicare guidelines define "an individual at high risk" as the following: "Screening colonoscopies are covered once every 24 months for Medicare beneficiaries that are considered at high risk based on the following: (1) close relative (sibling, parent, or child) who has had colorectal cancer or adenomatous polyp(s); (2) family history of adenomatous polyp(s); (3) family history of hereditary nonpolyposis colorectal cancer; (4) personal history of adenomatous polyp(s); (5) personal history of colorectal cancer; (6) personal history of inflammatory bowel disease, including Crohn's disease or ulcerative colitis" (*Medicare Claims Processing Manual*, Chapter 13).

G0121 Colorectal cancer screening; colonoscopy on individual not meeting criteria for high risk

Several other services such as the above are included in this section. The appendixes included in the HCPCS level II book typically define the circumstances under which services would or would not be covered. This information is also available on the Medicare Web site (www.medicare.gov).

Alcohol and Drug Abuse Treatment Services (H0001-H2037)

Alcohol and drug abuse treatments are contained in this category, including individual therapy, group therapy, and crisis intervention. Behavioral health prevention education is also provided in this category.

STOP AND PRACTICE

Following are some practice exercises for the HCPCS level II codes covered so far.

	HCPCS Level II Code(s)
1. Implantable vascular access device, external access	____________
2. Replace battery, ventilator, heavy duty	____________
3. Respiratory tubing used with suction pump	____________
4. Intraocular lens	____________
5. Limited oral dental examination	____________
6. Pair crutches, wood, underarm with pads, grips, tips	____________
7. Behavior health hotline service	____________
8. High-risk colorectal colonoscopy	____________
9. Compression burn garment, lower trunk panty, custom fabricated	____________
10. Ambulance, basic life support, nonemergent, from home to hospital	____________

Drugs Administered Other Than Oral Method (J0120-J8999)

Medications administered subcutaneously (SC), intramuscularly (IM), and/or intravenously (IV) are included in this section. The drugs are listed alphabetically by the drug name. Drug names are often listed with generic names; therefore a drug reference manual, such as the *Physicians Desk Reference,* which is available in most medical facilities, may be an excellent reference.

As discussed in the tools previously presented in this chapter, medications are assigned codes based on the drug name and the administration amount. Unlike CPT, the "rounding" rule does not apply in HCPCS level II codes. Therefore it would be appropriate to code more than one unit of service if additional milligram(s) are administered. For example:

J1265 Injection, dopamine HCl, 40 mg

This code is intended for the SC, IM, and IV administration of dopamine. When more than 40 mg are administered, it would be appropriate to assign multiple units of service. Therefore a 45-mg injection of dopamine HCL would be assigned J1265/two units.

Chemotherapy Drugs (J9000-J9999)

The administration of antineoplastic drugs is included in this section rather than the drugs administered by other than oral means. Again, these drugs are in alphabetical order, by generic name; the drug reference manual would be helpful in this instance as well.

Durable Medical Equipment Supplies (K0001-K0899)

Codes from this section must be filed only with the appropriate DME Medicare Administrative Contract, known as a DME MAC, rather than the physician or professional carrier for services.

Orthotic Procedures (L0112-L4398)

Orthotics are devices used to control abnormal foot function. When the foot is not functioning correctly, painful areas result. An orthotics device can relieve that pain by providing support to the ligaments and the bone structures of the feet.

Codes in this section are arranged by anatomic area, such as upper limbs or lower limbs, as well as the specific body area, such as the elbow, wrist, or hand.

Prosthetic Procedures (L5000-L9900)

In medicine a prosthesis is an artificial extension that replaces a missing body part. Prostheses are typically used to replace parts lost as a result of injury (traumatic) or missing from birth (congenital) or to supplement defective body parts.

Codes in this section are presented by anatomic area and, more specifically, by specific body area.

Medical Services (M0064-M0301)

Codes for this section are primary for CMS designation of a specific services, such as the following:

M0064 Visit for monitoring or changing prescriptions for mental disorders
M0075 Cellular therapy
M0076 Prolotherapy
M0100 Intragastric hypothermia using gastric freezing
M0300 IV chelation therapy
M0301 Fabric wrapping of abdominal aneurysm

Laboratory and Pathology (P2028-P9615)

A number of laboratory and pathology services are not listed in the CPT (HCPCS level I) coding book, whereas others are specific to Medicare.

Codes P3000 and P3001 are used for Medicare patients for screening Papanicolaou (Pap) smears. One of these codes would be appropriate for a Medicare beneficiary rather than the CPT laboratory codes for Pap smears.

Temporary Codes (Q0034-G9967)

This section represents national codes assigned by CMS on a temporary basis. These codes would be considered for permanent adaptation either in HCPCS level II or HCPCS level I (CPT).

Diagnostic Radiology Services (R0070-R0076)

There are a limited number of codes in this section, limited to those for the transportation of x-ray equipment necessary to perform radiologic studies for a patient. Again, keep in mind that services included in HCPCS level II (as well as HCPCS level I CPT) are not necessarily reimbursable by carriers. They represent services that are commonly performed and serve as a tracking mechanism even in instances in which additional reimbursement may not be considered.

Temporary National Codes, Non-Medicare (S0012-S9999)

The codes in this section are not valid for Medicare submission and therefore should not be included on any claims to Medicare. Unlike the "Q" codes, these codes may be used for temporary codes that need to be established for non-Medicare carriers.

National Codes for State Medicaid Agencies (T1000-T5999)

Codes from this section were created solely for the purpose of reporting services to state Medicaid recipients and therefore would typically not be reported on any other claim forms. Types of services included in this section include such services as:

- Assessments
- Specialized medical equipment
- Hospice care
- Nonemergency transportation
- Incontinence products

Vision and Hearing Services (V2020-V5364)

Vision supplies such as spectacles (glasses), contact lenses, and other vision aids are included in this section as well as hearing evaluations and hearing aids, listening devices, and speech language services.

STOP AND PRACTICE

Practice assigning the appropriate HCPCS level II codes for the categories covered above.

	HCPCS Level II Code(s)
1. Leucovorin calcium, 75 mg	______
2. Ciprofloxacin, 300 mg IV use	______
3. Repair prosthetic device	______
4. Heel orthosis, leather	______
5. Lorazepam, 2 mg	______
6. Medicaid, incontinence pull-on protective underwear, youth, disposable	______
7. Hearing screening	______
8. Penicillin G benzathine, 1.2 million units	______
9. Knee orthosis, Swedish-type prefabricated	______
10. Partial hand prosthesis, Robin-Aids, thumb remaining	______

SYMBOLS

Symbols in HCPCS level II are similar to those located in HCPS level I CPT. Although different versions of the HCPCS level II manual differ slightly, the following symbols are consistent in each.

• New codes
▲ Revised codes
× Deleted codes

MODIFIERS

HCPCS modifiers were discussed in length during the introduction of CPT/HCPCS in Chapters 9 and 10. A complete listing is included in that material.

APPENDIXES TO HCPCS LEVEL II

Although the appendixes in each publication of HCPCS level II vary from publisher to publisher, many are similar. Some of the common appendixes are as follows:

- HCPCS level II modifiers.
- Medicare national coverage determinations describe in great detail specific Medicare coverage requirements for services in HCPCS level II. Information may include conditions covered, certification of medical necessity, and conditions under which the HCPCS level II item would be covered.
- Jurisdiction list of the services contained in HCPCS level II and the carrier that would be responsible for determining coverage and reimbursement for services. This list is commonly arranged in HCPCS sections.

Chapter in Review

Certification Review

- HCPCS codes and modifiers further define services not adequately addressed in CPT.
- The use of HCPCS codes and modifiers often eliminates the need for a report to specify the services or items provided.
- HCPCS codes and modifiers are accepted by specific carriers only. The coder must make certain they are used appropriately.
- HCPCS codes are all 5-digit alphanumeric codes.

Student Assignments

- Study Chapter 18.
- Review the Learning Objectives for Chapter 18.
- Review the Certification Review for Chapter 18.
- Complete the Chapter Review exercise to reinforce concepts learned in this chapter.
- Complete the practice exercises on the Evolve site for reinforcement of HCPCS coding concepts.
- Complete the Workbook exercises as assigned by your instructor or individually for additional practice.

Chapter Review Exercise

Locate the appropriate HCPCS code(s) for the following:

	HCPCS Code
1. Prosthetic partial foot with molded socket, ankle height	________
2. Cervical or vaginal cancer screening	________
3. Commode chair, mobile, with detachable arms	________
4. Hospital bed, semielectric, without mattress	________
5. Motorized wheelchair, fixed full-length arms	________
6. Injection, ceftazidime, 750 mg	________
7. Repair to broken denture base, complete	________
8. Replacement batteries for medically necessary transelectrical nerve stimulation unit	________
9. Gradient compression stocking, lymphedema	________
10. Breast prosthesis, mastectomy sleeve	________
11. Injection, cyclophosphamide, 4 g	________
12. Injection, methotrexate, 100 mg	________
13. Repair of orthotic device, 30 minutes	________
14. Prednisone, oral, 10 mg	________
15. Drug administered through metered-dose inhaler	________
16. Repair of durable medical equipment, 30 minutes	________
17. Crutches, underarm, pair, wood	________
18. Intraoral x-rays, complete	________
19. Injection, Rocephin, 50 mg IM	________
20. Injection, unlisted substance, 50 mg IM	________

Practical Application

Use the codes discussed in this chapter to assign the appropriate HCPCS level II codes as well as the codes for other services. If you are unable to determine the level of service (evaluation and management code assignment), indicate the type and location, such as office visit, established patient.

1. Patient presents with complaint of left lower knee pain. An expanded history and exam are performed, and moderate medical decision making. In addition, an arthrocentesis is performed with the injection of 10 mg of Kenalog.

   HCPCS code(s): ____________________
   CPT code assignment(s): ____________________
   ICD-9-CM code assignment(s): ____________________

2. 16-year-old with severe sore throat. An expanded problem-focused history and exam are performed, and 1.2 milliunits of Bicillin CR are administered IM.

   HCPCS code(s): ____________________
   CPT code assignment(s): ____________________
   ICD-9-CM code assignment(s): ____________________

3. 85-year-old woman tripped on some steps and fell; injury to the anterior aspects of both knees. She denies head injury or injury to the neck, back, chest. She has a history of heart disease and is on Coumadin.

   Exam reveals an alert, pleasant elderly woman. Swelling and ecchymosis of anterior aspects of knees. There is tenderness, more on the left. Function and sensation of both feet are intact. X-rays of both knees showed nondisplaced fracture of the left patella.

   A knee immobilizer was given to the patient for use once she returns home. Staff demonstrated the proper application and removal of the device.

   HCPCS code(s): ____________________
   CPT code assignment(s): ____________________
   ICD-9-CM code assignment(s): ____________________

4. Patient arrived in the emergency room in full cardiac arrest. He was working on converting a pickup truck into a dump truck and the truck fell off a lift on him. EMS intubated on the scene. He has obvious fractures of his left elbow and left wrist. CPR was continued. A needle thoracentesis was performed.

   The patient was administered epinephrine 3 mg IV at 10:00 am and 10:10 am and atropine at 10:15 am with no real response. He had no pulse. He was in asystole. Chest x-ray showed whiteout of the left lung, right thorax had multiple rib fractures. Patient had no response, and the code was stopped at 10:20 am.

   HCPCS code(s): ____________________
   CPT code assignment(s): ____________________
   ICD-9-CM code assignment(s): ____________________

5. Patient arrives at physiatrist's office to pick up heel orthotic only.

   HCPCS code(s): ____________________
   CPT code assignment(s): ____________________
   ICD-9-CM code assignment(s): ____________________

6. Established patient presents to the dentist's office for annual periodic dental evaluation.

   HCPCS code(s): ____________________
   CPT code assignment(s): ____________________
   ICD-9-CM code assignment(s): ____________________

7. Medicare patient with history of edematous polyps presents for periodic screening colonoscopy.

   HCPCS code(s): ____________________
   CPT code assignment(s): ____________________
   ICD-9-CM code assignment(s): ____________________

8. 85-year-old presents with leg pain. He was prescribed Keflex 500 mg bid for 10 days; however, it is worse since yesterday and he is not ambulating well. He is not short of breath. He has chronic dyspnea with activity, but that is unchanged. No fever, chills or chest discomfort.

   Exam included heart, abdomen, and lower extremities. He has 2+ edema below his knees. His labs were normal.

   PLAN:
   He was given 75 mg IM for his pain and prescribed Dilaudid 2 mg every 2 to 4 hours for pain. He is to follow-up in 2 to 3 days.

   HCPCS code(s): ____________________
   CPT code assignment(s): ____________________
   ICD-9-CM code assignment(s): ____________________

9. Delivery to the patients home of a heavy-duty transfer bench for tube or toilet transfer.

   HCPCS code(s): ____________________
   CPT code assignment(s): ____________________
   ICD-9-CM code assignment(s): ____________________

10. Delivery of over-door cervical traction equipment to patient's home.

    HCPCS code(s): ____________________
    CPT code assignment(s): ____________________
    ICD-9-CM code assignment(s): ____________________

SECTION 4

The Reimbursement Perspective

By this point, the student has learned the various coding methods and the guidelines needed to perform correct coding. As mentioned at the beginning of this text, the coding process is a continual building process of rules and guidelines.

These guidelines do not end at the conclusion of the discussion on coding. Although understanding and implementing the guidelines covered thus far are crucial to successful coding, additional guidelines provided by third-party carriers may change, eliminate, or deviate somewhat from these guidelines. Therefore Section IV consists of a discussion of the idiosyncrasies of third-party carriers in regard to coding systems.

The student will have the opportunity to review several documents outside the realm of the medical record documentation, such as claim forms and third-party explanations of benefits, to achieve a thorough understanding of the impact of coding on all aspects of the reimbursement process. ■

19

Coding from a Reimbursement Perspective

LEARNING OBJECTIVES

After completing this chapter, the student will be able to:

- Identify the different reimbursement methods.
- Comprehend the purpose of third-party contracts and their effects on coding.
- Grasp coding from the perspective of receiving proper reimbursement.
- Understand the forms used for coding and billing provider services compared with facility services.
- Know the areas in which third-party reimbursement differs.
- Describe the clean claim process.
- Apply concepts learned to billing case scenarios.

CODING REFERENCE TOOLS

Tool 19-1
Third-Party Contract Worksheet

Tool 19-2
Managed Care Contract Review

KEY TERMS

Advance Beneficiary Notice (ABN)
Charge Ticket
Clean Claim
CMS-1500
Explanation of Benefits (EOB)
Fiscal Intermediary (FI)
HCFA-1500
Resource-Based Relative Value Study (RBRVS)
Superbill
UB-04
Usual, Customary, and Reasonable (UCR)

Overview

Thus far, coding has been discussed from strictly a coding perspective, following the rules and guidelines outlined in CPT, ICD-9-CM, and other supporting coding books. This chapter discusses the "real world" of coding: what gets paid and what does not, how to code to carrier specifications, and the compilation of this information into a third-party contract worksheet.

This chapter is intended to address only coding issues that relate to reimbursement and to help the coder understand the complete cycle of coding and billing that must successfully be completed to obtain appropriate payment. It is not intended to cover all the topics and issues that relate to billing and the reimbursement process.

The coder must understand that third-party carriers are not required to strictly follow CPT, ICD-9-CM, HCPCS, DRG, or other coding guidelines as outlined in the universal coding books. Their only requirement is to accept these coding systems on claim forms (**CMS-1500** or **HCFA-1500** claim form for physician/provider and **UB-04** form for hospital inpatient facilities [Table 19-1]). Also, remember that inclusion of codes in any of these coding books does not imply coverage by third-party carriers; it only serves as a uniform mechanism for describing WHAT services were performed and WHY. Deviations and variations in the interpretation of the guidelines in these coding structures may be seen, as deemed appropriate by the individual third-party carrier. In this light, the coder/biller for the facility must be aware of these idiosyncrasies in coding for individual third-party carriers.

Third-Party Contracts

The best place to clarify the variances imposed by individual third-party carriers is in the contracts between the facility or provider and the individual third-party carrier. It is essential to review and keep these documents on hand and to make certain that the practice or facility needs are addressed in the third-party contract. The third-party contract should serve as the mutual understanding of how codes should be used for reimbursement and, if used correctly, what reimbursement will occur and when.

TABLE 19-1 CODES AND CLAIM FORMS USED IN DIFFERENT MEDICAL SETTINGS

	DIAGNOSIS	PROCEDURES	CLAIM FORM
Physician	ICD-9-CM	CPT	CMS-1500
Outpatient facility	ICD-9-CM	CPT/ICD-9 procedures	UB-04
Inpatient facility	ICD-9-CM	ICD-9 procedures	UB-04

DEFINITIONS

Third-party contracts are an agreement between the third-party carrier (typically an insurance carrier) and the provider (e.g., physician, physician group, supplier, facility) and should represent the terms of both parties, not just the third-party carrier. For instance, many third-party contracts outline the maximum time limits for a clean claim to be submitted. This period may vary from 15 days to 90 days, or it may last up to a year. After that time, the third-party carrier will not consider charges except possibly by an appeal process. The facility, however, also has the right to request imposition of some type of time frame for response of submitted claims and some type of penalty to the carrier for not upholding these guidelines.

GUIDELINES

This chapter discusses the most common and sometimes controversial interpretations of third-party contracts. With this information, a customized contract grid for use in the practice to convey this information to all appropriate staff may be developed. This can be used as guidelines as well as for the development of future contracts from this standardized format.

The coder should always keep in mind that coding must be accomplished according to guidelines from the appropriate coding sources (e.g., CPT, ICD-9-CM, HCPCS). Whether the carrier reimburses for a specific service, the service should be coded according to the appropriate guidelines. By coding and billing for all services, even though reimbursement may not be expected, the practice will be able to track services performed. In the event that the carrier determines that these services should have been paid during a specific period, the practice will possess the historical data necessary to refile for reimbursement.

If the practice believes that a specific service should be paid by the third-party carrier, denial by the carrier is not always the last word. The coder must establish the premise of why reimbursement should be made by using guidelines from the appropriate CPT, ICD-9-CM, or HCPCS coding book(s). For specialty services, the coder may also be guided by the coding guidelines recommended by the specialty organization (e.g., emergency department services based on the American College of Emergency Physicians). Care should be taken to use these resources in justifying request for reimbursement. Make certain not to use conference or seminar notes or guideline books other than those accepted by the third-party carrier.

Most third-party carriers have an appeals process established within their organizations. Appeals are best presented when a certified coder as the "expert" cites the references described above. If the initial decision of the third-party carrier is upheld, additional appeals may be made by the practice, perhaps with the physician involved, through the third-party carrier's medical director. Medicare and other governmental third parties have an elaborate appeals process that involves an initial appeal and a hearing process as well as an administrative judge to hear appeals by both the provider of service and the third-party carrier.

Remember that despite correct coding, not all services described with the use of proper codes will be reimbursed by all carriers. These coding books serve only as the mechanism to describe WHAT services were provided and WHY they were performed and to list all services that may be considered for reimbursement. The contract or regulations of the specific carrier determine whether a provider will be compensated for a specific service.

Reimbursement Method

It is important for the coder and biller to understand the reimbursement process and to know what reimbursement should be expected. This means the coder must understand some of the terminology of the reimbursement process to determine whether the coded services will be reimbursed and at what amount.

One of the most important factors to consider is whether the practice *participates* with the third-party carrier. When a practice or facility participates, that entity agrees to accept the amount contractually agreed on as payment in full. In some instances the third-party carrier will pay only a portion of the contracted amount, leaving the rest as patient responsibility. If the facility does not participate, it is under no contractual obligation to accept as payment in full the amount determined by the third-party carrier to be the allowed amount. This is important when services are coded according to appropriate guidelines yet the carrier elects to deny or reduce payment for these services.

When the facility participates with the third-party carrier and specific codes are not covered, the contract specifies whether the facility is required to write off these services, or if it may bill the patient. If the facility does not participate, it may bill the patient for these services after the appeals process has been exhausted. In these instances, the facility or practice must document the "reasonable" attempts made to receive payment from the carrier before patient billing.

Once the carrier makes a determination regarding payment for services, it is also important to make certain that services are paid according to the third-party contract.

USUAL, CUSTOMARY, AND REASONABLE

Most third-party carriers use one of two methods for determining the appropriate amount of reimbursement for physician services. The first of these reimbursement methods, the **usual, customary, and reasonable** (**UCR**) method, has been around for many years. This method is based on the following components:

Usual The facility/practice/provider's usual charge for the service performed.

Customary The amount usually charged by all providers or facilities for the service. An average or mean is then calculated, which represents the customary reimbursement for that service.

Reasonable Amount determined by the third party to represent data gathered on usual and customary fees and the assignment of a reasonable percentile of these data. For example, the reasonable allowance may be 80% of the customary fee.

Consider the importance of modifiers as they relate to the correct calculation of the previous numbers. When services are billed with modifiers because these modifiers signify unusual circumstances, they are not calculated in the UCR reimbursement method. Omission of the appropriate modifiers with varying charge amounts, however, has a significant effect on the calculation of these UCR reimbursements. The following example demonstrates this concept.

CPT code 99213: Usual charge for practice is $75

During a specified period, the practice submitted the charge a total of 50 times as follows:

99213 Office visit established, level 3
30 times @ $75.00 (usual charge) = $2250
20 times @ $60.00 (usual charge) = $1200
(Reduced charge for reduced service without modifier 52)
TOTAL CHARGES = $3450
Total charges $3450/50 patients = Average charge of $69

On the basis of these submissions by this provider, the customary reimbursement for this service would now be $69 rather than the $75 charge.

In some cases the coder or biller may notice a significantly reduced reimbursement compared with the charge amount because other providers are submitting charges at lesser amounts or without modifiers when appropriate.

In addition, third-party carriers often use data that have been compiled some time in the past, in some cases more than a year earlier. When this occurs, the customary calculation will reflect the providers charges from previous years, and reimbursement will be substantially less than the current charge information.

RESOURCE-BASED RELATIVE VALUE STUDY

Another reimbursement method used by third-party carriers for provider reimbursement is referred to as **resource-based relative value study** (**RBRVS**). Because of the growing number of complaints from providers and facilities regarding the "flaws" of the UCR method, the federal government commissioned Harvard University to develop this new method of reimbursement calculation. The RBRVS method takes into account the following components:

Geographic allowance — Consists of an index called the *Geographical Practice Cost Index* (GPCI). The GPCI measures the differences in physician costs for practice expenses and malpractice expenses in different geographic areas compared with the national average.

Work units — A value assigned to each CPT code that reflects the physician's or provider's work value.

Practice expense — The cost to the practice of providing the service based on geographic adjustment by area.

Malpractice expense — An assigned value based on the malpractice history and record on morbidity and mortality for the service.

RBRVS is used by Medicare and a number of other carriers to determine the "worth" or reimbursement they will consider for each CPT code. It is often used as well by providers to help determine fees for services as well.

Practice Reimbursement Mechanisms

The immediate job of the coder is to review or assign appropriate codes to the services provided. The long-term job of the coder encompasses a number of duties within the medical practice.

Obviously, coding is an integral part of the reimbursement process; however, this process extends from the time the patient schedules an appointment to the time the patient checks in and out for the appointment. The codes are then entered into the computerized or manual billing system.

It is imperative that the coder be involved in these processes. Coding correctly on the initial attempt is vital for prompt turnaround on claims submitted. Initial claims processing usually averages 30 to 60 days. Some states have passed legislation specifying the amount of time each carrier is allowed to process a **clean claim,** or claim that contains no errors or omissions. The term clean claim, however, can be ambiguous, and insurance carriers identify any minor problems with claims to avert processing and avoid paying claims within the defined period if possible. The goal of the practice should be that all initial claims are clean claims. This would afford prompt and accurate reimbursement without the need for additional work and intervention on the part of the practice.

If the initial claim cannot be processed as the result of error or if additional information is needed, either a corrected claim form or additional information must be forwarded to the carrier for consideration. Most states have not legislated time limits for processing these claims; therefore carriers may delay processing of these claims as long as possible. Some of the large carriers may take an average of an additional 6 to 12 weeks to process the resubmitted claim.

Discussion follows on medical office processes and the effect of coder involvement in these processes. It will become apparent that the coder also provides essential input or training in other areas that affect reimbursement as well.

FILE MAINTENANCE AND COMPUTER SETUP OF CODING NOMENCLATURE

This is an area in which errors can multiply quickly. When an erroneous code or amount is entered into the computer system, the error will multiply each time that code is used by the practice.

The addition of new procedure and diagnosis codes, as well as the review of previously entered codes, should be performed by an established coder. Once these codes are verified, data entry personnel with little coding knowledge will enter the correct codes. Access to adding, editing, or deleting these codes should be restricted to the coder and a limited number of knowledgeable administrative staff members.

OFFICE CHARGE TICKET AND HOSPITAL CHARGE DOCUMENT

In addition to verifying information entered into the computerized or manual billing system, the design of the practice **charge ticket** or **superbill** and the development of a hospital charge document aid greatly in ensuring that correct codes are being used for coding and billing the practices services.

The coder should be involved with this process, which should occur at least biannually. Service analyses or productivity reports available from the computerized billing system identify the most frequent procedures and diagnosis codes to be included on the charge documents. Other information needed to code appropriately, such as the following, should be preprinted on the charge ticket or hospital document:

- Referring physician (consultation codes)
- Modifier codes (those used for specific codes [e.g., evaluation and management (E & M) modifiers listed in that section of the charge document])
- A mechanism to "match" diagnosis codes and procedure codes for medical necessity (when multiple services are performed, which specific diagnoses match specified procedures)

The review and updating of charge documents should correlate with the yearly publication of CPT and ICD-9-CM/ICD-10-CM and with the time the practice updates most of its third-party contracts and the contract worksheet information. Figure 19-1 shows a sample hospital charge document intended to capture all necessary charge information for the practice.

One of the biggest mistakes made in conjunction with the use of a charge document is that services are often not reviewed for correct coding. An example is the office charge document or superbill, on which a provider may indicate the level of service (E & M code) and diagnosis(es). This informa-

HOSPITAL CHARGE WORKSHEET

Date Received: Info Taken By:

PROCEDURE(S): CARDIAC CATHETERIZATIONS/INJECTIONS/IMAGING

HEART	CATHS
93510-26	Left, Percutaneous
93511-26	Left, By Cutdown
93524-26	Left, Combined Transep/ Retrograde
93526-26	Combined Rt/Lt

OTHER	
93503	Swan-Ganz
93536	Insert Intra-Aortic Balloon Catheter

INJECTION PROC	
93539-26	Arterial Conduits, Sel Opacification
93540-26	Aortocoronary Venous Bypass Grafts, Sel Opacification
93541-26	Pulmonary Angiography
93542-26	Rt Ventricular/Right Atrial Angiography
93543-26	Lt Ventricular/Left Atrial Angiography
93544-26	Aortography
93545-26	Selective Coronary Angiography

IMAGING PROCEDURE	
93555	Ventricular/Atrial Angiography
93556	Pulm Angiography, Aortography and/or Sel Coronary Angio

DETERMINATION OF APPROPRIATE CODING:

Choose Approp Injection/Imaging Codes

VALID DIAGNOSIS CODE(S): FOR CATHS ONLY/OTHER PROCEDURES ON REVERSE

MITRAL VALVE	
394.0	Stenosis
394.1	Rheum Insuff
394.2	Stenosis w/Insuff
394.9	Other Diseases
AORTIC VALVE	
395.0	Rheum Stenosis
395.1	Rheum Insuff
395.2	Rheum Stenosis w/Insuff
395.9	Other Rheum Dz
MITRAL AND AORTIC VALVES	
396.0	Stenosis
396.1	Mitral Stenosis with Aortic Insuff
396.2	Mitral Insuff w/ Aortic Stenosis
396.3	Mitral/Aortic Insuff
396.8	Multiple Involve
396.9	Unspecified
MYOCARDIAL INFARCTION	
410.0*	Anterolateral Wall
410.1*	Oth Anterior Wall
410.2*	Inferolateral Wall
410.3*	Inferopost Wall
410.4*	Oth Inferior Wall
410.5*	Other Lat Wall
410.6*	True Post Wall
410.7*	Subendocardial
410.8*	Other Spec Sites
410.9*	Unspec Site
*5th digit for episode of care	
0-episode unspec	
1-initial	2-subsequent
411.0	Post MI Syndrome
411.1	Inter Coronary Sny Unstable Angina Impending MI
411.81	Coronary Occlus w/o MI
411.89	Other Isch Hrt Dz
412	Old MI
413.0	Angina Decubitus
413.1	Prinzmetal Angina
413.9	Unspec Angina
CORONARY ATHEROSCH	
414.00	Unspec Type Vess
414.01	Native Coronary
414.02	Auto Biol Bypass Gr
414.03	NonAuto Bypass Gr
414.04	Artery Bypass Graft
414.05	Unspec Byp Graft
414.10	Aneurysm Hrt Wall
414.11	Aneurysm Cor Vess
414.19	Aneurysm Other
421.0	Bact Endocarditis
421.1	In Dz Stated Else
421.9	Unspecified
424.0	Mitral Valve Dis
424.1	Aortic Valve Dis
424.90	Endocarditis,Valve
424.99	Other Endocarditis
429.71	Acq Card Septal Def Seq to MI
CONGENITAL DEFECTS	
746.3	Stenosis Aortic Valv
746.4	Insuff Aortic Valve
746.5	Mitral Stenosis
746.6	Mitral Insuff
746.7	Hypoplastic Lt Hrt Syndrome

CHARGE ENTRY INFORMATION:

Patient Name: ____________ Hospital: ________ Inpt ____ Outpt ____ Other: ____________

Date of Current Service: ____________ Admit Date: ____________ Other: ____________

Referring Phy Info: ____________

Attending Physician: ____________

	CPT	Mod	Dx #1	Dx #2	Dx #3	Dx #4	Other (Specify):
1-							
2-							
3-							
4-							
5-							

Date Entered: ____________ Initials: ________

Comments: ____________

FIGURE 19-1. A hospital charge ticket sample for a cardiology practice. All information must be included from a coding perspective so that the physician and coder may accurately reflect services provided.

tion may then be entered in the billing system without review or monitoring. As a result, a large percentage of errors may be made on these forms and significant reimbursement may be lost or potential fraud may be committed.

ANCILLARY SERVICE REQUEST FORMS

Ancillary services require the diagnosis to justify medical necessity of providing those services. If the facility provides ancillary services for outside facilities or providers (e.g., stress treadmills or radiology), the appropriate diagnostic information must be obtained from the ordering physician. Because the requesting physician is not a part of the practice, it is imperative to provide ordering physicians with the information needed to order, perform, code, and receive reimbursement for this service. Many practices provide ancillary services to outside providers as a supplement to their practice income. Many do not realize that a large percentage of these services may in fact not be paid because of insufficient diagnostic information from the ordering physician. For instance, highly comprehensive cardiac testing, such as thallium stress tests, may not be reimbursed for the diagnosis of "chest pain," but may be reimbursed for "angina" or "abnormal ECG."

It is imperative that the practice provide ordering physicians with the information needed to correctly code and bill for services performed. The practice may wish to design an ancillary request sheet with the needed information and the most common diagnosis codes, excluding diagnoses not covered by most insurance carriers. For Medicare patients, the performing provider must inform the patient in advance that the service may not be covered and must obtain a signed waiver form, known as the **advance beneficiary notice (ABN)**, from the patient. If the diagnostic information provided by the ordering or referring physician is not sufficient for reimbursement, the patient should be informed before his or her arrival at the facility. If the diagnosis is not covered, the ordering or referring physician can explain this to the patient in advance, thus avoiding an uncomfortable situation for all involved. The practice may wish to market ancillary services that it provides; an ancillary request form provides a convenient mechanism for referring patients, and it offers assistance in selecting the most appropriate diagnostic information and the most appropriate test for the presenting complaint. A sample of an ancillary request form is shown in Figure 19-2.

The Coder as Coding and Reimbursement Educator

Another crucial job of the coder in the medical practice is the job of educator. The business office or billing department may possess the expertise to bill the services for reimbursement; however, the coder has the knowledge to select the proper codes to place on the billing form to obtain appropriate reimbursement. Without that knowledge and the correct code on the claim form, the practice or facility will not be reimbursed appropriately. The billing staff may produce and file claims or UB-04s efficiently. If coding is not correct and if it does not completely describe the services and justify why they were performed, the practice or facility may not get paid.

As the coding expert in the facility, the coder must create mechanisms to spread coding information to other personnel who, at a minimum, need to understand the selection of codes, the purpose of justifying medical necessity, and the use of modifier codes. This does not mean that the practice or facility should expect all personnel to become proficient coders, but all should recognize inconsistencies and triggers that will result in denial or nonpayment of claims.

In the process of choosing procedure codes or modifier codes that a specific carrier does or does not recognize, information can be automatically loaded into the computerized billing system, thus guiding the practice or facility staff to select the correct code(s). For instance, a specific carrier does not use the preventive medicine codes for "well woman visits" but has developed a set code "99999" for this purpose. The computerized billing system can be programmed so that anytime that particular carrier code is entered and a preventive medicine code is entered by data entry personnel, the system converts that code to "99999." This eliminates the need for data entry personnel to manually override the billing system and helps avoid error.

When specific diagnosis codes are required in conjunction with certain procedure codes, the system can be programmed to reject other code combinations or to alert the data entry personnel of a potential error. For instance, when preventive medicine codes for a specific carrier require that all such services must be billed with diagnosis code "general medical examination," the system can be triggered to alert personnel when this combination is not used.

Review of the charge entry process also helps the billing office in the submission of payable claims. The best-spent 15 to 30 minutes of time during the coder's workday (or that of another trained individual) is used to review the charge tickets or charge entry documents before charge entry for incompleteness, coding deficiencies, or missing information such as modifiers and medical necessity diagnoses. An additional 15 to 30 minutes is well spent reviewing the paper claims and electronic claims register of claims prepared for transmittal. Despite the review of the charge document before data entry, errors are made, omissions do happen, and a clean claim may no longer be clean. The practice must now wait an additional 6 to 12 weeks for payment after initial rejection, and additional work must be done by staff to resubmit.

In addition, a review of the **explanation of benefits (EOB)** received from insurance carriers is imperative to identify claims that, despite programming of the computerized billing

DIAGNOSTIC CARDIOLOGY ORDER FORM

Practice Name/Address:
Practice Phone/Fax:

ECHOCARDIOGRAPHY (Please mark applicable diagnosis)

Diagnosis	Code	Diagnosis	Code
Angina	413.9	Heart Murmur	785.2
Aortic Valve Disorder	424.1	Mitral Valve Prolapse	424.0
Atrial Fibrillation	427.31	Mitral Stenosis	394.0
ASHD	414.00	Myocardial Infarc Old	412
Cardiomegaly	429.3	Pulmonary HTN	426.0
Cardiomyopathy	425.4	Pulmonary Valve Disorder	424.3
Chest Pain Unspec	786.50	Syncope	780.2
Chest Pain,Tightness	786.59	Tachycardia	427.2
Congenital Heart Dz	746.9	Tricuspid Valve Disorder	424.2
Coronary Artery Dz	414.00	Ventricular Fibrillation	427.41
		Other: CONTACT PRACTICE FOR ASSISTANCE	

HOLTER MONITORING (Please mark applicable diagnosis)

Diagnosis	Code	Diagnosis	Code
Angina, Unspecified	413.9	Mitral Valve Disorders	424.0
Angina, Unstable	411.1	Palpitations	785.1
ASHD	414.00	PVCs	427.69
Atrial Fibrillation	427.31	Premature Beats	427.61
Atrial Flutter	427.32	Syncope	780.2
Arrhythmia, Unspec	427.9	Tachycardia	427.81
Bradycardia	427.89	Ventricular Fibrillation	427.41
Cardiomegaly	429.3	Ventricular Flutter	427.42
Cardiomyopathy	425.4	Other: CONTACT PRACTICE FOR ASSISTANCE	

THALLIUM STRESS TEST (Please mark applicable diagnosis)

Diagnosis	Code	Diagnosis	Code
Atherosclerosis/Arteries	414.00	Heart Blocks:	426.3
Atherosclerosis/Unspec	440.20	Left Bundle Branch	426.4
Atherosclerosis/Inter Claudification	440.21	Right Bundle Branch	426.10
Abnormal ECG	794.31	Unspecified	428.9
Angina, Unstable	411.1	Heart Failure Unspec	414.9
Angina, Unspecified	413.9	Ischemic Heart Disease	424.0
Atrial Fibrillation	427.31	Mitral Valve Disorders	V67.0
Congestive Heart Failure	428.0	Postsurgical F/Up	
Coronary Artery Disease	414.9	Other: CONTACT PRACTICE FOR ASSISTANCE	

Patient Name: DOB:
Insurance Type: Auth #:

Ordering/Referring Physician: Phone:

In the event one of the above diagnoses is not applicable for the service requested, contact THE PRACTICE for assistance in selecting the correct test/diagnosis for the patient's condition.

FIGURE 19-2. An ancillary request form. This may be used to help referring physicians supply adequate information for coding and billing of services requested by outside physicians.

system and review of the charge document and claim, still did not receive proper reimbursement. Improperly paid or denied claims should not be dealt with on a one-on-one basis, but according to how the error occurred and how the correction is made. For instance, suppose that multiple units were placed on the charge document for medication, were entered into the system, and appeared to have been successfully printed on the claim, yet the carrier paid for only one unit. A review of the EOB indicates how the insurance carrier received the claim (paper or electronic), how many units were received on the claim, and so forth. Appropriate action can then be taken to correct this problem in the future.

If modifier codes are missing on the EOB, isolate the source of this error (e.g., charge ticket completion, data entry), educate staff, and correct the problem. Use the computerized billing system whenever possible to "foolproof" this system. When this is not possible, make sure staff members are aware of the problem and know how to address it.

General Third-Party Coding and Reimbursement Resources

Although third-party carriers have specific guidelines that they follow regarding coding, many follow CPT, ICD-9-CM, and DRG guidelines along with general guidelines that are published and are available to facilities and providers. Some of these common guidelines are the following:

Correct Coding Initiative	Indicates CPT code combinations considered bundled
Surgical cross-reference unbundling books	List each surgical code contained in CPT with CPT codes considered bundled or included in the global package for that specific surgical code. Remember that extenuating circumstances may allow coding of these services with the appropriate modifier for reimbursement consideration.
Coders' Desk Reference	Lists each procedure (CPT) and gives a detailed description about what the procedure is, what is included, and what may be coded separately.

Specific Third-Party Coding and Reimbursement Guidelines

In addition to general guidelines regarding coding and reimbursement, most carriers have specific guidelines they use for reviewing and determining reimbursement for coded services. Along with general guidelines and principles, these specific third-party guidelines should be incorporated into the third-party contract worksheet (see Tool 19-1). Areas that should be delineated are detailed below.

TIME LIMITS

Determine the time limit established by each third-party carrier for submission of claims as well as appeal and resubmission time limits. Make certain that claims are submitted within these guidelines. In some cases this means follow-up, not only for status, but for receipt of claim during the specified time limits.

Even though the practice has sent a claim during the specified time limits, this does not mean that the third party will acknowledge receipt within that same time frame. Dating the receipt of claims after the time limit is a common practice among third-party carriers for not paying claims. Claims that are "lost" and never received will also exceed time limits if they are not followed up expediently.

HCPCS VERSUS CPT CODES

Make certain the contract worksheet encompasses the coding nomenclature(s) used by each carrier. In some cases, carriers will not accept HCPCS procedure or modifier codes. In other instances, third-party carriers insist on the use of these codes when appropriate. Denial or payment sometimes rests on the appropriate use of these codes along carrier-specific guidelines. Third-party guidelines indicate that when both CPT and HCPCS codes are acceptable, the codes with the highest level of specificity (HCPCS) should be assigned.

CODING AND BILLING FOR NONPHYSICIAN SERVICES (MODIFIER FOR PHYSICIAN ASSISTANT OR OTHER PHYSICIAN EXTENDERS)

Make certain the practice determines whether services are reimbursable when they are provided by health professionals other than physicians. Determine whether the carrier recognizes these nonphysician entities as well as what services and providers they recognize.

Physician assistants and nurse practitioners may provide services under the direction of the physician or independently. Some carriers allow these services to be billed under the name of the provider; others require that these services be billed only under the name of the supervising physician.

Make certain that services requiring the supervision of a licensed physician are documented as such with the appropriate physician countersignatures for overseeing the care and concurring with the assessment and treatment plan. This typically requires a minimum notation of "reviewed and concur," the date, and the physician's "mark" of authentication.

In many instances the third-party carrier will require the use of a modifier code to indicate that services were performed with the use of a physician extender. Many carriers reimburse these services at a reduced rate from when the physician provides the services.

Specific HCPCS modifiers designate that services have been performed by a physician extender or in connection with a physician extender. These modifiers are located in the HCPCS modifier section on CPT coding.

Medicare has specific guidelines for "incident to" billing. If a practice employs physician extenders (i.e., physician assistants, nurse practitioners, other nonphysician providers), the practice should be familiar with these guidelines, which spell out under what circumstances nonphysician providers may see patients independently, under the supervision of the provider and the appropriate billing guidelines for these services. This information is available on the Centers for Medicare and Medicaid Services Web site (www.cms.gov).

TOOL 19-1

THIRD-PARTY CONTRACT WORKSHEET

	Cov Serv	Auth Req	Coverage Limits	Provide Serv In-House	Outside Facility Coding Considerations
OFFICE SERVICES					
Annual Exams					
Office Visits/Consults					
Diagnostic X-Rays					
Labs:					
Pap Smears					
Blood Draws					
Urinalysis					
Lab Work					
Other					
Other					
Other					
Other					
HOSPITAL SERVICES					
Hospital Admissions					
Hospital Visits					
Consultations					
Surgical Procedures					
Other					
Other					

INSURANCE NAMES:

HOSPITAL NETWORK:

PHARMACY NETWORK:

MANAGED CARE NAME:

HMO Plan
PPO Plan
Indemnity Plan

EVALUATION AND MANAGEMENT SERVICES GUIDELINES (DOWNCODING)

Many third-party carriers have instituted coding software that "downcodes" services based on the diagnostic coding provided on the claim form. The only information used for paying a large volume of services are ICD-9-CM diagnostic codes and CPT procedure codes. Often, however, these codes do not consider the large number of diagnostic options and other factors used to determine level of service. As a cost-saving measure, many third-party carriers have instituted the use of software that determines the level of service based simply on the diagnostic code(s) provided. If the provider has coded the service at a higher level, the claim will automatically be downcoded and the reimbursement will be significantly less than the original level submitted.

Medical service providers should watch for these downcoding practices on their explanation of benefits. The medical practice reserves the right to appeal the third-party decision, usually by submitting a copy of the physician documentation used to determine the correct level of service. Once again, the physician documentation will determine the proper reimbursement. Many medical practices and several medical societies representing physicians have begun to challenge this practice in the court system.

PREVENTIVE MEDICINE VISITS

Many insurance carriers still do not recognize the need for preventive medicine services and therefore do not reimburse for these services. Make certain the services are, in fact, preventive, meaning no treatment of complaints is provided during the visit; the diagnosis would be a "well" diagnosis such as "well woman" or "well baby."

Other third-party carriers do reimburse for these well visits but do not recognize the use of preventive medicine codes. Make sure to capture this information on the third-party contracts worksheet as well.

Despite the fact that CPT guidelines indicate a preventive medicine visit as well as a regular level of service (with modifier 25), there may be instances in which the patient presents for a well visit but with a number of problems; few carriers reimburse for more than one E & M service per day. If these two "significantly separately identifiable" E & M services do take place, they should be billed accordingly. The practice will want to code the most significant service (usually the preventive medicine service) first, followed by the level of office visit with modifier 25. If the third party disallows one of these services, it typically would be the second service; therefore the least significant service may not be reimbursed.

MODIFIERS (GENERAL)

CPT defines the modifier codes and their use and explains which sections of CPT these modifiers are used for; however, many third-party carriers interpret these guidelines differently. Some carriers do not recognize any modifier codes; others recognize certain modifier codes only in specific instances. For instance, Medicare's interpretation is that all surgical services have a minimum follow-up period of 10 days. Medicare may not recognize the use of modifier 57 (decision for surgery) for reimbursement of any E & M services. This can differ with each Medicare carrier or **fiscal intermediary** (**FI**) as well.

Check each of the practice's or facility's third-party carrier contracts, making sure the use of these modifiers is specifically spelled out. If this is not specified in the contract, third-party carriers are free to interpret these guidelines in whatever manner they wish. In most cases, their interpretation will NOT be to the practice's or facility's advantage.

GLOBAL (BUNDLED) SERVICES

Although CPT and several coding bundling and unbundling books specify services covered under the "global" concept, many third-party carriers interpret these guidelines differently. If the practice or facility provides specialty services that include global surgical services, make certain these guidelines are clarified in each carrier contract. For instance, if the practice provides global maternity care services, make certain guidelines for services outside the global package, such as high-risk pregnancies, and additional services over and above the global guidelines in CPT and the American College of Obstetrics and Gynecology are outlined by each carrier. Significant reimbursement may be lost if this information is not specified in the third-party contract.

COSURGEON OR TWO SURGEONS

Carriers usually have specific guidelines pertaining to cosurgeons that include whether these services will be reimbursed and what the effect is on reimbursement. The practice will want to make certain that their providers always include such information in the operative report because many third-party carriers request this information as proof that both surgeons were involved.

Reimbursement for cosurgeons or two surgeons is typically around 125% of the regular allowance for the service, with each provider receiving approximately 62.5%. This may vary from carrier to carrier, so the practice will need to determine the correct reimbursement for each carrier for these services.

ASSISTANT SURGEONS

Many hospital and outpatient facilities have specific bylaws that detail when the use of an assistant surgeon is required; however, third-party carrier guidelines will not necessarily coincide with these facility requirements.

The practice must determine both the surgical codes that will be reimbursable by each carrier for assistant surgeons and the reimbursable amount, which will dramatically differ from the primary surgeon fee. Some carriers reimburse as little as 10% to 20% of the surgery allowance for the assistant surgeon.

As a result, many assistant surgeons may request that the primary surgeon list them or allow them to bill as cosurgeons. Not only is this practice illegal and unethical, but it meets the definition of fraud for all parties involved. In addition, the primary surgeon would be paid only approximately 62.5% of the allowance for the service, rather than the 100% allowance for services coded and billed correctly.

MULTIPLE PROCEDURES

Reimbursement for multiple surgical procedures, with or without the proper use of modifier 51, may differ from carrier to carrier. The practice must make certain that the specific carrier's interpretation is included in the contract with each carrier. Significant differences in ultimate reimbursement may result from differences in interpretation.

Development of Third-Party Contract Worksheets

Perhaps the best tool for the coder to introduce into the practice is a third-party contract worksheet. Development of this involves review of each of the third-party contracts for specific requirements regarding codes, such as the following:

- Services the practice is contracted to perform
- Services the practice may or may NOT perform
- Locations where services may be referred or rendered
- Services requiring preauthorization
- Acceptable and unacceptable modifier codes
- Acceptable and unacceptable procedure codes
- Special carrier-specific procedure codes

After acquiring this information, the coder, with the assistance of the billing or business office, can develop information sheets for use by the staff. At a glance the scheduler and the data entry, clinical, and professional staff members can determine whether a service can be provided and whether the practice will be reimbursed.

This information will serve as a helpful tool to all practice employees for obtaining appropriate authorizations and using specific CPT codes, modifiers, or guidelines. A blank form of a third-party contract worksheet is shown in Tool 19-1. Figure 19-3 is a sample of such a worksheet. In development of this third-party contract worksheet, it will be necessary for the practice to read carefully through each contract, gather the needed information, and request clarification or modification of the contract when information is missing or ambiguous. This is the time for clarification, rather than when claims are denied or are not reimbursed to the practice's or facility's expectations because of a misunderstanding on contract issue(s).

Most third-party contracts include a fee schedule; however, they often include only the most frequently used CPT codes. Make certain the carrier clearly spells out reimbursement protocol (e.g., Medicare fee schedule, percent of charges) for all services not specified in the fee schedule provided.

Gather the information needed for a third-party contract worksheet by using an outline such as Tool 19-2. This same type of information can be gathered for hospital services as well. Hospitals may need to employ an individual or a group of individuals to research, update, and disburse this information to all employees and to present educational materials regarding this information.

MANAGED CARE NAME:

	Cov Serv			Auth Req			Coverage Limits			Provide Serv In-House			Outside Facility Coding Considerations
OFFICE SERVICES													
Annual Well-Woman Exams	Y	Y	Y	Y	N	N	1 YR	1 YR	1 YR	Y	Y	Y	Must use Preventive Med Codes, Dx V72.3 only
Office Visits/Consults	Y	Y	Y	Y	N	N	N	N	N	Y	Y	Y	Do not use Confirm Consult Codes
Diagnostic X-Rays	Y	Y	Y	Y	N	N	N	N	N	Y	Y	Y	Dx Rad Only/All Others Outside
Labs:													
Pap Smears	Y	Y	Y	N	N	N	N	N	N	N	N	N	SKL
Blood Draws	Y	Y	Y	N	N	N	N	N	N	Y	Y	Y	Use Code 99000 (No Modifier 90)
Urinalysis	Y	Y	Y	N	N	N	N	N	N	Y	Y	Y	Urinalysis 81000 In-House Only/All Others Out SKL
Lab Work	N	N	N	N	N	N	N	N	N	N	N	N	Blood Draws In-House Only/All Others Out SKL
Other:													
Other:													
Other:													
Other:													
HOSPITAL SERVICES	All inpatient services require preauthorizations												
Hospital Admissions	Y	Y	Y	Y	Y	Y	N	N	N	N	N	N	
Hospital Visits	Y	Y	Y	Y	Y	Y	N	N	N	N	N	N	
Consultations	Y	Y	Y	Y	Y	Y	N	N	N	N	N	N	
Surgical Procedures	Y	Y	Y	Y	Y	Y	N	N	N	N	N	N	
Other:													
Other:													

INSURANCE NAMES:
DDD Insurance
AAA Employers Group
Rad Centers:
XYZ Radiology (407) 888-8888
ABC Radiology (407) 777-7777

HOSPITAL NETWORK:
EEE Hospital
FFF Hospital

PHARMACY NETWORK:
Pharmacies Are Us (407) 222-2222

MANAGED CARE NAME:

HMO Plan
PPO Plan
Indemnity Plan

FIGURE 19-3. Sample contract worksheet. This worksheet shows the information included in the contract to which other office staff must have access on a daily basis.

TOOL 19-2

MANAGED CARE CONTRACT REVIEW

Managed Care Plan:________________________________
Plan #s:________________________________
(List)

HMO:________PPO:________Cap:________Other:________
Original Contract Date:________________________
Last Date Reviewed:____________By:____________

CONTRACT BENEFITS:
Termination Clause:________________________
Claims Filing Deadline:________________________

	Y	N	Comments	Other
Covered Services:				
ECG				
Lab				
X-ray				
Diag				
Other				
Other				
Authorizations:	Y	N	Comments	Other
ECG				
Lab				
X-ray				
Diag				
Hosp				
Hosp Proc				
Other				
Other				
Plan Limitations:	Y	N	Comments	Other
ECG				
Lab				
X-ray				
Diag				
Hosp				
Hosp Proc				
Other				
Bill Aboves:	Y	N	Comments	Other
(List)				
Modifiers:	Y	N	Comments	Other

Fee Schedule________________________
Last Date Reviewed____________By ____________
In Computer: Y_____N_____Reviewed Date____________
Adj Code_____ Payment Code_____ Reviewed Date____________

Chapter in Review

Certification Review

- Third-party carriers are not required to follow guidelines outlined in CPT, ICD-9-CM, and other coding books.
- Provider and physician services are reported on the CMS-1500 form.
- Facility and hospital services are reported on the UB-04 form.
- The third-party contract should serve as a mutual understanding of how codes should be used for reimbursement.
- The third-party contract should represent the terms of both parties: the third party and the provider of the service.
- Participation with a third-party carrier means the provider agrees to accept as payment in full the amount contractually allowed.
- The usual, customary, and reasonable (UCR) method involves the usual charge, the customary charge, and the amount considered reasonable by the carrier.
- The resource-based relative value study (RBRVS) method is based on geographic allowance, work units, practice expense, and malpractice expense.
- The coder serves as the office reimbursement educator.
- Third-party contracts should delineate items such as the following:
  - Time limits
  - HCPCS and CPT codes
  - Reimbursement for nonphysician services
  - E & M service guidelines
  - Preventive medicine guidelines
  - Modifiers
  - Global services
  - Cosurgeons and assistant surgeons
  - Multiple procedures
- Third-party contract worksheets should be developed by the practice to educate and inform office personnel of the specifics of each third-party contract.

Student Assignments

- Study Chapter 19.
- Review the Learning Objectives for Chapter 19.
- Review the Certification Review for Chapter 19.
- Complete the Chapter Review exercise to reinforce concepts learned in this chapter.
- Complete the practice exercises on the companion Evolve site for reinforcement of concepts learned In this chapter.
- Complete the Practical Application exercises.
- Complete the Workbook exercises as assigned by your instructor, or individually for additional practice.

Chapter Review Exercise

Obtain a third-party contract from a practice or facility. Review the contract, identifying the key elements to incorporate into the third-party contract worksheet as well as any clarification or missing information needed from the third-party carrier. Enter this information on the outline form before incorporating it into the actual third-party contract worksheet.

Remember that third-party contracts may be renegotiated, and addendums for clarification can be made at any time. The practice does not have to accept a third-party contract as presented. Approach the third-party carrier from the perspective of clarification rather than confrontation. The third-party carrier usually will be willing to clarify or provide any missing information.

Practical Application

For the following reports and notes, determine whether they will be paid as submitted or whether errors have been made. If the report is not correct, determine what corrections need to be made.

1. Office visit

OFFICE NOTE

Chief complaint: ______________________________

Date: ______________________

Vital signs: BP______ P______ R______

History:

DISPOSITION:
This 88-year-old new patient was lifting a pan, which fell on her right hand. She does have osteoporosis. Her medications are as listed. Her allergies are also as listed.

Reveals an alert, pleasant elderly woman. There is ecchymosis and tenderness of the base of the proximal phalanx of the right middle finger. The skin is intact. Motion of the finger is limited. Sensation is intact. There is good capillary refill. X-rays of the right hand show no fracture.

Exam:

Contusion, right hand. Possible fracture, right middle finger

Diagnosis/assessment:

She is to elevate the hand with ice. She may take ibuprofen as needed. If she develops increased pain or any other problem she is to follow up with her usual physician.

ICD-9-CM Codes:
816.00
923.20
E917.9

Willen Obst MD

Patient name: ______________________________

Date of service: ______________________

GODFREY MEDICAL ASSOCIATES
1532 Third Avenue, Suite 120 • Aldon, FL 77713 • (407) 555-4000

2. Office visit

OFFICE NOTE

Chief complaint: ____________________

Date: ____________

Vital signs: BP_____ P_____ R_____

History:

Exam:

Diagnosis/assessment:

PLAN: This 78-year-old female claims she woke up feeling short of breath and a little chest pain. She was here about 24 hours ago with dizziness, weakness, and emesis and was diagnosed with benign positional vertigo. She was prescribed Antivert that she says she is using, but it isn't helping. The patient agreed to be seen by me when she realized ambulance costs for transfer to another city wouldn't be covered.

Seems to be positive for a number of emergency visits for similar complaints. She does have an artificial porcine valve and apparently has had bypass surgery.

Vioxx, Tagament, Slow Iron, Norvasc, and the Antivert mentioned. Apparently intolerant to Tylenol, ASA, ibuprofen, and, I believe, sulfa.

She is afebrile. Vital signs are stable. She seems to be sleepy but is also anxious. Color is normal. She is not diaphoretic. NECK: supple. JVP is flat. Carotids are normal. CHEST: clear with good air entry bilaterally. Heart sounds are normal. She has aortic stenosis type murmur. ABDOMEN: soft and nontender, perhaps a little mild tenderness in the left upper quadrant. Pulses are normal.

ECG did not reveal any acute changes.

She was originally given sublingual nitro, which she said helped. By the time the lab results came back, she had talked to the nurse and came to the conclusion that she had overreacted when she woke up, was likely just anxious, but now was feeling fine.

She wants to go home.

1. Questionable anxiety

ICD-9-CM Codes:
300.00, 786.05, 786.50

CPT Codes:
99285
93010

Stacy Kraft, MD

Patient name: ____________________

Date of service: ____________

GODFREY MEDICAL ASSOCIATES
1532 Third Avenue, Suite 120 • Aldon, FL 77713 • (407) 555-4000

3. Progress note

PROGRESS NOTE

Date: 02/12/XX	Vital signs: T	R
Chief complaint: Cough for 2 weeks	P	BP

4-month-old is brought in with complaint he has been having a cough for over 2 weeks. Now he has a fever and coughs a lot. Also fussy. He is eating fair.

Examination:

Temperature 101, pulse 140, respirations 36. No use of accessory muscles. Throat: some congestion. Ears:
bilaterally does reveal red eardrum on the left with absent-like reflex. Normal vesicular breathing. No rhonchi or crackles.

Chest x-ray, PA & lateral is negative

CBC normal

Impression:

Bilateral otitis media. Probably pneumonia.

Plan:

Augmentin 125 mg per 5 ml.
1 tsp tid × 10 days

ICD-9-CM Codes:
486 Pneumonia
382.9 Otitis Media

Maurice Doates, MD

Patient name:
DOB: 10/08/20XX
MR/Chart #: 10084

GODFREY REGIONAL OUTPATIENT CLINIC
3122 Shannon Avenue • Aldon, FL 77712 • (407) 555-7654

4. Progress note

PROGRESS NOTE

Date: 03/08/XX **Chief complaint:** Sore throat/cough × 1 week	**Vital signs:** T R P BP

03/08/XX 9-year-old female with sore throat and cough which she has had now for about a week.

Examination:

Temperature in the office is 101.4
Skin is clear. Ear drums negative, pharynx red. Culture taken. Negative for strep. Chest clear to auscultation.
Heart tones regular w / 0 murmurs. Abdomen soft.

Impression:

URI with pharyngitis
Diabetes
Ingrown toenail

Plan:

Amoxicillin 250 mg tid for 20 days

CPT Code:
99284

Felix Washington MD

Patient name: Anita White
DOB: 7/28/19XX
MR/Chart #: 67777

GODFREY REGIONAL OUTPATIENT CLINIC
3122 Shannon Avenue • Aldon, FL 77712 • (407) 555-7654

5. Operative report

OPERATIVE REPORT

Patient information:

Patient name:
DOB:
MR#:

Date:
Surgeon:
Anesthetist:

Preoperative diagnosis:

Cholecystitis, cholelithiasis

Postoperative diagnosis:

Same

Procedure(s) performed:

Cholecystectomy with operative cholangiogram

Anesthesia:

Assistant surgeon:

Description of procedure:

31-year-old white female presented with mid-epigastric and right upper quadrant pain increasing in intensity. Evaluation revealed multiple gallstones, and surgery was recommended. The options, risks, alternative treatments, and exact nature of the procedure were described in detail, and she seemed to understand well. Patient was taken to the operating room; under adequate general anesthesia, the abdomen was prepped and draped in a sterile fashion. The stomach and bladder were drained and supraumbilical incision was made. The Veressneedle was used for institution of the pneumoperitoneum. A 10mm port was placed, as well as the usual upper paramedian 10mm port and lateral 5mm ports. Gallbladder was retracted up to its bed using blunt dissection and cautery. The cystic duct was identified, and an intraoperative cholangiogram was read as normal. The cystic duct and cystic artery were ligated and divided. The gallbladder was dissected free of surrounding tissue with cautery, and was removed through the upper paramedian port. The right upper quadrant was then irrigated. After hemostasis was assured, wounds were closed with 2-0 Vicryl and 4-0 Vicryl subcuticular. Skin incisions were then infiltrated with Marcaine, at which time the patient was taken to the recovery room in stable condition.

CPT Codes:
47605
Open Cholecystectomy with
Cholangiogram

Adam Westy MD

GODFREY REGIONAL HOSPITAL
123 Main Street • Aldon, FL 77714 • (407) 555-1234

6. Operative report

OPERATIVE REPORT

Patient information:

Patient name:
DOB:
MR#:

Date:
Surgeon:
Anesthetist:

Preoperative diagnosis:

Chronic adenotonsillitis
Bilateral chronic serous otitis media

Postoperative diagnosis:

Procedure(s) performed:

Tonsillectomy and adenoidectomy
Bilateral P. E. tube placement

Anesthesia:

Assistant surgeon:

Description of procedure:

9-year-old male with chronic adenotonsillitis along with bilateral chronic serous otitis media. The patient was taken to the operating room, where, under adequate general anesthesia, mouth gag inserted, the right tonsil was grasped, anterior and posterior pillars were incised. The tonsil was dissected free of surrounding tissue, removed with a snare. Identical procedure was then performed on the left side as well. Large amount of adenoid tissue was removed and after appropriate hemostasis, the pharynx was irrigated.

The patient was returned to the recovery room in satisfactory condition.

CPT Code:
42821 Tonsillectomy and Adenoidectomy
69436-50 Tympanostomy

Rachel Perez MD

GODFREY REGIONAL HOSPITAL
123 Main Street • Aldon, FL 77714 • (407) 555-1234

7. Operative report

OPERATIVE REPORT

Patient information:

Patient name:
DOB:
MR#:

Date:
Surgeon:
Anesthetist:

Preoperative diagnosis:

Displaced left ankle fracture; Salter II fracture distal fibula with disruption of deltoid Reduction and casting of left ankle

Postoperative diagnosis:

Procedure(s) performed:

Anesthesia:

Assistant surgeon:

Description of procedure:

The patient is a healthy 12-year-old who sustained an external rotation injury to his ankle. Diagnosis of displaced Salter II fracture of the distal fibula was made with noted displacement of the mortise. Patient was brought to the operating room and general anesthesia was administered via mask. He was kept in the supine position, while we performed a manipulation after removing the splint by internally rotating the foot relative to the tiba and applying pressure to the distal fibula. We confirmed reduction with C arm and applied a short leg cast. Once the cast was set, we confirmed the anatomic reduction with permanent images. Patient was taken to the post-anesthesia room, having tolerated the procedure well.

CPT Code:
27788-LT Fx Repair Closed Distal Fibula With Manipulation
29405-LT Short Leg Cast

Rachel Perez MD

GODFREY REGIONAL HOSPITAL
123 Main Street • Aldon, FL 77714 • (407) 555-1234

8. Emergency department record

EMERGENCY ROOM RECORD

Name:	Age:	ER physician:
	DOB:	
Allergies/type of reaction:	**Usual medications/dosages:**	

Triage/presenting complaint:

Patient is a 46-year-old who had hysterectomy performed approximately one week ago. She called our office this morning complaining of fever, nausea and vomiting over the past 24 hours.

Upon arrival, the patient relates a 24 hour history of nausea, vomiting and abdominal tenderness. Of note, the patient has an indwelling catheter which was inserted postoperatively due to her inability to void. She was to return to the office postoperatively on the 3rd postop day for possible removal of the catheter.

Initial assessment:

Time	T	P	R	BP	Other:					

Medication orders:

Lab work:

Urine sample taken from the catheter is positive for red and white blood cells. Urine culture is performed and the patient is given antibiotics.

X-ray:

Physician's report:

Diagnosis:

ASSESSMENT: Bladder infection due to indwelling catheter

Discharge **Transfer** **Admit** **Good** **Satisfactory** **Other:**

Physician sign/date

Nancy Connolly MD

CPT Code: 99283

GODFREY REGIONAL HOSPITAL
123 Main Street • Aldon, FL 77714 • (407) 555-1234

9. Operative report

OPERATIVE REPORT

Patient information:

Patient name:
DOB:
MR#:

Date:
Surgeon:
Anesthetist:

Preoperative diagnosis:

Mucus bloody stools

Postoperative diagnosis:

Procedure(s) performed:

Diverticula
Colonoscopy
Patient presents with change in bowel habits, intermittent rectal bleeding and some mucus. The procedure was described in detail to the patient and he seemed to understand the risks, alternative treatments.

Anesthesia:

Assistant surgeon:

Description of procedure:

The patient was taken to the endoscopy suite and in the left lateral position, the long colonoscope was inserted without incident. The perirectal area was normal. The rectal ampulla was normal. There were scattered diverticula of the left colon. The left colon, transverse colon were otherwise normal. The colonoscope was unable to be advanced to the cecum due to tortuous colon anatomy. The scope was removed and the patient returned to the recovery room in satisfactory condition.

CPT CODE:
45378

Rachel Perez MD

GODFREY REGIONAL HOSPITAL
123 Main Street • Aldon, FL 77714 • (407) 555-1234

10. Radiology report

RADIOLOGY REPORT

MR#:
DOB:
Dr.

Patient name: David Jones

Clinical summary:

Fever, rule out pneumonia

Abdomen:

Conclusion:

CHEST X-RAY
04/08/XX

Deep inspiration. No infiltrate seen in either lung. Infiltrate present previously in the right upper lobe has resolved since film of 02/01/XX.

Normal chest.

Ddt/mm

D:
T:

, M.D. Date 04/08/XX

CPT CODE: 71020
ICD-9-CM CODE: 780.6

GODFREY REGIONAL HOSPITAL
123 Main Street • Aldon, FL 77714 • (407) 555-1234

SECTION 5

Facility Coding and Reimbursement Processes

The facility coding process is similar to the coding processes discussed in previous sections of this text. The hospital facility coder faces additional challenges, however, that physician and provider coders do not encounter. The hospital coder has an additional volume of medical records to review so that appropriate ICD-9-CM diagnostic and procedure codes may be assigned. In addition, the outpatient hospital coder must possess the skills to code ICD-9-CM diagnostic and procedural codes as well as CPT codes.

Section V discusses the hospital coding processes as well as the reimbursement methods for facilities. Table 1 below summarizes the different codes used by the outpatient and inpatient facility coders as well as the physician coder. It also outlines the differences in the format in which services are reported to third-party carriers.

Chapter 20 covers the basic coding guidelines for inpatient and outpatient hospital coding, whereas Chapter 21 details the concept of diagnosis-related groups (DRGs) and provides guidelines for DRG assignments as well as Ambulatory Payment Classifications (APCs). The student will have the opportunity to identify the key components of hospital chart documentation for coding and to assign DRGs and APCs for hospitalizations. These chapters are included only as an overview to the hospital facility coding and billing process and are not intended to provide the level of training necessary to become a hospital coder. They also compare the coding duties and responsibilities of the physician coder with that of the facility coder. The physician coder must understand the differences in code assignment for facilities and physicians. In many instances the physician coder will receive documentation from the facility that includes the facility code assignments. Without understanding the basic differences in coding assignments, the physician coder may believe the facility codes are in error or, worse yet, use the codes assigned by the facility for the provider as well. As the facility process is reviewed, it will become apparent that facility coders and physician coders are distinctly different.

It is also important to understand that the physician coder is reporting codes for professional services performed by the provider, whereas the facility coder is reporting codes for the resources the facility used in providing care to the patient. ■

20

Hospital and Facility Coding

LEARNING OBJECTIVES

After completing this chapter, the student will be able to:

- Understand the rules for selecting the appropriate diagnosis for inpatient coding.
- Describe and apply the signs and symptoms rules for inpatient facility coding.
- Know the do's and don'ts for inpatient coding.
- Comprehend the importance of diagnostic coding order for inpatient coding.
- Understand the importance of assigning the principal diagnosis for inpatient coding.
- Comprehend the proper use of Volume 3 ICD-9-CM procedure codes for inpatient coding.
- Assign codes for significant inpatient procedures.
- Grasp the coding nomenclature for outpatient hospital coding.
- Identify and apply the basic steps for assigning outpatient facility codes.
- Understand the guidelines for assigning ICD-9-CM and CPT codes for outpatient facility coding.
- Apply inpatient and outpatient facility coding concepts to practical coding scenarios.

CODING REFERENCE TOOLS

Tool 20-1
Rules for Selecting Appropriate Diagnoses for Inpatient Hospital Coding

Tool 20-2
Signs and Symptoms Rules for Inpatient Hospital Coding

Tool 20-3
Diagnosis Do's and Don'ts for Inpatient Hospital Coding

Tool 20-4
Diagnostic Order Rules for Inpatient Hospital Coding

KEY TERMS

Ambulatory Payment Classifications (APCs)

Principal Diagnosis

Query Process

Significant Procedures

Volume 1 (Index to Diseases)

Volume 3 (Index to Procedures)

Documentation and Coding Guidelines

Although the documentation guidelines for facility coding are similar to those of physician coding, the depth and volume of the medical records are much more extensive. The coder must be capable of working through a significant volume of pages for each admission to assign codes appropriately.

Consider a typical inpatient chart. Keep in mind that only documents required for arriving at the appropriate diagnostic and procedural codes have been included. Because the inpatient chart is so voluminous, creating an outline of the components that comprise the hospital medical record may be advisable.

ADMISSION HISTORY AND PHYSICAL EXAMINATION

Commonly referred to as an *H&P* (history and physical) (Fig. 20-1), this portion of the record typically represents the initial evaluation of the patient, the plan for the admission, and the admitting diagnosis.

PROGRESS NOTES

Each day the patient is seen by the physician(s), an entry is made in the medical record (Figs. 20-2 and 20-3). Each date may be entered on a separate sheet or multiple entries made on the same page. Documentation may be dictated or handwritten by the physician. If several physicians see the patient on any given day, multiple entries may be made for that date of service by each individual provider.

ANCILLARY RECORDS AND REPORTS

Ancillary records such as radiology, laboratory, and diagnostic tests are included in the review of the hospital record (see Figs. 20-4 and 20-5). Interpretations of these data are codeable only when they are made by the physician or documented concurrence with the diagnosis is made. Many of these records contain information that reflects additional conditions treated or considered during the course of the hospitalization. The coder may only use information documented by the physician or may query the physician regarding the possibility of additional diagnoses. The query process is discussed later in this chapter.

NURSING NOTES

In addition to daily documentation by the physician regarding the patient's progress, nurses, technicians, and other staff document care provided to the patient as well as observations regarding the patient's progress (Figs. 20-6 to 20-9). This type of documentation can be used for assigning diagnostic or procedural codes only when the physician documents agree with the findings by other staff members. For instance, if the nurse records that "the patient appears in severe respiratory arrest," this information may be used in assigning diagnoses when documented by the physician.

The same would apply for nursing documentation of vital signs or interpretation of laboratory or other data. For example, nursing staff contact the physician because of an increase in the patient's temperature, recorded as "103.7" and documented by the nurse as "fever." The diagnosis of "fever" may not be used unless stated by the physician. However, these documents are vital in determining diagnoses that may be appropriate in final diagnostic code selection and identification of additional diagnoses or patient complications. The facility coder must often look for additional diagnostic statements through the use of nursing notes, ancillary reports, and other documentation to assign the most appropriate principal diagnosis and thus ensure the most appropriate reimbursement for the admission.

OPERATIVE RECORDS AND REPORTS

If the patient needs surgery during the hospitalization, the operative record will reflect the procedure performed and the reason for that procedure. Keep in mind that the reason for the surgical procedure may not be the primary or principal reason for the admission. Principal diagnosis is discussed later in this chapter.

MEDICATION RECORD

A record is typically made of medications given, the route of administration, and the dosage administered during the course of the hospitalization.

DISCHARGE SUMMARY OR RECORD

At the conclusion of the hospital admission, the admitting physician reports a summary of the hospitalization course, including reason for admission, progress during admission, and discharge status and instructions (Fig. 20-10). The figures on the following pages represent a typical inpatient hospital record. Keep in mind that this record only encompasses information that is useful in determining diagnoses and that many other documents and papers are contained within the hospital record.

Regarding the outpatient record, the documents will usually be similar and, in both instances, when a surgical procedure is performed an operative note should be included in the documents for documentation and coding purposes.

Text continued on p. 703

HISTORY AND PHYSICAL EXAMINATION

Admit date: 05/09/XXXX Jay Corman, MD

Admitting Diagnoses: 1) Intrinsic Asthma - History of Steroid Requirement 2) Penicillin Sensitivity 3) Hypertension 4) Elevated Creatinine 5) History of Gonococcal Urethritis 6) Status Post Bilateral Inguinal Herniorrhaphies

Patient is a 56-year-old black male with a history of asthma, admitted from the Emergency Room for an exacerbation of his bronchospastic disease. The patient's history is significant for admissions relevant to asthma in: 1) 1997 patient was admitted with room air arterial blood gas of pH 7.33, pCO2 52, pO2 55. He was subsequently intubated and treated with steroids. His hospital course was complicated by hyperglycemia and hypertension. 2) Patient admitted again in 1999 and treated with steroids. 3) Patient was admitted in 2001 and treated with steroids, where his prebronchodilator pulmonary function tests revealed an FEV1 of 1.3 liters and an FVC of 3.3 liters. The patient was seen by Allergy service, and recommended the patient return for skin testing and wear a mask for his job; however, he failed to show for follow-up.

Patient now gives a history of wheezing beginning three weeks ago, after being in a fried chicken store and being irritated by the burning grease. Ten days prior to admission the patient noted swelling around his face and eyes and went to see a private allergist who diagnosed contact dermatitis of the face. The patient was skin tested and found to be positive for mites and mold. The patient was given Kenalog 20 mg IM. He was later mailed a desensitization shot to be administered at home, which he did, five days prior to admission. The patient's wheezing was exacerbated by dust at work, and, two nights prior to admission he smelled some burning bacon at home and his shortness of breath became much worse and he reported to the hospital. The patient was held in the observation unit overnight and admitted the following morning. It should be noted that the patient finished a steroid taper dose of 5 mg qid twelve days prior to admission. The patient denies any history of aspirin sensitivity. PFT in the ER were significant for an FEV1 of 900 with an FVC of 2700 cc. Room air arterial blood gas was pH 7.43, pCO2 40, pO2 73.

Past medical history:

Patient gives a history of penicillin allergy, with an episode of anaphylaxis in 1986. Hypertension following initiation of steroid therapy. Asthma, see history of present illness, herniorrhaphy times two.

Family and social history:

Works as a forklift operator at a creosote company. The patient is exposed to creosote, sawdust from oak, pine, hickory, ash and gum and a lot of dusty conditions in general. Patient denies cigarette use, use of ethanol or illegal drugs. Family history significant for patient's father who died at age 70 for unknown kidney disease, two siblings who died from sudden death and a sister who also has asthma. The patient also has two children who have asthma. He lives at home with four sons and his wife. There are no house pets. The patient has a high school education and grew up in the area.

Review of systems:

Patient has experienced a weight loss from 190 to 170 pounds during the past two months secondary to diet. The patient has a history of gonococcal urethritis times three in the past. Also has a past history of rectal bleeding in 1988 and 1989.

Physical exam:

Revealed a well-developed, well-nourished middle-aged black male in no acute distress.

Vital Signs:	BP 160/120, Pulse 102 and regular, Respirations, 28, Patient afebrile.
Skin:	Hyperpigmented areas around the face and eyes
Lymphatic:	No adenopathy
HEENT:	Benign, Tympanic membranes clear bilaterally, no sinus tenderness, mouth without lesions, neck supple, without thyromegaly.
Lungs:	Revealed diffuse inspiratory and expiratory wheezes all lung fields
Cardiac:	Carotids were 2+, no murmurs heard.
Abdomen:	Benign, without bruits or hepatosplenomegaly.
GU:	Normal circumcised male, rectal exam normal tone, soft prostate, no masses
Extremities:	Without cyanosis, clubbing or edema
Neuro:	Within normal limits

Laboratory/radiology:

Admission of SMA-6 was significant for a glucose of 227 mg/dl. Admission CBC significant for hemoglobin of 13.8 gm/dl. Admitting urinalysis was unremarkable. Admission ECG and CXR reported as normal.

X-ray:

Assessment:

Asthma, will admit and treat with steroids

Plan:

Jay Corman MD

GODFREY REGIONAL HOSPITAL
123 Main Street • Aldon, FL 77714 • (407) 555-1234

FIGURE 20-1. History and physical examination form for a patient admitted through the emergency department. The patient has acute asthma symptoms.

PROGRESS NOTE

Date/time

05/10/XXXX

S:

56 yo BM

1) Asthma, required intubation in past
2) HTN
3) Glucose intolerance due to steroids

O:

Meds:
1) Theodur 600 bid
2) HCT 250
3) Minipress 2 tid

A:

Generally doing well. Has occasional episodes, pt dyspnea/wheezing, but overall feels good. PE 140/80, P72, reg, respirations 14. Chest, scattered expiratory wheezes.

P:

Will order respiratory therapy and IV steroids and check for improvement in the AM.

Jay Corman MD

PROGRESS NOTES

GODFREY REGIONAL HOSPITAL
123 Main Street • Aldon, FL 77714 • (407) 555-1234

FIGURE 20-2. Initial progress note for admitted patient. The physician has recommended respiratory therapy and IV steroids along with a recheck the following morning.

PROGRESS NOTE

Date/time

05/11/XXXX

S:

56-year-old BM

1) Asthma
2) HTN
3) Glucose intolerance due to steroids

O:

A:

P:

1. Still having bilateral expiratory wheezes despite respiratory treatment 2. Will check CXR for any improvement and continue IV steroid therapy.

Jay Corman MD

PROGRESS NOTES

GODFREY REGIONAL HOSPITAL
123 Main Street • Aldon, FL 77714 • (407) 555-1234

FIGURE 20-3. Additional progress note for admitted patient. The patient is still experiencing acute symptoms, and the physician will continue IV steroid therapy.

RADIOLOGY REPORT

MR#:
DOB:
Dr. Jay Corman

Clinical summary:

Wheezing

Abdomen:

PA AND LATERAL CHEST 05/09/XXXX

Conclusion:

Reveals infiltrates in the right and left lower lobes as well as signs of chronic pulmonary processes.

Ddt/mm

D:
T:

M.D. Date

GODFREY REGIONAL HOSPITAL
123 Main Street • Aldon, FL 77714 • (407) 555-1234

FIGURE 20-4. Radiology report. Posteroanterior and lateral chest x-rays revealed infiltrates in the right and left lower lobes of the patient's lungs.

RADIOLOGY REPORT

MR#:
DOB:
Dr. Jay Corman, MD

Clinical summary:

Follow up asthma

Abdomen:

PA AND LATERAL CHEST 05/11/XXXX

Conclusion:

Reveals some improvement over 05/09/XXXX x-ray. Infiltrates still present in the right and left lower lobes, however, not as prevalent as previous x-ray.

Ddt/mm

D:
T:

M.D. Date

GODFREY REGIONAL HOSPITAL
123 Main Street • Aldon, FL 77714 • (407) 555-1234

FIGURE 20-5. Radiology report for follow-up x-ray done 2 days after admission. The patient has shown improvement.

NURSING NOTES

Date/time

05/10/XXXX

S:

Patient experiencing extreme shortness of breath. Patient states "I had an asthma attack. I was in observation last night". Patient's chief complaint shortness of breath. Lungs with crackles throughout. White frothy sputum of moderate amounts produced. IV of 500 D5W at KVO with 500 D5W with 1 gm of Aminophylline. IV patent and infusing well. IV dressing applied. CXR performed tonight. Remained at bed most of evening. Appetite fair at dinner. Up to sink with assistance. Gait steady.

O:

A:

P:

Betty Jones RN

PROGRESS NOTES

GODFREY REGIONAL HOSPITAL
123 Main Street • Aldon, FL 77714 • (407) 555-1234

FIGURE 20-6. Nursing note from second day of admission. Patient still has acute symptoms.

NURSING NOTE

Date/time

05/10/XXXX

S:

Alteration in oxygenation with shortness of breath.

O:

VSS afebrile. Lungs with diffuse wheezes. Received bronchosol nebulizer ×2.

Cough productive, large amount of white sputum with plugs. PO intake excellent

A:

Asthmatic exacerbation

P:

Bronchodilators, steroids

Hydration

Betty Jones RN

PROGRESS NOTES

GODFREY REGIONAL HOSPITAL
123 Main Street • Aldon, FL 77714 • (407) 555-1234

FIGURE 20-7. Nursing note from second day of admission. Patient still has acute symptoms and treatment is continuing.

NURSING NOTES

Date/time

05/11/XXXX

S:

Alteration in oxygenation, shortness of breath

O:

Afebrile, P-84, RR-18, BP 150/95, 146/80.
Resting quietly in bed most of shift.
Lungs with diffuse wheezes, productive of small amount of semi-thin, white sputum.
Continues on bronchodilator, steroids. Increased Aminophylline drip to 35 gtts.
1740 denies shortness of breath, feeling better.
Repeat CXR this PM

A:

P:

Betty Jones RN

PROGRESS NOTES

GODFREY REGIONAL HOSPITAL
123 Main Street • Aldon, FL 77714 • (407) 555-1234

FIGURE 20-8. Nursing note from third day of admission. Patient has fewer symptoms and treatment is continuing.

NURSING NOTES/DISCHARGE NOTE

Date/time

05/12/XXXX

S:

Patient indicates feeling much better. Scattered few wheezes heard. Patient experiencing no shortness of breath. CXR indicated clearing infiltrates.

O:

A:

P:

Discharge instructions given and discharge medications include:

1) Prednisone 60 mg po q am tapering dose thereafter 50 mg po × 2 days, 40 mg × 2 days, 30 mg × 2 days, 20 mg × 2 days until seen in clinic

2) Theodur 600 mg po bid

3) Terbutaline 5 mg po q 8 hours

Betty Jones, RN

PROGRESS NOTES

GODFREY REGIONAL HOSPITAL
123 Main Street • Aldon, FL 77714 • (407) 555-1234

FIGURE 20-9. Nursing note from day of discharge. Patient has improved and is ready for discharge with proper medications.

DISCHARGE SUMMARY

Admitted: 05/09/XXXX
Discharged: 05/12/XXXX

Discharge diagnoses:

1. Extrinsic Asthma
2. Hypertension
3. Elevated Creatinine
4. Status Post Bilateral Inguinal Herniorrhaphy

History:

Patient is a 56-year-old black male who presented with shortness of breath to the emergency room on 05/08/XXXX where he was initially treated. He was transferred to observation during the evening, and subsequently admitted on the morning of 05/09/XXXX. The patient's history significant for previous admissions for asthma, one requiring intubation, and the other admissions requiring steroid administration.

History on admission was a three week history of wheezing, followed by increasing shortness of breath on the evening of 05/08/XXXX following the smell of burning food at home. The patient had just finished a steroid taper dose twelve days prior to admission.

Laboratory and radiology studies:

On admission, CXR indicated infiltrates in the right and lower lobes with signs of a chronic process. By 05/11/XXXX a repeat x-ray indicated improvement in infiltrates.

Hospital course:

1) Asthma: Patient was admitted with exacerbation of asthma and treated with the usual therapy of intravenous aminophylline, intravenous steroids, bronchodilator treatments and showed rapid improvement. At the time of discharge, pulmonary function studies showed FEV1 of 2.1 liters pre-treatment, 2.5 liters post-operative, FVC 4 liters pre-treatment and 4.3 liters post-treatment.
2) Hyperglycemia: History of steroid–induced hyperglycemia. Accu-checks were followed twice per day during the patient's hospitalization and all were under 200 mg/dl.
3) Hypertension: Patient's diastolic BPs were within the range of 80 to 90 mg Hg during this hospitalization on his current medications.

DISCHARGE MEDICATIONS:
Prednisone 60 mg po q am tapering dose thereafter 50 mg po × 2 days, 40 mg × 2 days, 30 mg × 2 days, 20 mg × 2 days until seen in clinic
Theodur 600 mg po bid
Terbutaline 5 mg po q 8 hours

Jay Corman MD

GODFREY REGIONAL HOSPITAL
123 Main Street • Aldon, FL 77714 • (407) 555-1234

FIGURE 20-10. Discharge summary for entire patient visit. The report includes information about all symptoms, inpatient treatment, and discharge instructions.

Steps in the Inpatient Facility Coding Process

Volume 1 (Index to Disease), Volume 2 (Tabular List of Diseases), and Volume 3 (Index to Procedures) of the ICD-9-CM coding book constitute the basis for inpatient hospital diagnostic coding and reimbursement. As with physician coding, the hospital coder must be accurate to justify medical necessity for services billed.

The process by which hospital diagnostic coding is performed is similar to that for physician diagnostic coding. Some of the guidelines, however, differ significantly.

Step 1: Identify key elements or words for possible use as diagnoses.
Step 2: Determine which diagnostic statements are necessary for proper diagnostic coding purposes.
Step 3: Determine the appropriate diagnostic code order.
Step 4: Assign diagnostic codes to diagnoses selected from ICD-9-CM.

Review these steps in detail, noting the differences in guidelines for hospital diagnostic coding from those learned in the physician diagnostic coding section.

Step 1: Identify key elements or words for possible use as diagnoses.

Terms such as "probable," "possible," "rule out," and "suspect" MAY be used in the inpatient hospital diagnostic coding environment, unlike with physician coding. Remember the differences between physician and hospital diagnostic coding.

	Physician Provider	Hospital Facility
Chief reason for encounter (WHY)	ICD-9-CM	ICD-9-CM
Procedure or service (WHAT)	CPT ICD-9-CM	ICD-9-CM Volume 3

Note that the hospital coder is also providing justification regarding the medical necessity for the charges billed, typically facility charges. The use of diagnostic statements that include words such as "possible," "probable," "suspect," or "rule out" is acceptable. The facility provides the same services for the patient tested for a specific condition as it does for the patient who, at the conclusion of the physician encounter, has that specific codeable diagnosis. This represents the biggest difference between physician and hospital diagnostic coding. Note, however, that when the diagnosis has been "ruled out" before the conclusion of the hospitalization, that diagnostic statement may NOT be used.

STOP AND PRACTICE

For the following scenarios, determine what signs, symptoms, or diagnosis(es) would be appropriate for inpatient facility coding. Indicate what diagnosis(es) would be appropriate for inpatient facility coding purposes.

	Diagnosis(es) to Assign
1. Abdominal pain, rule out rectal carcinoma	________
2. Abdominal pain/fever due to acute appendicitis	________
3. Elevated white blood cell count due to possible acute appendicitis	________
4. Pain and swelling due to ankle sprain	________
5. Pain and swelling due to possible ankle fracture	________
6. Abdominal pain, suspect diverticulitis	________
7. Eye pain, probable foreign body	________
8. Chest pain, rule out myocardial infarction	________
9. Nausea and vomiting, rule out diverticulitis	________
10. Fever and diarrhea	________

Step 2: Determine which diagnostic statements are necessary for proper diagnostic coding purposes.

The coder should identify diagnostic statements in the hospital setting that may or may not be used for coding purposes. Rules for selecting appropriate diagnoses are outlined in Tool 20-1; rules for identifying signs and symptoms are given in Tool 20-2. The do's and don'ts for inpatient hospital coding are listed in Tool 20-3. A detailed discussion regarding signs and symptoms rules was previously presented in Section 2, ICD-9-CM Diagnostic Coding.

Step 3: Determine the appropriate diagnostic code order.

The diagnostic order rules for inpatient hospital coding are listed in Tool 20-4.

Step 4: Assign diagnostic codes to diagnoses selected from ICD-9-CM.

The chart "10 Steps to Accurate Coding" from ICD-9-CM (see Tool 4-2) is accurate for hospital coding, as are the CMS Guidelines for ICD-9-CM Coding (see Tool 4-3), found in Section 2 of this text.

TOOL 20-1

RULES FOR SELECTING APPROPRIATE DIAGNOSES FOR INPATIENT HOSPITAL CODING

1. If it is not documented, it did not happen.
2. The condition, problem, or other circumstances chiefly responsible for the health encounter or visit are reported. This is referred to as the *chief reason for encounter.*
3. Unconfirmed diagnoses described as "possible," "probable," "questionable," "rule out," "ruled out," or "suspect(ed)" CAN BE USED for hospital inpatient diagnoses and coding purposes.
4. Code the condition to the highest level of specificity. In some cases this may be the sign, symptom, abnormal test, or reason for the visit or encounter.
5. If the encounter does not identify a definite condition or problem at its conclusion, the coder should select the documented chief complaint or chief reason for the encounter.
6. Never code a diagnosis that is not listed in the diagnostic statement.

TOOL 20-2

SIGNS AND SYMPTOMS RULES FOR INPATIENT HOSPITAL CODING

Signs and symptoms should be used ONLY when:

1. The principal diagnosis has not been established at the conclusion of the encounter.
2. No more specific diagnoses for the specific condition can be made at the end of the encounter or visit.
3. Presenting signs and symptoms are transient and no definitive diagnosis is made.
4. The symptom is treated in an outpatient setting without the additional workup necessary to arrive at a more definitive diagnosis at the conclusion of the encounter.

Signs and symptoms do NOT need to be used when they are an integral part of the underlying diagnosis or condition already coded.

V codes and E codes, which have previously been discussed, are also appropriate in hospital inpatient coding. Remember that these codes do not indicate the primary or principal diagnosis; they are important in determining liability for reimbursement purposes. When conditions are stated as "history of," V codes for those conditions should be used only when they contribute additional diagnostic information or explain the complexity of the inpatient stay. Chronic conditions should be clarified so that the appropriate diagnosis may be used.

As mentioned in Section 2, the 2008 ICD-9-CM Coding Guidelines serve as the basis for coding guidelines. In addition, *Coding Clinic,* published by the American Hospital Association (AHA), serves as an authoritative source for guidelines regarding ICD-9-CM coding. This publication is updated quarterly.

TOOL 20-3

DIAGNOSIS DO'S AND DONT'S FOR INPATIENT HOSPITAL CODING

1 For previous conditions stated as diagnosis when previous condition has no bearing on current visit—DO NOT CODE

Coder may use a "V" code (history of) if significant.

2 Chronic conditions not the thrust of treatment—DO CODE

Certain diseases such as hypertension, Parkinson's disease, diabetes, and chronic obstructive pulmonary disease are examples of systemic diseases that require continued clinical evaluation and monitoring during each visit.

If visit does not involve evaluation or treatment of condition—DO NOT CODE

3 Conditions that are an integral part of the disease—DO NOT CODE

Example: Patient with nausea and vomiting from infectious gastroenteritis. Nausea and vomiting are common symptoms of this disease process and need not be coded.

4 Conditions that are NOT an integral part of the disease—DO CODE

Example: A 5-year-old with 104° F fever associated with pneumonia also experienced convulsions. Pneumonia is coded (fever usually associated with pneumonia need not be coded) and convulsions are coded (not always associated with pneumonia or fever).

5 Diagnosis not listed in final diagnostic statement—CHECK WITH PHYSICIAN

If integral to correct coding, ask the physician to incorporate this information in the final diagnostic statement. This statement may appear in the discharge information or throughout the hospitalization notes.

6 Abnormal findings—CODE WHEN NECESSARY

Should be assigned only when the physician is unable to arrive at a diagnosis before the conclusion of the encounter. If an abnormal finding is the only diagnostic information available, the coder should check with the physician to make certain a codeable diagnosis is not available.

TOOL 20-4

DIAGNOSTIC ORDER RULES FOR INPATIENT HOSPITAL CODING

1 Signs and symptoms codes are assigned only after diagnosis and only when they were NOT an integral part of the diagnostic statement.

2 Acute conditions are coded as the primary diagnosis in most instances because it is assumed they are the primary reason for the encounter. The exception would be the case of a significantly more serious condition.

EXCEPTION: Myocardial infarction not listed as Acute, acute otitis media

Many serious conditions are automatically assumed as acute when coding from ICD-9-CM (the ICD-9-CM coding book lists "acute" in parentheses).

3 Chronic conditions (when coded by previous rules) are coded secondary to any acute conditions or primary reasons for the encounter. Make sure to use chronic codes.

4 The first diagnosis listed in hospital coding should be the principal or most important diagnosis, reason for encounter, or thrust of treatment.

STOP AND PRACTICE

Try coding some of the following diagnoses based on the inpatient hospital diagnostic coding rules given thus far. Code the following diagnoses appropriately according to hospital inpatient diagnostic rules.

		ICD-9-CM Code(s)
1.	Abdominal pain	______
	Possible appendicitis	______
2.	Cough	______
	Fever	______
	Probable pneumonia	______
3.	Anemia, probably due to chronic blood loss	______
4.	Angina, most likely unstable	______
5.	Acute bronchitis	______
	Cough	______
	COPD	______
6.	Elevated blood pressure, probably not hypertension	______
7.	Nausea and vomiting, probably due to either gastroenteritis or kidney stones	______
8.	Ankle pain, ankle fracture ruled out	______
9.	Abdominal pain, possibly due to ovarian cyst	______
	Pelvic inflammatory disease	______
10.	Confusional state	______
	Nausea and vomiting	______
	Dehydration	______
	Alzheimer's dementia	______
11.	Pneumonia	______
	Fever and cough due to pneumonia	______
	Hypokalemia	______
12.	Cholecystitis with cholelithiasis	______
	Abdominal pain	______
	Nausea and vomiting	______
13.	Abdominal pain	______
	Fever	______
	Possible appendicitis	______
14.	Fever	______
	Possible influenza	______
15.	Right scrotal swelling	______
	Right inguinal hernia/hydrocele	______
16.	Fever, vomiting, diarrhea	______
	Possible vital gastroenteritis	______
17.	Gastroenteritis, possible viral	______
18.	Confusion, possible Alzheimer's	______
19.	Diverticulosis, possible *H. pylori*	______
20.	Abnormal ECG, MI ruled out	______

Additional Inpatient Coding Guidelines

In addition to the steps that remain the same for hospital and physician coding, clarification needs to be made regarding some hospital-specific definitions and guidelines.

PRINCIPAL DIAGNOSIS

Principal diagnosis is defined as the condition chiefly responsible for the patient's admission to the hospital (after diagnostic or therapeutic studies). Remember that the chief reason for the encounter in hospital coding is the chief reason or medical necessity for the admission. Specific guidelines for determining principal diagnosis are as follows. The comprehension of this definition is essential to correct inpatient coding assignment, as shown in Chapter 20, which discusses reimbursement for inpatient coding assignments.

When More Than One Diagnosis Meets the Criteria for Principal Diagnosis

When more than one diagnosis meets the criteria for principal diagnosis, and ICD-9-CM guidelines do not specify the use of one code instead of another as primary or principal, either may be sequenced first (e.g., congestive heart failure, pneumonia).

The tendency is to code the diagnosis that accounts for the majority of services provided when both codes meet the qualifications for principal diagnosis (the more significant diagnosis).

When More Than One Condition Listed Pertains to Similar and Contrasting Conditions

In this instance the coder selects the diagnosis, which is the condition that resulted in hospital admission and for which most services were provided. If, during the course of the admission, one of the diagnoses possible for inclusion as the principal diagnosis is ruled out, the diagnosis not ruled out would be used.

When Symptom(s) Are Listed with Comparable Diagnosis, or When Symptoms Contrast with the Diagnosed Condition

When symptoms are NOT an integral part of one of the diagnoses, they are used in lieu of unestablished diagnoses.

Patient with abdominal pain due to either appendicitis or ovarian cyst

Because appendicitis and ovarian cyst are not confirmed diagnoses, abdominal pain should be selected as the primary diagnosis.

When Original Treatment Plan(s) Are Not Completed During the Course of the Encounter or Admission

In this case, the reason for the admission or encounter is still used as the principal or primary diagnosis. In addition to the principal and any contributing diagnoses, hospital coding requires that all significant procedures be coded. **Significant procedures** are defined as the following:

- Surgical procedures, including excisions, incisions, destructions, amputations, repairs, manipulations, insertions
- Those associated with anesthesia; all procedures requiring anesthesia other than topical anesthetic risk
- Those associated with trauma; all procedures that carry a risk of possible impairment, procedural risk, or physiologic disturbance
- Procedures that require specialized training

In the case of procedural diagnostic coding, the principal diagnosis is defined as the reason for definitive treatment or outpatient procedure. Review the medical chart at the beginning of the chapter (Figures 20-1 to 20-10) and determine the appropriate diagnoses as well as the principal diagnosis.

Although several problems were identified during the course of the hospitalization, the primary reason for the inpatient hospitalization was exacerbation of asthma. Contributing or secondary diagnosis included the following:

- Steroid-induced hyperglycemia
- Hypertension

Exacerbation of asthma was the chief reason for hospitalization, so it would be assigned as the principal diagnosis. The additional diagnoses would also be assigned appropriate ICD-9-CM codes.

STOP AND PRACTICE

Practice assigning ICD-9-CM diagnostic codes for the following inpatient coding scenarios. Assign codes only to conditions for which it would be appropriate to assign code(s) in the inpatient facility setting. Appropriate order for diagnosis is discussed later in this chapter.

	ICD-9-CM Code Assignment(s)
1. Abdominal pain, rule out appendicitis	________
Acute appendicitis	________
Hypertension	________
Hypothyroidism	________
2. Cough	________
Fever	________
Elevated white blood cell count	________
Possible pneumonia	________
Acute bronchitis	________
3. Elevated amylase	________
Workup acute pancreatitis	________
Hepatitis C	________
Alcoholic cirrhosis	________
4. Chest pain, rule out MI	________
Anterolateral myocardial infarction	________
Elevated troponin	________
Hypertension	________
Congestive heart failure	________
5. Anemia	________
Possible gastrointestinal bleed	________
Acute blood loss anemia	________
GERD	________
Gastritis	________
6. Shortness of breath	________
CXR, ABG indicate congestive heart failure	________
Patient also with history of hypertension, CAD, COPD	________
7. Lump, left breast	________
Admission for excision of lump, indicating breast carcinoma, left outer quadrant	________
Chemotherapy initiated prior to discharge	________
8. Low back pain	________
Urinary tract infection	________
Possible pyelonephritis	________
9. Metastatic breast cancer, admitted due to acute pain	________
Patient has history of HTN, IDDM	________
Admitted for control of intractable pain due to metastatic breast cancer	________
10. Admitted for amputation of gangrenous second toe, right foot	________
Patient has IDDM, HTN, and gout	________

USE OF VOLUME 3 ICD-9-CM

When a procedure has been identified as "significant" according to previous guidelines, the service and the reason for the procedure or encounter (diagnosis) should be coded. All procedures classified as significant based on these guidelines are coded for both outpatient and inpatient hospital services. Some carriers no longer require the use of ICD-9-CM procedure codes on outpatient facility claims.

Procedures in the ICD-9-CM procedure index are organized by the approach or type of surgical procedures, such as incision, excision, or repair. Volume 3 ICD-9-CM procedures should be assigned under the following conditions:

Procedure is surgical.
Procedure has an associated anesthetic risk.
Procedure has an associated procedural risk.
Procedure requires specialized training.

Some additional coding guidelines apply to the ICD-9-CM procedural index:

Bilateral procedures	If the procedure code descriptor does not specify bilateral, and therefore is not inherent in the code, the ICD-9-CM procedure code should be assigned twice.
Incomplete procedures	For purposes of ICD-9-CM procedural coding, assign procedures only to the extent they are completed.
Biopsy versus excision codes	Use biopsy code(s) when only a portion(s) of a lesion is removed and excision codes only when the entire lesion is removed.
Laparoscopic procedure converted to open surgery	When procedures are laparoscopic and converted, only the open or final definitive procedure is assigned an ICD-9-CM procedure code.
Endoscopy procedures	Only the most significant endoscopic procedure should be assigned an ICD-9-CM procedure code.

Layout

The layout of ICD-9-CM Volume 3 is identical to that used in the main sections of ICD-9-CM. Contained within Volume 3 is an Index to Procedures (alphabetical) and a numeric index. The guidelines discussed earlier apply to selecting the appropriate code from Volume 3. If the coder uses the same guidelines established for Volumes 1 and 2 of ICD-9-CM, Volume 3 is not difficult to use. Remember that this section of the ICD-9-CM diagnostic coding book is used by facility and hospital coders ONLY. Physician and provider coders use the CPT manual to code for services performed. If the coder requires information on provider and physician coding only, only Volumes 1 and 2 may be purchased.

The coder must select the appropriate code from the procedure index for the significant procedure(s) performed and must cross-reference or verify the selected code in the numeric index. The importance of this process and of the codes associated with these procedures is discussed in Chapter 19. As previously mentioned, some carriers have recently discontinued the requirement of ICD-9-CM procedural codes on outpatient hospital claims.

Box 20-1 lists the numeric categories for codes found in ICD-9-CM Volume 3. Note that ICD-9-CM procedural codes are based on services performed; they are indexed based on anatomic system and procedure.

STOP AND PRACTICE

Take the following scenarios and assign the appropriate ICD-9-CM procedure codes for the inpatient facility coding scenarios.

	ICD-9-CM Procedure Code(s)
1. Abdominal hysterectomy	______
2. Elective vasectomy	______
3. Laparoscopic cholecystectomy	______
4. Heart transplant	______
5. CABG, three-vessel vein grafts	______
6. Pacemaker insertion, dual chamber	______
7. Tonsillectomy	______
8. Gastric bypass	______
9. ORIF femur fracture	______
10. Arthrodesis, ankle	______
11. Amputation, finger	______
12. Bronchoscopic alveolar lavage	______
13. Transbronchial bronchoscopic biopsy	______
14. Colectomy	______
15. TURP	______
16. Left heart catheterization with coronary and left ventricular angiography	______
17. Endotracheal intubation	______
18. Laminectomy lumbar herniated disk	______
19. Craniotomy with high-speed drill with burr holes	______
20. Arthroscopic carpal tunnel release	______

The Query Process

With the large volume of inpatient (and sometimes outpatient) documentation that must be reviewed, the coder will likely identify potential diagnoses and procedures that would add to the complexity of the hospital admission. Coders are not free to add these diagnostic statements, but they can query the physician regarding whether additional diagnoses would be appropriate. The coder must be careful not to lead the physician to a diagnostic statement solely because that particular diagnosis would increase the reimbursement. This query process is typically in place at all hospitals and facilities and is used for both inpatient and outpatient care.

STOP AND PRACTICE

Write an appropriate query to the physician for the following exercises. Keep in mind that the inquiry cannot be leading and should be direct, with as little physician documentation as possible needed.

1. Colonoscopy performed with removal of colonic polyp.
   Documentation deficiency: method of removal
   Query: ______________________________
2. Lesion removed from left arm
   Documentation deficiency: nature (benign/malignant), size
   Query: ______________________________
3. Laceration repair 2.5 cm of arm
   Documentation deficiency: complexity (simple/intermediate/complex)
   Query: ______________________________
4. Multiple lesions removed from back
   Documentation deficiency: size, nature of each lesion
   Query: ______________________________
5. Fracture repair of the distal radius
   Documentation deficiency: closed/open, with or without fixation/manipulation
   Query: ______________________________

Outpatient Hospital Facility Coding

The outpatient hospital diagnostic coder should follow the rules for the physician and provider coder. The outpatient hospital coder may also need to include the Volume 3 procedure code for procedures performed when required by the carrier. Outpatient coding requires assignment of applicable CPT codes, ICD-9-CM Volume 1 and 2 codes, and Volume 3 procedure codes when applicable. Although the outpatient hospital coder typically is employed by the facility, the physician or provider roles for coding apply because the services are not reimbursed based on DRGs.

BOX 20-1 INDEX OF ICD-9-CM VOLUME 3 (PROCEDURE CODES)

Operations on the nervous system	01-05
Operations on the endocrine system	05-07
Operations on the eye	08-16
Operations on the ear	18-20
Operations on the nose, mouth, pharynx	21-29
Operations on the respiratory system	30-34
Operations on the cardiovascular system	35-39
Operations on the hemic/lymphatic system	40-41
Operations on the digestive system	42-54
Operations on the urinary system	55-59
Operations on the male genital system	60-64
Operations on the female genital system	65-71
Obstetric procedures	72-75
Operations on the musculoskeletal system	76-84
Operations on the integumentary system	85-86
Miscellaneous diagnostic or therapeutic procedures	87-99

When the student undertakes diagnostic coding for outpatient surgery, reference should be made to the diagnostic rules presented in Section 2.

Steps in the Outpatient Hospital Facility Coding Process

Coding rules differ for inpatient and outpatient hospital facility coding. Inpatient and DRG coding were discussed earlier in this chapter. Outpatient hospital facility coding uses the following systems:

- CPT codes for all services rendered
- ICD-9-CM diagnostic codes to justify the medical necessity of services provided
- ICD-9-CM procedural codes for all services performed

Outpatient hospital facility coding is the only area that requires all three concurrent code types for all services for reimbursement. In addition to ICD-9-CM diagnostic and procedural codes, the outpatient facility coder must also assign CPT codes. Because the CPT manual was originally written with the intent of providing terminology for physician or provider coding, outpatient facility coders are instructed to ignore any terminology in the CPT book that refers to provider or physician when selecting the most appropriate CPT code(s). The outpatient facility coder should also pay close attention to National Correct Coding Initiative edits because they also differ somewhat from provider guidelines. Another significant difference is the use of the CPT manual for outpatient facility coding if there are no follow-up days or a "global" period for surgical procedures. Many patients may not have their follow-up care provided at the same facility where the procedure was provided or may only have follow-up care in the provider's office. Therefore when additional services are provided on any date other than the original date of service, no modifier code is required for that service. In instances in which surgical services are performed on the same date of service, the applicable modifier codes such as modifier 58 would be appropriate. The coding assignments for outpatient facility obviously may differ from the physician coding assignments.

MODIFIER CODES

Perhaps the most significant difference in provider CPT coding and outpatient facility is the appropriate use of CPT modifiers. The outpatient hospital coder is limited to a smaller number of modifier codes than the physician or provider coder. The modifier codes most commonly applicable to the outpatient hospital setting are listed in Tool 20-1. Specifically, the outpatient hospital coder does not use modifier 51 for multiple surgical procedures. This issue is addressed by the payment status indicators used in the Ambulatory Patient Classifications (APC) reimbursement system (see Chapter 21).

Two new modifier codes, modifiers 73 and 74, used by the hospital outpatient coder are not used by the physician or professional coder. Modifier 73 is used in the outpatient hospital setting when a surgical procedure is terminated after the preparation for surgery has been completed but before the administration of anesthesia. The facility is reimbursed proportionally for the completed part of the procedure. Modifier 74 is used when the surgical procedure is terminated after the administration of anesthesia; with the proper documentation, the facility is reimbursed a proportionate amount for the expended resources.

In addition, modifier 27 is amended when two visits are performed on the same day at the same facility.

Modifier 25 is used on the outpatient facility side to denote significantly separately identifiable evaluation and management services and assigned whenever significant or surgical procedures are performed (see Chapter 21).

Table 20-1 illustrates all the modifiers applicable for outpatient hospital facility coding—both CPT modifiers as well as HCPCS level II modifiers.

When using CPT descriptors for assigning service codes for outpatient facility coding, any inferences to "physician" are ignored. Keep in mind that when assigning CPT codes for services for an outpatient facility, the code is intended to represent the resources the facility has sed (not the physician resources) in performing that service. This includes modifiers as well as CPT codes.

EVALUATION AND MANAGEMENT ACUITY SERVICES

Unlike physician coding, evaluation and management codes are not assigned the same as for physician guidelines. In 2000, when the outpatient prospective payment system was

TABLE 20-1 OUTPATIENT FACILITY MODIFIERS

25	Significantly, separately identifiable E & M at the time of another procedure or service
27	Multiple outpatient E & M encounters on the same date
50	Bilateral
52	Reduced services
58	Staged/related
59	Distinct and separate
73	Discontinued procedure before induction of anesthesia/preparation of patient for surgery
74	Discontinued procedure after induction of anesthesia/preparation of patient for surgery
76	Repeat procedure, same physician
77	Repeat procedure, different physician
78	Return to the OR for related procedure
79	Unrelated procedure or service
CA	Inpatient-only procedure performed as emergency outpatient when patient dies before admission
GA	Waiver of liability form on file (ABN)
GG	Screening and diagnostic mammogram on same patient, same date
GH	Diagnostic mammogram converted from screening mammogram same date
GY	Services excludes, does not meet Medicare guidelines or non-Medicare contract benefit
GZ	Service expected to be denied as not reasonable or necessary
QL	Patient pronounced dead after ambulance called
QM	Ambulance service provided under arrangement with provider of services
QN	Ambulance service provided directly by provider of services
RT	Right side
LT	Left side
FA	Thumb, left hand
F1	Second digit, left hand
F2	Third digit, left hand
F3	Fourth digit, left hand
F4	Fifth digit, left hand
F5	Thumb, right hand
F6	Second digit, right hand
F7	Third digit, right hand
F8	Fourth digit, right hand
F9	Fifth digit, right hand
TA	Great toe, left foot
T1	Second digit, left foot
T2	Third digit, left foot
T3	Fourth digit, left foot
T4	Fifth digit, left foot
T5	Great toe, right foot
T6	Second digit, right foot
T7	Third digit, right foot
T8	Fourth digit, right foot
T9	Fifth digit, right foot
LC	Left circumflex artery
LD	Left anterior descending artery
RC	Right coronary artery

E & M, Evaluation and management; *ABN,* advance beneficiary notice.

introduced, facilities were given the opportunity to formulate their own methods for assigned levels of services, known as *acuity levels.* Although a number of methods are used by facilities for this purpose, the CPT codes are still used and levels assigned must meet the intention of the CPT descriptors. For example, code 99281, emergency room level 1 visit, must still meet the "problem focused" evaluation and management criteria.

Critical care services are interpreted and paid differently for outpatient facilities. Critical care, for instance, is only reimbursed for the first hour (CPT code 99291). Unlike outpatient facility services, the physician is reimbursed for critical care patients based on time (both code 99291 and 99292 are reimbursed) for medically necessary conditions.

For evaluation and management services that contain numerous levels, the CPT definition of levels of service is not applicable. Per CMS, each facility is free to design its own acuity system, by which the facility determines the level of acuity provided to the patient. This acuity level should be based on the amount of facility resources expended in treating, evaluating, and managing the patient. An example of an acuity sheet is illustrated in Table 20-2.

Consider the following outpatient facility chart (Figs. 20-11 to 20-13) and determine the appropriate diagnosis and procedures that will be reimbursed for the encounters.

From the outpatient documentation, the following diagnoses would be appropriate, as well as the assignment of the following procedure code(s):

Hydrocele
  Unilateral inguinal hernia
  Procedures: Repair inguinal hernia, initial, reducible
  Surgical pathology, level II

It would not be appropriate to assign code(s) for the surgical operating room, hospital room, and board during the preoperative and postoperative period; these are included in the reimbursement under APCs for the procedure. It would also be inappropriate to assign code(s) for the anesthesia and any of the supplies or materials required because they are covered by reimbursement for the surgical procedure under outpatient hospital coding guidelines.

The outpatient hospital facility coder uses ICD-9-CM coding guidelines as outlined in Section 2 and the CPT guidelines outlined in Section 3 of this text, with some exceptions such as modifier 51 usage. Keep in mind that the word "physician," when referenced in the CPT manual, should be ignored for the purpose of assigning codes for services rendered by the facility in the outpatient hospital setting.

With these guidelines in mind, examine the following outpatient hospital facility scenarios.

TABLE 20-2 SAMPLE FACILITY ACUITY SHEET

99281 ER Level 1	99282 ER Level 2	99283 ER Level 3	99284 ER Level 4	99285 ER Level 5
Insect bite	X-rays	Foley catheter	Thoracentesis	Central line
Prescription	Ace wrap	ECG	IV infusion	TPA
Rechecks	Bandages	Dermabond	ABGs	Code
Suture removal	Fetal heart tones	Slit lamp	Epistaxis with cautery	Admit to observation
DOA, no treatment	STD cultures	Pelvic exam	IVPs	Trauma
Suture removal	Fetal heart tones	Slit lamp	Breathing treatment	Automobile accident with multiple injuries
Recheck	Urine specimen	Enema	Paracentesis	Conscious sedation
Catheter removal	Blood work	FB removal	Intraabdominal symptoms	

ECG, Electrocardiogram; *IV,* intravenous; *TPA,* tissue plasminogen activator; *ABGs,* arterial blood gases; *DOA,* dead on arrival; *STD,* sexually transmitted disease; *IVP,* intravenous pyelography; *FB,* foreign body.

STOP AND PRACTICE

Assign the appropriate ICD-9-CM diagnostic and procedure codes as well as the appropriate CPT codes for the following outpatient hospital facility scenarios.

1. Excision of multiple lesions of the back, neck and arm, all determined to be benign back lesion 2.0 cm, neck lesion 1.0 cm and arm lesion 2.5 cm excised and closed.
   ICD-9-CM code(s): ______
   ICD-9-CM procedure code(s): ______
   CPT code(s): ______
2. Excisional breast biopsy. Lesion is identified with preoperative radiologic marker and the complete lesion is removed by excision. Surgical path indicates lesion is benign.
   ICD-9-CM code(s): ______
   ICD-9-CM procedure code(s): ______
   CPT code(s): ______
3. Diagnostic knee arthroscopy following 3 months of knee popping and catching. Arthroscopic access is made, lateral meniscus shows fraying and tear, which are debrided back to a stable rim.
   ICD-9-CM code(s): ______
   ICD-9-CM procedure code(s): ______
   CPT code(s): ______
4. Patient presents to emergency room for laceration check and re-dressing of wound to left forehead.
   ICD-9-CM code(s): ______
   ICD-9-CM procedure code(s): ______
   CPT code(s): ______
5. Placement of central venous access catheter with subcutaneous port for 65-year-old with breast cancer needing chemotherapy. Tunneling device was used.
   ICD-9-CM code(s): ______
   ICD-9-CM procedure code(s): ______
   CPT code(s): ______
6. Patient presents to emergency room for problems with central venous catheter. The catheter is examined and it is determined that it should be removed as it is no longer being used and appears to be infected.
   ICD-9-CM code(s): ______
   ICD-9-CM procedure code(s): ______
   CPT code(s): ______
7. 54-year-old presents for screening colonoscopy. Colonoscope is advanced to the cecum, with removal of multiple polyps, two by snare technique, one by hot biopsy forceps. An additional polyp was also biopsied.
   ICD-9-CM code(s): ______
   ICD-9-CM procedure code(s): ______
   CPT code(s): ______
8. Patient with external hemorrhoids with hemorrhoidal banding completed.
   ICD-9-CM code(s): ______
   ICD-9-CM procedure code(s): ______
   CPT code(s): ______
9. Extracapsular cataract extraction on an 84-year-old with IOL implant to be performed at a later date.
   ICD-9-CM code(s): ______
   ICD-9-CM procedure code(s): ______
   CPT code(s): ______
10. CT of the abdomen performed for abdominal pain. CT is performed using oral and IV contrast.
    ICD-9-CM code(s): ______
    ICD-9-CM procedure code(s): ______
    CPT code(s): ______

HISTORY AND PHYSICAL EXAMINATION

Rachel Perez, MD

Chief Complaint: Right scrotal swelling

25-year-old who previously underwent circumcision at birth, however, right scrotal swelling on and off since birth. Scrotal ultrasound obtained notes both testicles of normal size in the absence of solid testicular mass or testicular torsion. Right testicle displaced inferiorly secondary to 2.5–3.5 cm right hydrocele which is not septated or present internal debris noted.

Past medical history:

Noncontributory
PAST SURGICAL HISTORY: Circumcision at birth
ALLERGIES: No known drug allergies

Family and social history:

Review of systems:

Constitutional, negative for recent fever, weight loss, decreased appetite. HEENT: Positive for rhinitis. Negative for sore throat, earache. Cardiovascular: Negative for hypertension or congenital heart disease. Respiratory: Negative for asthma, bronchitis, productive cough. GI: negative for emesis, diarrhea, jaundice, constipation or melena. Hematological: Negative for bleeding disorder, bruising, anemia. Musculoskeletal: negative for congenital connective tissue disorder, recent joint swelling. Neuro: Negative for seizure disorder, meningitis, neurological disorder.

Physical exam:

In general, well developed, well nourished, 25-year-old male alert and in no acute distress:

HEENT: Normocephalic, atraumatic, EOM intact.
Neck: Supple without palpable lymphadenopathy.
Lungs: Clear to auscultation bilaterally without labored respirations or wheezing.
Heart: Regular rate and rhythm.
Abdomen: Soft, flat, nontender, nondistended, urinary bladder not palpable. No palpable abdominal organomegaly.
GU: Circumcised phallus without penile mass or lesion. Urethra meatus patent without evidence of gross blood or penile discharge. Left testicle descended and displaced laterally secondary to large right hemoscrotal mass effect due to hydrocele. Large right hydrocele present which does transilluminate for which the right testicle is not physically palpable. No scrotal fixation. No palpable inguinal adenopathy or any inguinal hernia appreciated bilaterally.
Extremities: No cyanosis, clubbing or edema.
Neuro: Alert and cooperative with no focal motor deficit

Laboratory/radiology:

White count 7.3. Hemoglobin 11.9. Platelets 323,000. PT 11.4. PTT 31.4. Urinanalysis on void; color yellow, clarity clear, no red cells, trace bacteria. Sodium 137, Potassium 4.0. BUN 14, Creatinine 0.4. Glucose 85, Calcium 9.6

X-ray:

Assessment:

IMPRESSION: Right inguinal hernia/hydrocele

Plan:

Patient scheduled for outpatient surgery consisting of right hydrocelectomy through inguinal approach with possible ligation of inguinal hernia if present under anesthesia.

Rachel Perez MD

GODFREY REGIONAL HOSPITAL
123 Main Street • Aldon, FL 77714 • (407) 555-1234

FIGURE 20-11. History and physical examination form for a patient with right scrotal swelling.

OPERATIVE REPORT

Patient information:
Patient name: DOB: MR#:
Preoperative diagnosis:
Right hydrocele
Postoperative diagnosis:
Right inguinal hernia/hydrocele
Procedure(s) performed:
Right inguinal hernia repair with excision of right hydrocele
Anesthesia:
General
Assistant surgeon:
Description of procedure:

After informed consent, patient was taken to the Operating Room, placed in supine position, and given general endotracheal anesthesia per protocol. The external genitalia and lower abdomen were prepped with betadine solution, draped in the usual sterile fashion. Patient did receive one dose of IV antibiotic consisting of 150 mg Ancef prior to initiation of the surgical procedure.

A left oblique incision was made approximately one finger-breadth above the right pubic tubercle in order to allow appropriate access to the right inguinal canal. The subcutaneous tissue and Scarpa's fascia were incised sharply to the level of the aponeurosis of the external oblique. Hemostasis of small perforating vessels was obtained with electrocautery. The external inguinal ring was identified where the overlying fascia of the external oblique was sharply incised in the direction of its fibers to expose and open the right inguinal canal.

The ileoinguinal nerve was identified and sharply excised from overlying tissue of the spermatic cord and retracted laterally to prevent future injury. Self-retaining retractors were placed to assist with exposure of the spermatic cord.

The spermatic cord was bluntly freed from the external oblique aponeurosis in the entire inguinal canal. A Penrose drain was placed in the area around the spermatic cord to assist with retraction.

Cremasteric fibers were sharply taken down to the level of the spermatic cord near the internal inguinal ring. The hernia sac was bluntly dissected free of the spermatic cord fascia and adjacent vascular structures.

The vas deferens was identified posterior to the hernia sac and likewise dissected free of the surface of the hernia sac. Once the vas deferens and vascular structures were dissected free of the hernia sac, a straight clamp was placed across the hernia sac and transsected distal to the clamp.

The hernia sac was then dissected free of cord structures to the level of the internal inguinal ring. High ligation was performed at this level by placement of 2 silk ties of 2-0 silk. The hernia sac was excised and sent to Pathology for analysis.

The distal edges of the tunic vaginalis were grasped with mosquito clamps and subsequently opened with electrocautery where a noncommunicating hydrocele was evident. The right testicle could not be delivered into the surgical field secondary to associated hydrocele component. Aspiration of hydrocele through the scrotal sac using a 22-gauge needle was performed with the return of straw-colored fluid. Subsequent delivery of the right testicle into the surgical field was performed for which it was left attached to the gubernaculums.

Wound was then thoroughly irrigated with saline and edges of the external oblique reapproximated with a running 3-0 Vicryl suture. The Scarpa's fascia was then reapproximated with running 3-0 Vicryl. Skin edges were reapproximated with a running 4-0 Vicryl suture and Benzoin and steri-strips were applied and a sterile dressing placed.

Final needle, sponge, and instrument count were correct. The patient tolerated the procedure well.

Rachel Perez MD

GODFREY REGIONAL HOSPITAL
123 Main Street • Aldon, FL 77714 • (407) 555-1234

FIGURE 20-12. Operative report for hernia repair.

SURGICAL PATHOLOGY REPORT

Name:_____ Hosp. No.:_____ Path. No.:_____

Date:_____ Room:_____ Age:_____ Sex:_____ Surgeon:_____ M.D.

Operation: Excision of Hydrocele, Inguinal Hernia Repair

Material submitted: Hernia Sac, Surgical Excision

Pre-op diagnosis: Right hydrocele

Post-op diagnosis: Right inguinal hernia/hydrocele

Previous material:_____ Pertinent history:_____

Diagnosis:

Hernia sac, (clinically right), excision:
Benign fibroadipose tissue consistent with hernia sac

Gross description:

The specimen is labeled hernia sac. Received is a 6 mm in greatest diameter tan-grey portion of membranous-appearing tissue. The specimen is totally submitted in one cassette.

Micro description:

Slides reviewed

Maria Callingmo M.D.
Surgical Pathologist

GODFREY CLINICAL LABORATORIES
465 Dogwood Court • Aldon, FL 77712 • (407) 555-9876

FIGURE 20-13. Surgical pathology report for the hernia sac.

Chapter in Review

Certification Review

- The basis for inpatient coding assignment differs from physician coding in that the encounter includes everything from admission to discharge.
- Volumes 1, 2, and 3 of the ICD-9-CM diagnostic coding book are used for inpatient diagnostic coding.
- Statements such as "probable," "possible," and "rule out" are used for coding purposes with inpatient diagnostic coding.
- Principal diagnosis is defined as the condition chiefly responsible for the patient's admission to the hospital after diagnostic or therapeutic studies.
- Outpatient hospital diagnostic coding follows the rules for physician coding.
- Outpatient hospital diagnostic coding uses ICD-9-CM Volume 3 to report significant procedures when applicable.

Student Assignments

- Study Chapter 20.
- Review the Learning Objectives for Chapter 20.
- Complete the Stop and Practice exercises for Chapter 20.
- Study the Certification Review for Chapter 20.
- Complete the Chapter Review exercise to reinforce concepts learned in this chapter.
- Complete the practice exercises on the companion Evolve site for reinforcement of facility coding concepts.
- Complete the Practical Application exercise for real-life coding scenarios.
- Complete the Workbook exercises as assigned by your instructor, or individually for additional practice.

Chapter Review Exercise

Look up and code these procedures from Volume 3 of the ICD-9-CM.

	Volume 3 ICD-9-CM Code
1. Exploratory laparotomy	________
2. Repair of fractured clavicle	________
3. Appendectomy	________
4. Cholecystectomy	________
5. Cystourethroscopy	________
6. Tonsillectomy with adenoidectomy	________
7. Insertion of PE tubes for otitis media	________
8. Knee arthroscopy	________
9. Blood transfusion, packed red blood cells	________
10. Colonoscopy with biopsy	________
11. Bone scan	________
12. Flexible sigmoidoscopy	________
13. Pacemaker implant	________
14. Cardiac catheterization	________
15. Physical therapy	________
16. Esophageal speech training	________
17. Kidney transplant	________
18. Clavicular osteotomy	________
19. Wound dressing	________
20. Amputation, below the knee	________
21. Abdominal ultrasound	________
22. CPAP ventilation	________
23. Vasectomy	________
24. Vaginal delivery with episiotomy	________
25. Corneal transplant	________

On the basis of the guidelines established for hospital inpatient diagnostic coding and for physician coding, determine which of these diagnoses would be used for inpatient versus physician coding. Designate by indicating inpatient (I), physician (P), or both (IP) and assign the appropriate ICD-9-CM code. Assign ICD-9-CM codes only to those that are appropriate.

		ICD-9-CM Code	Designation (I, P, or IP)
26.	Rule out pneumonia	______	______
27.	Acute bronchitis	______	______
28.	Myocardial infarction	______	______
29.	Ruled out ankle fracture	______	______
	Ankle pain	______	______
30.	Acute respiratory failure	______	______
	COPD	______	______

Given the following diagnostic information, indicate what diagnostic statement would be used for physician and inpatient purposes.

		Physician	Inpatient
31.	Myocardial infarction	______	______
	COPD	______	______
32.	Abdominal pain	______	______
	Rule out appendicitis	______	______
33.	Urinary tract infection, most likely streptococcal	______	______
34.	Anemia, possibly due to chronic blood loss	______	______
35.	Anemia due to GI bleed	______	______

Practical Application

Following the appropriate steps for coding, assign ICD-9-CM diagnosis or procedure codes as well as CPT codes when appropriate for the following exercises. Assign code(s) based on outpatient hospital facility coding guidelines.

1. Chest pain, rule out MI, no procedures performed, inpatient

   ICD-9-CM diagnostic code(s): ______________

   ICD-9-CM procedure code(s): ______________

   CPT code(s) (if applicable): ______________

2. Angina, rule out MI, CABG performed, inpatient

   ICD-9-CM diagnostic code(s): ______________

   ICD-9-CM procedure code(s): ______________

   CPT code(s) (if applicable): ______________

3. Colonoscopy with snare polypectomy performed outpatient

   ICD-9-CM diagnostic code(s): ______________

   ICD-9-CM procedure code(s): ______________

   CPT code(s) (if applicable): ______________

4. ER visit, level 4, chest X-ray, ECG for chest pain, rule out MI

   ICD-9-CM diagnostic code(s): ______________

   ICD-9-CM procedure code(s): ______________

   CPT code(s) (if applicable): ______________

5. Seizure disorder in 22-year-old with CHF, inpatient 7 days

   ICD-9-CM diagnostic code(s): ______________

   ICD-9-CM procedure code(s): ______________

   CPT code(s) (if applicable): ______________

6. Patient presents to ER with urinary retention, diagnosed with UTI

   ICD-9-CM diagnostic code(s): ______________

   ICD-9-CM procedure code(s): ______________

   CPT code(s) (if applicable): ______________

7. 14-year-old with chronic tonsillitis presents for outpatient tonsillectomy with possible adenoidectomy. Tonsils were grasped and excised along with hypertrophic adenoidal tissue.

   ICD-9-CM diagnostic code(s): ______________

   ICD-9-CM procedure code(s): ______________

   CPT code(s) (if applicable): ______________

8. Patient admitted with fatigue, cough, and fever that has persisted for several weeks. CXR, culture demonstrates *E. coli* pneumonia. Treated with IV antibiotics and nebulizer treatments for 4 days and discharged on oral antibiotics on day 5.

   ICD-9-CM diagnostic code(s): ______________

   ICD-9-CM procedure code(s): ______________

   CPT code(s) (if applicable): ______________

9. Patient admitted with chest pain, SOB. MI ruled out. Repeat ECG, cardiac enzymes are normal and patient is discharged on the second day.

   ICD-9-CM diagnostic code(s): ______________

   ICD-9-CM procedure code(s): ______________

   CPT code(s) (if applicable): ______________

10. Patient presents with shortness of breath, history of COPD. Diagnosed with acute exacerbation of COPD, given steroids PO and nebulizer treatment and discharged from ER.

    ICD-9-CM diagnostic code(s): ______________

    ICD-9-CM procedure code(s): ______________

    CPT code(s) (if applicable): ______________

21

Hospital and Facility Reimbursement Process

LEARNING OBJECTIVES

After completing this chapter, the student will be able to:

- Understand the different methods for hospital inpatient and outpatient reimbursement.
- Delineate the significant differences between inpatient and outpatient and physician coding.
- Understand and apply the coding guidelines for assigning Diagnosis-Related Group (DRG)/ Ambulatory Payment Classification (APC) codes.
- Comprehend the significance of the correct assignment of principal diagnosis for the purpose of determining the correct DRG code.
- Grasp the importance of identifying the presence or absence of complications and/or comorbidities that may present additional risk consideration for inpatient hospital cases.
- Understand the grouping of DRGs into categories known as major diagnostic categories.
- Understand the assignment of APC codes under the Outpatient Prospective Payment System.
- Apply facility billing concepts to practical billing scenarios.

CODING REFERENCE TOOLS

Tool 21-1
DRG Coding Guidelines

Tool 21-2
MDCs Listing

KEY TERMS

Ambulatory Payment Classification (APC)
Complications and Comorbidities
Diagnosis-Related Group (DRG)
Fee-for-Service
Major Diagnostic Category (MDC)
New Technology and Pass-Through Services
Outpatient Prospective Payment System (OPPS)
Payment Status Indicators
Per Diem
Principal Diagnosis
Prospective Payment System (PPS)
Secondary Diagnosis

Documentation and Coding Guidelines

The documentation needs for inpatient and outpatient hospital coding and billing are discussed in Chapter 20. Keep in mind that for facility coding and billing, all documentation may be reviewed and used in the assignment of codes for billing and reimbursement purposes. Also remember that the principal diagnosis for inpatient facility coding and billing is determined only at the conclusion of the encounter (admission), after the completion of all studies and ancillary services.

Although reimbursement processes are discussed in this chapter, it is important to remember that the Diagnosis-Related Group (DRG) or Ambulatory Payment Classification (APC) assignments are not made at the facility, but are assigned by the carrier based on the ICD-9-CM codes and CPT codes submitted by the facility as appropriate. It is important, however, to understand the process to comprehend the need for appropriate diagnostic order and code assignments.

Inpatient Facility Billing and Reimbursement Methods

The most significant differences in hospital and physician coding involve the methods for coding the *what,* or the services performed. The coder must remember that these methods differ because of the reimbursement philosophies for providers and physicians compared with hospitals and facilities. Facility reimbursement is typically accomplished with a collection of all services required to provide care, or "facility services," rather than with individual itemization. A look at the three main methods for reimbursement of inpatient or facility care helps in understanding the coding systems for inpatient coding.

Three basic inpatient methods are used for inpatient reimbursement: pay for service, per diem, and the prospective payment system.

FEE FOR SERVICE

Fee for service coding is based on the expenses incurred by the facility in providing services to a specific patient for a specific admission. Under this method of reimbursement all services are covered, including items such as room, meals, surgical suites, nursing care, surgical procedures, pharmaceuticals, supplies, and other items necessary for the treatment of the patient's condition or illness.

PER DIEM

Per diem charges are based on a fixed payment amount per day for all services provided by the hospital or facility. This fixed amount may vary according to type of admission or level of service. For instance, per diem reimbursement for a patient in a critical care bed would be greater than that for a regular medical bed.

PROSPECTIVE PAYMENT SYSTEM

The **prospective payment system** (**PPS**) of reimbursement agrees to a set amount of reimbursement according to the type of case (diagnosis, illness, symptom, or injury). The most familiar prospective payment system is the **Diagnosis-Related Group** (**DRG**) system used by the federal government for Medicare claims. This system is used by many other third-party carriers as well.

DRGs reimburse a set amount based on the patient's diagnosis and treatment during the admission. This method assumes that patients with similar illnesses or symptoms undergo similar procedures and testing, and each of these illnesses or symptoms is assigned a specific reimbursement amount as specified by the assignment of a DRG code.

Facilities are now able to formulate their reimbursement according to the DRG assignment because the dollar amount for reimbursement has *prospectively* been determined and agreed on.

The original DRG system, which was developed at Yale University, divided all principal diagnoses into similar categories, referred to as **major diagnostic categories** (**MDCs**). The primary purposes of the DRG system are reimbursement, evaluation of quality of care, and use of services. Congress mandated the use of the DRG system for all inpatient Medicare care in 1983, making it necessary for all hospitals providing care to Medicare recipients to follow this method for submitting services to Medicare Part A.

In addition to the obvious purpose of determining reimbursement, DRGs serve other important functions for hospitals because they provide a means of evaluating quality of care and use of services. Because the cases "grouped" together under one DRG assignment are similar in their treatment protocols and related conditions and treatments, the hospital has the ability to use these data for outcome analysis and quality review. In addition, the data derived from the DRG assignment are analyzed in evaluating the use of services. Each DRG represents the "average" services provided for similar patients with similar treatments, so the data give the hospital the ability to detect overuse by the facility or by a particular provider. DRGs also provide the necessary data to ensure that the quality standards of the hospital are met.

From the reimbursement perspective, each DRG is intended to represent the average resources or services necessary to treat patients placed in that group. The DRG assigned also relates to the hospital case mix and the types of patients the particular hospital treats. Each hospital calculates a hospital case mix index (CMI), which is determined by dividing all provided DRG relative weights by the total number of Medicare encounters at that particular hospital.

Reimbursement is based on the weight assigned to that DRG multiplied by the base rate for that particular hospital. The hospital can calculate its payment based on the following formula:

DRG Relative Weight × Hospital Base Rate
= Hospital Payment

The DRG system currently is composed of more than 500 valid groups that classify patients and correlate the services used and length of stay based on the following:

- Principal and secondary diagnoses
- Procedure codes
- Sex
- Age
- Discharge status
- Presence or absence of complications and comorbidities
- Birth weights for neonates

Components of DRG Code Assignments

Further discussion follows regarding the components that determine the correct assignment of DRG codes under this system.

PRINCIPAL AND SECONDARY DIAGNOSES

The assignment of a DRG is based primarily on the principal diagnosis and includes up to eight additional diagnoses. The DRG code is based on diagnoses and procedures designated by the use of ICD-9-CM codes. The rules for coding diagnoses from the inpatient perspective differ from those previously discussed for physician and outpatient use. Chapter 20 presents the inpatient ICD-9-CM codes.

Principal diagnosis is defined as the condition determined to have caused the hospital admission of the patient after studies were completed. After assignment of the appropriate ICD-9-CM diagnostic codes with the inpatient hospital coding rules, the coder must determine the principal diagnosis. Contributing or **secondary diagnoses** are assigned as well when they contribute to either the complexity of the case or the medical decision-making process of the principal diagnosis. The assignment of principal and supporting diagnoses would be made only at the conclusion of the encounter or admission and only after all diagnostic studies are completed.

PRESENT ON ADMISSION INDICATORS

Medicare now requires facilities to report conditions that are present on admission (POA) to distinguish conditions that were present at the time the patient is admitted to the hospital from conditions acquired during the hospitalization. Medicare will no longer consider additional payment for conditions that are hospital acquired. General requirements are as follows:

- Required for all claims involving Medicare inpatient admissions to acute care hospitals
- Defined as present at the time the order for inpatient admission occurs
- Issues of inconsistencies must be resolved by the provider
- Conditions not reportable under ICD-9-CM diagnostic guidelines are not reportable as POA

This information is reported on the UB-04 claim form in Form Locator 67. It is reported as follows:

Y	Diagnosis was present at time of inpatient admission
N	Diagnosis NOT present at time of inpatient admission
U	Unknown whether condition was present at time of inpatient admission
W	Clinically undetermined whether present at time of inpatient admission
1	Exempt from POA reporting

For additional information regarding current guidelines for POA, refer to the *ICD-9-CM Official Guidelines for Coding and Reporting.*

PROCEDURE CODES

The coder must determine whether specific surgical procedures that affect the DRG are performed during the admission. All procedures must be coded for use in DRG assignment. The coder must also use the Volume 3, Procedure Coding section of ICD-9-CM for assignment of these codes, as previously discussed.

SEX

Several DRG codes are based on the sex of the patient. Obviously, DRG assignment for prostate conditions should be assigned to male patients only, and vaginal delivery codes would be specific to female patients, classified by reproductive age only.

AGE

After the selection of diagnostic codes, the case should be reviewed for patient age because many DRG assignments are based on age, such as the following:

Simple pneumonia and pleurisy age >17
Simple pneumonia and pleurisy age 0-17

Obviously, components such as birth weights of neonates would be appropriate only for neonates.

DISCHARGE STATUS

Some DRG codes depend on whether the patient has been discharged alive or deceased. The coder must ascertain this information from the chart as well.

PRESENCE OR ABSENCE OF COMPLICATIONS AND COMORBIDITIES

The system of assigning conditions and diagnoses that present an additional risk consideration in inpatient cases was completely restructured and implemented in 2007. Before October 2007, Centers for Medicare and Medicaid Services (CMS) defined these conditions as **complications and comorbidities,** or *CCs*. However, this method allowed additional payment consideration all complications and comorbidities regardless of their severity, or lack thereof. The assignment of a CC typically increased the length of stay by at least 1 day in more than 75% of the patient cases. The introduction of the Medicare Severity (MS)-DRG system primarily changed the structure of the CCs, leaving the basic DRG structure the same.

With the MS-DRG system, additional CCs are based on resources used, not length of stay, through the creation of major CCs (MCCs). Significant conditions such as serious open fractures, underlying infections, and obstetric or neonatal complications are examples of conditions that allow the assignment of an MS-DRG rather than a regular DRG.

Table 21-1 illustrates some conditions that qualify for the assignment of MS-DRGs. An entire listing of MS-DRGs can be found at www.cms.gov.

TABLE 21-1 EXCERPT FROM MS-DRG LIST

MS-DRG	FY09 FINAL RULE POST-ACUTE DRG	FY09 FINAL RULE SPECIAL PAY DRG	MDC	TYPE	MS-DRG TITLE	WEIGHTS	GEOMETRIC MEAN LOS	ARITHMETIC MEAN LOS
020	No	No	01	Surg	Intracranial vascular procedures w/PDX hemorrhage w/MCC	8.2920	14.8	18.3
021	No	No	01	Surg	Intracranial vascular procedures w/PDX hemorrhage w/CC	6.3596	13.7	15.5
022	No	No	01	Surg	Intracranial vascular procedures w/PDX hemorrhage w/o CC/MCC	4.1535	7.6	9.3
023	No	No	01	Surg	Craniotomy w/major dev impl/acute complex CNS PDX w/MCC or chemo implant	5.0584	8.9	12.7
024	No	No	01	Surg	Craniotomy w/ major dev impl/acute complex CNS PDX w/o MCC	3.4597	6.2	9.0
025	Yes	No	01	Surg	Craniotomy and endovascular intracranial procedures w/MCC	5.0109	9.9	13.0
026	Yes	No	01	Surg	Craniotomy and endovascular intracranial procedures w/CC	3.0058	6.4	8.2
027	Yes	No	01	Surg	Craniotomy and endovascular intracranial procedures w/o CC/MCC	2.1029	3.5	4.5
028	Yes	Yes	01	Surg	Spinal procedures w/ MCC	5.1919	10.7	14.3
029	Yes	Yes	01	Surg	Spinal procedures w/CC or spinal neurostimulators	2.7943	5.1	7.1
030	Yes	Yes	01	Surg	Spinal procedures w/o CC/MCC	1.5385	2.8	3.7

FY, Fiscal year; *PDX*, primary diagnosis; *MDC*, major diagnostic category; *LOS*, length of stay; *MCC*, major complications and comorbidities; *CC*, complications and comorbidities; *CNS*, central nervous system; *dev impl*, device implant; *chemo*, chemotherapy.

BIRTH WEIGHTS FOR NEONATES

In the treatment of a neonate, specific DRG assignments are made for low birth weight neonates. For example, DRG 386 applies to birth weights of less than 1500 g, gestation less than 28 weeks, or both.

DRG Coding Process

When the coder must determine a DRG assignment, he or she can refer to the steps in Tool 21-1 to determine DRG assignment. In most instances the assignment of DRG codes is accomplished by computerized encoder software at the facility. Software has been developed that leads the coder through a series of questions; it then assigns DRGs and diagnostic codes. Despite the convenience and ease of use of inpatient encoder systems, the hospital inpatient coder must have the knowledge and skills to determine principal diagnosis, secondary diagnoses, and patient severity.

Although approximately 25 major diagnostic categories are used for inpatient DRG assignment, the subcategory DRG codes number more than 500. A listing of the MDCs is provided in Tool 21-2. In addition, Box 21-1 contains a sample of DRG assignments for one MDC category. The listing of DRG assignments is extensive and encompasses an entire book; therefore this text has provided only samples as an illustration of the DRG system. A complete list of DRG assignments is available on the CMS Web site (www.cms.gov).

Hospital DRG coding may seem more challenging because it encompasses many records rather than just a specific visit note or operative note. The coder should remember that for coding of hospital DRG services, the encounter begins at admission and ends at discharge. Therefore, compared with physician coding, any properly documented information during the hospital encounter may be used for selecting and coding the DRG.

The coder probably will not be exposed to manual coding of DRG codes; therefore this text contains only a limited number of DRG coding exercises. If necessary, use the hospital inpatient DRG coding worksheet (Figure 21-1) and review the chart example (Figure 21-2). Keep in mind that inpatient charts are usually voluminous; this example is only long enough to meet the student's needs for demonstrating the appropriate assignment of a DRG.

In looking at the sample chart in Figure 21-2, consider only components necessary for proper coding.

Steps in DRG Assignment Process

- **Step 1: Identify the appropriate diagnosis.**
  First, identify the elements that make up the diagnosis:

> The patient came from a nursing home and felt weak on the right side. Workers there thought she was alert but confused. When seen in the ED she was able to answer questions appropriately and follow commands but was unable to lift her right leg. She had some motion in her right arm but was unable to squeeze her right hand. When evaluated by the ED physician, she was determined to be confused and was difficult to understand. CT was obtained, with initial impression of a large, left hemispheric bleed.

TOOL 21-1

DRG CODING GUIDELINES

1. Establish principal diagnosis and secondary diagnoses.
2. Determine all significant procedures and code accordingly.
3. Determine whether a surgical procedure was performed.
4. Based on the principal diagnosis, assign the correct MDC category.
5. Determine whether to use the medical or surgical partition.
6. Check for contributing factors that affect DRG assignment and assign correct DRG within the appropriate MCD category:
   - Age
   - Sex
   - Discharge status
   - Presence or absence of complications or comorbidities
   - Birth weight for neonates

TOOL 21-2

MDC LISTING

MDC	Category	DRG Range
1	Diseases/Disorders Nervous System	1-35
2	Diseases/Disorders Eye	36-48
3	Diseases/Disorders Ears, Nose, Mouth, Throat	49-74, 168-169, 185-187
4	Diseases/Disorders Respiratory System	75-102, 475
5	Diseases/Disorders Circulatory System	103-145, 478-479
6	Diseases/Disorders Digestive System	146-167, 170-184, 188-190
7	Diseases/Disorders Hepatobiliary System/Pancreas	191-208, 493-494
8	Diseases/Disorders Musculoskeletal System/Connective Tissue	209-256, 471, 491, 496-503
9	Disease/Disorders Skin, Subcutaneous Tissue, Breast	257-284
10	Endocrine, Nutritional, Metabolic Diseases/Disorders	285-301
11	Diseases/Disorders of the Kidney/Urinary Tract	302-333
12	Diseases/Disorders Male Reproductive System	334-352
13	Diseases/Disorders Female Reproductive System	353-369
14	Pregnancy, Childbirth, Puerperium	370-384, 469
15	Newborns, Neonates with Conditions Originating in Perinatal Period	385-391, 469-470
16	Diseases/Disorders Blood, Blood-Forming Organs/Immunological Diseases	392-399
17	Myeloproliferative Diseases/Disorders and Poorly Differentiated Neoplasms	400-414, 473, 492
18	Infectious/Parasitic Diseases	415-423
19	Mental Diseases/Disorders	424-432
20	Alcohol/Drug Use/Drug-Induced Organic Mental Disorders	433-437
21	Injuries, Poisonings, Toxic Effect Drugs	439-455
22	Burns	456-460, 472
23	Factors Influencing Health Status, Other Contact Health Services	461-467
24	Multiple Significant Trauma	484-487
25	Human Immunodeficiency Virus Infections	488-490

DRG Codes Associated with all MDC classifications

DRG	Description
468	Extensive Operative Room Procedure Unrelated to Principal Diagnosis
476	Prostatic Operating Room Procedure Unrelated to Principal Diagnosis
477	Nonextensive Operative Room Procedure Unrelated to Principal Diagnosis
480	Liver Transplant
481	Bone Marrow Transplant
482	Tracheostomy
483	Tracheostomy
495	Lung Transplant

BOX 21-1 DRG LISTING (BY MDC)

MDC 1: Diseases and Disorders of the Nervous System

DRG	
1	Craniotomy except Trauma, age 18 or older
2	Craniotomy for Trauma, age 18 or older
3	Craniotomy, age 17 or younger
4	Spinal Procedures
5	Extracranial Vascular Procedures
6	Carpal Tunnel Release
7	Peripheral and Cranial Nerve and Other Nervous System Procedures with CC
8	Peripheral and Cranial Nerve and Other Nervous System Procedures without CC
9	Spinal Disorders and Injuries
10	Nervous System Neoplasms with CC
11	Nervous System Neoplasms without CC
12	Degenerative Nervous System Disorders
13	Multiple Sclerosis and Cerebellar Ataxia
14	Specific Cerebrovascular Disorders except TIA
15	TIA and Precerebral Occlusions
16	Nonspecific Cerebrovascular Disorders with CC
17	Nonspecific Cerebrovascular Disorders without CC
18	Cranial and Peripheral Nerve Disorders with CC
19	Cranial and Peripheral Nerve Disorders without CC
20	Nervous System Infection except Viral Meningitis
21	Viral Meningitis
22	Hypertensive Encephalopathy
23	Nontraumatic Stupor and Coma
24	Seizure and Headache, Age >17 with CC
25	Seizure and Headache, Age >17 without CC
26	Seizure and Headache, Ages 0-17
27	Traumatic Stupor and Coma, Coma >1 Hour
28	Traumatic Stupor and Coma, Coma <1 Hour, Age >17 with CC
29	Traumatic Stupor and Coma, Coma <1 Hour, Age >17 without CC
30	Traumatic Stupor and Coma, Coma <1 Hour, Ages 0-17
31	Concussion, Age >17 with CC
32	Concussion, Age >17 without CC
33	Concussion, Ages 0-17
34	Other Disorders of Nervous System with CC
35	Other Disorders of Nervous System without CC

MDC 4: Respiratory System

DRG	
075	Major Chest Procedures
076	Other Respiratory System or Procedures with CC
077	Other Respiratory System or Procedures without CC
078	Pulmonary Embolism
079	Respiratory Infections/Inflammations Age >17 with CC
080	Respiratory Infections/Inflammations Age >17 without CC
081	Respiratory Infections/Inflammations Ages 0-17
082	Respiratory Neoplasms
083	Major Chest Trauma with CC
084	Major Chest Trauma without CC
085	Pleural Effusion with CC
086	Pleural Effusion without CC
087	Pulmonary Edema and Respiratory Failure
088	Chronic Obstructive Pulmonary Disease
089	Simple Pneumonia/Pleurisy Age >17 with CC
090	Simple Pneumonia/Pleurisy Age >17 without CC
091	Simple Pneumonia/Pleurisy Ages 0-17
092	Interstitial Lung Disease with CC
093	Interstitial Lung Disease without CC
094	Pneumothorax with CC
095	Pneumothorax without CC
096	Bronchitis/Asthma Age >17 with CC
097	Bronchitis/Asthma Age >17 without CC
098	Bronchitis/Asthma Ages 0-17
099	Respiratory Signs/Symptoms with CC
100	Respiratory Signs/Symptoms without CC
101	Other Respiratory System Diagnoses with CC
102	Other Respiratory System Diagnoses without CC
475	Respiratory System Diagnosis with Ventilator Support

CC, Complications and comorbidities; *TIA*, transient ischemic attack.

HOSPITAL INPATIENT DRG CODING WORKSHEET

Chart#/Patient Name:

	List Components Here		Assign Codes Here	
Step 1 - Principal/Secondary Diagnosis 1A - List diagnosis 1B - Determine primary diagnosis "Condition established after study to be chiefly responsible for admission to hospital for care" Number diagnoses in appropriate order				
Step 2 - Significant Procedures				
Step 3 - Determine whether surgical procedure performed Yes/No				
Step 4 - Assign the MDC Based on principal diagnosis				
Step 5 - Determine whether medical or surgical partition Med/Surg				
Step 6 - Check for Contributing Factors Age Sex Discharge status Presence/absence of complications or comorbidities Birthweight for neonates				
ASSIGNMENT **DRG:** **Principal Dx:** **Addtl Dx:**				

FIGURE 21-1. Diagnosis-Related Group (DRG) coding worksheet used for coding hospital DRG charts.

HISTORY AND PHYSICAL EXAMINATION

Godfrey Regional Hospital History & Physical
Admission: 12/01/00

The patient came from a nursing home and felt weak on the right side. Workers there thought she was alert, but confused. When seen in the ER, she was able to answer questions appropriately and to follow commands but was unable to lift her right leg. She had some motion in her right arm but was unable to squeeze her right hand. When evaluated by the ER physician, she was determined to be confused, and was difficult to understand. CT was obtained, with initial impression of a large, left hemispheric bleed.

Past medical history:

Remarkable for polymyalgia, GERD, hyperthyroid, DJD of the knees. Hospitalizations for pneumonia, gout, situational depression. CURRENT MEDICATION: Prilosec 20 mg qd, Synthroid .125 mg daily, Propulsid 10 mg bid, Prednisone 20 mg daily, Cardizem CD 120 mg daily.

Family and social history:

Unobtainable from patient.

Review of systems:

Unobtainable from patient.

Physical exam:

Patient is alert but confused. She is not dysarthric. PERRLA. Extraocular movements are normal. Sclera is clear. TMs normal. No skull lacerations noted. Slight right VII nerve weakness. Lungs clear. Abdomen is soft, nontender, without guarding or rebound. Neuro/MS: Full ROM except right arm and leg. Unable to raise her left leg or to move it at all with positive Babinski's on right. Normal labs.

Laboratory/radiology:

X-ray:

Assessment:

Intracranial bleed.

Plan:

GODFREY REGIONAL HOSPITAL
123 Main Street • Aldon, FL 77714 • (407) 555-1234

FIGURE 21-2. Sample history and physical examination form.

Current medication: Prilosec 20 mg qd, Synthroid 0.125 mg daily, Propulsid 10 mg bid, prednisone 20 mg daily, Cardizem CD 120 mg daily.

Review of systems/family history: Unobtainable from patient.

Medical history: Remarkable for polymyalgia, GERD, hyperthyroidism, DJD of the knees; hospitalizations for pneumonia, gout, situational depression.

Physical examination: Patient is alert but confused. She is not dysarthric. PERRL. Extraocular movements are normal. Sclera is clear. TMs normal. No skull lacerations noted. Slight right VII nerve weakness. Lungs clear. Abdomen is soft, nontender, without guarding or rebound. *Neuro/MSK:* Full ROM except right arm and leg. Unable to raise her left leg or move it at all with positive Babinski's on right. Normal labs.

Assessment: Intracranial bleed.

List appropriate components and determine which diagnosis(es) should be included in the diagnostic statement:

1. Weak
2. Confused
3. Large, left hemispheric bleed
4. PMH polymyalgia
5. PMH GERD
6. PMH hyperthyroidism
7. PMH DJD knees
8. Intracranial bleed

(1) "Weak" and (2) "confused" are signs and symptoms of (3) "large, left hemispheric bleed" and (8) "intracranial bleed" and therefore may be eliminated. Medical histories, as long as they describe chronic continuing disorders, may be coded as existing in hospital coding, unlike physician or provider coding. Therefore the final diagnostic statement would look like the following:

1. Left hemispheric bleed, intracranial bleed
2. Polymyalgia
3. GERD
4. Hyperthyroidism
5. DJD knees

The principal diagnosis would be "the condition established after study to be chiefly responsible for admission to hospital for care." Because the four diagnoses listed as medical history were only considered for therapeutic ongoing treatment and were not the thrust of treatment, "left hemispheric bleed, intracranial bleed" is considered the *principal diagnosis.*

ICD-9-CM codes would be assigned as follows:

1. Intracranial bleed	Hemorrhage, intracranial	432.9
2. Polymyalgia	Polymyalgia	725
3. GERD	Reflux, gastroesophageal	530.81
4. Hyperthyroidism	Hyperthyroidism	242.90
5. DJD knees	DJD, knees	719.96

- **Step 2: Determine whether significant procedures were performed.**

The second step in DRG coding is to determine whether significant procedures were performed. They are not documented, so it must be assumed they did not occur.

- **Step 3: Assign the MDC according to the principal diagnosis.**

The third step in DRG coding is to assign the MDC according to the principal diagnosis. The principal diagnosis of intracranial bleed leads to an MDC in the nervous system section, which narrows selection to the DRG range of 1 through 35.

- **Step 4: Assign appropriate DRG code within specific MDC category.**

According to the MDC 1 listing included in this chapter, the assignment of DRG 14, "specific cerebrovascular disorders except transient ischemic attack," would be an appropriate assignment for this chart.

- **Step 5: Determine whether the partition should be medical or surgical.**

The fifth step in DRG coding is to determine whether the partition should be medical or surgical. Because no surgical services were identified, the medical partition would be appropriate.

- **Step 6: Check for contributing factors.**

The sixth step checks for contributing factors such as the following:

- Age (0 to 17 years) (>17 years)—DRG not age specific
- Sex (diagnosis is not sex specified)
- Discharge status (patient discharged "alive"): no separate DRG in this category for alive or deceased—N/A
- Presence or absence of severity conditions (none of the contributing diagnoses are considered MS-DRGs)—N/A
- Birth weight of neonates—N/A

The original assignment of DRG 14 is still appropriate. He coder must use all the skills he or she has developed in ICD-9-CM coding, procedural coding with Volume 3 of the ICD-9-CM (as well as Volumes 1 and 2), and DRG inpatient hospital coding.

A few inpatient coding exercises have been included in the Chapter Review Exercises to help the student work through the first inpatient exercises. If necessary, use Figure 20-1 to code step by step for the first DRG cases.

Outpatient Billing and Reimbursement Methods

Although some third-party carriers continue to reimburse outpatient hospital services on a line item basis, a large number of carriers have implemented the use of the **Ambulatory Payment Classification** (**APC**) method for the reimbursement of outpatient hospital services.

The APC was implemented in August 2000 in the hospital outpatient setting under the **Outpatient Prospective Payment System** (**OPPS**), following the model of DRG codes introduced decades before under a similar payment method. After successful implementation in this setting, the plan is to implement a similar reimbursement method in other settings, possibly including physician or provider services.

The APC system was originally based on diagnostic codes, resulting in the formulation of approximately 80 APC groups that cover every body system. After the formulation of the original ambulatory payment system groups, CMS determined that several inconsistencies existed within the system, and therefore the APC system was developed.

The primary objectives of the APC system are the following:

1. To simplify the outpatient hospital payment system
2. To ensure that payments adequately compensate hospital costs
3. To implement CMS' goals of deficit reduction

At this time, more than 700 APC groups are organized into four major categories: significant procedure APC, surgical services APC, ancillary services APC, and medical visits APC.

SIGNIFICANT PROCEDURE AMBULATORY PAYMENT CLASSIFICATION

Some procedures are considered significant and therefore should receive separate reimbursement. Examples include the following:

- Psychotherapy
- Dialysis
- Mammography
- Pulmonary tests
- Nuclear medicine
- Chemotherapy administration

SURGICAL SERVICES AMBULATORY PAYMENT CLASSIFICATION

This category includes major surgical procedures for which multiple-procedure payment reduction applies. This is similar to the current method of "reducing" the payment for multiple procedures because they are considered global, and only one procedure deserves global payment. Examples include the following:

- Arthroplasty
- Laparoscopy
- Cardiac catheterization
- Fracture treatment
- Endoscopy

ANCILLARY SERVICES AMBULATORY PAYMENT CLASSIFICATION

This group includes ancillary services for which a separate reimbursement should be made. Examples include the following:

- Radiology
- Electrocardiogram
- Immunization
- Infusion therapy (except chemotherapy)

MEDICAL VISIT AMBULATORY PAYMENT CLASSIFICATION

The assignment of a visit APC should be based on the location of service (e.g., emergency department or outpatient clinic only). Originally, the medical visit APC was to be based on diagnostic information as well as location of service. For simplicity, after the implementation of APCs in August 2000, the decision was made to assign these codes on the basis of only location and level of service.

CMS also allows levels of service to be assigned according to acuity levels. These acuity levels are facility determined; each facility may have different acuity levels for services performed. These levels may be assigned according to evaluation and management guidelines for levels of service, levels based on the complexity of the presenting problem or symptom, or levels designated on the basis of points assigned for the different facility resources expended in providing the visit. Currently CMS requires only that the levels are "distributive" between the five levels of services, namely 99281 through 99285 (e.g., emergency department visits), and that the facility is consistent in assigning these codes. CMS is expected to announce a more concrete standardized method of assigning these levels of service sometime in the future.

Critical care under OPPS is currently reimbursable only for the first hour.

NEW TECHNOLOGY AND PASS-THROUGH PAYMENTS

For new services that have not been assigned a current CPT code, temporary Healthcare Common Procedure Coding System (HCPCS) codes are assigned to allow reimbursement for new biologicals, new medications, and new technology devices that are above and beyond the usual scope of devices or drugs used in performing a service reimbursable under the OPPS reimbursement method. These items are typically priced significantly above the usual supplies required to provide a service. After their assignment of HCPCS codes, these items are reviewed on a regular basis for the possibility of a regular HCPCS or CPT code assignment.

GENERAL AMBULATORY PAYMENT CLASSIFICATION GUIDELINES

Not all services reimbursable under OPPS are also reimbursable under APC. Many services may be reimbursable only as an inpatient service or under another method other than APC or not reimbursable at all.

Payment status indicators are assigned to each CPT code to indicate how and whether the procedure performed will be reimbursed under the APC system of reimbursement or another payment method. Keep in mind that multiple CPT codes may be assigned for an encounter and may be considered reimbursable, although this is not the case with inpatient hospital coding.

The following are the most common payment status indicators:

A	Services paid under another method
C	Inpatient services not payable under APC method
E	Services not covered or allowed by Medicare program
F	Acquisition of corneal tissue
G	Current drug or biological pass-through
H	Device pass-through
J	New drug or biological pass-through
N	Incidental services, payment packaged into another APC service
P	Services paid only in partial hospitalization programs
S	Significant procedures with no reduction in multiple procedures
T	Surgical procedures with multiple procedure discount taken
V	Medical visits
X	Ancillary services payable under APC

TABLE 21-2 COMMON APC ASSIGNMENTS

ASSIGNMENT	CPT	APC
Outpatient Level 1/New	99201	0604
Outpatient Level 2/New	99202	0605
Outpatient Level 1/Established	99211	0604
Outpatient Level 2/Established	99212	0605
Emergency Room Level 1	99281	0609
Emergency Room Level 2	99282	0613
Outpatient Level 3/New	99203	0606
Outpatient Level 3/Established	99213	0605
Emergency Room Level 3	99283	0614
Outpatient Level 4/New	99204	0607
Outpatient Level 4/Established	99214	0606
Outpatient Level 5/New	99205	0608
Outpatient Level 5/Established	99215	0607
Emergency Room Level 4	99284	0615
Emergency Room Level 5	99285	0616
X-Ray, Ankle, AP and Lateral	73600	0260
X-Ray, Chest, PA and Lateral	71020	0260
X-Ray, Finger, 2 Views	73140	0260
X-Ray, Foot, AP and Lateral	73620	0260
X-Ray, Forearm, 2 V	73090	0260
X-Ray, Hand, 2 V	73120	0260
Electrocardiogram	93005	0099
Laceration Repair, Simple, Other Than Facial, <2.5 cm	12001	0024
IV Hydration, First Hour	90760	0440
IV Hydration, Ea Addtl Hour	90761	0437
IV Infusion, Ther/Diagnostic, First Hour	90765	0440
IV Infusion, Ther/Diagnostic, Each Addtl Hour	90766	0437
IM/SQ Injection	90772	0437

AP, Anteroposterior; *PA,* posteroanterior; *V,* views; *Ea Addtl,* each additional, *Ther,* therapeutic; *IM,* intramuscular; *SQ,* subcutaneous.

STEPS IN AMBULATORY PAYMENT CLASSIFICATION ASSIGNMENT PROCESS

Although the assignment of DRGs for inpatient and APCs for outpatient services is not made at the facility but at the time the services are submitted for payment to the third-party carrier, it is important for the facility to determine the appropriate assignment of DRG codes or APC assignments to determine appropriate reimbursement.

Table 21-2 lists the most common APC assignments for the coding scenarios contained in this text. This is not intended to be a complete listing because there is an APC assignment for every CPT and HCPCS code, and the list is extensive. The most current and complete listing of APC assignments can be found on the CMS Web site at www.cms.gov. The student may need to refer to that listing to complete some of the exercises contained in this text.

Determine appropriate coding and APC assignments for the following typical encounter in the outpatient facility (Figure 21-3). From the report the following can be determined:

Services:	ED visit
	X-ray, forearm
	Laceration repair, arm, 1.75 cm
Diagnoses:	Open wound, arm
	Automobile accident, driver, loss of control
Procedural:	X-ray, forearm
Services:	Laceration repair

Assign codes for the services/diagnoses outlined:

ICD-9-CM diagnostic code(s): ____________________

ICD-9-CM procedure code(s): ____________________

CPT code(s): ____________________

APC code(s) assignments: ____________________

EMERGENCY ROOM RECORD

Name:	Age:	ER physician:
	DOB:	
Allergies/type of reaction:	**Usual medications/dosages:**	

Triage/presenting complaint: Patient presents to the emergency room following a minor automobile accident in which the patient was the driver of a vehicle that lost control and hit a bridge abutment. Patient experiences an open wound to the arm, approximately 1.75 cm in length.

Initial assessment:

Time	T	P	R	BP	Other:				

Medication orders:

Lab work:

X-Ray:

Physician's report:

The patient is seen by the ER physician who evaluates the wound, x-rays the forearm, and sutures the wound and the patient is discharged for follow-up in 7–10 days.

Indicates:
Procedures/Services Diagnostic Statements

Diagnosis:	Physician sign/date
Discharge Transfer Admit Good Satisfactory Other:	

GODFREY REGIONAL HOSPITAL
123 Main Street • Aldon, FL 77714 • (407) 555-1234

FIGURE 21-3. Services performed on a patient in the emergency department, an outpatient hospital setting.

Chapter in Review

Certification Review

- Three different reimbursement methods exist for coding inpatient services.
- The fee for service reimbursement method reimburses all services necessary for treatment of the patient's condition or illness.
- The per diem method of reimbursement assigns a set rate per day for services, according to the level of service and the type of admission.
- The prospective payment system (PPS) reimbursement method uses the diagnosis-related group (DRG) system for determining appropriate reimbursement for services.
- The DRG method of reimbursement sets a reimbursement amount based on the patient's diagnosis and treatment during admission.
- Inpatient coding allows the coder to assign one principal diagnosis and up to eight additional diagnoses.
- When significant procedures are performed during the inpatient stay, Volume 3 of the ICD-9-CM is used for assigning an appropriate code.
- DRG code categories are based on patient age, sex, discharge status, presence or absence of comorbidities or complications, and birth weights of neonates.
- Outpatient reimbursement is based on Ambulatory Payment Classification (APC).
- Multiple APC assignments may be designated per encounter in the outpatient setting.

Student Assignments

- Study Chapter 21.
- Review the Learning Objectives for Chapter 21.
- Review the Certification Review for Chapter 21.
- Complete the Chapter Review exercise to reinforce concepts learned in this chapter.
- Complete the practice exercises on the companion Evolve site for reinforcement of inpatient and outpatient billing concepts.
- Complete the Practical Application exercise for real-life coding scenarios.
- Complete the Workbook exercises as assigned by your instructor, or individually for additional practice.

Chapter Review Exercise

Using the concepts discussed in this chapter, assign DRG codes or APC assignments as appropriate. It will be necessary to assign the appropriate diagnosis(es) and/or CPT code(s) to arrive at the correct DRG/APC for these facility encounters.

1. Chest pain, rule out MI, no procedures performed, inpatient
   APC/DRG assignment(s): ____________________
2. Angina, rule out MI, CABG performed, inpatient
   APC/DRG assignment(s): ____________________
3. Colonoscopy with snare polypectomy performed, outpatient
   APC/DRG assignment(s): ____________________
4. ER visit, level 4, chest X-ray, ECG for chest pain
   APC/DRG assignment(s): ____________________
   ____
5. Seizure disorder in 22-year-old with congestive heart failure. Admitted to 7 days, no surgical interventions
   APC/DRG assignment(s): ____________________
6. Patient presents to ER with urinary retention, diagnosed with UTI
   APC/DRG assignment(s): ____________________
7. 14-year-old with chronic tonsillitis presents for outpatient tonsillectomy with possible adenoidectomy. Tonsils were grasped and excised along with hypertrophic adenoidal tissue.
   APC/DRG assignment(s): ____________________
8. Patient admitted with fatigue, cough, and fever that has persisted for several weeks. CXR, culture demonstrates *E. coli* pneumonia. Treated with IV antibiotics and nebulizer treatments for 4 days and discharged on oral antibiotics on day 5.
   APC/DRG assignment(s): ____________________
9. Patient admitted with chest pain, SOB. MI ruled out. Repeat ECG, cardiac enzymes are normal, patient is discharged on the second day.
   APC/DRG assignment(s): ____________________
10. Patient presents with shortness of breath, history of COPD. Diagnosed with acute exacerbation of COPD, given steroids PO and nebulizer treatment and discharged from ED.
    APC/DRG assignment(s): ____________________

Practical Application

Apply DRG or APC codes for the following charts. Keep in mind that the number of lines provided for diagnoses and procedure codes is not necessarily indicative of the number needed. It is

necessary to determine the appropriate ICD-9-CM diagnostic codes, procedure codes, and CPT codes (when appropriate) before selecting the appropriate APC/DRG.

NOTE: A DRG guide or encoder may be needed to code some of the inpatient facility cases because they do not fall into the MDC categories listed as examples in this book.

1. History and physical

HISTORY AND PHYSICAL EXAMINATION

Godfrey Regional Hospital History & Physical
Admission:

HISTORY:
29-year-old gravida 0, para 0 woman with RUQ pain for several months. Pain was described as severe and sharp without radiation. The pain reoccurred and patient visited her PCP. A sonogram performed and gallstones were diagnosed.

The patient has had no pain over the past couple months after starting a no-fat diet. No history of jaundice, dark urine or difficult stools. No fever or chills.

Past medical history:

Unremarkable
Allergies: None

Family and social history

Social history: Patient does not smoke or take drugs. Does take an alcoholic drink occasionally
Family history: Unremarkable

Review of systems:

Negative

Physical exam

Physical examination reveals slight overweight female in no acute distress. Head, eyes, ears, nose and throat are normocephalic and atraumatic. Lungs are clear to auscultation. Breasts without masses. Rectal exam guaiac negative with no masses. Abdomen is soft and slightly tender to palpation in the right upper quadrant.

Laboratory/radiology:

X-ray:

Assessment:

RECOMMENDATION:
Patient admitted for further evaluation and possible cholecystectomy

Plan:

DICHARGE SUMMARY:
Patient was admitted and cholecystectomy was performed on day 2. The patient recovered satisfactorily without complications and was discharged on day 3 for follow-up in my office in 7-10 days.

Patrick Adams MD

GODFREY REGIONAL HOSPITAL
123 Main Street • Aldon, FL 77714 • (407) 555-1234

ICD-9-CM diagnostic code(s): ____________________

ICD-9-CM procedure code(s): ____________________

MDC assignment: ____________________

DRG assignment: ____________________

2. Discharge summary

DISCHARGE SUMMARY

Admitted:
Discharged:

Discharge diagnoses:

Admitting diagnosis: Fracture of right tibia, closed
Discharge diagnosis: Fracture of right tibia, closed
Operation: Closed reduction, internal fixation with Lottes nail, right tibia

History:

The patient was playing baseball on the day of admission. He was hit at second base and sustained an injury to his right leg with immediate pain and swelling. He was brought to the emergency room and diagnosed as having fractured his right tibia.

PHYSICAL EXAM: The fracture site was tender to palpation. He had good sensation and circulation to the leg, but marked swelling was present.

Laboratory and radiology studies:

X-RAYS: Multiple views of the tibia revealed a stairstep-type fracture at the distal portion of the middle third of the tibia.

Hospital course:

On the day of admission, the patient was taken to surgery and a Lottes nail was inserted to fix the fracture. The patient's postoperative course was essentially benign. He was placed in a long leg cast and gradually ambulated on crutches.

DISCHARGE PLAN:
The patient will remain on crutches for the next 6 weeks. At that time another set of x-rays will be taken to assess the progress of healing. The patient is to call the office if he experiences increased pain, swelling or duskiness of the toes.

Discharge Meds: Tylenol #3, one po q 4h, prn pain.

GODFREY REGIONAL HOSPITAL
123 Main Street • Aldon, FL 77714 • (407) 555-1234

ICD-9-CM diagnostic code(s): ____________________ MDC assignment: ____________________

ICD-9-CM procedure code(s): ____________________ DRG assignment: ____________________

3. Discharge summary

DISCHARGE SUMMARY

Admitted:
Discharged:

Discharge diagnoses:

History:

This is a 56-year-old female with a history of metastatic breast carcinoma since 1992 and of severe bone pain which has worsened recently. The patient presents now for insertion of a Mediport catheter.

Patient has history of polycystic kidney disease. Denies lung disease, myocardial Infarction, cardiovascular accident, diabetes or hypertension.

Patient has a long history of multiple chemotherapeutic regimens.

Past Surgery: Right modified radical mastectomy 1992

Allergies: None

Medications: Inderal 40 mg daily am, Capoten and Dilaudid

Social History: Nonsmoker, nondrinker and non IV drug abuser

PHYSICAL EXAM: Temperature 98.7, pulse 72, respirations 18, blood pressure 120/80
HEENT: Normal Lungs: Clear
Heart: Regular rhythm, S1 and S2
Chest: Mastectomy noted.
Abdomen: Soft, nontender, positive bowel sounds
Extremities: Edema 1+ in right upper extremity.
Neuro: Normal

Laboratory and radiology studies:

Laboratory Studies: Within normal limits

Hospital course:

Patient underwent central venous catheter placement with port without any complications. She also received three (3) units of packed red blood cells and was deemed stable for discharge on day two.

Adam Westy MD

GODFREY REGIONAL HOSPITAL
123 Main Street • Aldon, FL 77714 • (407) 555-1234

ICD-9-CM diagnostic code(s): ____________________ MDC assignment: ____________________

ICD-9-CM procedure code(s): ____________________ DRG assignment: ____________________

4. Discharge summary

DISCHARGE SUMMARY

Admitted:
Discharged:

Discharge diagnoses:

Postoperatively, the patient did well. She was discharged on day three to follow up in the surgery clinic. A bone scan, done while in the hospital, showed abnormal areas of increased activity in the thoracic spine. Tomograms of the sacroiliac region are recommended for further evaluation

History:

This 72-year-old female was admitted with left breast mass. She presented to the surgical clinic after she noted the mass several weeks ago. The patient consented to a lumpectomy and axillary lymph node dissection.

She is gravida VI, para VI, menarche age 15, first child at 28 years old. The patient used oral contraceptives for approximately 7 years in the past and is presently postmenopausal. She has no family history of breast cancer.

Past Medical/Surgical History:
Cholecystectomy In 1986, Hypertension, currently on Aldomet

PHYSICAL EXAMINATION:
Patient had a large, left upper outer quadrant breast mass as well as matted axillary lymph nodes. Breast mass measured approximately 3 × 4 as well as the axillary mass.

Laboratory and radiology studies:

Hospital course:

Patient was taken to operating room and had a lumpectomy. Frozen section revealed ductal carcinoma, and axillary dissection, which included axillary nodes, was positive for metastatic carcinoma.

Willem Obert MD

GODFREY REGIONAL HOSPITAL
123 Main Street • Aldon, FL 77714 • (407) 555-1234

ICD-9-CM diagnostic code(s): ____________________ MDC assignment: ____________________

ICD-9-CM procedure code(s): ____________________ DRG assignment: ____________________

5. Discharge summary

DISCHARGE SUMMARY

Admitted:
Discharged:

Discharge diagnoses:

History:

89-year-old male presented with abdominal pain, crampy and gradual in onset, for the previous 5 days. He denied nausea, vomiting, fever, or chills. He had multiple bowel movements for the 3 days prior to admission. Pain was not radiating.

PHYSICAL EXAM:
Temperature on admission was 98.0, pulse 102, respirations 18, blood pressure 120/70.

He had a softly distended abdomen, tender with minimal bowel sounds. Patient had a small hernia, obvious only when coughing and it was easily reducible. Stool was heme positive.

Laboratory and radiology studies:

WBC 13,700, hemoglobin 17.7, hematocrit 54.9, electrolytes normal and amylase 61

Hospital course:

Patient admitted with diagnosis of small bowel obstruction and NG tube was placed. He was kept NPO. X-rays showed feces through the large bowel in the midabdomen and two dilated loops of small bowel with probable air fluid levels.

The patient was hydrated with decompression. On repeat exam, there was no improvement. Taken to the OR and underwent exploratory laparotomy. Lysis of adhesions was performed. Patient was noted to have diverticulosis of the sigmoid and transverse colon.

An angiogram was performed and viability was questionable. Decision was made to take the patient back to the OR for an additional look. Exploration revealed a collection of fluid in the bowel and good pulsations.

Postoperative course was complicated by intermittent poor appetite and difficulty with bowel movements. Patient was finally discharged on day 17 to be followed up in the surgery clinic.

Patrick Adams MD

GODFREY REGIONAL HOSPITAL
123 Main Street • Aldon, FL 77714 • (407) 555-1234

ICD-9-CM diagnostic code(s): ____________________ MDC assignment: ____________________

ICD-9-CM procedure code(s): ____________________ DRG assignment: ____________________

6. Emergency department record

EMERGENCY ROOM RECORD

Name:	Age:	ER physician:
	DOB:	
Allergies/type of reaction:	**Usual medications/dosages:**	

Triage/presenting complaint:

Initial assessment:

Time	T	P	R	BP	Other:					

Medication orders:

Lab work:

X-ray:

X-ray shows a fracture of the 5th metacarpal bone, a small to moderate amount of displacement to that joint.

Physician's report:

SUBJECTIVE:
27-year-old male who comes to the ER after slipping and falling last night while walking down some stairs. He fell with his knuckles down on the stairs. He states it has been quite painful despite applying ice intermittently since the accident. He has not taken any medication but indicates this is one of the most painful things he has experienced. He has noticed quite a bit of swelling and bruising as well over the right hand.

OBJECTIVE:
Vital signs are stable, BP Is 100/80, temperature 97, pulse 72. Pain is currently 5 out of 10. On exam, there is a great deal of swelling of the region of the 4th and 5th metacarpal region of the right hand. There is pinpoint tenderness over the 5th metacarpal as well.

PLAN:
Patient placed in short arm spica cast of the right arm and hand. Advised to follow-up in two weeks to recheck.

Diagnosis:	**Physician sign/date**
ASSESSMENT: Fracture 5th metacarpal bone or Boxer's fracture	Robert Rai MD
Discharge Transfer Admit Good Satisfactory Other:	

GODFREY REGIONAL HOSPITAL
123 Main Street • Aldon, FL 77714 • (407) 555-1234

ICD-9-CM diagnostic code(s): ____________________

ICD-9-CM procedure code(s): ____________________

CPT code(s): ____________________

APC assignment(s): ____________________

7. Emergency department record

EMERGENCY ROOM RECORD

Name:	Age:	ER physician:
	DOB:	
Allergies/type of reaction:	Usual medications/dosages:	

Triage/presenting complaint:

Initial assessment:

Time	T	P	R	BP	Other:				

Medication orders:

Lab work:

X-ray:

Physician's report:

SUBJECTIVE:
34-year-old complaining of tooth pain. He does have a cavity that extends quite deep. He states it swells when it hurts. He has no fever or chills. Some nights it keeps him up. He has tried a number of tooth analgesics but none of them have helped. He currently has an appointment with the dentist in one week but just cannot take the pain.

Past Medical History: None

OBJECTIVE:
Vital signs normal, afebrile with temperature of 98.6

PHYSICAL EXAMINATION:
There is a cavity noted on one of the back molar teeth. No pus or green drainage are noted. There was moderate swelling noted on the left cheek in comparison to the right.

PLAN:
Place patient on Penicillin, 500 mg po tid for ten days. For pain, he was given IM Injection of Demorol 75 mg and Vistaril 25 mg. He was given Vicoden for pain prn until he sees the dentist.

Diagnosis:	Physician sign/date
ASSESSMENT: Tooth pain secondary to decay	Nancy Connolly MD
Discharge Transfer Admit Good Satisfactory Other:	

GODFREY REGIONAL HOSPITAL
123 Main Street • Aldon, FL 77714 • (407) 555-1234

ICD-9-CM diagnostic code(s): ______________________

ICD-9-CM procedure code(s): ______________________

CPT code(s): ______________________

APC Assignment(s): ______________________

8. Operative report

OPERATIVE REPORT

Patient information:

Patient name:
DOB:
MR#:

Date:
Surgeon:
Anesthetist:

Preoperative diagnosis:

Postoperative diagnosis:

Procedure(s) performed:

Screening Colonoscopy

Anesthesia:

Assistant surgeon:

Description of procedure:

After adequate sedation, the Olympus colonoscopy was introduced and passed into the rectal vault which clearly had residual stool. Following irrigation and further examination, it was apparent poor bowel prep would preclude us from completely the evaluation. There were certainly no large mass lesions however polypoid lesions could not be ruled out. At the level of the hepatic flexure, a large amount of stool was visualized and the procedure was aborted at this time. The colonoscope was withdrawn without complications.

Attempted colonoscopy aborted due to extremely poor bowel prep. Patient will require re-prep and possible barium enema given screening needed.

Adam Westgate MD

GODFREY REGIONAL HOSPITAL
123 Main Street • Aldon, FL 77714 • (407) 555-1234

ICD-9-CM diagnostic code(s): ____________________ CPT code(s): ____________________

ICD-9-CM procedure code(s): ____________________ APC assignment(s): ____________________

9. Operative report

OPERATIVE REPORT

Patient information:

Patient name:
DOB:
MR#:

Date:
Surgeon:
Anesthetist:

Preoperative diagnosis:

Carcinoma of right breast

Postoperative diagnosis:

Same

Procedure(s) performed:

Right lumpectomy with sentinel node dissection followed by complete axillary node dissection

Anesthesia:

Assistant surgeon:

Description of procedure:

Patient was preoperatively injected with Technetium 99 in the right subareolar area. Incision was made at the right axilla at the lower hairline between pectoralis major and the latissimus dorsi muscle. We extended the incision in the axilla towards the chest wall. A large blue and hot node was found against the chest wall, medial to the edge of the pectoralis major muscle. We used the cutting current of the Bovie to dissect the node. This node was submitted as a sentinel node for further evaluation.

While we awaited the results of the sentinel node biopsy, we started a lumpectomy which was done using an elliptical transverse incision in the upper breast. We extended the dissection towards the chest wall and then posteriorly we included the pectoralis major muscle fascia.

The axillary dissection was carried out starting at the distal axilla and going upwards in between the long thoracic nerve and thoracodorasal nerve.

The wound was irrigated, hemostasis was obtained and the wound was closed.

Rachel Perez MD

GODFREY REGIONAL HOSPITAL
123 Main Street • Aldon, FL 77714 • (407) 555-1234

ICD-9-CM diagnostic code(s): ____________________

ICD-9-CM procedure code(s): ____________________

CPT code(s): ____________________

APC assignment(s): ____________________

10. Operative report

OPERATIVE REPORT

Patient information:	
Patient name: DOB: MR#:	Date: Surgeon: Anesthetist:

Preoperative diagnosis:

Malignant melanoma of chest

Postoperative diagnosis:

Malignant melanoma of chest

Procedure(s) performed:

Wide excision of malig melanoma chest
Complex closure

Anesthesia:

Assistant surgeon:

Description of procedure:

Chest was prepped and draped in the standard surgical manner. Skin was incised in an elliptical manner around the melanoma taking 2 cm of margin in all directions. Full thickness of skin was excised. The skin was then closed with deep fascial layer taking the pectoralis fascia on both sides, a subcutaneous layer of Interrupted Vicryl and then a running 4-0 Monocryl subcuticular suture layer.

Adam Westgy MD

GODFREY REGIONAL HOSPITAL
123 Main Street • Aldon, FL 77714 • (407) 555-1234

ICD-9-CM diagnostic code(s): ____________________

ICD-9-CM procedure code(s): ____________________

CPT code(s): ____________________

APC assignment(s): ____________________

SECTION 6

Monitoring, Compliance, Certification, and Career Development

Monitoring and compliance of the coding process is perhaps the culmination of successful coding. Coding begins and ends with documentation, so it is appropriate to end this text with a reemphasis on the importance of documentation in the coding process. The coder must understand the coding systems and their differences from a third-party carrier perspective and must ensure that all coding processes have been completely successful. A comprehensive monitoring process ensures compliance and decreases a facility's risk of accusations of fraudulent activity.

Section 6 encompasses legislation regarding fraud and abuse as well as processes that ensure compliance. The student will have the opportunity to complete a chart audit and prepare a report of those findings. This section also includes review information for the coding certification examination. Reviews of medical terminology and sample coding questions provide the opportunity for certification examination preparation. ■

22

Monitoring and Compliance Process

LEARNING OBJECTIVES

After completing this chapter, the student will be able to:

- Define, identify, and compare fraud and abuse.
- Know the implications of fraudulent or abusive activities.
- Understand the mechanisms of the practice monitoring process.
- Describe the steps to follow when completing a chart audit.
- Comprehend the importance of a compliance program.
- Identify the events that typically trigger a third-party audit.
- Apply coding concepts to practical coding and compliance scenarios.

CODING REFERENCE TOOLS

Tool 22-1
Data Entry Review Form

Tool 22-2
Claims Review Process

Tool 22-3
Chart Audit Logsheet

Tool 22-4
Chart Audit: E & M Worksheet

Tool 22-5
Practice Protocol Logsheet

KEY TERMS

Abuse

Compliance Programs

False Claims Act

Fraud

Health Insurance Portability and Accountability Act (HIPAA)

The Joint Commission

Line Item

Manual Review and Flag

Office of the Inspector General (OIG)

Qui Tam Provision

Whistleblower Protection Act

Fraud and Abuse Legislation

Many practices do not employ a full-time coder. Instead, they rely on office staff or the provider(s) to determine levels of service provided. This typically subjects the practice to reduced reimbursement and substantially increases the potential for fraud and abuse.

A number of years ago the federal government investigated only a small number of these practices and facilities for potential fraud and abuse. In most cases the practice or facility was unaware of potentially fraudulent activity, either because of ignorance or as a result of inadequate involvement in the billing and coding process.

Increased legislation over the past several years, however, has made all individuals involved in the coding and billing process potentially liable for fraudulent billing activity. In addition, the "ignorance excuse" is no longer a defense with federal or third-party carriers. Fraud and abuse are widespread in the health care industry today, and virtually all third-party carriers have increased resources devoted to recovering monies paid for fraudulent claims.

Fines, penalties, and potential imprisonment can be the outcome of fraudulent activity in the health care industry today. These punishments may be imposed on any individual involved in the fraudulent activity and any individual who is aware of a potentially fraudulent activity but does not take action. This could even include the office receptionist if he or she were aware of inappropriate billing practices.

The Centers for Medicare & Medicaid Services (CMS) and the **Office of the Inspector General (OIG)** have the authority to suspend, exclude, terminate, and impose fines and penalties on providers, practitioners, and suppliers who commit acts in direct violation of one of the many antifraud and antiabuse amendments enacted since the mid-1970s. Penalties may involve fines, imprisonment, and exclusion from the Medicare program on a permanent basis.

The OIG annually publishes and distributes a "Work Plan for the Fiscal Year," with 100 items targeted for review for potential fraud and abuse. Many of the items discussed in this text have been targeted on an annual basis since the inception of this list because of the inability of providers to comply with government regulations for documentation and coding guidelines. Both evaluation and management (E & M) levels of service and documented medical necessity have remained top items on this list as a direct result of completed audits in which physicians have been unable to comply with E & M guidelines as well as physician charts lacking diagnostic documentation to substantiate services performed and billed.

There have been many newspaper articles regarding large facilities that were fined millions of dollars for services billed and not provided. In reality, many of these services were performed. Documentation did not, however, substantiate those services. In these circumstances the government had the authority to penalize the facility with fines and, in some cases, imprisonment of high-level employees.

Following are some of the major legislative actions and amendments passed in response to the rising practice of fraud and abuse in the United States.

MEDICARE-MEDICAID ANTI-FRAUD AND ABUSE AMENDMENTS

Anyone who knowingly and willfully makes or causes another to make false statements regarding services performed is guilty of a felony and may be fined up to $25,000, imprisoned for up to 5 years, or both. These amendments apply to beneficiaries who commit such an act, punishable by a fine of up to $20,000, imprisonment for up to 1 year, or both.

AMENDMENT TO MEDICARE-MEDICAID ANTI-FRAUD AND ABUSE AMENDMENTS

This addition to the amendments states that any person who knowingly and willfully solicits or receives payment or remuneration, such as a kickback, bribe, or rebate, is guilty of a felony with fines up to $25,000, imprisonment for up to 5 years, or both.

MEDICARE AND MEDICAID PATIENT AND PROGRAM PROTECTION ACT AND FALSE CLAIMS ACT AMENDMENTS

The Medicare and Medicaid Patient and Program Protection Act provides authority to impose civil monetary penalties under Section 1128A of the Social Security Act for the following:

- Fraudulent or false claims presented for payment
- Fraudulent or false records used to file a claim
- False or fraudulent claims paid as a result of conspiracy to defraud the government

The penalties under the **False Claims Act** call for fines of $5000 to $10,000 per false claim, plus damages up to three times the total amount of false payments. Under this act the government is not required to prove specific intent to defraud. The civil standard of proof under this act is "by the preponderance of evidence," not the criminal criterion of "beyond a reasonable doubt." Actions under the False Claims Act may be taken within 6 years of the violation or within 3 years of the date when material facts are known. The time may not extend past a 10-year period after the violation.

False Claim Act cases may be initiated either by the Department of Justice or private citizens under the **qui tam provision** of the **Whistleblower Protection Act** of 1989. Under this provision private citizens are entitled to a percentage of monies recovered from the fraudulent activities.

ADDITIONAL COMPLIANCE LEGISLATION: STARK LAW, ANTIKICKBACK STATUTE, AND SELF-REFERRAL LAWS

Under more recent legislation, the federal government has dictated that it is illegal to knowingly and willfully solicit payment in return for referrals, purchasing, leasing, or arranging for the purchasing of referrals, purchasing, or leasing. A physician or other entity may not refer to an individual with which the physician or any immediate member of his or her family has a financial relationship. There is an extensive list of exceptions. Some common areas included under the antikickback and self-referral mandates include clinical laboratory services, occupational and physical therapy, radiology services, durable medical equipment, and home health services. Under the self-referral guidelines of the Stark Law, the physician who has a financial relationship with an entity may only refer to that entity with the express permission and consent of the patient.

Many other legislative amendments and orders address the prosecution of fraudulent activities. The coder must remain current on legislative amendments and proposals in this arena. The coder must understand what constitutes fraud and abuse as well as what can be done to comply with governmental and third-party guidelines.

As a result of the increased investigative efforts of governmental and third-party agencies against potential fraud and abuse, the field of compliance within the health care industry has grown immensely. The coder must be aware of the need for compliance and understand the processes in place to ensure such compliance at his or her practice or facility.

The coder and other office staff should understand the definitions of fraud and abuse. They also must be aware of the consequences when such activities take place within the practice.

Fraud and Abuse

Specific federal guidelines exist regarding the definitions of **fraud** and **abuse**. As previously mentioned, ignorance of such activities in a particular practice or facility is no longer a legitimate defense. Typically, most practices first insist that no such events occur within their organizations. However, after review, they realize that fraud and abuse may be taking place. Keep in mind that the definitions of fraud and abuse may differ from one third-party carrier to another. Therefore the practice or facility should have such information accessible for each contract in which it participates.

FRAUD

Fraud is a felony punishable by imprisonment, fines, and interest for all parties involved or for those who have knowledge that such acts have taken place. Fraud is defined as follows.

Making false statements or misrepresentation of facts on claims. This may occur in the form of incorrect information submitted on the claim form or submission to the carrier in error of services that were not performed (e.g., urinalysis was ordered by physician, was unable to be completed, yet was billed to third-party carrier).

Having knowledge that false statements or representation was made with the intent to gain a greater amount than due or to receive payment when none is due. This involves filing claims for services that are noncovered in a manner that may make them payable or submitting a diagnosis code in such a way as to make a noncovered service a payable service. Whether this practice is initiated by the provider or at a patient's request (e.g., having knowledge that the practice or facility changes diagnoses or dates of services at the request of patients so charges will be covered by their carriers) does not change the fact that it constitutes fraud.

Receiving benefits on behalf of one person and putting them to use other than for the benefit of that person. Prescribing a piece of durable medical equipment or another item for a Medicare recipient when that item will be used by the spouse, who may not be covered, constitutes fraud—whether it is an oversight by the provider or is at the patient's request.

Presenting a bill for medical items or services while knowing or having reason to know that the claim is false or fraudulent. Because ignorance is no longer a defense, if an individual has a reason to know that a claim is false, such as the facility does not provide the service or medical item—and perhaps does not stock a specific item that is being billed—the individual involved in the billing and the others who had knowledge that this item could not be billed are liable.

Presenting a claim on behalf of a person excluded from the Medicare or Medicaid program. It is the responsibility of the billing entity to know which providers or facilities have been excluded from the Medicare or Medicaid program and to submit no billing on their behalf. This information is readily available at http://www.medicare.gov.

Presenting claims of physician services under a provider number other than that physician's provider number or an appropriate group provider number. If a practice bills for services not provided by that specific practice, then this act is also fraud. In the past it was acceptable for a practice to enter into arrangements in which it would bill for the services of another provider in exchange for a billing fee. Federal laws have been passed since that time prohibiting billing for any services not provided by the billing entity.

Presenting a claim for physician services when the person who provided or supervised the services was not an appropriately licensed physician or when the physician was misrepresented as being specialty certified when he or she was not. This most commonly occurs when a physician extender (e.g., nurse practitioner, physician assistant) provides a service without meeting the guidelines under the

Medicare program for proper supervision by the supervising physician.

Providing items or services and soliciting, offering, or receiving kickbacks, bribes, or rebates of a fee. An entity receiving any financial incentive for services referred or received meets the definition of fraud as defined by federal guidelines.

ABUSE

Abuse is a misdemeanor punishable by fines, interest, jail time, or all three. Abuse is defined as follows.

Overuse of medical and health services. This occurs when more than the services usually necessary are ordered, such as unnecessary "rechecks." Again, the coder sees the need for medical documentation of the medical necessity. If this documentation is included, the definition of abuse has not been met.

Billing excessive charges for services or supplies. This refers to billing for services or supplies in excess of fair market value plus the cost of administration. The practice should establish a charge formula for supplies and medications that is part of the organization's compliance manual as well as the policies and procedures manual. This formula should establish the method used for determining both practice or facility fees for these services and the percentage of increase justified by the costs for stocking supplies, spoilage, and so forth.

Filing claims for services deemed "not medically necessary" or, if medically necessary, not to the extent rendered. This includes excessive office visits or ancillary services not justified by medical documentation as medically necessary and repeat procedures for which no justification or documentation exists regarding the need to repeat.

Breaching assignment agreements, resulting in the beneficiary being billed for amounts disallowed by the carrier on the basis that such charges exceed "reasonable charge" criteria. This may occur as the result of contractuals not being properly taken at the time the Medicare Explanation of Benefits is received. This may be an oversight; however, as previously discussed, ignorance is not a defense in fraud and abuse cases. There is an obvious need for the individual responsible for posting payments to understand the coding concepts and the contractual obligations of the third party and the practice so that a breach of assignment agreement does not take place.

Using a separate schedule of charges for Medicare charges that is higher than non-Medicare charges. Medicare legislation prohibits the use of multiple-tier fee schedules. In other words, Medicare law prohibits non-Medicare patients from receiving services for less than a Medicare patient. The practice should make certain not to offer self-pay discounts to patients at the time of service that are lower than those allowed by Medicare. Practice policy and procedure should dictate that no discounts can be quoted or given at the time of service. Any discounts to be offered should be given after the patient's financial agreement is completed (i.e., the patient pays the agreed-on portion).

Exceeding the limiting charge imposed on nonparticipating providers for specific services. In the event the practice is "nonparticipating" with Medicare, it may not collect from a patient more than 115% of the limiting nonparticipating allowance. (This is stated in the yearly Medicare Fee Allowance information, which is available from the carrier or on its Web site.)

Using improper billing practices, including submission of bills to Medicare instead of third-party payers that are primary insurers for Medicare beneficiaries. When Medicare beneficiaries have other primary insurance or insurance that is responsible for services (e.g., workers' compensation, liability or auto insurance, or other primary insurance under the "Working Aged"), the provider or practice must bill that insurance carrier or payer first. The practice or provider is expected to determine the other third-party coverage and bill the appropriate primary insurance carrier for services. Attempting to bill or collect from Medicare when other coverage should be primary is considered abuse.

Ordering procedures or services more frequently than good standard medical practice allows. Documentation of medical necessity would eliminate any accusations of abuse because the services would be documented as justified. All ancillary services ordered should include documentation of both an ordering physician and medical necessity.

Ordering a battery of diagnostic tests when diagnosis indicates the need for only a few tests. When medical documentation supports the need for a specific test as opposed to a number of ancillary tests performed, investigation of abuse would be appropriate. This definition of abuse came about as the result of physicians and providers who would automatically order specific "screening" tests on the basis of a patient's age, sex, and presenting complaint without determining which tests were, in fact, medically necessary for that particular patient. Many times these tests were ordered and performed before the patient was even seen by the physician or provider. As long as the medical necessity for each ordered test can be substantiated from the medical documentation, this will not be an issue for the practice.

Some additional facts about determination and prosecution of fraudulent or abusive practices should be considered, as discussed in the following paragraphs.

IMPORTANT CONSIDERATIONS REGARDING FRAUD AND ABUSE

Fraud and abuse are punishable regardless of intent. Even when a provider or practice commits fraudulent acts in error, charges may still result. In most instances, when a practice or provider has been found responsible for fraudulent billing, the OIG, as part of the audit process, requires that entity to implement a compliance program in the event that one has not already been put into place.

Ignorance is no longer a defense for fraud or abuse. Ignorance, or the lack of knowing what constitutes fraud or abuse, or the oversight that fraudulent or abusive activities are taking place in the practice is no longer a defense.

All parties who have knowledge of fraudulent or abusive activity are punishable. This includes any staff member who is party to, participates in, or should be aware of the occurrence or potential occurrence of fraudulent or abusive activity. Billers, coders, clerical and administrative staff, physicians, and owners can all be liable. No one is exempt if his or her responsibilities involve the billing or coding and reimbursement process within the practice. For this reason liability insurance is now available for these individuals. Certified coders are particularly vulnerable in a fraudulent situation because they are considered experts. The coder should be involved in the reimbursement and coding process and should be able to determine whether these types of activities are taking place.

Fraud and abuse are charged by the line item. The assessment for fraudulent and abusive activity is charged on the basis of each line item, averaging between $3000 and $10,000 per line. The third party auditing the practice has the right to perform an audit of additional items and to determine percentage of error based on the sampling. The number of fraudulent or abusive claims will be determined according to the error percentage. This number will be charged the $3000 to $10,000 line item fine.

A **line item** represents one "line" of the claim form. For instance, if the claim form lists five "lines" or five CPT codes on a given claim, this represents five line items, and each fraudulent line item would be assessed.

The practice, provider, or facility has the responsibility of challenging and disproving any error percentage of fraudulent or abusive activity through the appeal and legal processes. If the practice believes that the representative sampling chosen by the third-party carrier is erroneous, it has the responsibility to gather the data to disprove the finding. This typically will involve much research on the part of the practice, often requiring the employment of a consulting firm to gather the facts. In addition, the practice may need to employ legal representation to contest the charges. Even in the event that no fraud or abuse is proven, the financial effect of challenging these charges is astronomical.

Medicare and other third-party carriers have the right to exclude physicians or providers from their programs as the result of fraudulent or abusive activity. When fraudulent activity is confirmed, the third-party carrier may exclude the billing entity, which may be the physician, the group provider, or the facility. This means the practice or facility must notify many of its patients that it no longer participates and cannot continue to treat them. This, of course, will have a significant financial impact on the entity as well. In addition, many third-party carriers now communicate this information through a network to other third-party carriers who may choose to disqualify the provider or practice from their programs.

The third-party carrier may place the practice or provider on "manual review" for an indeterminate amount of time. Medicare refers to this process as "flagging" the physician. Third-party carriers often require that all claims for a provider or practice found guilty of fraudulent or abusive activity must undergo a **manual review and flag** process. This includes all claims, even those that typically would be processed automatically. Unfortunately, most third-party carriers do not set a time limit for this process, and the third-party carrier is left to determine when the provider or practice will be reviewed and the flag possibly removed.

Providers or practices have sometimes stayed in the flagged status for years before the carrier returned them to their previous status. Obviously, the financial impact of this status is overwhelming because no claims will be paid for approximately 60 to 90 days, the time required to manually review all claims. If the third-party carrier represents a large portion of the practice's patient population, the loss of revenue for this carrier for a 90-day period will be significant.

Financial impact to the practice or provider is significant regardless of the findings. The financial impact from a fraud or abuse investigation is monumental, even to large practices. In addition to the potential loss from fines, penalties, and possible imprisonment, the practice typically must hire legal representation and health care consultants to assist in defense of the allegations. If the practice or provider survives the financial penalties imposed, additional financial impact will result if the carrier decides to impose the manual review process on all claims submitted by the practice or provider.

Therefore it is in the best interest of the practice to identify any activities that might be construed as fraudulent and to act on them immediately. The coder is probably vulnerable and is in a good position to identify any such activity.

STEPS FOR REPORTING FRAUD AND ABUSE

If the coder identifies activities he or she believes to be fraudulent, the following steps should be taken.

Report the information to the direct supervisor. Initially this may be done verbally; however, if no action seems forthcoming, the coder should document his or her concern in writing.

Notify the carrier about any error and be willing to correct the error. Determine the extent of the error and the financial impact. Prepare a response to the carrier, including identification of the error(s), the explanation of benefits for each error, and a check in the total amount of the error(s) made. Send the detailed information to the carrier with a certified return receipt.

In many instances the carrier will respond by returning the check; however, if the carrier wants to prosecute at a later time, the legal system probably will not find the practice or provider guilty of any intent and the financial impact will be significantly less.

Keep in mind that if the carrier identifies the potential fraud or abuse before the practice or provider does, the practice and anyone who was aware of the issues can be held accountable.

Request a response in writing from the supervisor. Indicate a willingness to help prepare a response to the carrier. Insist on receiving a written response from the supervisor. If the immediate supervisor does not respond, put any concerns in writing to the administrator, CEO, or CFO and ask to receive a response in writing.

Contact the compliance officer or director. If the practice has a compliance officer, make certain that the individual is informed. Do not rely on the direct supervisor or the administrator to inform the compliance officer.

Make certain the practice owners or physicians are aware of the information. Do not rely on others to inform all responsible parties.

Contact the practice attorney or legal representative if no action is taken by those previously contacted. Document all contacts concerning the issue, requests for response, and subsequent findings. In the event the practice is investigated for fraud or abuse, any actions that have been taken in notifying the practice of the situation will need to be defended.

Use the "whistleblower" program to anonymously report fraud and abuse. Most third-party carriers have a program for offering information regarding suspected fraud or abuse activities. Many of these programs offer an incentive to the individual who reports the activity in an effort to encourage reporting.

If coding ethics are significantly compromised, discuss whether resignation is necessary. Make certain that all entities that have been contacted previously are informed by *you, the coder,* about the decision. Address why it is necessary to consider resignation and what actions should be taken to correct the problems within the practice.

The coder will want to maintain copies of all correspondence sent to practice supervisors, administrators, legal representatives, and any other individuals. If the carrier decides to prosecute the practice or provider, the coder may need the written documentation to prove to the carrier that he or she attempted to resolve the problem without success. Fraudulent and abusive activities will have a profound effect on the coder as well as the provider and the practice.

The remainder of this chapter is dedicated to monitoring processes that may identify or eliminate any fraudulent or abusive activity or accusations of such activity. The implementation of these processes may save the practice from fraudulent and abusive activities. Alternatively, the use of such processes may prove to the third-party carrier that the errors were without intent, and the resulting penalties may be less extensive. In addition, these monitoring processes ensure maximum revenue coding and ensure that the practice is cognizant of reimbursement for all services rendered. This is extremely important in the health care industry because third-party carriers continue to reimburse less and less.

Monitoring Processes

In the section on coding from a reimbursement perspective, the importance of monitoring is briefly discussed. The coder will find that his or her involvement in the monitoring process is imperative to ensure the correctness of documents and their appropriate preparation for third-party carriers.

Many coders believe their responsibilities begin at the point at which codes are assigned to services and diagnoses; however, the importance of everyone's participation in the coding process has been demonstrated. Also demonstrated is the importance of the physician's documentation and the information gathered from the charge documents by other clerical and clinical staff in the office. The monitoring process for the coder involves the following elements.

DATA ENTRY PROCESS AND MONITORING TECHNIQUES

From the moment the data enter the practice's computerized billing system, the accuracy of information determines the number of clean claims the practice will send to third-party carriers. The clean claim process has already been discussed, along with the delays or denials that occur as a result of what might seem small and insignificant oversights.

The data entry personnel in the practice typically are not educated as coders, so the coding staff will need to teach data entry personnel and provide them with educational reference tools for correctly entering data. Many of these "tools" can be built into the computerized billing system by programming; other issues must be manually identified by data entry personnel.

Most computerized billing systems have much potential for gathering the correct information for specific services. Critical data, such as referring physician names and national provider identification numbers (NPIs) for consultations, may be preloaded into the computer. The billing system may then be programmed to require a referring physician name when any CPT code identified as a "consultation" is entered. Many such safety catches can be preprogrammed into the computer system to help data entry and other personnel successfully enter data for a clean claim.

The coder should work with the systems administrator or information specialist in the practice and identify which of the following options are available for use in the practice's computerized billing system. Use as many of these as possible; they will prevent unneeded errors and delays in reimbursement.

"Macro Codes" for Multiple Services Performed Together

When the provision of a surgical service always allows for a special supply item to be billed in addition to the service, these may be entered into many billing systems with one code, which will actually print the two or more codes necessary to completely describe and bill the services performed. For example, when performing colonoscopy, the physician may bill the services for the colonoscopy as well as the provision of a surgical tray. Rather than leaving the entry of two procedure codes to data entry personnel, allowing the possibility that one will be overlooked, most billing systems are capable of building a "macro" code. This is similar to a mechanism in word processing software—when one particular word or phrase is entered, a standardized group of words appears. In this instance, for the colonoscopy service and surgical tray, the macro will be entitled COLON. When the data entry personnel enter the procedure code COLON, the system will automatically enter two charges, one for the colonoscopy and one for the surgical tray, thus eliminating the possibility of oversight.

Macro codes may also be useful for injections that require a code for the administration as well as the medication itself.

Multiple Units

Another error that commonly occurs when data entry personnel enter charges is multiple units of service. Typically, either the computerized billing system does not ask for number of units, or the data entry operator is not familiar with the service and does not realize that multiple units of service may occur for a particular code.

Modifier Code Usage

When modifier codes are necessary for certain procedures, the computerized billing system can be used to enter these codes with their respective modifier codes; it can also offer a selection of modifier codes on charge documents.

A frequent review of the charges entered into the computerized billing system will reflect whether services are being entered as intended or if errors are being made that may implicate the practice for fraud or abuse.

A data entry audit process should be a part of the facility or practice review plan for compliance. Tool 22-1 provides guidelines for completing a data entry audit. Specified guidelines for performing this data entry audit process should be incorporated into the policy and procedures manual or compliance plan. Set time intervals for performing this review should be defined in this documentation as well, along with a log recording the performance of this function.

CLAIMS REVIEW PROCESS

The coder should also be directly involved in the claims review process. After completion of the charge document and data entry, **all claims should be reviewed electronically and on paper before they are forwarded to the third-party carrier(s).**

The "clean claim" process and its importance in receiving proper reimbursement on a timely basis have been discussed. Errors that have occurred up to the point the claim is generated should be detected before mailing. Keep in mind that many of the staff involved in the recording of these charges and subsequent claims are not coders and therefore may not realize that coding errors have occurred.

Electronic claims may also be reviewed before transmission by an audit trail programmed into the computerized billing system or by the generation of a claims worksheet or similar report of each claim as it will be transmitted to the carrier.

Claims may be reviewed by noncoding personnel for the most common errors, such as incomplete insurance information, incorrect identification numbers, and relationship discrepancies.

Coding information that should be reviewed includes the following:

- CPT codes that require a modifier
- ICD-9-CM codes matched correctly to the appropriate CPT codes
- CPT codes requiring specific ICD-9-CM diagnostic codes
- High-level procedures requiring specialized diagnostic codes

The practice may wish to develop some type of "model claim" for use when reviewing claim forms. If the practice deals with a carrier that has unusual guidelines specific to that carrier only, it may wish to develop a separate model claim for that carrier.

One suggestion for doing this is to make an overhead transparency of a blank CMS insurance claim form and mark fields that must be completed by highlighting or other designation. Mark fields requiring specialized information, using notations such as "correct number of digits" or "leave blank." This transparency may then be placed over paper claims for this specific carrier for review of completeness.

When errors are encountered the problem can be identified and the root corrected, and not only for that specific claim. For instance, if a specific diagnosis code requires five digits and the claim has a code with only four, identify the origin of the problem in the computerized billing system and correct it—but not just for that specific claim. This will eliminate that error in the future and prevent the chance that the error will not be captured on subsequent claims.

If errors occur as the result of data entry mistakes, the individual responsible for those errors should be notified and retrained appropriately so the errors do not occur in the future.

Errors may also occur as the result of misprints or mistakes on the charge documents. These must be corrected immediately by reprinting the document or, if necessary, making a temporary correction in the computerized billing system that takes out the wrong code and directs the system to print the correct code until reprinting of the charge document occurs.

Most importantly, when errors are encountered during the claims review process, they should be recorded over time for review. During the month-end process, these categories of errors can be totaled and reviewed and the appropriate action

TOOL 22-1

DATA ENTRY REVIEW FORM

DATE: ____________		DATA ENTRY REVIEW FORM				PRACTICE NAME: ____________		
OPERATOR	DATE OF SERVICE	PHYSICIAN/ PROVIDER	PATIENT NAME	CHT# PT#	LINE ITEM SUBMITTED	LINE ITEM KEYED	EXPLANATION	CALCULATION +/–
Page______ of ________							TOTAL	

taken to avoid them in the future. This process should be incorporated into the policy and procedures manual or compliance plan, with set time intervals for performance established. Tool 22-2 shows a sample claims review form.

CODING AND CHART REVIEW PROCESS

Whether charges are coded by a practice coder or a physician or are determined by other office staff, all coding should be reviewed on a regular basis. Many practices and facilities, especially smaller ones, do not employ a full-time coder and instead depend on other office staff or the physician(s) to select the proper codes for billing and reimbursement. Coding must be reviewed on a regular basis by the practice coder or an outside coder or coding group. Chart audits or reviews should be conducted by the practice, both internally and by an external source, to ascertain whether appropriate coding protocols are being followed. If a compliance program is in

TOOL 22-2

CLAIMS REVIEW PROCESS

DATE: ______________________

CLAIMS PROCESSED	# CLAIMS	$ BILLED	COMMENTS
ELECTRONIC			
Medicare			
Commercial			
TOTALS			
PAPER			
Medicare			
Medicaid			
Commercial			
TOTALS			
GRAND TOTAL			

BILLING ERRORS	# CLAIMS	$ BILLED	COMMENTS
REGISTRATION			
ID#			
Wrong Insurance			
Other			
TOTALS			
CHARGE DOCUMENT			
Referring Physician			
Other			
Auth #			
TOTALS			
CODING			
Diagnosis			
Procedure Code			
Place of Service			
Other			
TOTALS			
OTHER (Specify):			
TOTALS			
GRAND TOTAL			

Completed by:______________________ Date:____________________

place for the practice, the chart audit should also determine whether compliance guidelines are being followed. In the event of a third-party audit, if the practice has a compliance program in place the third party will want to determine whether that compliance plan is being followed (discussed later in this chapter).

Tools 22-3 and 22-4 show examples of typical chart audit forms. These forms may vary according to services typically performed in the practice but should include evaluation and management, surgical procedure review, and medical documentation review.

The need for the chart review process has already been discussed. The primary purpose is to review and recommend enhancements to medical record documentation to prevent third-party audit; to identify undercoding and overcoding; and to detect documentation deficiencies that may result in

TOOL 22-3

CHART AUDIT LOGSHEET

DATE: ________		CHART AUDIT LOGSHEET				PRACTICE: ________			
DATE OF SERVICE	PHYSICIAN/ PROVIDER	PT NAME	CHARTS PT#	CODE SUBMITTED	CODE REVIEW	CHANGE		REASON	CALCULATION +/–
						UP	DOWN		
Page _______ of____								TOTAL	

TOOL 22-4

CHART AUDIT: E & M WORKSHEET

Patient:____________________ Date of Service:____________________

Location of Service:	Off/Output ☐	Off/Consult ☐	ER ☐	Prev Med ☐
	Init/Hosp ☐	Sub Hosp ☐	Discharge ☐	
	Init NH ☐	Sub NH ☐		
Patient Status:	New ☐	Established ☐		
Referring Physician:	Yes ☐	No ☐		

HISTORY

Problem Focused	☐ Chief complaint; brief history of problem
Expanded Problem Focused	☐ + Problem pertinent system review
Detailed	☐ CC; extended history; extended ROS; pertinent PMH/FH/SH
Comprehensive	☐ CC; extended history; complete ROS; complete PMH/FH/SH

EXAM

Problem Focused	☐ Affected body area or organ system
Expanded Problem Focused	☐ + other related systems
Detailed	☐ Extended exam of affected/extended body area/organ system
Comprehensive	☐ Complete single system specialty exam/complete multisystem exam

MEDICAL DECISION MAKING Elements	A	B	C	D
Number of diagnosis and management options	Minimal	Limited	Multiple	Extensive
Amount/complexity of data reviewed	Minimal	Limited	Multiple	Extensive
Risk complications/morbidity/mortality	Minimal	Low	Moderate	High

Straightforward	☐ 2/3 Column A elements met
Low Complexity	☐ 2/3 Column B elements met
Moderate Complexity	☐ 2/3 Column C elements met
High Complexity	☐ 2/3 Column D elements met

TIME Only if >50% of face-to-face time with patient in counseling/coordination of care
Total time documented:____________

E & M code assigned:____________________ ICD-9-CM code assigned:____________
Recommendations:____

Reviewer:____________________ Date:____________________

third-party targeting for audit, disciplinary action by third parties, or legal action from a fraud, abuse, or liability standpoint.

What Should Be Included in the Chart Audit

A representative sampling of the chart activity for the practice should be included in the audit. If multiple physicians belong to the practice, a representative sampling for each provider, including any physician extenders (e.g., physician assistants, nurse practitioners), should be completed. There is no specific formula for identifying the number of charts that should be reviewed; however, the volume for each provider should be proportionate to the volume or percentage of patients each provider sees. At a minimum, the number of patients seen in a typical day per physician should be pulled; the same protocol should be followed for surgical procedures.

Although the number of charts pulled would be equal to one day's service by each provider, the charts typically should be pulled from different dates and months to make certain that results are based on a true random sampling. In addition, the chart audit or review may be extended to a billing audit or review as well. This would involve reviewing the medical record documentation process as well as the charge documentation process. In this process charges are reviewed as they are submitted from the provider or the charge document, to charge entry, then to billing and final adjudication of the claim. Hospitals and other facilities are required to perform such audits for their services as the result of standards set by **The Joint Commission (TJC)**. TJC requires that these types of activities be performed and recorded on a regular basis.

Preparing Charts for the Audit

Typically, the auditing entity (e.g., the practice or outside auditor) is responsible for randomly pulling the medical charts necessary for the chart audit. The practice or facility, however, may pull the charts for the audit, making certain the charts remain a random sample for accurate auditing. A small number of charts may be pulled from medical records at one time, or all charts may be pulled at one time. Keep in mind, however, that typically the practice continues to see patients during the audit. Some of the charts pulled for the random sampling may need to be put back if the patient(s) selected must be seen during the audit period. If this occurs, each of these charts should be replaced with a different randomly selected chart. The audit process should occur with as little disruption to the practice as possible. For this reason many chart audits are performed in increments.

Tools Needed for the Chart Audit or Review Process

In addition to the current CPT and ICD-9-CM or current coding books, the chart auditor must use the appropriate forms to complete the audit. The forms differ according to the type and extent of the review. Samples of the most common review documents are included in this chapter discussion. Worksheets similar to those used for initial coding of CPT and diagnosis-related group services may also be helpful in this process.

What Is Reviewed in the Chart Audit

Because each chart audit may be performed for various reasons, the chart auditor should meet with the requesting party of the audit to determine if there are specific concerns or areas of concentration. Some of the most common reasons the chart audit is performed are as follows.

Undercodes or Overcodes

When medical record documentation substantiates a higher or lower level of service than that reported, these services are termed *overcoded* or *undercoded.* Many practices undercode to be "safe" from fraud and abuse. Significant revenue is lost as the result of this unnecessary practice.

Obviously, overcoding may result in third-party audit and the possibility of fraud and abuse allegations. The goal of the practice should be to code and bill services at the level they are performed. When overcoding or undercoding occurs, the chart auditor determines the significance and identity of medical documentation that may be missing or deficient in maximizing the coding level.

Missing Documentation or Signatures

As has been emphasized throughout this text, if it is not documented, it did not happen. In many instances the service provided probably achieves the level of service billed. If the documentation to substantiate that level of service, ancillary service, or procedure is not present, however, it should not be coded or billed. This includes the completion of the medical documentation by acknowledging that statements are complete and accurate with a signature or authentication mark as well as a date.

If physician extenders are responsible for providing services or portions of service, the attending or overseeing physician must review and document the report with a signature or mark and the date.

Levels of Service Distribution

For the practice to determine whether the volume of each level of service is "within the norm" for its specialty, level of service distribution is determined by the volume of each level of service calculated as a percentage of the total number of visits. The practice may monitor its percentage level of service distributions before a chart audit by contacting any of the medical management associations to which it belongs. This information is gathered for the past year through a process of practice surveys by specialty.

Ancillary Service Documentation and Signature Requirements

Every service that requires a physician order MUST have certain information documented for that service to be coded and billed. The required documentation includes the following:

- Physician order to provide the service
- Documentation of service provided
- Interpretation of test by physician
- Signature and countersignature of physician when services are provided by nursing or physician extender staff

The inclusion of laboratory slips or electrocardiogram printouts, for instance, does not constitute proof that the service was completed unless the physician has read, interpreted, and documented his or her interpretation by signing and dating the results. Services such as medications, injections, and immunizations require documentation of the order for services as well as review by the ordering physician that they were completed as ordered and confirmation of physician review by signature and date.

Compliance with Practice or Facility Chart Protocol

If practice protocols call for charts to be dictated, filed in a certain order, signed, and dated in specific locations, these procedures should be reviewed in relation to compliance with practice or facility protocols. If the practice has adopted a compliance program, this portion of the review should also encompass whether the practice is adhering to the guidelines of its compliance program. Tool 22-5 shows the types of issues the practice should review.

Documenting Chart Deficiencies

When deficiencies are noted in the elements discussed, the chart auditor should note those deficiencies. Additional notations can also be made of enhancements that might be made to achieve compliance. Documentation of the following deficiencies should be noted with details:

- Changes in level of service
- Documentation deficiencies
- Signature deficiencies

Compiling Audit Data

On completion of the actual chart review, a compilation of results is necessary along with a report back to the requesting party. For the financial impact of the results to be calculated, pricing information should be obtained for services audited from the office. Overcoded or undercoded items should be recorded on a chart audit logsheet. The auditor will then need to calculate the difference between actual reimbursement and the correct reimbursement for services as documented. Services that have been coded and billed, but were audited as not sufficiently documented to warrant coding, should be entered on the chart audit logsheet as well. If the chart audit extends into a billing audit as well, a charge capturing review should also be completed.

The charge capturing review requires several randomly sampled day schedules or appointment logs from the practice or facility. A review of coding and billing records should be conducted to determine whether the patients seen were billed and whether other procedures performed were coded as well.

Preparation of the Audit Report

When the results of the chart audit are prepared, the report must not sound offensive to the practice. The auditor should keep in mind that the practice apparently identified the need for the audit and therefore has taken the first step in determining the extent of discrepancies and correcting them. For this reason, the auditor should eliminate the use of words such as "errors" and replace them with words such as "recommendations." The auditor will also want to assure the practice that the purposes of the audit are to prevent third-party audit, enhance documentation, and work with the practice toward that end. The chart auditor should make certain that the chart audit is not construed as an attempt to find all the "errors" or "mistakes" made by the practice staff. The auditor must make sure to include positives along with the negatives. For instance, if practice coding is deficient but charts are all dictated, well written, signed, and efficiently organized, the auditor must be sure to mention the positive findings as well. Even if the extensive effort made by staff to achieve chart or documentation completion falls short of the needs as evidenced by the chart audit, their efforts should be praised.

The chart auditor should prepare written documentation of findings, referencing documentation from the coding reference books (CPT and ICD-9-CM).

Level of Service Deficiencies

The level of service distribution curve for the practice's particular specialty should be stated. The practice's level of service curve based on the charts audited must be calculated and compared with that standard.

Remember that the level of service curve for the audited practice may, in fact, be different from the norm, even if the levels of services are documented and coded correctly. Thus the practice has the opportunity and should be prepared to substantiate that its levels of service have been coded correctly. At a minimum the practice can be confident in the event of an audit that its levels of service distribution have already been substantiated.

Documentation Deficiencies

All documentation deficiencies relating to the practice should be identified and information provided on how these deficiencies may be corrected easily and efficiently without a great deal of additional work on the part of the practice. The need for complete documentation should be emphasized from both a fraud and an abuse perspective as well as from a liability standpoint.

Calculation of Deficiencies

After each deficiency and the resultant increase or decrease in reimbursement has been documented, this increase or decrease should be calculated on a monthly and annualized basis.

One of the most common complaints from coders is that the staff and physicians do not seem to comprehend the extent of their documentation and coding deficiencies. Communicating to the physician on a daily basis that a $100 discrepancy exists would seem nominal and of little consequence. Multiplying that $100 discrepancy by 22 working days, however, results in a $2200 loss per month; multiplying that figure by 12 months results in an annual loss of $26,400. Deficiencies must be put in terms that will draw needed attention and result in a simple resolution. Providers are more willing to make simple adjustments to documentation deficiencies rather than major changes to maximize levels of all services performed.

Summarizing Audit Findings

The auditor should make sure to reinforce the purpose of the audit, address concerns discussed with the practice before the audit, follow up on results, and determine how the practice can implement any needed corrections. It should be emphasized that the auditor will be available to help make the changes necessary to achieve maximum-effect documentation and coding.

Every type of deficiency should be identified as well as the extent of these deficiencies and the corrective steps needed.

TOOL 22-5

PRACTICE PROTOCOL LOGSHEET

DATE: ____________			PRACTICE PROTOCOL LOGSHEET				PRACTICE: ______________________								
			DOCUMENTATION STYLE				CHART CONTENTS			DOCUMENTATION OF REVIEW					
PATIENT NAME	DOS	MR/ CHT#	DICTATED	WRITTEN	SOAP	NARRATIVE	DATED	SIGNED	LEGIBLE	VITAL SIGNS	PT HX	LABS	X-RAY	OTHER ANCILL.	
Y = Yes N = No Page _______ of____					Totals No.										
					Grand Totals										
					% Error										

The impact on the practice, uncorrected and corrected, should be explained. Define step-by-step processes to correct the problems and prioritize a list of deficiencies to address first. Priorities should be based on the cost to the practice in increased or decreased reimbursement as well as the potential risks for fraud and abuse and the calculated financial impact.

Both an in-depth detailed analysis of the audit and a quick reference one-page summary should be prepared so that individuals who may lack time to read the details can, at a minimum, read the bottom line. The financial impact of each error and the total impact of all items identified should be given, including the annualized numbers. This often encourages review of the more detailed information.

Compliance Programs

Compliance programs are well-defined written policies and procedures outlining a specific set of guidelines to ensure that the practice adheres to third-party standards. These standards may involve areas such as medical documentation, coding, billing, or other defined processes.

At this time no laws require physicians to implement compliance programs. If a provider is audited by the federal government, however, the government reserves the right to mandate that a compliance plan be put into place within a set period if it believes that this step is appropriate.

Even though a corporate or practice compliance plan is not required, federal regulations mandate that **Health Insurance Portability and Accountability Act (HIPAA)** guidelines be monitored and followed.

HIPAA REQUIREMENTS

Under HIPAA, which was enacted in 1996, set standards are required for the confidentiality of patient records and the processing of health care claims, including but not limited to the following:

- Standards for electronic claims transactions such as common codes, identifiers, and security methods to ensure consumer records are protected from inappropriate use and disclosure. This affects health plans, health care clearinghouses, and health care providers conducting financial and administrative transactions electronically.
- Creating privacy standards for patient records such as limiting the use and release of medical records and other personal health insurance information and patients' access to their records.
- Establishing an employer identification number that will be effective no later than July 30, 2004 (this requirement has been put on hold).
- Establishing common code sets to be used for assigning codes to all claim forms. These common code sets were established as ICD-9-CM and CPT.

Current changes or additions to HIPAA legislation are available from the CMS Web site at http://www.cms.gov/hipaa.

THE JOINT COMMISSION ACCREDITATION REQUIREMENTS

As previously discussed, hospitals are mandated by organizations such as TJC to comply with standards to receive and maintain accreditation. This accreditation process is necessary for the following reasons:

- It is required for reimbursement by many third-party carriers.
- It validates quality of care.
- It provides a competitive edge over facilities that are not accredited.

At a minimum, TJC (and other accrediting authorities) requires the following review criteria:

- Each department must have a quality assessment plan.
- Results of documentation monitoring or clinical pertinence reviews must be reviewed in the appropriate committees with interdisciplinary input.
- Qualified personnel must perform all tasks of documentation and all documentation reviews.
- Overall content of the medical record must be sufficient to provide continuity of care.
- Basic documentation elements must be present, such as the following:
  - Patient informed consent
  - Patient education
  - Diagnoses and procedures
  - Pertinent history
  - Observations, assessments, and plans
  - Diagnostic data
  - Therapeutic data
- Reviews must focus on the following:
  1. Problem cases
  2. High-volume cases
  3. Sampling across cases
- Departments responsible for entries into the record must have written policies on timeliness and data distribution.
- Evidence of morbidity and mortality measurements and indicators, health information management, transcription, and quality assurance must show pertinent policies and examples of documentation reviews.
- There must be evidence of policies relating to data correction, revisions, and editing.

Policies and procedures are maintained in the hospital facility that outline exactly how all these guidelines will be implemented, monitored, and maintained. These documents are reviewed at the time the facility is reviewed for accreditation.

Practice compliance programs are not right for all providers and practices. Most importantly, if the practice decides to implement such a program, it will be obligated to enforce the guidelines outlined in the compliance program.

The following should be considered when determining whether a practice should institute a compliance program.

DETERMINING PRACTICE NEED FOR A COMPLIANCE PROGRAM

The practice's vulnerability for fraud and audit is based on the following elements:

Coding practices and practice size	The third party performing the audit is interested in identifying some of the largest offenders and those that, because of their size, will press smaller practices into compliance.
Specialty	Certain specialties may be more prone to investigation because past audits in such practices have revealed a high degree of fraudulent activity.
E & M levels of distribution	Levels of service distribution and volume of high-ticket items are identified for potential fraud investigation.

ELEMENTS THAT TRIGGER AN INVESTIGATION OR AUDIT

Keep in mind the three main reasons practices and facilities are investigated for fraud and abuse:

1. Patient complaint
2. Employee complaint
3. Level of service distribution inconsistencies

In addition to the previous components, the following reasons can be added:

4. Information from other investigations (referral patterns, other services already under investigation)
5. Data gathered from processed claims:
   - Abnormal distribution of levels of service
   - Billing errors
   - Repetitive care protocols
   - Copayment or deductible violations

The implementation of a practice compliance program is time consuming and detail oriented. The compliance program ensures quality of care, documentation, coding, and other services provided by the practice in much the same way that the accreditation of hospitals attempts to ensure quality of care for patients in those facilities. Having a written, enforced compliance program in place has a number of advantages; however, a compliance plan that has no follow-up or is not enforced may actually be more of a threat to the practice than no compliance plan at all. Box 22-1 lists seven federal guidelines for compliance programs.

ADVANTAGES TO HAVING A COMPLIANCE PROGRAM IN PLACE

The advantages to implementing a compliance program proactively are the following:

- Identification of potential problems within the practice before those outside the practice investigate and possibly prosecute.
- Ability to show consistency in coding protocols. (Consistently wrong is better than no consistency. Consistency shows effort and eliminates the possibilities of intent to defraud.)
- Consistency of data for statistical purposes within the practice. These data may be used for contracting as well as in revenue projections and budgeting for the practice.
- Ability to deal consistently with patient inquiries and complaints regarding level of service questions. All personnel can interpret how the levels of service were determined and can explain in a consistent manner to the satisfaction of the patient or third-party inquiry.

BOX 22-1 SEVEN FEDERAL GUIDELINES FOR COMPLIANCE PROGRAMS

For a compliance program to be implemented, several elements must be present so that it conforms to federal guidelines. Following are the seven main components required for a federally approved compliance program:

1. The organization has established compliance standards reasonably capable of reducing the prospect of criminal conduct.
2. High-level personnel have overall responsibility to oversee compliance.
3. Substantial discretionary authority is not delegated to individuals with a propensity to engage in illegal activities.
4. The organization has communicated standards and procedures to employees and agents.
5. The organization has taken reasonable steps to achieve compliance with its standards and to publicize a reporting system for employees without fear of retribution.
6. Standards are consistently enforced through appropriate disciplinary measures.
7. The organization takes all reasonable steps to respond appropriately to offenses and to prevent recurrences.

Chapter in Review

Certification Review

- CMS and OIG have the authority to suspend, exclude, terminate, and impose fines and penalties on providers, practitioners, and suppliers who commit acts in direct violation of antifraud and antiabuse legislation.
- Fines and penalties for fraud and abuse are imposed by line item charged rather than claim form.
- *Fraud* is requesting payment for services that should not be paid according to third-party guidelines.
- *Abuse* is defined as provision of excessive services that are not medically necessary.
- Variations on the definitions of fraud and abuse exist with each third-party carrier.
- Fraud and abuse are punishable regardless of intent.
- All parties involved with or who had knowledge of fraudulent activity are liable for charges.
- Costs to the practice from fraud and abuse charges are significant, regardless of the findings.
- All suspected fraudulent and abusive activities should be reported in writing.
- Data entry personnel should be monitored for efficiency as well as errors in data entry of codes.
- Claims should be reviewed by an individual knowledgeable in coding to determine whether the claims are clean and the codes are appropriate.
- Coding and chart reviews should take place in the practice on a regularly scheduled basis. Coding trends or problems can be identified internally before third-party carriers identify, audit, and impose fines and penalties.
- Compliance programs are important for ensuring consistency in coding and billing.
- The three main reasons providers are investigated for fraud and abuse are patient complaints, employee complaints, and level of service distribution inconsistencies.

Student Assignments

- Study Chapter 22.
- Review the Learning Objectives for Chapter 22.
- Review the Certification Review for Chapter 22.
- Complete the Chapter Review exercise to reinforce concepts learned in this chapter.
- Complete the practice exercises on the companion Evolve site for reinforcement of concepts on monitoring and compliance.
- Complete the Practical Application exercise for real-life scenarios in coding compliance.
- Complete the Workbook exercises that simulate an actual provider office or physician chart audit.

Chapter Review Exercise

Complete the following exercises.

1. Give examples of fraud.

____

____

____

2. Give examples of abuse.

____

____

____

3. Outline the proper steps in reporting fraud and abuse.

____

____

____

4. Identify and explain what elements should be identified in a chart audit process.

____

____

____

5. Define the seven components that make up a compliance program.

____

____

____

Practical Application

For the charts and the code(s) assigned on the following pages, identify potential compliance issues for Godfrey Regional Outpatient Clinic. Then suggest how policies and procedures within the clinic could be changed to avoid these issues in the future. These issues may represent potential fraud or abuse situations or undercodes with potential for additional reimbursement.

1. Outpatient office note

OFFICE NOTE

Chief complaint: ______

Date: ______

Vital signs: BP______ P______ R______

History:

Five months S/P total abdominal colectomy with ileorectal anastomosis for a carcinoma of the colon located 20 cm above the ileocecal valve. The patient was referred to me for surgical intervention following findings on a colonoscopy. She now presents for her first post-operative visit and further discussions for therapy.

Exam:

Liver is not enlarged to palpation or percussion. The incision is well healed. The inguinal regions are normal, and there is evidence of tenderness or discomfort on the left side. Rectal exam was normal.

Diagnosis/assessment:

Patient was advised regarding the options of treatment including no further treatment, aggressive surgical resection, systemic chemotherapy and/or regional chemotherapy.

She is advised to review her options and will get back with us in the next week or so.

Patrick Olson MD

Patient name: ______

Date of service: ______

GODFREY MEDICAL ASSOCIATES
1532 Third Avenue, Suite 120 • Aldon, FL 77713 • (407) 555-4000

CPT code assignment: 99242

Problem(s) identified: ______

Future resolution: ______

2. Consultation

OFFICE NOTE

Chief complaint: ____________________

Date: 08/23/XX

Vital signs: BP______ P______ R______

History:

Attending Physician: Samuel Jones, MD

The patient is seen in consultation due to chest pain and cardiac irregularity. Patient indicates he had a severe episode of chest pain and was hospitalized for a heart attack.

Approximately 3 days ago, he started having more shortness of breath. He also began having chest pain plus nausea and vomiting. His breathing was quite difficult, therefore he came to the Emergency Department and was found to have congestive heart failure with cardiac irregularities.

The Emergency Room physician, Dr. Samuel Jones, requested a cardiac consultation in the Emergency Department.

Exam:

On physical exam, the patient's BP is 186/80, pulse 100, and he runs paroxysmal atrial tachycardia, frequent premature ventricular contractions. His neck veins are distended, he has moist rales in his lungs. The heart has a systolic murmur at the apex. His abdomen is soft, no masses can be felt. He has 2+ edema in the lower extremities.

Diagnosis/assessment:

It is my impression he has a combination of arteriosclerotic and hypertensive cardiovascular disease. He also appears to have pulmonary emphysema secondary to his smoking with COPD.

I have recommended admission to the ER physician and would be happy to follow this patient further on an inpatient basis if requested.

Thank you for your request for a consultation.

cc: Dr. Samuel Jones, ED

Patient name: ____________________

Date of service: ____________________

GODFREY MEDICAL ASSOCIATES
1532 Third Avenue, Suite 120 • Aldon, FL 77713 • (407) 555-4000

CPT code assignment: 99284

Problem(s) identified: ____________________

Future resolution: ____________________

3. Emergency room record

EMERGENCY ROOM RECORD

Name:	**Age:**	**ER physician:**
	DOB:	

Allergies/type of reaction:	**Usual medications/dosages:**

Triage/presenting complaint:

This is an 18-year-old presenting to the emergency department with complaint of ear pain. She states only experienced in right ear, no drainage or discharge. She has placed a cotton ball in the ear for some relief.

Initial assessment:

Time	**T**	**P**	**R**	**BP**	**Other:**				

Medication orders:

Lab work:

X-Ray:

Physician's report:

OBJECTIVE:
Vital signs are stable. Examination of the left ear shows good light reflex. No erthyema present. Right ear shows TM which is erythematous and bulging. No discharge appreciated. Neck: Positive lymph node on the right side of the neck. No other masses noted. Posterior pharynx was visualized, no erythema noted.

ASSESSMENT:
Right otitis media

PLAN:
Placed on Augmentin 875 mg po bid for ten days

Diagnosis:	**Physician sign/date**
	Robert Rai MD
Discharge **Transfer** **Admit** **Good** **Satisfactory** **Other:**	

GODFREY REGIONAL HOSPITAL
123 Main Street • Aldon, FL 77714 • (407) 555-1234

CPT code assignment: 99284

Problem(s) identified: ____________________

Future resolution: ____________________

4. Operative report

OPERATIVE REPORT

Patient information:

Patient name:
DOB:
MR#:

Preoperative diagnosis:

Right shoulder rotator cuff tear

Postoperative diagnosis:

Procedure(s) performed:

Anesthesia:

Assistant surgeon:

Description of procedure:

Patient was taken to OR, placed in a beach chair position. Standard posterior portal was made and an arthroscope was inserted. An anterior accessory portal was made. The posterior labrum had significant fraying and debridement was completed.

There was a rotator cuff tear of the supraspinatus that measured approximately 1.5 cm. A parachute suture anchor was inserted and the suture placed through the cuff and the cuff was then repaired using sliding notch.

The joint was then irrigated and drained and the wounds were closed with Biosyn and steri-strips.

GODFREY REGIONAL HOSPITAL
123 Main Street • Aldon, FL 77714 • (407) 555-1234

CPT code assignment: 29827-RT

Problem(s) identified: ______________________________

Future resolution: ______________________________

5. Operative report

OPERATIVE REPORT

Patient information:

Patient name:
DOB:
MR#:

Preoperative diagnosis:

Family History of Colon Cancer

Postoperative diagnosis:

Cecal Polyp
Colon Polyps
Internal Hemorrhoids

Procedure(s) performed:

Anesthesia:

Assistant surgeon:

Description of procedure:

Colonoscope was introduced and advanced all the way up to the cecum identified by the ileocecal valve, appendical orifice and light reflex. In the cecum there was a flat polypoid lesion which was removed by snare. The lesion could not be completely removed because of its thin walled cecum and may cause perforation. The scope was retracted. In the transverse colon, there was a large polyp which was removed by snare and sent to histopathology. Another small polyp was removed in the transverse colon by snare. She had diverticulosis of the left side and small sized internal hemorrhoids. No other abnormalities were noted.

Rachel Perez MD

GODFREY REGIONAL HOSPITAL
123 Main Street • Aldon, FL 77714 • (407) 555-1234

CPT code assignment: 45385 × 3

Problem(s) identified: ______________________________

Future resolution: ______________________________

6. Consultation

OFFICE NOTE Gastroenterology Consultation

Chief complaint: ____________________

Date: ____________

Vital signs: BP______ P______ R______

History:

The patient has a history of receiving multiple blood transfusions for his multiple vascular surgeries. There was no history of any jaundice following any of these transfusions, although he does relate some jaundice many years ago, etiology unknown. He has manifested no symptoms referable to liver disease and remains asymptomatic. No history of significant alcohol intake and only one drug could implicate Hepatitis, Aldomet, which he has been on for approximately one year.

Exam:

His physical exam revealed his liver extended 3-4 fingerbreaths below his right costal margin and was firm. We found his SGOT elevated, several repeat blood tests have shown varying degrees of elevation of bilirubin and transaminases. Additionally, his globulins have been elevated and his pro time has been mildly prolonged.

Diagnosis/assessment:

It seems likely he has chronic liver disease from his transfusions, the etiology being Hepatitis C. It is unlikely his Aldomet is contributing to his condition.

In view of his mild enzyme elevations, I would not recommend treating him in view of his age and general medical condition with immunosuppressive therapy. We will simply watch him and have repeat liver tests in the next 2-3 months.

Please let me know if I can further assist with the diagnosis and treatment of this very pleasant gentleman.

Patrick Olsen MD

Patient name: ____________________

Date of service: ____________

GODFREY MEDICAL ASSOCIATES
1532 Third Avenue, Suite 120 • Aldon, FL 77713 • (407) 555-4000

CPT code assignment: 99245

Problem(s) identified: ____________________

Future resolution: ____________________

7. Operative report

OPERATIVE REPORT

Patient information:

Patient name:
DOB:
MR#:

Preoperative diagnosis:

Left knee medial femoral condyle avascular necrosis

Postoperative diagnosis:

Same

Procedure(s) performed:

Arthroscopy w/drilling of medial femoral avascular necrosis
Synovectomy of the patellofemoral compartment

Anesthesia:

Assistant surgeon:

Description of procedure:

The patient is a 45-year-old female with Addison's disease and chronic history of steroid usage who presents with left knee pain, swelling and catching. Physical exam and radiographic studies consistent with left knee medial femoral condyle avascular necrosis.

Patient was brought to the operating room and a left knee arthroscopy was performing placing the arthroscope in the medial joint line portal. Exam of the patellofemoral compartment revealed
articular cartilage intact but patient noted to have abundant synovitis of the patellofemoral compartment. This was debrided using a shaver. Exam of the medial compartment revealed
The medial meniscus was intact, however, patient noted to have chondromalacia as well as softening of the cartilage over the area of the medial femoral condyle avascular necrosis. These areas were drilled using a K wire in order to stimulate blood flow to these areas. Exam of the intercondylar notch revealed that the ACL was intact. A non-Q pain pump was inserted for postoperative pain control. Arthroscope along with all the instrumentation was removed.

GODFREY REGIONAL HOSPITAL
123 Main Street • Aldon, FL 77714 • (407) 555-1234

CPT code assignments: 29879-LT, 29875-59-LT, 29899-59-LT

Problem(s) identified: ____________________

Future resolution: ____________________

8. Operative report

OPERATIVE REPORT

Patient information:

Patient name:
DOB:
MR#:

Preoperative diagnosis:

Subcutaneous mass of posterior shoulder

Postoperative diagnosis:

Subcutaneous mass of posterior shoulder

Procedure(s) performed:

Excision of right shoulder lipoma

Anesthesia:

Assistant surgeon:

Description of procedure:

78-year-old gentleman with gradually enlarging subcutaneous mass in the posterior shoulder. It has recently become enlarged and become symptomatic.

Presence of 5 × 8 cm lipoma present at the posterior fold of the right axilla. Lesion noted to be submuscular. These muscles were reflected and muscle division was minimized during the excision.

Following the excision, the skin edges were approximated using a running 3-0 Monocryl suture placed in the subcuticular layer.

GODFREY REGIONAL HOSPITAL
123 Main Street • Aldon, FL 77714 • (407) 555-1234

CPT code assignment: 11406

Problem(s) identified: ______________________________

Future resolution: ______________________________

9. Office visit

OFFICE NOTE

Chief complaint: ______________________________

Date: ______________

Vital signs: BP 140/80 P 85 R 22 T 99.3

History:

32-year-old male, lifelong smoker, referred to me for 2 week history of dry cough associated with dull substernal discomfort and dyspnea, particularly on exertion. Otherwise, he has been remarkably free of any other associated symptoms. Denies fever, chills, night sweats, weight loss.

Admits to childhood asthma. Traveled extensively throughout the US including travel to California Deserts and Central Valley. He had a TB skin test 10 years ago and flu vaccine 3 years ago.

Past Medical History remarkably negative.

Exam:

Chest exam completely normal. No rales, wheezes, rhonchi or rubs. No cough. Cardiac exam showed a regular rate and rhythm with no murmur or gallop.

Laboratory Data:
PA chest x-ray is striking for new interstitial infiltrate seen in both mid-lung zones with some
Shagging of the cardiac borders.

Spirometry before and after bronchodilator shows vital capacity of 3.79 or 69% after an 11% improvement with bronchodilator. The FEV1 achieves 3.24 liters or 72% of predicted after 12% improvement with bronchodilator. The FEV1/FVC ratio was mildly increased at 85 instead of predicted 82.

Diagnosis/assessment:

Differential diagnosis include the following:
Hypersensitivity pneumonia
Mycoplasmal pneumonia

Will treat with Amoxil for next 10 days. Would suggest reevaluation at that time with repeat
Chest x-ray. Can be followed up with PCP or additional evaluation by myself at that time.

Stanley Krantz, MD

Patient name: ______________________________

Date of service: ______________

GODFREY MEDICAL ASSOCIATES
1532 Third Avenue, Suite 120 • Aldon, FL 77713 • (407) 555-4000

CPT code assignments: 99242-25, 94060, 71020

Problem(s) identified: ______________________________

Future resolution: ______________________________

10. Operative report

OPERATIVE REPORT

Patient information:
Patient name: DOB: MR#:
Preoperative diagnosis:
Right inguinal hernia
Postoperative diagnosis:
Right inguinal hernia
Procedure(s) performed:
Right inguinal herniorrhaphy with mesh plus
Anesthesia:
Assistant surgeon:
Description of procedure:
45-year-old patient for hernia repair. After IV sedation an oblique incision was made in the right groin. Skin and subcutaneous tissue was divided sharply. A large defect was found in the floor of Hesselbach's Triangle. Preperitoneal space was entered and the direct bulge was reduced back into the peritoneum. An extra larage Marlex plug was inserted into the defect and anchored into place. The area was closed with 4-0 Monopril subcuticular sutures. Adm Wketz MD

GODFREY REGIONAL HOSPITAL
123 Main Street • Aldon, FL 77714 • (407) 555-1234

CPT code assignments: 49505, 49568

Problem(s) identified: ____________________

Future resolution: ____________________

23

The Certification Process

Congratulations on your decision to take one of the coding certification examinations. Coding certifications are designed to recognize and reward mastery in clinical coding as well as provide a first-line defense against fraud and abuse. Certified coders are recognized and acknowledged across the country as a valuable source of professional expertise.

The demand for credentialed coders continues to skyrocket as physicians and facilities continue to undergo increased fraud and abuse investigation by third-party carriers and the Office of the Inspector General. The inability to find qualified coders, unacceptable chart audit error rates, and an increased focus on coding compliance have resulted in an increased demand for certified coders.

Now that you have completed the learning process, it is time to consider the different organizations that certify coders and the types of certification that are possible. Consideration should be given to all organizations and the tests they offer to best meet the needs of the coder. Obviously, the choice to become a physician or professional coder instead of a facility coder (inpatient or outpatient) will help make that decision. A comparison of the different coding certification examinations offered by the American Academy of Professional Coders (AAPC) and American Health Information Management Association (AHIMA) are outlined in Table 23-1. Note that all certification examinations require registration some time in advance, so register early!

Preparing for the certification examination should not be taken lightly. It involves significant preparation time and practice, practice, and more practice. Use materials in the Workbook or on the Evolve site that accompanies this text for additional review and coding practice.

Following are some suggested strategies for preparing for certification examination:

- Set a specific study schedule. If not preparing for the certification examinations as part of an academic program, set aside time a minimum of 4 to 6 weeks in advance of the actual examination to review materials, practice coding, and re-review. A sample 6-week schedule is outlined in Figure 23-1.
- Remember that examinations are time restricted, so make certain when taking practice examinations and exercises to set the specific time allotted for the number of exercises that have been chosen. Keep in mind the following:
  1. Do not spend a great deal of time on any one question.
  2. Each question, regardless of length or complexity, is worth the same amount.
  3. If pressed for time, try skipping an extremely time-consuming or complex question to answer other questions that may be easier to answer.
- Review practice examination materials, including the answers and rationales for the correct answer. If you miss a key coding concept, check the CPT, ICD-9-CM, or Healthcare Common Procedure Coding System (HCPCS) level II manual to review the concept and perhaps make notes to refer to during the actual examination.
- Only CPT, ICD-9-CM, and HCPCS books are allowed in the examination. Note that the AAPC examinations require the use of the American Medical Association (AMA) edition of the CPT manual only. The AHIMA examinations allow use of a medical dictionary for a portion of the examination; the AAPC examinations do not. It is imperative that *the student's* additional notes for coding guidelines and tips be appropriately marked or written in these code books. Your

TABLE 23-1 CODING CERTIFICATION EXAMINATIONS

CERTIFICATION	CERTIFYING BODY	EXAM TYPE	SCHEDULE	BOOKS REQUIRED	NO. OF QUESTIONS/ TIME	FORMAT	COMPETENCIES EVALUATED
Certified professional hospital coder (CPC-H)	AAPC	Hospital outpatient	Quarterly by local AAPC	CPT, ICD-9, vols. 1-3, HCPCS level II	150/5.5 hours	Multiple choice	Medical terminology, ASC facility, CPT/ICD-9 guidelines, HCPCS level II, human anatomy, UB-04 claims, Medicare guidelines, APCs, revenue codes
Certified coding specialist (CCS)	AHIMA	Hospital inpatient, ambulatory care	Electronic	CPT, ICD-9, vols. 1-3, medical dictionary (optional)*	81/4 hours	60 multiple choice, 21 coding	Health information documentation, ICD-9-CM guidelines, procedure guidelines, inpatient hospital guidelines, outpatient hospital, data quality, data management
Certified professional coder (CPC)	AAPC	Physician-based, office, group practice, multispecialty, specialty	Quarterly by local AAPC	CPT, ICD-9, vols. 1-3, HCPCS level II	150/5.5 hours	Multiple choice	Medical, human anatomy, CPT coding guidelines, ICD-9 coding guidelines, HCPCS level II, evaluation and management, anesthesia, surgery, modifier use
Certified coding specialist, physician-based setting (CCS-P)	AHIMA	Physician setting	Electronic	CPT, ICD-9, vols. 1-3, medical	81/4 hours	60 multiple choice, 21 coding	Health information, documentation, reimbursement methods, regulatory guidelines

*Books used in Section II only.
AAPC, American Academy of Professional Coders; *AHIMA,* American Health Information Management Association; *ASC,* ambulatory surgical center; *HCPCS,* Health Care Common Procedure Coding System; *APC,* ambulatory payment classification.

Suggested Six-Week Study Schedule		
Week	**Number of Hours**	**Concentration**
1	2 hours	• Prepare medical terminology cards
	3 hours	• Review medical terminology
	2 hours	• Review ICD-9-CM guidelines
	4 hours	• ICD-9-CM practice exercises
	2 hours	• Mock exam (available in workbook) composed of medical terminology/A & P ICD-9-CM coding
Total	13 hours	
2	2 hours	• Review medical terminology cards
	2 hours	• Review general surgery guidelines integumentary, musculoskeletal, respiratory, cardiovascular, digestive systems guidelines
	1 hour	• Addition of coding notes to book
	6 hours	• Surgery practice exercises integumentary, musculoskeletal, respiratory, cardiovascular, digestive systems
Total	11 hours	
3	1 hour	• Review medical terminology
	2 hours	• Review surgery guidelines urinary/male/female
	1 hour	• Addition of coding notes to book
	6 hours	• Surgery practice exercises urinary/male/female
Total	10 hours	
4	1 hour	• Review medical terminology
	2 hours	• Review surgery guidelines nervous/eye/ear
	1 hour	• Addition of coding notes to book
	6 hours	• Surgery practice exercises nervous/eye/ear
Total	10 hours	
5	1 hour	• Review medical terminology
	1 hour	• Review surgery guidelines
	2 hours	• Mock surgery exam (all sections) available in workbook
	1 hour	• Review/addition of coding notes
	2 hours	• Review radiology, pathology, medicine, HCPCS guidelines
	1 hour	• Addition of coding notes to book
Total	8 hours	
6	2 hours	• Mock exam radiology, pathology, medicine, HCPCS sections
	1 hour	• Exam review/addition of notes
	2 hours	• Mock exam (all sections) available in workbook
	1 hour	• Exam review/addition of notes
	5 hours	• 5 hour complete mock exam
	2 hours	• Exam review/additional review
Total	13 hours	
Grand total:	65 hours	

FIGURE 23-1. Sample 6-week study schedule for prearing for a certification examination. *A & P,* Anatomy and physiology.

instructor should have stressed the need for students to make notes in these books during the program. If you have made notes in other textbooks, notebooks, or other locations, you may want to incorporate those notes into your coding books. This will allow you to "test" the correctness of this material as you prepare, take mock examinations, and practice exercises. You should know where to locate appropriate information needed during the actual certification examination.

Following are some additional suggestions regarding notes in code books:

- Items may not be taped, glued, or pasted into coding reference books; copy needed information into the texts themselves.

- If you have made voluminous notes during the course of the coding program, resulting in a lot of handwritten "clutter," use a highlighter to specifically mark notes needed for the test so they will stand out.
- Keep notes brief, perhaps in bullet format rather than in narrative format, so they are easy to find and reference. Remember that time is an element in successfully completing the examination. Summaries needed for coding are included in this text.
- Flag frequently referenced information. The professional editions of the coding books typically are already tabbed; however, additional tabs may be added to areas you cannot locate easily.
- Keep in mind that examinations are based on the student's comprehension of coding rules and concepts and that many of the correct answers on the examinations are based on the student's comprehension and application of coding guidelines.
- Additional study materials are available in the Workbook that supplements this text. Additional outside materials are available for preparation for the certification examination from a number of organizations. Assess whether these materials are necessary or whether the current textbook, Workbook, and Evolve materials are sufficient.
- Several short mock examinations are located in the Workbook, with time specifications indicated for completion. Also included is a final examination that tests comprehension of all examination sections. Do not attempt the practice examinations or final practice examination until you complete a full review.
- All examinations require knowledge of medical terminology, anatomy, and physiology. This material is tested either through specific questions on these categories or in the student's application of this knowledge in reading and extrapolating information from operative reports and other medical record notes. Do not forget to review combining forms, suffixes, prefixes, and abbreviations in preparation for the examination as well as coding principles. If you have not used this text as part of a medical coding program and therefore have not studied medical terminology, you may want to purchase a medical terminology text for this purpose. Also note that the introduction to the professional edition of CPT includes some medical terms and medical illustrations that may be modified as necessary for key words lists.

Each student should evaluate his or her knowledge level to plan the amount of time necessary to prepare for a certification examination. Following are two short medical terminology examinations with 25 questions each to help assess your knowledge of medical terminology. Take time to evaluate your performance on the practice examinations. Determine areas that need additional study. Additional review and practice exercises are available in the Workbook and Evolve site that accompany this text.

This review begins with the areas of medical terminology, anatomy, ICD-9-CM, HCPCS, and coding concepts. These comprise the first section of the AAPC certification examination. These areas are covered in comparable exams, such as the CCS-P exam, as well. The format may be multiple choice or fill in the blank.

A review of your medical terminology or anatomy textbook would be beneficial for the medical terminology portion of the exam. A review of Chapter 1 of this text may be helpful as well. If you used study cards during the medical terminology module of your coursework, use this same technique for review.

Study hard, review coding concepts, take the mock examinations, and practice, practice, practice and you, too, can become a professional certified coder. Good luck!

Medical Terminology Practice Examination 1 (Time Alloted: 45-50 Minutes)

1. *Histo* is defined as
   a. fat
   b. nucleus
   c. organ
   d. tissue
2. *Onco* is defined as
   a. cancer
   b. disease
   c. tumor
   d. organ
3. The term *lateral* describes movement toward the
   a. front
   b. side
   c. top
   d. back
4. The outer layer of skin is called the
   a. dermis
   b. corium
   c. epidermis
   d. keratin
5. The combining form that means *nail* is
   a. unguo
   b. onycho
   c. tricho
   d. a and b
6. The combining form that means *hidden* is
   a. conio
   b. rhytido
   c. xero
   d. crypto
7. *Ortho* is defined as
   a. straight
   b. oxygen
   c. incomplete
   d. breathe

8. The word root that means *kidney* is
   a. nephro
   b. vesico
   c. reno
   d. a and c
9. The combining form *pyelo* is defined as
   a. bladder
   b. renal pelvis
   c. urethral meatus
   d. ureter
10. *Tomo* is defined as
   a. cut, section
   b. sound
   c. scanty
   d. night
11. The combining form meaning *sugar* is
   a. glycoso
   b. hydro
   c. glycol
   d. a and c
12. The definition of *trans* is
   a. around
   b. before
   c. through
   d. after
13. To give birth is denoted by the word part
   a. paro
   b. nato
   c. parto
   d. either a or c
14. The upper chambers of the heart are the
   a. atrium
   b. ventricles
   c. pericardium
   d. epicardium
15. The function of the ear is
   a. hearing
   b. equilibrium
   c. speech
   d. a and b
16. The combining form *acouo* means
   a. balance
   b. ear
   c. hearing
   d. a and b
17. The set of vertebrae that forms the inward curve of the spine is the
   a. thoracic
   b. sacral
   c. lumbar
   d. b and c
18. The first vertebra in the neck is abbreviated as
   a. C1
   b. T1
   c. L1
   d. S1
19. The upper jawbone is called the
   a. maxilla
   b. mandible
   c. clavicle
   d. ulna
20. The combining form *myelo* is defined as
   a. spinal cord
   b. gray matter
   c. brain
   d. nerve root
21. The combining form *encephalo* is defined as
   a. spinal cord
   b. brain
   c. nerve root
   d. cerebellum
22. The combining form *phaso* means
   a. one
   b. mind
   c. speech
   d. sensation
23. The combining form that means *mind* is
   a. mento
   b. phreno
   c. psycho
   d. all the above
24. The combining form that means *gray matter* is
   a. polio
   b. myelo
   c. meningo
   d. rhizo
25. The suffix *paresis* is defined as
   a. slight paralysis
   b. sensitivity
   c. seizure
   d. softening

Medical Terminology Practice Examination 2 (Time Alloted: 45-50 Minutes)

1. The suffix that means *control, stop,* or *standing* is
   a. osis
   b. plasm
   c. genesis
   d. stasis
2. The term meaning *pertaining to below* is
   a. posterior
   b. dorsal
   c. inferior
   d. distal
3. The combining form *myco* is defined as
   a. fungus
   b. muscle
   c. oil
   d. dust

4. *Adeno* means
   a. wrinkles
   b. life
   c. gland
   d. scaly
5. *Ostomy* is a suffix that means
   a. creation of an artificial opening
   b. cut into, incision
   c. for visual examination
   d. stretching out, dilation, expansion
6. The suffix that means *surgical puncture to aspirate fluid* is
   a. capnia
   b. centesis
   c. otomy
   d. either b or c
7. The prefix *poly* is defined as
   a. many
   b. without
   c. through
   d. few
8. The suffix that means *suturing* or *repairing* is
   a. megaly
   b. trophy
   c. orrhaphy
   d. esis
9. The term *cystocele* is defined as
   a. stone in the bladder
   b. drooping in the bladder
   c. protrusion of the bladder
   d. inflammation of the bladder
10. *Orchidopexy* is defined as
    a. surgical fixation of a testicle
    b. excision of the seminal vesicles
    c. incision into a testis
    d. surgical repair of the glans penis
11. Painful menstrual discharge is the definition of
    a. metrorrhea
    b. amenorrhea
    c. dysmenorrhea
    d. metrorrhagia
12. The prefix *ante* means
    a. against
    b. after
    c. before
    d. without
13. The suffix meaning *hardening* is
    a. malacia
    b. sclerosis
    c. penia
    d. crit
14. *Cholecystectomy* refers to
    a. excision of bile
    b. excision of gallbladder
    c. excision of stones from gallbladder
    d. repair of gallbladder
15. The suffix *pepsia* means
    a. opening
    b. small growth
    c. tumor
    d. digestion
16. The term *rectocele* is defined as
    a. inflammation of the uvula
    b. prolapse of the rectum
    c. protrusion of the rectum
    d. disturbance of bowel function
17. The combining form for *cornea* is
    a. kerato
    b. corneo
    c. core
    d. a and b
18. The combining form *cryo* means
    a. cold
    b. light
    c. vision
    d. cornea
19. The wrist bone is called the
    a. radius
    b. phalange
    c. carpal
    d. calcaneus
20. The foot bones are called the
    a. phalanges
    b. metacarpals
    c. tarsals
    d. metatarsals
21. When a person is lying flat on his or her back, face up, the position is known as
    a. supination
    b. extension
    c. inversion
    d. pronation
22. The combining form that means *rib* is
    a. chondro
    b. clavico
    c. claviculo
    d. costo
23. Inflammation of the membranous coverings of the brain and spinal cord is called
    a. duritis
    b. poliomyelitis
    c. polyneuritis
    d. meningitis
24. The term that means *blood tumor below the dura mater* is
    a. neuroblast
    b. neuroma
    c. cerebral thrombosis
    d. subdural hematoma

25. *Spondylo* is defined as
    a. scapula
    b. vertebra
    c. cranium
    d. symphysis pubis

Basics of ICD-9-CM Coding

For the ICD-9-CM portion of the exam review, take a look at the basic ICD-9-CM concepts learned during this portion of the coding program. Following is a basic review.

1. Always code the primary reason for the encounter or service to the highest level of specificity.
2. If signs and symptoms are an integral part of a coded diagnosis, they do not need to be coded.
3. Code all diagnoses, signs, and symptoms involved in the diagnosis and treatment for that encounter (including chronic systemic diseases).
4. Do not code diagnoses that are no longer applicable (although "history of" may be coded if applicable).
5. Only definitive diagnostic statements may be used. Do not use statements with suffixes or prefixes that include "rule out," "possible," or "probable."

PREPARING TO BE AN EFFICIENT ICD-9-CM CODER

1. Review the symbols used in the ICD-9-CM book and understand their meanings.
2. Identify the correct code selected and make certain the diagnosis is from the appropriate section or subsection of ICD-9-CM. For example, you have selected code 300.9 for an upper respiratory infection; however, in checking the chapter, you find that the 300 series of codes is for psychiatry and this diagnosis is not psychiatric in nature. The most common mistakes on ICD-9-CM codes are made on the first digit (usually transposition errors) or the fourth and fifth digits (omission or wrong selection).
3. Always cross-reference your section from the alphabetical to the tabular section. Never rely on one section for selecting the correct code. Remember that the test is based on coding principles; therefore one or more of the answer selections may appear correct if you do not cross-reference.
4. Always read the codes included in the same section above and below your selection to make certain a more correct code has not been missed.
5. E codes are NOT used as primary diagnosis codes; they identify how the diagnosis (illness) occurred.
6. V codes MAY be used for a primary diagnosis when they are the chief reason for the encounter (e.g., patient visit for chemotherapy).
7. After preliminary selection of the code, read all the exclusions, inclusions, and other notes to make certain additional information is not needed to correctly code.
8. If an index of E codes and V codes does not already exist in your copy of ICD-9-CM, consider making your own index. This will help when selecting the appropriate E codes and V codes because the average coder is not familiar with the individual categories for these services. This can be an invaluable tool and save a great deal of time.

Tools are already located in your coding textbook. They may be copied by hand into your coding books, but you may not physically insert them (e.g., tape, staple, clip).

Take a moment to test your knowledge of ICD-9-CM and determine what additional time you should spend on preparing for this section of the examination.

ICD-9-CM Practice Exercises (Time Alloted: 45-50 Minutes)

1. When locating a laceration in ICD-9-CM, the coder should look under
   a. laceration
   b. wound, open
   c. abrasion
   d. contusion
2. Fractures not specified as open or closed would be coded as
   a. open
   b. closed
   c. not otherwise specified
   d. open or closed
3. When both chronic conditions and acute conditions are coded, which is coded first?
   a. acute condition
   b. chronic condition
   c. whichever is listed first in the documentation
   d. either can be coded first
4. Masses are coded as
   a. neoplasms, unspecified
   b. neoplasms, undetermined
   c. neoplasms, benign
   d. masses
5. Determination of primary and secondary neoplasms is by
   a. the primary site
   b. where the neoplasm started
   c. a and b
   d. the site currently being treated
6. The code for a migraine headache with aura is
   a. 784.0
   b. 346.00
   c. 346.90
   d. 346.0
7. The code for an old, healed myocardial infarction is
   a. 412
   b. 410.90
   c. 410.20
   d. 410.9

8. The code(s) for malignant hypertension with CHF is
   a. 403.91
   b. 401.0, 428.0
   c. 403.01
   d. 402.01
9. The code(s) for COPD with acute respiratory failure is
   a. 518.81, 496
   b. 496, 518.81
   c. 496
   d. 518.81
10. The code for a threatened abortion is
   a. 640.90
   b. 640.00
   c. 640.0
   d. 640.9
11. The code(s) for bleeding esophageal varices due to alcoholic cirrhosis of the liver is
   a. 456.20
   b. 571.2, 456.20
   c. 571.5, 456.20
   d. 571.5, 456.21
12. The code for an abnormal chest x-ray is
   a. 793.10
   b. 793.1
   c. 793.9
   d. 794.31
13. The code(s) for painful scarring of the hands due to old full-thickness burns is
   a. 709.2
   b. 944.30
   c. 709.2, 906.6
   d. 906.6
14. The code for a laceration of a finger with infection is
   a. 884.0
   b. 883.1
   c. 883.0
   d. 881.0
15. The code(s) for superficial, partial thickness, or full-thickness burns of the arm is
   a. 944.30
   b. 943.30
   c. 943.30, 943.20, 943.10
   d. 944.30, 944.20, 944.10
16. The code for myocardial infarction is
   a. 412
   b. 410.90
   c. 410.9
   d. 410.8
17. The code for abdominal pain; gastroenteritis, probably viral is
   a. 558.9
   b. 008.8
   c. 008.69
   d. 535.00
18. The code(s) for nausea; vomiting; fever; possible appendicitis is
   a. 787.02, 780.6
   b. 787.0
   c. 541
   d. 787.01, 780.6
19. The code for greenstick femur fracture is
   a. 821.39
   b. 821.00
   c. 821.0
   d. 821.3
20. The code for closed fracture, radius and ulna is
   a. 813.83
   b. 813.93
   c. 813.18
   d. 813.81
21. The code for postpartum hypertension presenting during pregnancy is
   a. 642.xx
   b. 401.9
   c. 401.0
   d. 643.xx
22. A patient with a history of colonic polyps presents for colonoscopy with symptoms of bloody stools and abdominal pain. The applicable code(s) is
   a. V12.72
   b. 578.2
   c. 578.1, 789.00
   d. 578.1, 789.00, V12.72
23. A patient presents with wrist pain from a fall on stairs. X-rays suggest a spiral radial fracture. The applicable code(s) is
   a. 719.43
   b. 719.43, E880.9
   c. 814.01
   d. 814.00, E880.9
24. The code for atherosclerotic heart disease is
   a. 414.01
   b. 414.0
   c. 414.00
   d. 414.9
25. The code for hypertensive heart disease is
   a. 402.00
   b. 402.90
   c. 402.0
   d. 402.10

ICD-9-CM Review

Now that you have begun to assess your ICD-9-CM coding skills, let's do some additional review. These additional guidelines are written in bulleted format so you may review them and make notations in your coding books when appropriate or necessary.

- Determine the main the diagnosis, condition, or problem that is the chief reason for the encounter.
- Determine the correct order for diagnosis for each procedure or encounter.
- Assign ICD-9-CM code(s), watching for fourth and/or fifth digit requirements.
- Code to the highest level of specificity.
- When signs and symptoms are an integral part of the diagnosis, no additional code is necessary for the signs and symptoms.
- Assign code(s) for all diagnoses, signs, and symptoms involved in the diagnosis or treatment for the encounter (including chronic systemic diseases).
- Do NOT assign diagnoses no longer applicable (if relevant, may use history of).
- Assign least significant diagnosis if not further clarified (e.g., closed vs. open fracture).
- Acute conditions are considered primary over other conditions.
- Only definitive diagnostic statements may be used. Words such as "rule out," "suspect," and "possible/probable" may not be used.

ICD-9-CM CODING TIPS

- Review symbols and terms.
- Understand appropriate use of manifestation codes (must have disease before manifestation; both codes are necessary).
- Identify the correct chapter of code assignment (incorporate ICD-9-CM index).
- Read all codes above and below selection for best choice.
- Read all notes ("includes," "excludes," "see also").
- Always cross-reference your selection from the alphabetical section with the numeric section of ICD-9-CM.

SPECIFIC ICD-9-CM CODING GUIDELINES

V Codes

- Encounter for circumstances influencing health status, not illness or injury.
- If chief reason for encounter, may be coded as primary code.
- Postoperative encounters may be coded as primary, preoperative diagnoses as secondary.
- May be used as primary if chief reason for encounter (e.g., chemotherapy).
- Incorporate V code index in ICD-9-CM coding book.

E Codes

- Are NEVER used as a primary diagnosis.
- Describe environmental events or circumstances that are the CAUSE of the problem.
- Incorporate E code index in ICD-9-CM coding book.

Hypertension Table

- Categorized as malignant, benign, specified.
- Unspecified if documented only as hypertension.
- Code 796.2 for elevated blood pressure not documented as hypertension.
- No relation can be assumed for conditions such as hypertension and heart disease EXCEPT *chronic* renal failure (not acute renal failure).

Neoplasm Table

- Categorized as malignant: primary, secondary, in situ.
- Other categories: benign, uncertain, unspecified.
- Metastatic to/metastatic from indicates point of origin/point spread.
- Codes listed in order of reason for encounter rather than primary, secondary.
- Neoplasms removed in remission: use history of.

Drugs and Chemicals Table

- Use adverse effects of drugs/poisoning decision tree.
- Therapeutic used only when drug is prescribed, given as directed, and no contraindications.
- Suicide attempts only coded when documented as such by physician.
- Requires at least two codes for each.

Injuries, Traumas, Burns

- Make sure diagnoses are matched to appropriate procedures.
- Most severe injury is coded first.
- Assign V codes for aftercare (e.g., pins, screws, plates).
- Assign E codes for accidents and injuries.
- Open/closed fracture codes do not necessarily agree with procedures performed.
- Assume closed fracture unless otherwise indicated.
- Multiple burns, same site: code only highest degree of burn.
- Rule of nines: evaluation of body surface area.
- Abrasions diagnosed as "deep": code as open wounds.
- Delayed healing or treatment, foreign body, major infection documented = complicated.
- Late effects: primary with cause/etiology coded secondary.

Maternity and Pregnancy Codes

- Problems unrelated to pregnancy: code condition and V22.2.
- Problems related to pregnancy become 600 series codes.
- Almost all pregnancy codes require fifth digits (except a handful of codes).
- Code 650, normal delivery, only when delivery is completely normal.
- V27.X is assigned to designate delivery on mother's encounter.

HCPCS Review

- Determine whether services should be coded with CPT or HCPCS.
- When multiple units of service are performed:
  - Rounding rules do not apply.
  - Days and units should be used.
- Incorporate HCPCS index into HCPCS book.

Coding Concepts

- Modifiers:
  - Used for further explanation; usually not paid under other circumstances.
  - Assigned by categories of service (e.g., evaluation and management [E & M], surgery).
  - Multiple modifier 99 use.
- Global procedures:
  - Package concept: services necessary to provide service, normal uncomplicated follow-up care.
  - Services outside normal follow-up require modifier.
- Symbols
  - •: New procedures
  - +: Add-on procedures

Review all the above guidelines, referencing the appropriate chapters in this text when clarification or additional information is needed. Make notes in the appropriate code book for guidelines you have not retained and try the sample examination for medical terminology, ICD-9-CM, HCPCS, and coding concepts.

Medical Terminology, ICD-9-CM, HCPCS, and Coding Concepts Practice Examination (Time Alloted: 1 Hour, 30 Minutes)

Medical Terminology

1. *Carcinoma in situ* refers to
   a. cancer contained within the original site, not spreading
   b. cancer that has spread or progressed outside the original site
   c. any neoplasm contained within the original site
   d. none of the above
2. *Cyano* refers to
   a. dying, death
   b. blue
   c. red
   d. white
3. The abbreviation ORIF refers to
   a. fracture care
   b. fracture repair with fixation
   c. open fracture repair with internal fixation
   d. open fracture repair without internal fixation
4. An *esophagoduodenoscopy* would encompass
   a. endoscopic examination of the esophagus
   b. endoscopic examination of the esophagus and small intestine
   c. endoscopic examination of the esophagus and duodenum
   d. surgical examination of the esophagus and small intestine
5. *Bronchitis* refers to
   a. an upper respiratory infection
   b. inflammation of the lungs
   c. inflammation of the bronchus
   d. any inflammatory process relating to the respiratory system
6. *Neoplasm* literally means
   a. new growth
   b. cancerous growth
   c. skin growth
   d. none of the above
7. *Rhinoplasty* indicates
   a. any surgical procedure connected with the nose
   b. surgical repair of the nose
   c. surgical excision of the nose
   d. creation of an artificial opening in the nose
8. The abbreviation *BID* indicates
   a. bedtime in doses
   b. two times per day
   c. bathing it daily
   d. three times per day
9. *Cholecystitis* refers to
   a. inflammation of the bladder
   b. inflammation of the gallbladder
   c. inflammation of the bladder and gallbladder
   d. diseases of the gallbladder
10. The prefix *coron* refers to
    a. cardiac
    b. coronary
    c. coronosis
    d. coronocentesis
11. *Amniocentesis* refers to
    a. surgical puncture to aspirate amniotic fluid
    b. incision into the amniotic cavity to remove amniotic fluid
    c. ultrasound to determine amniotic fluid level of the amniotic sac
    d. none of the above
12. An *esophagogastroduodenoscopy* encompasses
    a. scope inserted to examine the lower intestinal tract
    b. scope inserted to examine the esophagus, stomach, and small intestine
    c. scope inserted to examine the esophagus, stomach, and duodenum/jejunum
    d. scope inserted to evaluate the esophageal tract

13. The abbreviation *NKA* means
    a. no knee amputation
    b. no known asthma
    c. no known allergies
    d. no allergies

Anatomy

14. The *clavicle* refers to
    a. the long bone of the arm
    b. the collar bone
    c. the scapula
    d. the humerus
15. The *pleura* refers to
    a. the chest wall
    b. the layer of tissue lining the pleural cavity
    c. the layer of chest within the rib area
    d. the lungs
16. The *phalanges* refer to
    a. the fingers
    b. the toes
    c. both a and b
    d. long bone of the leg
17. The *femur, tibia, and fibula* all refer to
    a. leg bones
    b. arm bones
    c. primary bones of the arms and legs
    d. hip bones
18. The *cecum* refers to
    a. the proximal end of the large intestine
    b. a portion of the small intestine
    c. a portion of the stomach
    d. a portion of the duodenum
19. The term *cervical* refers to
    a. the neck and cervix
    b. the neck
    c. the cervix
    d. any portion of the female reproductive system
20. The *jejunum and duodenum* are
    a. portions of the small intestine
    b. portions of the large intestine
    c. portions of the esophagus
    d. portions of the ureters
21. The term *thoracic* pertains to
    a. the lower portion of the spinal column
    b. the uppermost portion of the spinal column
    c. the middle portion of the spinal column
    d. any portion of the spinal column
22. The tubes located in the urinary system are known as
    a. the urethra
    b. the ureters
    c. the fallopian tubes
    d. the bladders

ICD-9-CM

23. The code(s) for fracture of the tibia as the result of a fall is
    a. 823.80
    b. 823.80/E888.9
    c. 823.92
    d. 823.00
24. Malignant neoplasm of the breast with metastasis to the uterus. Primary site has been treated and is no longer present. Patient presents for chemotherapy. The codes should be
    a. 174.9, 198.82
    b. V58.11, 179, 174.9
    c. V58.11, 198.82, V10.3
    d. V58.11, 198.82, 199.0
25. The code(s) for upper respiratory infection with acute bronchitis is
    a. 465.9, 466.0
    b. 465.9, 490
    c. 466.0, 465.9
    d. 465.9
26. A child presents to the physician with no complaints; however, mom wants the child to be "checked out" after an auto accident. The code should be
    a. V71.4
    b. 924.9
    c. V65.5
    d. Either a or c
27. A child presents to the physician with exposure to chickenpox. The code should be
    a. 052.9
    b. V01.71
    c. V05.4
    d. V05.9
28. A child presents with a painful ear and diagnosis of possible otitis media. The code(s) should be
    a. 382.9
    b. 382.0/388.70
    c. 388.70
    d. 380.10
29. When a fracture is not specified as open or closed, it should be coded as
    a. open
    b. closed
    c. refer to the surgical procedure to determine
    d. do not code
30. The abbreviation NOS refers to
    a. not otherwise specified in the ICD-9-CM book
    b. not specified by the physician further
    c. both a and b
    d. either a or b

31. A patient presents to the hospital for normal delivery of a single newborn. The code(s) should be
   a. V22.2
   b. 650, V27.0
   c. V22.1
   d. 650
32. The abbreviation CAD would be coded as
   a. 414.0
   b. 414.00
   c. 414.01
   d. 429.2
33. Chest pain, R/O MI would be coded as
   a. 786.50
   b. 786.59
   c. 786.50/410.9
   d. 410.9

HCPCS

34. HCPCS level II codes are all represented as
   a. five-digit numeric codes
   b. five-digit codes, some alpha, some numeric
   c. five-digit alpha-numeric codes
   d. five-digit alpha codes
35. When coding drugs from HCPCS level II and multiple increments of service are provided,
   a. each unit of service is billed separately
   b. all units are coded or billed under "days/units"
   c. all units that are met by one half or more are coded as separate line items
   d. all units that are met by one half or more are coded as "days/units"
36. Injection of testosterone suspension, 12 mg IM, would be coded as
   a. J3150 × 2 units
   b. J3140 × 3 units
   c. J3140 × 2 units
   d. J3140 one unit
37. Radiopharmaceutical diagnostic imaging agent, sestamibi, TC99M would be coded as
   a. A9500
   b. A9503
   c. A9504
   d. A9150
38. Hospital bed, with rails and mattress, would be coded as
   a. E0260
   b. E0250
   c. E0251
   d. E0261

Coding Concepts

39. Evaluation and management services may not be used by anesthesiologists, pathologists, or radiologists.
   a. true
   b. false
40. When two surgical procedures are performed at the same time, during the same surgical session, through the same surgical site, and using the same approach, they are coded with
   a. modifier 51 appended to the secondary code(s)
   b. modifier 59 appended to the secondary code(s)
   c. modifier 51 appended to all codes involved
   d. modifier 59 appended to all codes involved
41. What is the significance of appending a modifier to a service?
   a. it makes certain that a service is considered for payment
   b. it decreases the charge
   c. it increases the charge
   d. all the above
42. Normal postoperative follow-up periods are determined by
   a. RBRVS guidelines
   b. carrier guidelines
   c. Medicare guidelines
   d. all the above
43. Global procedures include all services performed during the postoperative period.
   a. true
   b. false

Assess your skills in the above areas and review areas that need additional work before progressing to the surgical coding section. This mock examination contains the same number of questions in the AAPC CPC certification examination. The number of questions differs for the AHIMA CCS-P examination; however, the examination encompasses the same material and concepts. Let's start the review of CPT coding with a brief overview of CPT coding guidelines.

Basics of CPT Coding Concepts

Suggestion: The professional edition of CPT offers additional notations and illustrations of medical procedures. If you are unfamiliar with a number of procedures or procedures not specific to the specialty you currently code, the professional edition may prove helpful.

- Always identify what section the service will be coded from and follow the guidelines and modifiers for that section of CPT only.
- Use the index to identify the general area to reference for CPT coding only. The index in CPT is NOT intended as a cross-reference mechanism, as is ICD-9-CM.
- Always code the highest level of specificity (e.g., open versus closed, complicated versus simple).
- Use the "narrowing down" principle at all times by determining:
  1. Section in CPT for the code
  2. Anatomic progression of the code in the section

3. Modifiers appropriate for the section
4. Individual guidelines for code series selected

PREPARING TO BECOME AN EFFICIENT CPT CODER

- Make sure guidelines and modifiers are specific to the coding section selected. For example, some anesthesia modifiers are used only for anesthesia. Use the modifier listing on the inside cover of the CPT and mark the section(s) for which each modifier is applicable.
- If a guideline pertains to a specific coding section, you may want to make a note in that section as well as a cross-reference. For example, guidelines for operative visits code 99024 are listed in the medicine section; however, you may be more inclined to use these when coding E & M services. Note the page number in the medicine section to refer to or highlight the most important information.
- When more than one CPT code is necessary to code a specific encounter, consider whether a modifier is necessary.
- If coding a procedure from the surgery section and visit is involved, check the guidelines for preoperative and postoperative visits and/or use a modifier. If the E & M visit is significantly separately identifiable, a modifier will be necessary.
- If tabs are available for your CPT book, use them if they are not already inserted. You may insert additional tabs as you feel appropriate and subdivide the most commonly used sections.
- Read and review guidelines in each chapter as well as guidelines given at the beginning of each subsection. Highlight these narrative sections so the most important "do's and don'ts" will be readily accessible without reading the narrative data each time.

SURGICAL CODING CONCEPTS

Following is a basic outline of surgery coding. It is not intended to capture all the information on surgery coding, but to review the basics learned during your comprehensive study of surgery coding. As you review these guidelines, refer to the appropriate chapters in this text and study the more comprehensive material available. Practice additional coding exercises in the text and Workbook or on the Evolve site. The more you practice, the more familiar and comfortable you will become with the surgery section of CPT. This section is essential to passing the certification examination because a large portion of the test encompasses surgical coding, surgical concepts, and surgery modifiers on both the AAPC and AHIMA physician certification examinations.

General Guidelines

- Global concept
- Normal uncomplicated postoperative periods

Understanding what components are included in the surgical procedure is integral to the overall concept of surgical coding.

Modifier Codes

21	Unusual procedure services
50	Bilateral
	List one line for first procedure, second identical service with modifier 50
51	Multiple procedures
	Same session, same approach, same anatomic site (one session, one approach, one anatomic site)
52	Reduced services
53	Discontinued services
	Physician decision based on patient's well-being
54	Surgical care only
55	Postoperative care only
56	Preoperative care only
57	Decision for surgery (usually E & M)
58	Staged/related services
	Staged *or* related
59	Distinct procedures
	Distinct session, distinct approach, distinct anatomic site(s)
62	Two surgeons
63	Procedure on infant <4 kg
66	Surgical team
78	Return to operating room
79	Unrelated procedure/service same physician during postoperative period
80	Assistant surgeon
81	Minimum assistant surgeon
82	Assistant surgeon (qualified resident not available)

Integumentary System

Lesions

- Benign/malignant
- Location (anatomic group)
- Size (in centimeters; includes margins)
- Cannot be combined
- Closure other than simple may be coded
- Reexcision same session, code only final excision
- Reexcision later, code with modifier 58

Repairs

- Complexity (simple/intermediate/complex)
- Location (anatomic grouping)
- Size (in centimeters)
- Same complexity/grouping can be combined
- Staples, adhesive glues coded, adhesive strips not coded

Skin Grafts

- Extent (pinch/split/full)
- Location (anatomic grouping)
- Size (in square centimeters)
- Extensive preparation of graft site codes

Adjacent Tissue Transfers

- Rotation/advancement flaps
- W/Y/Z plasties

- Size (in square centimeters)
- Removal of lesion included

Destruction Lesions

- Benign/premalignant versus malignant

Mohs' Micrographic Surgery

- Physician must perform two components: surgery and pathology

Breast

- Incision/excision/introduction/repair/reconstruction
- Biopsies versus excisions
- Preoperative markers
- Mastectomies: partial/subcutaneous/radical/modified radical
- Insertion of breast prosthesis: during/after mastectomy

Musculoskeletal System

General Guidelines

- By anatomic site
- Incision/excision/repair/revision/reconstruction/fracture/dislocation
- Specific site
- Specific procedure technique: open/closed, with/without manipulation, fixation

Cast Application

- Included in global allowance
- Additional/replacements may be coded
- May be coded if surgical/definitive treatment not provided

Arthroscopy

- Last section in musculoskeletal system
- Least/most significant
- Anatomic order
- Separate compartments are considered distinct (for knees)

Respiratory System

General Guidelines

- By anatomic site (anatomic order)
- Incision/excision/endoscopy/removal foreign body/repair/revision/reconstruction
- Specific site
- Specific procedure technique
- Endoscopic introduction included in any endoscopic procedure
- Endoscopic versus open

Cardiovascular System

Pacemakers and Defibrillators

- Permanent/temporary/replacement
- Single/dual
- Battery is generator (pulse generator)

Coronary Artery Bypass Grafting (CABG)

- Venous (one word/one code)
- Arterial (one word/one code)
- Venous/arterial (two words/two codes)
- Obtaining vein included except for upper extremity vein and femoropopliteal
- Redos: code 33530

Vascular Catheters

- Central venous versus peripheral
- Tunneled/nontunneled
- Ports/pumps
- By age

Endovascular Repair and Abdominal Aortic Aneurysm

- + Insertion guidewires/catheters
- + Fluoroscopic guidance
- + Other interventions

Angioplasty and Atherectomy (not Coronary)

Vascular Injection Procedures

- Selective: needle/catheter moved/repositioned/manipulated/guides
- Nonselective: directed in vessel/not moved
- Code used must accurately reflect puncture site and final catheter position
- Highest order catheterization coded, not lesser ones

Digestive System

General Guidelines

- By anatomic site (anatomic order)
- Incision/excision/endoscopy/repair/revision/reconstruction
- Specific site
- Specific procedure technique
- Endoscopic technique included in any endoscopic surgical procedure

Tonsillectomy and Adenoidectomy

- By age/areas removed

Hernia Repairs

- Types of repair (inguinal/lumbar/femoral/ventral/incisional/umbilical)
- Initial/recurrent
- Age
- Open/laparoscopic

Endoscopies: Colon

- Proctosigmoidoscopy
- Sigmoidoscopy
- Colonoscopy
- Use of modifiers 52 and 53

Endoscopies: Upper Gastrointestinal

- Esophagogastroduodenoscopy
- Multiple endoscopic procedures
- Use of modifier 51 versus 59

Appendectomies and Cholecystectomies

- Laparoscopic/open
- Incidental appendectomy
- Dilation without direct visualization: 43450 series
- Only successful dilation is coded

Genitourinary System

Urinary System

- Diagnostic endoscopies included in surgical
- Watch "separate procedures"
- Urodynamics: modifier 51 for multiple procedures

Male Genital System

- Circumcisions: newborn/other, method
- Vasectomy: excision/vas deferens
- Prostatectomy (both male genital and urinary)

Female Genital System

- Hysterectomy (vaginal vs. abdominal)
- Tubal ligation
    - Laparoscopic
    - Time of cesarean section
    - During same hospitalization
    - Surgical

Maternity Care

- Antepartum, delivery, postpartum
- Categorized by type delivery (vaginal/cesarean section, vaginal birth after cesarean section [VBAC])
- Each portion of package has separate codes when split
- Abortion includes spontaneous
- Missed abortion: dead fetus retained
- Incomplete abortion: products of conception retained

Nervous System and Sense Organs

Nervous System

- Skull base: approach/definitive/repair codeable
- Carpal tunnel
    - Nonlaparoscopic is transection of carpal nerve
- Laminectomy: excision of lamina
- Laminotomy: incision of lamina
- Code 95990 for refilling or maintenance of spinal infusion pump
- Percutaneous placement of epidural or intrathecal catheter
    - Codes 62270-73, 62280-84, 62310-19
- Spinal cord neurostimulator implantations by site stimulated, not approach

Eye and Ocular Adnexa

- Strabismus surgery: horizontal/vertical, number of muscles
- Cataract: extracapsular or intracapsular, with or without intraocular lens
- Radiokeratotomy

Auditory

- Myringotomy versus tympanoplasty
- Use of operating microscope: not modifier 51

After you have reviewed the above information and additional information in the surgery section of this text, try the following surgery practice exercises.

Surgery Practice Examination: Part 1 (Time Alloted: 55 to 60 Minutes)

Chose the correct codes for the following encounters.

1. Extensive basal cell carcinoma of the left retroauricular area. Wide excision of basal cell carcinoma of the left auricular area with harvesting skin graft of the left thigh and skin graft application to the area of excisional lesion removal.
    a. 11640, 15120
    b. 11640, 15000, 15120
    c. 15120
    d. 11440
2. The right breast was markedly enlarged consistent with gynecomastia and benign. The incision was made and the breast tissue that was marked out was dissected free. The breast tissue was then closed in layers.
    a. 19100-RT
    b. 19120-RT
    c. 19300-RT
    d. 19160-RT
3. Arthroscope was inserted into the shoulder and the surfaces of the humeral head and glenoid were intact without evidence of cracking or tears. The rotator cuff showed fraying and the decision was made to perform an arthroscopic acromioplasty. A rotary shaver was used to perform a bursectomy with debris removed via shaver. A rotary burr was then used to perform an anterior inferior acromioplasty with debris produced removed via suction. Because of the location of the tear, the decision was made to repair the rotator cuff through a mini-arthrotomy. This was accomplished and the procedure was completed.
    a. 29826
    b. 23410, 29826-51
    c. 23412
    d. 23415

4. After general anesthesia was obtained, the knee was easily flexed to about 85 degrees. It was then gently manipulated so that it flexed to about 125 degrees. Scar tissue bands were heard popping with gentle manipulation. Following this the knee passively flexed to 115 degrees. Full extension was achieved and the knee was then injected with 80 mg of Kenalog and Marcaine.
   a. 27570
   b. 27570, 20610-51
   c. 20610
   d. 27580
5. Left knee arthroscopy is done under four portals: anterolateral, anteromedial, superolateral, and posteromedial. The diagnostic arthroscopy was started, placing the arthroscope in the anterolateral portal. There is severe fibrosis and hypertrophy of the fat pad and grade II and III chondromalacia of the femoral condyle. A partial medial meniscectomy is performed as well as a partial lateral meniscectomy after which a chondroplasty of the patellofemoral joint was performed.
   a. 29880-LT
   b. 29880-LT, 29877-59-LT, 29870-50-LT
   c. 29880-LT, 29877-59-LT
   d. 29881-LT
6. The right posterior chest was prepped with Betadine, sterile technique. A Pharmaseal catheter was instilled into the right posterior clavicular line, two spaces below the scapula and 1.2 L of serosanguineous fluid was removed without difficulty. Once the thoracentesis was completed, the patient had decreased shortness of breath.
   a. 32095
   b. 32421
   c. 31899
   d. 32422
7. Patient was prepped in the usual manner and the scope was advanced through the cecum. There was an area that appeared to be flat and had an almost flat lesion, where I took a few biopsies. The rest of the colon appeared normal. In the sigmoid colon two polyps were identified and both were snared in toto and retrieved.
   a. 45385, 45380-51, 45378-51
   b. 45385
   c. 45385, 45378-51
   d. 45385, 45380-51
8. A guide wire was inserted into the right orifice (urethra) via the cystoscopy, advanced all the way to the right renal pelvis, following which the distal right ureter was dilated using a balloon dilator, size 10 cm and a #9 rigid ureteroscopy was introduced transurethrally.
   a. 52341
   b. 52341, 52000-51
   c. 52000
   d. 52282
9. Chronic wound of the left thigh. FTSG was obtained from the right thigh and placed on a 4 × 4 cm chronic wound on the left thigh after appropriate flushing and irrigation.
   a. 15100, 15002
   b. 15002
   c. 15220
   d. 15100
10. On admission, the patient was taken to the x-ray suite where the radiologist, with ultrasonic guidance, localized a breast lump with a needle. The patient was then taken to the surgical suite, where the right breast was cleaned with DuraPrep and draped. The entry point was at about the 3 o'clock position. The needle was localized and followed to its termination. The area in question was identified, a generous margin was achieved and encompassing the needle and node in question; all of this was taken in one piece and sent to pathology.
    a. 19100
    b. 19120
    c. 19125
    d. 19125, 19290
11. Closed reduction with manipulation of a metacarpal fracture of the thumb and index finger. Under general anesthesia, the patient was placed in position and lateral incision made distal to the fractures. Guidewires and pins were inserted and screws inserted to percutaneous fixate the fractures. Closure performed with 2-0 and 3-0 Dexon and a short arm splint applied.
    a. 26605 × 2
    b. 26608 × 2
    c. 26608
    d. 26650
12. Patient jumped a fence and twisted his knee when he fell. The orthopedic surgeon performed a diagnostic arthroscopy. It was found that the patient had torn his medial meniscus and a meniscal repair was performed.
    a. 29882
    b. 29882, 29870-51
    c. 29881
    d. 29881, 29870-51
13. Colonoscopy with biopsy of polyp, excision of another polyp, snare technique and fulguration of bleeding.
    a. 45385, 45382-51, 45380-51
    b. 45385, 45382-51
    c. 45385
    d. 45382, 45385-51, 45380-51

14. Digital rectal examination was done and no masses palpable. Scope was introduced, advanced to the cecum identified by the ileocecal valve. The scope was withdrawn watching for AV malformations, masses, polyps. In the sigmoid colon two polyps were identified, both of them less than 5 mm, which were hot biopsied and sent to histopathology.
    a. 45380
    b. 45384
    c. 45380, 45378-51
    d. 45384, 45382-51, 45380-51
15. Patient prepped and draped in the dorsal lithotomy; using the resectoscope the urethra and bladder were inspected with a significant bladder contraction. Guide wire was inserted through the contraction using Collins knife cutting. At the two, ten, seven and five o'clock positions the bladder neck was opened.
    a. 52400
    b. 52500
    c. 52510
    d. 52000
16. Cystoscope was inserted and bladder shows trabeculation but no mucosal lesions, no erythema, and no stones were identified. The bladder was emptied and cystoscope removed. Finger was inserted into the rectum; the prostate was large along the posterolateral ridge toward the apex.
    a. 52005
    b. 52255
    c. 52000
    d. 52001
17. A 2-cm infraumbilical incision was performed and peritoneum was insufflated and trocar and scope introduced. Liver, bowel, appendix, bladder, and uterus appeared normal. There were multiple cysts on the left ovary consistent with benign follicular cysts which were aspirated. Chromotubation was then performed and bilateral tubal patency was documented.
    a. 49322
    b. 58350
    c. 49322, 58350-51
    d. 58679
18. Veress needle was inserted and large trocar was inserted followed by insertion of the laparoscope. There was no evidence that an IUD had perforated the uterus. The IUD was noted to be embedded in the omental pad anteriorly. Using the grasper through the scope, the IUD was freed up and pulled in toto through the portal. The IUD was removed and the CO_2 allowed to escape and the incision was closed.
    a. 58100
    b. 58301
    c. 58300
    d. 58552
19. A 65-year-old undergoing chemotherapy, poor peripheral IV access, presents for insertion of Infuse-A-Port. Guide wire was placed into the right internal jugular vein to the superior vena cava. A pocket was made under the right anterior chest. The catheter was threaded into the superior vena cava. A tunneling device was used to tunnel the catheter, hooked to the Infuse-A-Port, and the pocket was then closed.
    a. 36560
    b. 36561
    c. 36558
    d. 36571
20. Patient presents for liver biopsy due to elevated liver enzymes. The area of the biopsy site was chosen, and a small nick was made on the skin and advanced all the way into the liver capsule. The patient was told to hold her breath and the biopsy gun was inserted into the liver. Obtained a biopsy, which was taken the pathology.
    a. 47100
    b. 47000
    c. 47010
    d. 47999
21. Patient with serous otitis media presents for replacement of right ventilation tube and placement of left myringotomy tube. Following the administration of general anesthesia, the right tube was examined and determined to need removal. A replacement tube was placed in the right ear. A myringotomy was performed and fluid was aspirated. A modified T-grommet tube was placed in the left ear.
    a. 69436-LT, 69436-76-52-RT
    b. 69436-50
    c. 69421-50
    d. 69436-LT, 69424-RT
22. A semicircular incision was given in the margin of the umbilicus of this 7-year-old, dividing the skin and subcutaneous tissue and lifting the skin. Dissection was carried down to the fascia. Posterior part of the umbilical skin was detached and exam showed a pinpoint opening in which the omentum was stuck. This opening was enlarged transversely and the omentum, which was adhesed to the umbilical opening, was released and put back into the abdominal cavity.
    a. 49600
    b. 49587
    c. 49585
    d. 49582
23. Redundant skin of the superior eyelids was demarcated with a marking pen. The skin and orbicularis were incised, elevated, and excised. The orbital septum was opened. Protruding fat hernia pads were

isolated, clamped, and excised. An identical procedure was performed on the opposite eye.
a. 15820-50
b. 15823-50
c. 15822-50
d. 15821-50

24. Patient presents with left axillary swelling. Left axilla was prepped and incision was made. Axillary contents were removed and there were some enlarged lymph nodes.
a. 38530
b. 38500
c. 38520
d. 38525

25. Patient with 2 × 2 cm mass in the right ovary presents for exploratory laparoscopy. The left ovary had a 1 × 4 cm simple cyst filled with old purple fluid consistent with old endometrioma. The right ovary pulled up the pelvic side wall into the cul-de-sac area and there were a lot of fibrinous exudates. The round remnants on each side were grasped and dissection was performed into the broad ligaments. The cyst and its contents were aspirated.
a. 58800
b. 58805
c. 58820
d. 49322

Review the questions missed in the practice examination, the CPT surgery guidelines, and concepts that were missed or not applied appropriately. Then try the practice examination below. Keep in mind that each of these tests should be timed so that you experience a realistic testing scenario. The Section II, Surgery examination has 60 questions and should be completed in 1 hour and 45 minutes or less.

Surgery Practice Examination: Part 2 (Alloted Time: 2 Hours)

Choose the correct codes for the following encounters.

1. Chronic wound of left arm. STSG was obtained from the right thigh and placed on a 4 × 4 inch chronic wound on the left arm after appropriate flushing and irrigation.
a. 15200
b. 15220
c. 15120
d. 15100

2. Right subcutaneous mastectomy, skin tag removal. Inscribed a circumareolar incision and the dermis and subcutaneous breast tissue was infiltrated. Areola was elevated off the breast tissue. Breast tissue was excised with electrocautery and removed. Right groin was exposed and prepped. Dermis at the base of the skin tag was infiltrated and the skin tag was removed by shave excision.
a. 19303-RT
b. 19300-RT
c. 19304-RT, 11200
d. 19304-RT, 11200

3. Wide excision of basal cell carcinoma, 1.5 cm of left nares. Harvesting of split-thickness graft from left neck and application of graft to the site of the excision of the left nares.
a. 11642
b. 11642, 15120
c. 15120
d. 11442, 15120

4. Excision biopsy of left foot mass, 1.5 cm, identified as ganglion cyst on pathology, closed, simple.
a. 28090
b. 11402
c. 28090, 12001
d. 11402, 12002

5. Laceration repairs as follows:
1.5 cm arm, simple
2.5 cm arm, simple
1.5 cm arm, intermediate
a. 12001, 12001-51, 12031
b. 12001 × 2, 12031
c. 12031, 12002-51
d. none of the above

6. Skin graft, split, from thigh to the arm to cover a defect 3 × 4 cm.
a. 15120
b. 15220
c. 15002, 15220
d. 15100

7. Excision of breast mass, 2.5 cm identified by preoperative radiologic marker.
a. 19100
b. 19120
c. 19125, 19290
d. 19125

8. A 1.3-cm nasal lesion was excised from the nasal labial area. Following this, a pedicle flap was elevated along the nasal labial area and rotated into anatomic position. This was sutured into placed and excellent coverage was noted.
a. 11641, 14060
b. 14060
c. 11641
d. 11640

9. On admission, the patient was taken to the x-ray suite where the radiologist, with ultrasonic guidance, localized a breast lump with a needle. The patient was then taken to the surgical suite, where the right breast was cleaned with DuraPrep and draped; the entry point was at about the 3 o'clock

position. The needle was localized and followed to its termination. The area in question was identified, a generous margin was achieved and encompassing the needle and the node in question. All of this was taken in one piece and sent to radiology for evaluation. (NOTE: Code the surgeon's procedure.)

a. 19120
b. 19125
c. 19125, 19290
d. 19101

10. The ulcer at the second MJP was circumscribed and removed in toto. The tourniquet was let down and a Apligraf skin graft was prepared and cut to size and stitched into place with 4-0 Nylon simple interrupted sutures.

a. 15340
b. 15341
c. 15220
d. 15240

11. Open reduction with internal fixation of a metacarpal fracture of the thumb and index finger. The patient, under general anesthesia, was placed in position and a lateral incision made and with manipulation the metacarpal fractures were identified. Guide wires were inserted and a screw inserted. Closure was performed with 0, 2-0, and 3-0 Dexon and a short arm splint was applied.

a. 26600
b. 26607
c. 26615 × 2
d. 26608 × 2

12. Patient fell from a tree house and fractured his right fibula/tibia. Closed treatment of these shaft fractures after manipulation and placement of traction was performed.

a. 27758
b. 27760
c. 27750
d. 27752

13. Patient tripped and hit foot on chair last night. His toes continued to have pain and the next day he visited his physician. Radiologic exam found he had fractures his great and second toe. The physician strapped his toes and patient was released.

a. 28456
b. 29550
c. 29550, 29550-51
d. none of the above

14. 68-year-old female had a total hip replacement 4 years ago. When she was getting out of her chair today, she noticed severe pain in her hip and was unable to move. Examination revealed she had dislocated her prosthetic hip. Orthopedic surgeon manipulated her hip back into place.

a. 27250-54
b. 27253
c. 27265
d. none of the above

15. Patient arrives for visit 3 weeks after repair of a fracture. He is returning to the physician to have a new short leg walking cast applied due to the initial cast being damaged in the shower.

a. 29305-58
b. 29425-58
c. postoperative charge, no charge
d. 99024

16. Patient arrives to have long arm cast removed following a fracture repair done approximately 6 weeks previous.

a. no charge
b. 99024
c. 29075
d. none of the above

17. Patient with patellofemoral arthritis of the left knee. Introduction of the Stryker shaver up to the patella and chondroplasty performed, smoothing down some of the chondromalacia.

a. 29870-LT
b. 29870-LT, 29877-59-LT
c. 29883-LT
d. 29877-LT

18. Internal derangement of the left knee with operative arthroscopy of the left knee with chondroplasty of the patellofemoral joint and medial compartment with partial medial meniscectomy of the left knee.

a. 29877-LT
b. 29881-LT, 29877-59-LT
c. 29881-LT
d. 29881-LT, 29877-LT

19. Syndesmotic screw status post pons fracture with left proximal fibular fracture with removal of hardware.

a. 20680
b. 20670
c. 20694
d. 20680-LT

20. Anterior instability of right shoulder with open Bankard repair with open right capsular shift. Shoulder capsule was elevated with bone and roughened up on the surface. Loose fragments were irrigated and removed. Advanced capsule into position tying sutures down over the capsule itself. Pushed humeral head back into place and closed with pants-over-vest fashion.

a. 23455-RT
b. 23455-RT, 23460-RT
c. 23460-RT
d. 23929

21. Bronchoscope was passed into the tracheobronchial tree. Right upper lobe, right middle lobe, right lower lobe were all patent as well as left lower and upper. The bronchoscope was taken through the right upper lobe. Brushings and two biopsies were obtained of the density in the right upper lobe.
   a. 31625
   b. 31628
   c. 31628, 31629
   d. 31628, 31632
22. Anterior laryngoscope was entered into the oral cavity and passed down to the level of the vocal cords. Polyps were identified on the left false vocal cord as well as the right true vocal cord in the anterior-most region. CO2 laser was used to excise the polyps, identified as papillomas, without injuring the vocal cords.
   a. 31536
   b. 31540
   c. 31570
   d. 31541
23. A thoracentesis kit with aspirating catheter was advanced into the intercostal space, and 1 liter of cloudy amber fluid was removed. The patient had some mild chest tightness and the catheter was removed at that time.
   a. 32421
   b. 32000
   c. 32422
   d. 32310
24. Utilizing a 5-inch sinuscope and microdebrider, the right concha bullosa was resected in its lateral portion. Subsequently, the anterior wall of the ethmoids was removed with the microdebrider and the hypertrophic mucosa and anterior ethmoid cells were cleared with the microdebrider. The maxillary sinus ostia was cleared of hypertrophic mucosa on the right side followed by the same procedures on the left.
   a. 31267-50, 31254-51/50
   b. 31267-50, 31254-51/50, 31240-51
   c. 31254-50
   d. 31267-50
25. Hypertrophic mucosa of the lateral nasal wall and anterior wall of the ethmoid bulla were removed with microdebrider. The maxillary sinus was then addressed and thickened polypoid mucosa was removed from the ostia and sinus.
   a. 31267, 31254-51
   b. 31254, 31267
   c. 31267
   d. 31254
26. Using Seldinger technique, a guide wire was placed into the right internal jugular vein to the superior vena cava of a 65-year-old female. Then made a pocket under the right anterior chest wall and created it so the Infuse-A-Port would fit into the pocket. The guide wire was removed and the catheter threaded into the superior vena cava. Then using the tunneling device, the catheter was tunneled onto the anterior chest wall and the port placed in the pocket, at which time the pocket was closed.
   a. 36560
   b. 36561
   c. 36563
   d. 36565
27. Traumatic external nasal and internal nasal septal defect. There were several fractures in the septum. Portions of the cartilaginous septum were missing. There were several tears in the mucoperichondrium. Remnants were removed as well as spurs off the maxillary crest. A tip support was reconstructed with cartilaginous graft obtained from removed cartilaginous septum remnants.
   a. 30540
   b. 30520
   c. 30620
   d. 30630
28. An 18-gauge spring-loaded needle was inserted into the lung and three cores of tissue were removed using the coaxial spring-loaded biopsy needle.
   a. 32400 × 3
   b. 32405
   c. 32405 × 3
   d. 32400
29. An area in the right posterior chest was punctured using an 18-gauge needle and a 8.5 French drainage catheter was inserted. Approximately 100 cc of yellowish pus without odor was withdrawn. Catheter was secured and left in position.
   a. 32000
   b. 32002
   c. 32020
   d. 32035
30. Incision was made over the previous pacemaker scar and the pulse generator was extruded and the leads disconnected. Atrial lead is #4058, serial #02500, ventricular lead is #4262, serial #060719. The new pacemaker was model Meridiem DR, Model #1276, serial #415811. The leads were reconnected, the pocket irrigated, and closure done in layers.
   a. 33208
   b. 33212
   c. 33233, 33213
   d. 33213
31. Patient is a 7-year-old with adenoidotonsillitis. With patient under general anesthesia, tonsils were grasped with Allis forceps and an incision was made around the anterior tonsillar pillar. The tonsillar capsule was identified and the tonsil bluntly dis-

sected free. Identical procedure performed on the other tonsil as well. All bleeding was controlled, and at close of the tonsillectomy no bleeding was present. The nasopharynx was viewed indirectly, and a considerable amount of adenoid tissue was removed. It was curetted and all nubbins of adenoid tissue were removed. No bleeding was present at the end of the procedure, and the postoperative condition of the patient was good.
a. 42821
b. 42860
c. 42825
d. none of the above

32. ERCP with sphincterotomy and stent placement.
a. 43262
b. 43262, 43268-51
c. 43268, 43262-51
d. 52332

33. Hernia, initial, inguinal, age 4 years.
a. 49495
b. 49500
c. 49520
d. 49501

34. Laparoscopic appendectomy.
a. 44970
b. 44950
c. 44955
d. 44979

35. Colonoscopy completed to the cecum, visualizing the splenic flexure.
a. 45380
b. 45378-53
c. 45378-52
d. 45378

36. A 3-year-old swallowed a quarter and x-ray confirms position in the high esophagus. Patient was brought to the endoscopy suite and the endoscope was introduced through the pharynx without difficulty. The coin was noted immediately upon entering the esophagus. This was grasped with a tooth tenaculum and then pulled intact from the esophagus.
a. 43215
b. 43235
c. 43247
d. 43247, 43235-51

37. Digital rectal examination was done and no masses palpable. The scope was introduced and advanced all the way up to the cecum, identified by the ileocecal valve and appendical orifice. The scope was withdrawn watching all of the colonic mucosa. There were several pockets of liquid stools at various stages. No AV malformations noticed, no masses, no polyps. In the sigmoid region there were two polyps adjacent to each other, one a little larger than the other, both of them less than 5 mm, which were hot biopsied and sent for histopathology. The scope was straightened and pulled out.
a. 45384
b. 45380
c. 45384 × 2
d. 45380, 45384

38. Patient with left inguinal pain following inguinal hernia repair 5 years ago. The old incision was reopened and dissection carried down to the external oblique. The external ring was located and the external oblique opened in line with its fiber. Spermatic cord was isolated, and the mesh placed previously was palpable. Patient was set upright and instructed to cough; however, no defect could be identified even with straining. The incision was closed.
a. 49000
b. 49010
c. 49329
d. 49320

39. Colonoscope introduced and advanced to the cecum. Beyond the cecal valve was an area that appeared to be flat with cauliflower-looking appearance. Took a few biopsies, hot and cold, from the area in question. In the area of the sigmoid colon, two polyps were identified which were snared in toto and retrieved.
a. 45385
b. 45380
c. 45385, 45380-51
d. 45383

40. Colonoscope was introduced through all flexures of the cecum. One polyp was identified in the splenic flexure and was removed with biopsy forceps. The patient had minimal AV malformation and bleeding was cauterized.
a. 45382
b. 45380, 45382-51
c. 45382, 45380-51
d. 45380

41. Patient prepped and draped in the dorsal lithotomy position and the urethra and bladder were inspected using the resectoscope. He had about a 10 French bladder neck contraction. Guide wire was inserted through the contraction, and then using the Collins knife cutting at the 2, 10, 7, and 5 o'clock positions the bladder neck was opened. Electrical cautery was used to obtain hemostasis.
a. 52601
b. 52500
c. 52510
d. 52500-59

42. The patient was positioned in the dorsolithotomy position and the abdomen, vulva, and vagina were prepped with Betadine. The cervix was extending

outside the vagina. The cervix was grasped with a tenaculum. The anterior incision was made approximately 2 cm from the cervix and anteriorly up to 5 cm from the urethral meatus. The denuded strip was approximately 2 to 3 cm in width. The denuded strip was grasped with a clamp, a posterior incision was made, and the procedure was then completed by suturing the anterior vaginal mucosa to the posterior vaginal mucosa and then successive suturing to elevate the uterus and anterior bladder wall. The vaginal epithelium was then closed with a continuous suture of Vicryl.

a. 57110
b. 57100
c. 57120
d. 57130

43. Cystoscope was inserted and the bladder showed trabeculation but no mucosal lesions, no erythema, no stones. The bladder was emptied and cystoscope removed. Finger was inserted into the rectum and the prostate was large. There was a hard, but not rock hard ridge posterolateral prostate toward the apex. The rest of the prostate was just very large and firm.

a. 52000
b. 55700
c. 52000, 55700
d. 55705

44. Evaluation under anesthesia revealed a normal uterus and no adnexal masses. Weighted speculum placed in the vagina. Cervix grasped with single-tooth tenaculum. There was a small polyp or redundant cervix, which was removed. Cervix had been dilated to a #21 French Bratt dilator and an endometrial curettage revealed scant tissue. The single-tooth tenaculum was removed, as was the weighted vaginal speculum.

a. 57505-51, 58120
b. 57505
c. 57505, 58120
d. 58120

45. A 2-cm infraumbilical incision was performed and the peritoneum was insufflated, and the trocar and the scope were introduced under direct vision. The liver, bowel, appendix, bladder, and uterus appeared normal. The cul-de-sac showed evidence of endometriosis, as did the right ovary. There were multiple cysts on the left ovary consistent with benign follicular cysts. The laser apparatus was used to laser ablate the endometriotic implants on the left uterosacral and cul-de-sac area as well as on the right salpinx and the right ovary. Chromotubation was then performed and bilateral tubal patency was documented. The incision was reapproximated using 4-0 Vicryl and the tenaculum was removed.

a. 49329, 58350-51
b. 58662, 58350-51
c. 58662, 58350
d. 58350

46. Enlarged lymph node in the left groin. Transverse skin incision was made in the left groin just above the inguinal ligament. Enlarged lymph node was identified, isolated, and removed.

a. 38500
b. 38505
c. 38510
d. 38520

47. A subumbilical incision was made and a blunt cannula placed. The liver, bowel, and appendix appeared normal. The patient's previous tubal ligation was noted. There were a few adhesions to the side wall that were taken down by sharp dissection. The left ovary was normal; the right ovary had a 5-cm cyst that was marsupialized with scissors and allowed to drain with clear fluid. It should be noted that there were large varicosities of the pelvic wall bilaterally. Thus we had to remove the adhesions, open up the ovarian cyst, and marsupialize. The previous subumbilical incision was closed with 2-0 Vicryl.

a. 58679-22
b. 58679
c. 58679, 58660-51
d. 49322

48. A 74-year-old male with suprapubic abdominal pressure. Catheter was placed and left indwelling until drained completely. He will follow up with urologist.

a. 51701
b. 51703
c. 51702
d. 51700

49. Cervix was dilated and a #10 suction cannula was introduced. The walls of the anterior, posterior, and lateral endometrial cavity were curetted, yielding moderate amounts of retained products of conception. Additional tissue was removed and a Foley catheter was used to fill the bladder for proper visualization during the procedure.

a. 59820
b. 59841
c. 59812
d. 59840

The remainder of the exercises require you to assign the appropriate CPT codes and ICD-9-CM codes. Assign modifiers as appropriate.

50. Cystoscope was inserted into the bladder and the bladder shows diffuse erythema throughout. No specific lesions were located and a 5 French stent was advanced into the right ureteral orifice. A Foley catheter placed previously was removed and the stent left in place.

CPT code(s): ____________________
ICD-9-CM code(s): ____________________

51. Patient was placed in the sitting position and palpation of the longissimus muscle and multifidus muscle revealed eight trigger points. These trigger points were marked, skin prepped, and each trigger point injected with Marcaine 0.25%.
CPT code(s): ____________________
ICD-9-CM code(s): ____________________

52. Patient has intrathecal pump and PCP has requested an increase in the patient's dosage of morphine. Patient was placed supine and analysis indicated reserve volume of 14.5 cc with continuous rate of 0.45 mg per hour. His pump was increased to provide a continuous rate of 0.495 mg per hour to a total of 11.882 mg per day.
CPT code(s): ____________________
ICD-9-CM code(s): ____________________

53. The medial right elbow was approached through a curving posteromedial incision The ulnar nerve was identified in the wrist and freed and dissected. Next a palmar incision was made in line with the fourth ray, the palmar aponeurosis was divided. The carpal ligament was divided well into the distal forearm to ensure complete incision of the transverse carpal tunnel. External neurolysis was performed.
CPT code(s): ____________________
ICD-9-CM code(s): ____________________

54. C7-C8 was identified and 0.25% bupivacaine was injected as a test dose. Then 40 mg of Depo-Medrol was injected into the epidural space and the needle removed.
CPT code(s): ____________________
ICD-9-CM code(s): ____________________

55. A 22-gauge needle was used to inject 0.125% bupivacaine plain along with Kenalog, approximately 6 mg per cc. The patient's wrists were injected on the dorsal side. She received an injection near the articular fossa of the ulna and the pisiform bone. 1 cc was injected in a fanlike manner in that area and another 1 cc injected between the lunate and radius, and this was done at the radius and the scaphoid bone. This was done on both wrists.
CPT code(s): ____________________
ICD-9-CM code(s): ____________________

56. A 15 blade was used to make a stab incision at 2 o'clock on the left. The nucleus of the lens was hydrodissected with balanced salt solution. Phacoemulsification of the nucleus of the lens was carried out and the residual cortex aspirated from the cul-de-sac. The capsular bag was filled with BioLon and an Allergan model AR40, 20 diopter lens was introduced and placed in the eye.
CPT code(s): ____________________
ICD-9-CM code(s): ____________________

57. The globe of the eye was anesthetized and scissors were used to resect a large-base triangular wedge between the medial and lateral thirds of the lower lid close to the end of the tarsal plate. The defect was then closed.
CPT code(s): ____________________
ICD-9-CM code(s): ____________________

58. After the administration of general anesthesia, the external canal was cleared of cerumen. The tympanic membrane was very sclerotic and, as such, a myringotomy incision was placed and a Bobbin tympanostomy was placed with difficulty.
CPT code(s): ____________________
ICD-9-CM code(s): ____________________

59. 51-year-old with severe mental retardation and cerumen impactions unable to be cleared in the office. Utilizing the ear speculum, the external canal was cleared with similar findings on the opposite site. Following cerumen removal, Cortisporin otic suspension and cotton ball were placed in each ear.
CPT code(s): ____________________
ICD-9-CM code(s):.____________________

60. Utilizing the ear speculum after general anesthesia, the left external ear canal was cleared of cerumen and then the retained PE tube was freed and removed. A myringotomy incision was placed in the anterior inferior quadrant and a tympanostomy tube was placed without difficulty. Same procedure was performed on the right ear.
CPT code(s):____________________
ICD-9-CM code(s): ____________________

OTHER CPT SECTIONS

The last review section will encompass evaluation and management, anesthesia, radiology, pathology, and medicine coding. If you are taking the AAPC CPC examination, these areas encompass Section III of the test. If you are studying for another certification examination, these areas will be included on those tests as well.

Review the following material and practice additional exercises from the text, Workbook, and Evolve site. Keep in mind that a final coding practice examination for each area is included in the Workbook for this text as well as an examination that encompasses all the areas and guidelines in ICD-9-CM, HCPCS, and CPT.

General Guidelines

- New patient: no services from physician or practice (same specialty) 3 years
- New or initial visit (three of three components)
- Established/subsequent/follow-up (two of three components)

- Test does NOT encompass levels based on element counts
- Breakdown as follows:
  Step 1: Type and location of services
  Step 2: Status of patient (new or established)
  Step 3: Level of service
  Step 4: Modifier (if applicable)
- Time (unit/floor time)
  When used for determining level

Office and Outpatient Visits

- Outpatient facilities as well as office
- Code 99211 may be used for nonphysician E & M services only when (1) the physician is in suite, (2) there is an existing treatment plan, and (3) service is provided by a contracted employee.

Observation Visits

- Same date admit/discharge (99234-99236 series)
- Different dates (99217-99220 series)
- Does not have to be in observation area
- Only admitting physician may code
- If admitted same dates, most significant E & M (admit) will be coded

Hospital Inpatient

- Initial (admit) for admitting physician only
- Admit always most significant E & M for day (can use documentation from other visits)

Consultations

- Determine location or type (inpatient/outpatient/confirmatory)
- Need three elements:
  1. Written request
  2. Referring physician
  3. Written report
- When care is assumed, visits are no longer consultations
- May initiate treatment

Emergency Department

- All new patients (three of three components)
- Level 5 coded if history and examination are not documented because of patient's condition
- ED physician may bill interpret if providing services without the assistance of another physician and documents that service

Critical Care

- Based on documented time by physician
- Devotes full attention to patient; cannot provide care to other patients
- Critically ill or unstable patient
- May or may not be continuous
- Not based on location of service

Neonatal Intensive Care

- Per day
- Initial code 99295
- Subsequent days vary based on status of critically ill unstable, critically ill stable, low birth weight

Nursing Facility Services (Skilled Nursing Facility/Long-Term Care)

- Admission, subsequent, annual, discharge

Domiciliary, Rest Home, Custodial Care (Assisted Living)

- New patients/established patients

Home Services

- Place of residence at time of service
- New patients/established patients

Prolonged Services

- Face to face/non–face to face
- Time based
- In addition to original E & M

Care Plan Oversight Services

- Home health/hospice/nursing facility
- Based on time during calendar month
- Must be services beyond physician communication

Preventive Medicine Services

- No complaints
- Based on age and new/established
- Treatment/evaluation of "sick" problem in addition to preventive with modifier 25

Newborn Care

Designed only for use for the care of a newborn infant in the newborn nursery.

Special E & M Services

- Life/disability
- Work related/medical disability
- Not for treatment, only for evaluation

Modifier Codes

22	Prolonged E & M
24	Unrelated E & M during Global Period
25	Significantly Separately Identifiable
32	Mandated Services
52	Reduced Services
57	Decision for Surgery

Anesthesia Coding

- Arranged by anatomic site
- Begins with zero
- Used only by anesthesia providers

- Time used based on 10- or 15-minute increments depending on carrier
- Time begins when provider begins preparing and when no longer in attendance
- Time units + based relative units

Physical Status Modifiers (Mandatory)	Qualifying Circumstances (if Applicable)
P1: Normal healthy	Addition procedure code, not modifier
P2: Mild systemic	99100 Under 1/Over 70
P3: Severe systemic	99116 Total body hypothermia
P4: With constant threat to life	99135 Controlled hypotension
P5: Moribund patient not expected to live without surgery	99140 Emergency (defined as such)
P6: Brain-dead, harvesting organs	

HCPCS Modifiers

AA	Anesthesia performed
AD	Supervision by physician/more than four procedures
G8	Monitored anesthesia care (MAC) deep, complex, complicated, invasive
G9	MAC history of severe cardiopulmonary condition
QB	Rural health professional shortage area (HPSA)
QK	Medical direction two to four procedures
QS	MAC
QX	Certified registered nurse anesthetist (CRNA) with medical direction
QY	Medical direction CRNA
QZ	CRNA without direction

Radiology

General Guidelines

- Modifier 26 use
- Modifier 76/77 use
- Contrast material coded if other than oral or rectal
- Use of modifier 50 for radiology bilateral procedures
- Ultrasounds: complete or limited
- CT/MRI: With/without/with and without

Pathology

General Guidelines

- Disease-oriented panels
- Consultations versus E & M consultations
- Surgical pathology: specimen guidelines
- Automated versus manual
- Modifier 90: reference lab
- Modifier 91: repeat procedure
- Urinalysis: dipstick/automated/manual
- Drug screens

Medicine

Injection Codes

Injection	Medication
Immune globulin	90765-90768, 90772, 90774, 90775 immune globulin
Medications	90765-90775 medication name
Immunizations	90471-90474 immunization name
Chemotherapy	96401-96549 chemotherapy drug

- IV therapy by time
- Drugs coded with CPT/HCPCS depend on carrier

Psychiatry Codes

- Time/location
- Insight oriented/interactive

Dialysis (End-Stage Renal Disease [ESRD])

- Age
- Per day/per month

Ophthalmology

- New or established patients
- Level of service by testing performed
- Contact lens services
- Lens services

Cardiovascular

- Services by global, interpretation, technical only
- Not invasive, invasive in surgical section
- Heart catheterization:
  - Access site: vein/right, artery/left
  - Injection codes: by vessel
  - Imaging codes: by vessel
  - Percutaneous transluminal coronary angioplasty (PTCA)/stent/atherectomy: by vessel, not number of procedures
  - Use of LC/LD/RC modifiers

Vascular Procedures

- Extremity artery/vein-penile/venous

Pulmonary Function

- Pulmonary function test with/without bronchodilators

Allergy

- Testing type: scratch, puncture, intradermal (watch "each")
- Allergy immunotherapy with/without provision of extract
- Use of E & M codes

Electroencephalography (ECG) and Electromyography (EMG)

- EEG: sleep, cerebral death, other method
- EMG: muscles, nerves, number

Health and Behavior Assessments

- Modify behavior, not already established problem

Physical Therapy and Occupational Therapy

- By modality (supervised/constant attendance)
- By time

Wound Care Codes

- Chronic wounds
- Selective: specific treatment to specific area of wound
- Nonselective: treatment to entire wound

Medical Nutrition Therapy

- Group or single
- By minutes
- Nutritional therapy for medical conditions

Miscellaneous

99070 Special supplies	Drug/supplies not part of regular encounter
99024 Postoperative visit	Included in global fee
99000 Specimen handling	

Home Health Codes and Home Infusion Codes

- Used for services performed by home health personnel in the patient's home

Once you have reviewed the above information and studied the appropriate chapters in this text, try your knowledge of evaluation and management, anesthesia, radiology, pathology, and medicine coding with the following practice examination.

Evaluation and Management, Anesthesia, Radiology, Pathology, and Medicine Practice Examination (Alloted Time: 55-60 Minutes)

Choose the appropriate code for each scenario.

1. Office visit, established patient
   Problem-focused history
   Problem-focused exam
   Straightforward medical decision making
   a. 99212
   b. 99201
   c. 99213
   d. 99211
2. Emergency department visit
   Detailed history
   Expanded problem-focused exam
   Moderate medical decision making
   a. 99284
   b. 99285
   c. 99283
   d. 99282
3. Outpatient consultation, established
   Comprehensive history
   Comprehensive exam
   Moderate medical decision making
   a. 99263
   b. 99244
   c. 99243
   d. 99245
4. A premature newborn is admitted to the hospital neonatal intensive care unit. The baby remains unstable and critical for 2 days after admission. On the third day the baby is stable but still critical. The appropriate code(s) would be
   a. 99295, 99296 × 2
   b. 99295, 99231 × 2
   c. 99295
   d. 99295 × 3
5. A patient complaining of chest pain is met in the emergency department by his regular physician. After a comprehensive history and exam, high medical decision making, the patient is admitted by his physician to rule out myocardial infarction. The appropriate E & M code would be
   a. 99285
   b. 99284
   c. 99221
   d. 99223
6. A patient arrives at the physician's office for exacerbation of asthma. During the wait to see the physician, the patient experiences extreme difficulty breathing and goes into respiratory arrest. The patient is seen immediately, intravenous medications are started, and the physician continues to treat the patient until stabilized and an ambulance arrives. Time documented is 45 minutes. The appropriate code would be
   a. 99291
   b. 99215
   c. 99289
   d. 99288
7. Chest x-ray, posteroanterior only
   a. 71030
   b. 71010
   c. 71020
   d. 71015
8. Gallbladder ultrasound
   a. 76700
   b. 76705
   c. 76770
   d. 76775
9. Computed tomography scan, brain, with and without contrast
   a. 70480
   b. 70450
   c. 70470
   d. 70460
10. Allergy immunotherapy, single injection, patient provides own allergy extract
    a. 95117
    b. 95115

c. 95120
d. 95145

11. Psychotherapy, 45 minutes, outpatient office, behavior modifying
a. 90804
b. 90806
c. 90807
d. 90812

12. End-stage renal disease services, February 1 to 16, age 7 years
a. 90968 × 16
b. 90969 × 16
c. 90964 × 16
d. 90965

13. Injection of penicillin, 50 mg, intramuscular, administration only
a. 90774
b. 90775
c. 90776
d. 90772

14. Specimen handling charge for blood specimen prepared for delivery to laboratory
a. 99000
b. 99070
c. 99080
d. 99091

15. Nonselective wound treatment
a. 97597
b. 97602
c. 97598
d. 97605

16. IV infusion methotrexate, 50 mg (antineoplastic drug), 1 hour 30 minutes
a. 96545
b. 96413, 96416, chemotherapy HCPCS code
c. 96413, chemotherapy HCPCS code or 99070
d. 96412

17. Electrocardiogram, interpretation and report only
a. 93000
b. 93010
c. 93005
d. 93015

18. Cardiac stress test, interpretation and report only
a. 93018
b. 93000
c. 93015
d. 93010

19. Left heart catheter performed in conjunction with the following: left ventriculogram, coronary angiogram, pulmonary angiography, injections and imaging
a. 93510, 93543-51, 93545-51, 93541-51, 93556-51, 93555-51
b. 93501, 93543, 93545, 93541, 93556, 93555
c. 93510, 93543, 93545, 93541, 93555, 93556
d. 93510, 93543, 93545, 93541, 93555, 93556, 93556

20. PTCA right coronary, three balloons
PTCA left circumflex, two balloons
a. 92982-RC, 92984-LC
b. 92982 × 6
c. 92980-RC, 92982-LC
d. 92982-RC × 3, 92984-LC × 2

21. Left heart catheterization
Left ventriculogram injection and imaging
Right coronary injection and imaging
Right coronary vessel: PTCA
Left circumflex: PTCA
Right coronary vessel: stent × 3
Left circumflex: stent × 1
Left descending vessel: stent × 1
a. 93510, 93543, 93545, 93555, 93556, 92982-RC, 92984-LC, 92980-RC, 92981-LC, 92981-LD
b. 93501, 93543, 93545, 93555, 93556, 92980-RC, 92981-LD, 92981-LC
c. 93501, 93545-51, 93545-51, 93555-51, 93556-51, 92980, 92981-LC, 92981-LD
d. 93510, 93543, 93545, 93555, 93556, 92980-RC, 92981 × 2 (LC/LD)

22. Pulmonary function test
a. 94010
b. 94060
c. 94620
d. 94070

23. Digoxin level
a. 80100
b. 80101
c. 80102
d. 80162

24. Drug testing, barbiturates
a. 80100
b. 80100 × 2
c. 80102
d. 80184

25. Hematocrit
a. 85013
b. 85014
c. 85018
d. 85025

Congratulations! You have studied hard and ideally feel much more comfortable in your preparations for certification examination.

It is important that you take additional time to focus on areas in which you did not perform well and determine whether additional studying or additional practice is necessary. Also determine where careless errors were made and why.

The purpose for taking several practice tests is to experience the test mode, experience the amount of time allotted for the examination, and learn from your mistakes. Be sure to allot sufficient time to study and learn from your errors. Do not be surprised if during the mock examination in the Workbook or the actual certification examination you recall some of your previous errors. These will prevent you from making the same mistakes on the real certification examination.

Each sample test included in this chapter is intended for practice purposes only. The Workbook includes actual mock examinations for which you should be certain to time yourself; consider them comparable to a real certification exam. Each of the 25-question tests included in the section should be completed within 30 to 35 minutes to fall within the time allotted on the actual certification exams. If time permits, your instructor may chose to hold a mock examination during class time so you may experience some of the test anxiety that may occur during the actual certification examination.

Do not become discouraged if you do not receive a passing grade for each of the practice examinations. They are intended to show you areas where you need additional study or practice. Although the passing score for each section of the AAPC CPC certification examination differs, the average passing score is approximately 70%. The AHIMA guidelines differ as well; however, expect to need at least a 70% to 80% score to pass that examination.

Becoming certified is an important part of becoming a professional coder; it represents mastery of your coding skills and knowledge.

24

You Learned It, You Earned It: Get That Coding Job!

LEARNING OBJECTIVES

After completing this chapter, the student will be able to:

- Understand the importance of transferable skills and job-related skills.
- Use appropriate techniques in preparing a resume.
- Comprehend the effectiveness of a coding and billing portfolio.
- Understand where to look for coding positions.
- Comprehend appropriate interview techniques.

You have finished your coursework and you should be proud! Perhaps you were top (or near the top) in your class. However, being an "A" student is not the most important factor to your prospective employer.

Transferable Skills

Prospective employers are, of course, looking for job-related skills for specific positions. However, employers are also looking for these top 10 qualities in the employees they hire:

1. Teamwork
2. Problem solving
3. Interpersonal skills
4. Oral communication
5. Listening
6. Personal and career development
7. Creative thinking
8. Leadership
9. Goal setting and motivation
10. Writing skills

These skills are not concrete skills or ones that are learned from instruction, but are referred to as *adaptive skills*—skills that are inherent in one's personality and are transferable to any circumstance or job setting.

These skills are invaluable to an employer; without some or all of these skills, the job seeker is not marketable. Although average students may not believe they possess any of these skills, or believe that their personal skills in these areas do not relate to the coding profession, everyone possesses some of these skills.

Take a few moments to reflect on the above list and how your personal skills in these areas relate to your professional acumen.

STOP AND PRACTICE

Take a look at the above list of desired skills. Ask your friends, loved ones, and others who are familiar with your traits and personality which of the above skills you demonstrate regularly. Identify skills from that list that you feel you demonstrate best. It does not matter whether these skills are as a parent, a volunteer, or an employee—these traits are considered transferable. For example, if you are a problem solver in your personal life or current job, you will be a problem solver in your new career as well.

Once you have identified two to three of your skills that stand out, write a brief summary of how these skills could be brought forward and used in your new career field.

1. Skill:
____
Action: ___________________________________
How have you used this skill in the past? Give an example.
____
____
Result: ___________________________________
What was the result of using this trait?
____
Potential result: ___________________________
How can applying this skill relate to your new career field?
____

2. Skill: ___________________________________
Action: ___________________________________
How have you used this skill in the past? Give an example.
____
____
Result: ___________________________________
What was the result of using this trait?
____
Potential result: ___________________________
How can applying this skill relate to your new career field?
____

3. Skill: ___________________________________
Action: ___________________________________
How you used this skill in the past? Give an example.
____
____
Result: ___________________________________
What was the result of using this trait?
____
Potential result: ___________________________
How can applying this skill relate to your new career field?
____

Choose one of the above and present this skill or trait to the class. It is important to become confident that you possess the skills the prospective employer is seeking.

Most of the job applicants competing for the same position will likely meet these requirements; what will set *you* apart will be your confidence and how you demonstrate those inherent skills the market is seeking. Make sure these skills are listed on your resume and be prepared to give a scenario such as the above to prove your expertise.

Job-Related Skills

Probably the biggest stumbling block the coding student meets in an attempt to obtain a coding position is a lack of self-confidence. Often students indicate they have no job-related skills, yet when asked about their last two to three jobs they indicate they have worked in facilities where they excelled in areas such as customer service, financial management, telephone techniques, and other areas common in the medical practice. You must convince the potential employer you already possess many of the required skills and have work-related experience despite the fact you may not have worked in a medical office or facility.

STOP AND PRACTICE

Take a few moments to make a list of the job-related skills a potential coding and billing employer would look for. Make a list of the skills you already have or have acquired during your training that match this list. Make certain these skills are included on your resume.

____

____

____

____

____

____

____

____

Now that you have developed a list of your job-related and transferable skills, you need to make certain your potential employer is aware of your expertise. This can be accomplished in a number of ways.

Resume Preparation

Your resume is the first opportunity for your potential employer to get to know you. Typographical errors, poor layout, and poor overall appearance will put your resume in the rejection pile very quickly. Demonstrating some of the transferable skills noted above is important. What better place to demonstrate your writing skills and communicate your goals and motivation than on your resume?

Many acceptable formats for resumes can be found on the Internet relatively easily. However, keep the following rules in mind:

- Keep it short (one page if possible). Make sure your objective is in line with the job you are applying for.
- Modify your objective to fit a specific job when appropriate.
- If your education is the most valuable asset on your resume, list educational experience first. If job-related experience is your greatest attribute, list job experience first.
- Be precise. If your job title is "cashier," it is not necessary to indicate you handled money because this in inherent in the job description.
- Do not be repetitive. It is not necessary to describe skills multiple times.
- List all job experience; do not leave time gaps if possible.
- Do not list references on the resume; be prepared to offer them when requested, typically later in the hiring process.
- Do not include personal information (e.g., hobbies, health, age, children).
- Make sure to incorporate any externship, internship, or volunteer work in the field.

STOP AND PRACTICE

Write a first draft of your resume. Exchange the resume with another student in your class and have that person proof for errors and give suggestions for improvement.

Coding and Billing Portfolio

One of the best tools for a new coder or biller is a portfolio that demonstrates some of the real-world skills acquired in the classroom. For example, the coding charts in *Mastering Medical Coding* are real charts taken from real medical records. If a prospective employer indicates you lack the experience necessary for the job, select a few of the coding cases for the specialty and include them in your portfolio to demonstrate you have experience coding cases similar to their practice.

This will require changing the composition of your portfolio to meet the specialty for which you are applying, so keep in mind that the materials may need to change. Therefore your portfolio should be composed of pages with pockets to insert materials and change them when necessary. Look closely at the skills required based on the job description or posting and tailor your portfolio to encompass all of those skills. For example, a classified ad reads:

> Wanted: experienced coder familiar with E & M coding, ICD-9-CM coding. Must be knowledgeable in medical billing software and possess computer skills.

The ideal portfolio would include:

- Sample "tools" for E & M coding
- Sample exercises in E & M coding
- Printouts of reports, claims, or other materials prepared from the computerized billing system in the classroom
- Samples of documents prepared in Word, Excel, or Power Point that would represent materials prepared for a medical office
- Extra copies of your resume
- Reference list (available on request)

Where to Search

Now that you have assessed your skills and prepared materials to market your skills, you are ready to begin the job search.

Sources indicate that only 15% to 20% of all jobs are obtained from the classified section of the newspaper. The remaining 80% to 85% of jobs are found in the following ways:

- Employers constantly looking for good employees, even when openings do not exist
- Need for additional staff is recognized, and referrals are made before position has been approved
- Referrals and applications accepted before position is advertised

Because the majority of job openings are never advertised, the job seeker must know how and where to find these jobs. As time goes by more and more individuals become aware of openings, which decreases the chances of landing the job offer.

Other areas for job searching include:

—Networking

Anyone can be a source for a potential job. Students have found jobs through friends, relatives, acquaintances, fellow students, current employers, and their own physicians' offices. The more extensively you network, the more people become aware of your desire for a position, and the more likely you will come in contact with someone who can assist you in your job search.

Networking also includes attending professional meetings that may take place in your area. Job announcements are usually made at these meetings, and informal conversations may include mention of specific openings.

—Internet

Some Web sites are devoted exclusively to job seekers in the medical and health care fields, such as the following:

www.hiremedical.com
www.healthjobsusa.com
www.medicaljobsonline.com
www.medhunters.com

Web sites designed specifically for job searching in general are also useful, such as www.monster.com and www.careerbuilder.com.

In addition, a search engine such as www.google.com or www.yahoo.com can be effective for locating sites with job opportunities when using key words such as *health information, health care, coding,* or *billing.*

—Career fairs

In a single day you can meet dozens of potential employers at a job fair, usually sponsored by community agencies or large health care facilities. Be prepared to interview and bring clean, up-to-date copies of your resume. Make sure you look professional, as if you were going on an interview.

—Cold contacts

Make a list of potential employers and specialties you would be interested in. Schedule time for visiting these facilities and speaking with those responsible for making hiring decisions. Be prepared to interview, test, and have copies of your resume and portfolio available. You demonstrate many of the skills previously discussed when you show motivation, professionalism, and oral and written communication skills in your job search.

Classified advertisements in newspapers are still a resource for locating potential jobs or job markets. Some tips for reviewing the classified ads include the following:

- Look for associated job titles such as biller, coder, collections, front desk, insurance, and insurance verification.
- Watch the wording of the job ad; send your resume to the fax number, e-mail address, or mailing address or call only as directed in the ad.
- Remember that the ad is for the "perfect" applicant, so do not be turned away by ads that mention "1 year of experience" or "certified." You *do* have experience, as previously discussed, and you can certainly request 6 months to 1 year to prepare and pass the certification examination.

STOP AND PRACTICE

Take your resume and portfolio and prepare for a job interview day. Your instructor will give you the requirements, which may include dressing for the interview.

At the beginning of the day, two to three jobs will be posted in the classroom; choose to apply to one job posting. Your instructor will share your resume on an overhead transparency or projector screen in the classroom for the class to review.

You will be interviewed by your peers, so be prepared for some frank questions. Often your fellow students know you better than your instructor or the school faculty.

Interview Techniques

Before your practice interviews, prepare by reviewing the list of the most common interview mistakes:

- Looking disheveled or inappropriately dressed
- Poor posture
- Not maintaining eye contact
- Not making the connection between your skills and the employer's needs
- Bragging about how good you are and neglecting to back up your claims with evidence
- Displaying no enthusiasm regarding the job
- Badmouthing your current employer
- Appearing desperate for a job
- Responding in an unfocused, disorganized, or rambling manner
- Expecting your resume to speak for itself without referring to a specific job or training when answering questions
- Talking money before you receive at least a tentative job offer

- Being late
- Interrupting

Fellow students will be asked to score you in several areas throughout the interview, such as the following:

- First appearance
- Resume presentation
- Portfolio presentation and use
- Training and experience
- Interview skills

Your instructor will assign a point system to the scoring and announce the successful applicant for each position.

A multitude of questions may be asked during the interview process. Keep in mind that some are asked solely for the purpose of demonstrating your critical thinking or oral communication skills. Therefore a response such as "I don't know" or "no" tends to make the potential employer think you have not demonstrated these needed skills. Remember that if you need a few moments to prepare a response, you can respond with "Let me think about that for a moment," which will give you a few moments to prepare a response.

Some common interview questions include the following:

- Tell me about yourself.
- What are your strengths and weaknesses?
- Describe your ideal job.
- Why should we hire you?
- What are your goals? Where do you see yourself in 5 years?
- Tell me about your work experience.
- What will your references say about you?
- How does your previous employment or experience relate to this position?
- Tell me about a difficult or frustrating problem or situation and how you handled it.
- What are your salary requirements?
- Why do you want to work here?

STOP AND PRACTICE

Take a few moments to have a class discussion about correct and incorrect responses to each of the questions listed above.

Improving Your Chances of Employment

Your resume is flawless and your interviews appeared to go extremely well, yet you have not been offered a job. What can you do to improve your odds?

Certification is an important asset to the job seeker. For the student who has little or no on-the-job experience, certification is the positive that neutralizes the negative. A coding certification demonstrates your commitment to the coding profession as well as your coding skills. Chapter 23 discusses the various certification examinations and preparation for taking these tests.

Other suggestions for improving your odds include the following:

—Offer to "volunteer" or "shadow" to prove your skills to a prospective employer.

If you have not secured a job yet, spending a few hours a week demonstrating how your skills could be invaluable. Even if the prospective employer does not hire you, a letter of recommendation can go a long way in securing a position elsewhere.

—Recruit the assistance of your externship or internship site.

Your supervisor at your site has already established connections in the industry. During the exit interview process, or as you prepare to finish your externship, ask your supervisor for some direction or contact names. He or she may be willing to make a few calls to fellow professionals if you have done a good job for the organization. Respectfully request a written letter of recommendation as well.

—Offer to take a test to demonstrate your skills.

This will demonstrate your skills as well as your self-confidence.

—Network with fellow and past students.

Contact past students or students from your class who have secured positions to discuss tips on successful job-seeking techniques.

—Attend professional meetings in your area.

Make frequent contacts, especially during your job-seeking period, to make certain everyone is aware of your desire to secure a position.

—Finalize the coder's toolkit you developed in the classroom.

Prepare the materials in a professional manner and take this information with you on interviews to demonstrate your preparedness, professionalism, and dedication to the coding field.

—Review your resume and portfolio to make certain they are error free.

Have other coding professionals, your externship supervisor, and others in the field review and make additional suggestions for improvement.

As with any job search, be patient, continue to look for positions and possibilities, and make contacts. Your hard efforts in the classroom and during interviews will pay off.

Job seeking should be an organized process to schedule time for follow-ups, testing, preparing your portfolio, researching potential employers, and searching for additional job opportunities. Allot adequate amounts of time for these activities to be successful in your search.

Keep in mind that you may not secure a full-time coding position at first. Be realistic when job searching; realize that securing a position in the office or facility of your choice will give you an opportunity to demonstrate your skills and proficiencies. Soon you, too, will be a coder!

Chapter in Review

Student Assignments

- Study Chapter 24.
- Complete all the Stop and Practice exercises.
- Incorporate all the completed "projects" into an applicant (student) portfolio.

Credits

Figs. 1-1 to 1-29, 14-1 to 14-27, and 15-1: Shiland BJ: *Mastering healthcare terminology*, ed 2, St Louis, 2006, Mosby.

Figs. 2-11 and 17-3: Chester GA: *Modern medical assisting*, Philadelphia, 1998, WB Saunders.

Figs. 2-21 to 2-27: Courtesy Piermed, Inc., Lewisville, NC.

Figs. 3-3 to 3-4, 4-1, 19-1 to 19-3, and 21-1; Tables 8-3 and 13-1; and Tool 7-4: Courtesy MD Consultative Services, Orlando, FL.

Figs. 5-1 to 5-3: U.S. Department of Health and Human Services, Centers for Medicare and Medicaid Services.

Index

Page numbers followed by f indicate figures; t, tables; b, boxes.

D

E

N